Human Papillomavirus Infections in Dermatovenereology

CRC Series in
DERMATOLOGY: CLINICAL AND BASIC SCIENCE
Edited by Dr. Howard I. Maibach

The CRC Dermatology Series combines scholarship, basic science, and clinical relevance. These comprehensive references focus on dermal absorption, dermabiology, dermatopharmacology, dermatotoxicology, and occupational and clinical dermatology.

The intellectual theme emphasizes in-depth, easy to comprehend surveys that blend advances in basic science and clinical research with practical aspects of clinical medicine.

Published Titles:

Bioengineering of the Skin: Cutaneous Blood Flow and Erythema
Enzo Berardesca, Peter Elsner, and Howard I. Maibach

Bioengineering of the Skin: Water and the Stratum Corneum
Peter Elsner, Enzo Berardesca, and Howard I. Maibach

Bioengineering of the Skin: Methods and Instrumentation
Enzo Berardesca, Peter Elsner, Klaus-P. Wilhelm, and Howard I. Maibach

Bioengineering of the Skin: Skin Surface Imaging, and Analysis
Klaus-P. Wilhelm, Peter Elsner, Enzo Berardesca, and Howard I. Maibach

Dermatologic Research Techniques
Howard I. Maibach

Hand Eczema
Torkil Menne and Howard I. Maibach

Handbook of Mouse Mutations with Skin and Hair Abnormalities:
Animal Models and Biomedical Tools
John P. Sundberg

Health Risk Assessment: Dermal and Inhalation Exposure and Absorption of Toxicants
Rhoda G. M. Wang, James B. Knaak, and Howard I. Maibach

Pigmentation and Pigmentary Disorders
Norman Levine

Protective Gloves for Occupational Use
Gunh Mellström, J.E. Walhberg, and Howard I. Maibach

Skin Cancer: Mechanisms and Human Relevance
Hasan Mukhtar

Human Papillomavirus Infections in Dermatovenereology
Gerd Gross and Geo von Krogh

Forthcoming Titles:

The Contact Urticaria Syndrome
Smita Amin, Arto Lahti and Howard I. Maibach

Handbook of Contact Dermatitis
Christopher J. Dannaker, Daniel J. Hogan, and Howard I. Maibach

Human Papillomavirus Infections in Dermatovenereology

Edited by

Gerd Gross
Geo von Krogh

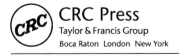

CRC Press
Taylor & Francis Group
Boca Raton London New York

CRC Press is an imprint of the
Taylor & Francis Group, an **informa** business

Senior Editor: Paul Petralia
Editorial Assistant: Cindy Carelli
Project Editor: Debbie Didier
Marketing Manager: Susie Carlisle
Direct Marketing Manager: Becky McEldowney
Cover Design: Dawn Boyd
PrePress: Kevin Luong
Manufacturing: Sheri Schwartz

Library of Congress Cataloging-in-Publication Data

Human papillomavirus infections in dermatovenereology / edited by Gerd
    Gross, Geo von Krogh.
        p.   cm. — (Dermatology)
    Includes bibliographical references and index.
    ISBN 0-8493-7356-5
    1. Papillomavirus diseases.   2. Skin—Diseases.   3. Sexually
transmitted diseases.   I. Gross, G. (Gerd)   II. Krogh, Geo von.
III. Series: CRC series in dermatology.
    [DNLM: 1. Papovaviridae Infections.   2. Tumor Virus Infections.
3. Neoplasms, Squamous Cell.   WC 500 H9188 1996]
RC168.P15H86 1996
616.5′0194—dc20
DNLM/DLC
for Library of Congress   96-8779
                                                                      CIP

The Editors

Gerd Gross, M.D., is Professor of Dermatology and Venereology at the University Hospital of Hamburg, Federal Republic of Germany. Dr. Gross obtained his training at the University of Freiburg, Federal Republic of Germany, receiving his M.D. degree in 1976 and his Dr. habil in 1986. He also qualified in medicine (1976) and in Dermatology and Venereology (1984). In 1986 he was awarded a Heisenberg-scholarship. Dr. Gross assumed his present position in 1987. In 1995 he was offered chair of the Department of Dermatology and Venereology at the University of Rostock, Federal Republic of Germany. He accepted this position in July 1996.

Dr. Gross is a member of several scientific societies, including Deutsche Dermatologische Gesellschaft, Arbeitsgemeinschaft Dermatologische Forschung, European Society for Dermatological Research, Deutsche Krebsgesellschaft, Arbeitsgemeinschaft Dermatologische Onkologie, European Academy of Dermatology and Venereology, Deutsche STD-Gesellschaft (ehemals Deutsche Gesellschaft zur Bekämpfung der Geschléchtskrankheiten), Medical Society for the Study of Venereal Diseases, Paul Ehrlich Gesellschaft, Deutsche Gesellschaft für Hygiene und Mikrobiologie, European Society of Clinical Microbiology and Infectious Diseases, and International Society for Interferon Research.

He is an editor of 4 scientific books and author of more than 80 papers. Furthermore, he has co-authored more than 30 books. His special interests are virus-induced diseases and the role of viruses in benign and malignant tumors of the skin and mucosae. Another current focus is dermatotherapy, especially therapy of viral infections and virus-associated tumors.

Geo von Krogh, M.D., Ph.D., is Associate Professor of Dermatology and Venereology at the Karolinska University Hospital (Karolinska Institute) in Stockholm, Sweden. Dr. von Krogh obtained his training at the University of Oslo and Bergen, Norway, receiving his M.D. degree in 1967. Further training in Norway and Sweden includes general surgery, internal medicine, diving medicine, and psychiatry. von Krogh qualified in Dermatology and Venereology in 1978 after training at the Southern University Hospital of Stockholm. Following a scholarship spent at the Department of Dermatology at the University of California in San Francisco, he acquired his Ph.D. in 1981. He has been affiliated as an Associate Professor at the Karolinska Hospital since 1988.

von Krogh is a scientific board member of the International Union against the Veneral Diseases and Treponematoses (IUVDT). He is also a member of the following scientific societies: Swedish Academy of Dermatology, The International Society for the Study of Vulvar Diseases, The International Papillomavirus Workshop Group, The European Academy of Dermatology and Venerology, The International AIDS Society, The International Society for STD Research (ISSTDR), The Medical Society for the Study of Venereal Diseases, and The American Venereal Disease Association. von Krogh served as the president for European Course on HPV-Associated Pathology from 1993 to 1996.

He has co-editorial merits of 4 scientific volumes and is the author and co-author of 90 papers. His special interest is venereology, with an emphasis on the clinical challenges of anogenital HPV-associated disease.

Contributors

Renzo Barrasso, M.D.
The Colposcopy Unit
Obstetrics and Gynecology Department
Hôpital Bichat
Paris, France

Robert D. Burk, M.D.
Departments of Pediatrics, Microbiology, and
  Immunology
The Albert Einstein College of
  Medicine
Bronx, New York

Hajo Delius
Forschungschwerpunkt Angewandte
  Tumorvirologie
Deutsches Krebsforschungszentrum
Heidelberg, Germany

Ethel-Michele de Villiers, Ph.D.
Abteilung für Tumorvirus-Charakterisierung
Forschungschwerpunkt Angewandte
  Tumorvirologie
Deutsches Krebsforschungszentrum
Heidelberg, Germany

Joakim Dillner, M.D.
The Microbiology and Tumor
  Biology Center
Karolinska Institute
Stockholm, Sweden

Pawel G. Fuchs, Ph.D.
Institut für Virologie der Universität zu Köln
Köln, Germany

Denise A. Galloway, Ph.D.
Program in Cancer Biology
Fred Hutchinson Cancer Research Center
and
Department of Microbiology
University of Washington
Seattle, Washington

Lutz Gissmann
Department of Obstetrics and Gynecology
Loyola University Medical Center
Maywood, Illinois

Gerd Gross, M.D.
Department of Dermatology and Venereology
University of Rostock
Rostock, Germany

Elke-Ingrid Grussendorf-Conen
Department of Dermatology
University of Aachen
Aachen, Germany

Stefania Jablonska, M.D.
Department of Dermatology
Warsaw School of Medicine
Warsaw, Poland

M. V. Jacobs, M.Sc.
Department of Pathology
Section of Molecular Pathology
Free University Hospital
Amsterdam, The Netherlands

A. Bennett Jenson, M.D.
Georgetown University School of Medicine
Department of Pathology
Washington, D.C.

Haskins K. Kashima, M.D., F.A.C.S.
Department of Otolaryngology — Head and
  Neck Surgery
The Johns Hopkins Medical Institutions
Baltimore, Maryland

Laura A. Koutsky, Ph.D.
Department of Epidemiology
School of Public Health and Community
  Medicine
Seattle, Washington

Brigid G. Leventhal, M.D. (Deceased)
Department of Oncology
Section of Pediatric Oncology
The Johns Hopkins Medical Institutions
Baltimore, Maryland

Slawomir Majewski, M.D.
Department of Dermatology
Warsaw School of Medicine
Warsaw, Poland

Jackek Malejczyk, Ph.D.
Department of Histology and Embryology
Warsaw School of Medicine
Warsaw, Poland

Chris J. L. M. Meijer, M.D., Ph.D.
Department of Pathology
Section of Molecular Pathology
Free University Hospital
Amsterdam, The Netherlands

Alexander Meisels, M.D., F.R.C.P.C., F.I.A.C.
Department of Pathology
Hôpital du Saint-Sacrement
Québec, Canada

Phoebe Mounts, Ph.D.
Department of Molecular Microbiology and
    Immunology
The Johns Hopkins Medical Institutions
Baltimore, Maryland

Slavomir Obalek, M.D.
Department of Dermatology
Warsaw School of Medicine
Warsaw, Poland

J. David Oriel, M.D.
University College and Middlesex School of
    Medicine
London, England

Gerard Orth, M.D.
Unité Des Papillomavirus
Institut Pasteur
Paris, France

Joel Palefsky, M.D., C.M.
Departments of Laboratory Medicine and
    Stomatology
University of California
San Francisco, California

Herbert Pfister, Ph.D.
Institut für Virologie der Universität zu Köln
Köln, Germany

Keerti V. Shah, M.D., D.R.P.H.
Department of Molecular Microbiology and
    Immunology
The Johns Hopkins Medical Institutions
Baltimore, Maryland

David A. Shoultz, M.S.
Department of Epidemiology
School of Public Health and Community
    Medicine
Seattle, Washington

P. J. F. Snijders, Ph.D.
Department of Pathology
Section of Molecular Pathology
Free University Hospital
Amsterdam, The Netherlands

John P. Sundberg, D.V.M., Ph.D.
The Jackson Laboratory
Bar Harbor, Maine

Kari J. Syrjänen, M.D., Ph.D.
Department of Pathology and Forensic Medicine
University of Kuopio
Kuopio, Finland

Stina Syrjänen, D.D.S., Ph.D.
Department of Oral Pathology and Forensic
    Dentistry
Institute of Dentistry
University of Turku
Finland

Ruth Tachezy
Institute of Hematology and Blood
    Transfusion
Department of Experimental Virology
Prague, Czech Republic

A. J. C. van den Brule, Ph.D.
Department of Pathology
Section of Molecular Pathology
Free University Hospital
Amsterdam, The Netherlands

J. W. van Oostveen, Ph.D.
Department of Pathology
Section of Molecular Pathology
Free University Hospital
Amsterdam, The Netherlands

Marc A. Van Ranst, M.D., Ph.D.
Rega Institute for Medical Records
Department of Microbiology and
    Immunology
University of Leuven
Leuven, Belgium

Geo von Krogh, M.D., Ph.D.
Department of Dermatovenereology
Karolinska Hospital
Stockholm, Sweden

Jan M. M. Walboomers, Ph.D.
Department of Pathology
Section of Molecular Pathology
Free University Hospital
Amsterdam, The Netherlands

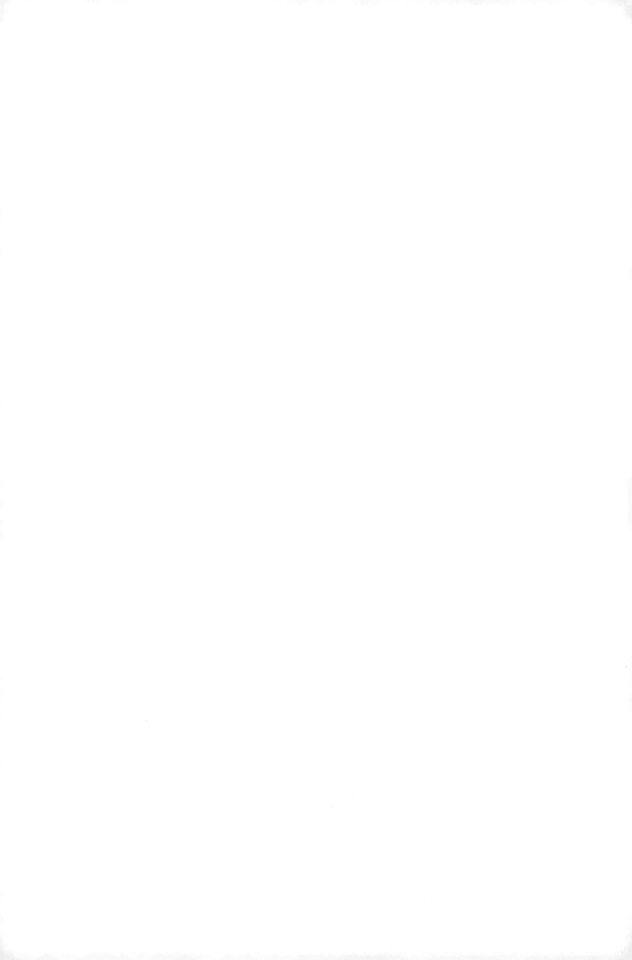

Table of Contents

VII. THERAPY

Introduction

Gerd Gross and Geo von Krogh

The recognition of human papillomaviruses (HPVs) as a major cause of various forms of human cancers, especially those of the uterine cervix in women, has represented the forerunner of a very rapidly expanding multidisciplinary field of clinical, molecular biological, socio-epidemiological, and immunological research during recent years.

Warts were already regarded as infectious by the end of the 19th century and a viral etiology was suggested in 1907 by Ciuffo demonstrating transmission of warts by a sterile, cell-free filtrate of wart tissue. Shope described the first papillomavirus more than 50 years ago as the infectious agent of infectious papillomatosis in rabbits. Some years later, studies performed by Rous showed that benign rabbit papillomas induced by Shope papillomavirus could progress to cancer when treated with specific nonviral cofactors. In 1949, Strauss and coworkers isolated virus-like particles from human skin papillomas. The systematic evaluation of the biology of both human and animal papillomaviruses, however, did not begin until the late 1970s when the application of molecular cloning performed by paramount researchers such as zur Hausen, Gissmann, and Howley helped to circumvent the obstacle that these viruses could not be propagated successfully in culture.

Today the plurality of HPV is well-established. More than 70 different HPV types have been identified and characterized by means of further developed refined, sensitive, and specific DNA hybridization assays. By convention, the original classification was based on the principle that viruses that hybridize by less than 50% with other known types are classified as a new type. For HPVs, more refined classification systems have developed based on less than 10% sequence homology for the L1 region of the ORF (open reading frame) of these viruses. Such analysis has been performed for most of the currently known HPV types, especially those associated with a significant risk of malignant transformation.

In this respect, HPVs appear to play a dual role, both as infectious agents and as carcinogenic factors both in the origin and in the development of benign, dysplastic, and malignant squamous cell tumors of the skin, the upper respiratory tract, the upper und lower gastrointestinal tract, the genitourinary tract, and in particular the cervix uteri (high risk HPV types). It appears that papillomaviruses are ubiquitous and very conservative agents. Almost identically structured viruses have been found in skin biopsies of individuals from isolated tribes from both Asia and South America.

Human papillomaviruses are strictly intraepithelial, slow-growing pathogens which establish chronic infections in the skin or internal mucosae as visible lesions, subclinical lesions, or even as latent infections. The latter state of infection, which is identifiable neither macroscopically nor by means of light-microscopy, is solely detectable by use of refined and sensitive modern DNA and /or RNA hybridization methods.

In humans, viral gene expression seems to be strictly confined to keratinocytes and linked to the differentiating epithelial cells. Alteration of the host cell's growth pattern may lead to cell proliferation and finally induce wart formation.Virion assembly occurs exclusively in terminally diffentiating cells, i.e., in cells which still have not yet converted to malignancy. Transformation of a wart to cancer is paralleled by loss of virus particle production. Viral DNA, however, persists at low copy number in the transformed cells either partially or completely integrated into the cellular chromosome. Integration of viral sequences may result in modification of human genes or even in oncogene activation, which in turn plays a role in malignant conversion and development of cancer. Latent infections are characterized by presence of episomal HPV DNA in morphologically normal epithelium. Such viral genomes either may derive from warts which have previously regressed or may represent persistent infection transmitted silently from cell to cell.

HPV infection can take place at different ages. The peak incidence of benign skin warts is clearly during childhood.Transmission of cutaneous warts is due to close contacts to infected material or to close skin-to-skin contacts. Cutaneous warts arising in adult individuals often reflect recurrent disease due to a certain degree of cellular immune deficiency and reactivation of silent HPV genomes.

The predominant mode of transmission for the genital HPV types appears to be via genital-to-genital contacts. Apparently rates of infection are similar for men and women. The fact that HPV infection is very prevalent among young sexually active populations suggests that transmission is relatively efficient. Moisture and abrasion potentially enhance transmission of virus. As in women, HPV 16 is the most frequently detected HPV type in men. The frequency with which HPV is transmitted perinatally is still unclear. HPV-associated recurrent respiratory papillomatosis appears to arise after perinatal transmission of HPV 11, or to a lesser degree of HPV 6. However, the risk of transmission to an infant from a pregnant woman with clinical or DNA evidence of HPV 11 or HPV 6 remains extremely low. Numerous studies designed to determine the frequency of HPV DNA detection in nasopharyngeal, orobuccal mucosal, or anogenital specimens obtained from newborn or young children lead to inconsistent results. The same is true for anogenital warts in young children. The cause of such lesions may either be genital HPV types or nongenital HPV types. The latter may have been transferred to this area by autoinoculation or heteroinoculation. Nevertheless, a not yet clearly defined number of infections by genital HPV-types are most likely the result of sexual abuse. To which extent visible anogenital HPV infections seen in young children are due to perinatal transmission remains still an unanswered question. Apparently vertical transmission of HPV from infected mothers to their babies and persistance of the virus within the genital area in childhood is possible. Furthermore it is of interest to perform studies to confirm recently published data demonstrating HPV DNA in amniotic fluids of pregnant women.

Anogenital HPV-induced lesions are usually multicentric, multiform, biological expressions occuring predominantly in areas submitted to microtraumatization during sexual activity, on epithelial transformational zones (cervix, anal canal), and on inflamed or irritated epithelia. Comprehension that subclinical infection is extremely common has created ambiguity on what level of ambition it should be considered as optimal for patient management, a clinical dilemma that might not be solved until more specific antiviral or immunotherapeutic modalities are available. For genital papillomavirus infection, some principles regarding contagiousness, infectivity, and therapeutic challenges are quite similar to other sexually transmitted viral diseases such as genital herpes. Therapy is only helpful to remove the visible part of the lesions; the infection itself, however, is not yet treatable. Upcoming efforts in the development of type-specific vaccines could potentially help either to completely prevent the infection or could at least be used therapeutically. This will become of clinical significance in particular for the management of lesions related to oncogenic virus types such as HPV 16 and HPV 18, and thus will hopefully prevent development of cervical cancer and other types of genital cancer.

Nevertheless, some progress in therapy especially of HPV infections of the urogenital tract can be recognized by now. Although there is no once-only therapy, early and circumscribed lesions can be treated easily using local therapies. Therapeutic options comprise primarily the use of podophyllotoxin solution or podophyllotoxin cream available recently. Alternative local treatments are trichloroacetic acid, 5-fluorouracil, interferon intralesionally, or cryotherapy. Surgery, even the simple scissor-snip excision which may be useful if lesions are small or solitary, requires local anaesthesia. The same is true for diathermy and laser treatment. In case of recurrent and progressive disease, combinations of surgical therapy and immune therapies such as interferon as well as a combination of interferon with retinoids have lead to optimistic results.

The aim of this textbook is to give an overview of the scientific and clinical data of papillomaviruses in general and of HPV-associated diseases which are of relevance for the dermatologist and venereologist. As papillomaviruses are wide-ranging pathogens, it may well be that this virus group holds further surprises in terms of human disease especially of the skin and the genitoanal tract. However, so much progress has been made recently in our understanding of this subject that a volume detailing current knowledge seems very timely. This is especially true with regard to the data related to molecular biology and immunology.

I. Historical Overview

1

Historical Overview

J. D. Oriel

CONTENTS

Human papillomaviruses (HPV) have been infecting people for a very long time. In the world of the ancient Greeks and Romans, warts were well known.[1] *Condyloma* is derived from the Greek word for a knob or knuckle, and *myrmecia*, still sometimes used to describe painful plantar warts, came from the Greek word for an anthill. Genital warts were called *thymia*, because they resembled the leaves of wild thyme, and colloquially were known as *ficus*, which means figs. In his *De medicina*, the Roman writer Celsus (1st century A.D.) described myrmeciae, thymia, and some lesions he called *acrochordon* which may have been common, or possibly filiform, warts. In ancient Rome it was widely believed that *ficus* were the result of promiscuous sexual behavior, and many satirical poems were written about them. The word *condyloma* has survived until today; *condyloma acuminatum* came into use at the end of the 19th century. *Thymus* and *acrochordon* dropped out of medical literature at an early date, but the English term *fig warts*, the German *Feigwarze*, the french *fic*, and the Spanish *higo* were still being used at the beginning of the 20th century. The word *verruca*, from the Latin for a hill, was introduced by a German physician, Daniel Sennert (Sennertus, 1572–1637).

I. AETIOLOGY

The cause of warts was unknown until the 20th century. Some strange suggestions were made by the earlier physicians. Under the heading "Peculiar sign" an annotation in *The Lancet* in 1849 reads:

> Dr. Durr maintained many years ago in Hufeland's journal that young females addicted to solitary habits often present warts on the index and middle finger...Dr. Van Oye adduces two recent cases in his practice where, by this sign, he was able to ascertain the cause of abnormal and extraordinary symptoms in young girls.[2]

In 1874, the Viennese dermatologist Ferdinand von Hebra mentioned various other theories—association with animals, manual work, repeated moistening and dirtying of the hands, and so on—and concluded that "the influences causing warts are still very obscure."

There was a widespread popular belief that common warts were contagious, but according to Joseph Payne, a physician at St. Thomas' Hospital, London, this was treated by writers on dermatology with "silence or contempt." In a paper published in 1891,[3] he described how he developed a wart on his own thumb after scraping lesions from a child with extensive skin warts, and stated that he believed that "common warts are due to the implantation of infected matter." He added that the origin of "pointed condylomas" was "not so clear," but soon after he wrote, ideas on the aetiology of *condylomata acuminata* and common skin warts were to converge.

Genital warts survived the Dark Ages. Some medieval writers mentioned them, and they were often described after the outbreak of syphilis began in Europe at the end of the 15th century. Unfortunately, many genital infections—notably syphilis, gonorrhea, and chancroid—were all attributed to the same "venereal poison," and this led many authorities, including John Hunter, to state that anogenital warts were due to syphilis. Hunter's contemporary, the Scottish surgeon Benjamin Bell, maintained that syphilis and gonorrhea were different diseases; he did not believe that syphilis caused warts, and he explained how syphilitic papular lesions and anogenital warts could be differentiated. Slowly this mistaken belief was abandoned, but only to be replaced by another, that the warts were due to gonorrhea. They often seemed to develop towards the end of an attack of gonorrhea—often very prolonged in those days—and for a time they were actually called "gonorrheal warts." But after Neisser discovered the gonococcus in 1879 it became clear that many patients with anogenital warts showed no signs of gonorrhea, so this explanation of the origin of warts was also abandoned. It was now maintained that gonorrheal pus was simply one of many irritants which, if prolonged, could provoke the formation of anogenital warts. Other irritants were held to include dirt, decomposed sebaceous material, and secretions "disordered through venery," hence the term "venereal warts" which is still sometimes used. This hypothesis was accepted without question by such eminent physicians as Hebra, Kaposi, and Hutchinson.

A turning point in the long disputes over aetiology was reached when, in 1893, the French dermatologist Gémy suggested that *condylomata acuminata* might be related to common skin warts; there were histological resemblances, and many patients with genital warts had warts on their hands. He suggested that the two diseases might be caused by the same parasite.[4] This proposal was made at a good time, because in the following year experiments on the contagiousness of common warts began. Variot and Licht independently induced skin warts in volunteers by injecting extracts of wart tissue.[5,6]

Other investigators obtained the same results, and in 1907 Ciuffo took the experiments further by successfully inoculating himself with an extract of skin warts which had been passed through a Berkefeld filter.[7] This at once suggested that the infecting agent might be a virus, and indicated a way in which the relationship between skin and genital warts could be explored by the inoculation of material from warts at both sites. Not surprisingly, it was difficult to find volunteers for these studies, but some prostitutes were persuaded to participate and in one disgraceful episode infected material was injected into the vulva of a virgin. In a few cases, the inoculation of filtered and unfiltered extracts of penile warts into nongenital skin was followed by the appearance of common warts, and the inoculation of extracts of common skin warts produced warts on the genitals. These results were enough to convince the investigators not only that genital warts were caused by a virus but that this virus was identical to that which caused common skin warts; this has been called the unitary theory.[8] After these experiments ended in the early 1920s, there was no serious study of papillomaviruses for more than 20 years.

In 1949, the viral origin of skin warts was confirmed when Strauss et al. demonstrated undoubted virus particles in extracts of palmar and plantar warts examined by electron microscopy,[9] and a few years later this virus was found to be localized in the nuclei of some cells in the stratum granulosum. These discoveries made it possible to resolve a dispute about the various inclusions which has been described in the cells of human warts. The early workers had seen eosinophilic cytoplasmic inclusions in sections of common warts, and subsequently eosinophilic nuclear inclusions were also described. On the other hand, in 1924 Lipschütz had shown the presence of basophilic intranuclear inclusions.[10] The significance of these various bodies was finally settled in 1962, when Almeida et al. showed that the formation of aggregates of virus particles always correlated with the development of basophilic nuclear inclusions; eosinophilic inclusions were nonviral, and probably consisted of keratin-like material.[11]

It proved difficult to demonstrate virus particles in extracts of anogenital warts because their concentration in these lesions is low, but it was eventually achieved in 1969.[12] The identical morphology of the particles present in skin and anogenital warts was regarded as supporting the unitary theory, although a study by immune electron microscopy raised the possibility that there might be differences between the viruses present in genital and nongenital sites.[13] The difficulty in studying this matter came from the fact that papillomaviruses could not be propagated in cell culture, so could not be studied by the methods of classical virology. In the late 1970s, developments in molecular virology made it possible to prepare cloned viral genomes and compare viral DNA extracted from a wide variety of conditions.[14] When this was done it was discovered that there were many viral types, and that some were repeatedly found in certain sites and lesions: HPV 1–4 in skin warts, HPV 6 and 11 in anogenital warts, and HPV 16, 18, and some others in cervical intraepithelial lesions and genital tract cancers. The association of some genotypes with genital cancers was of major importance, because until then HPV had not been linked to any major disease process. The unitary theory, which had been accepted for so many years, was discarded and the modern era of the study of HPV infection began.

II.   EPIDEMIOLOGY

During the first half of this century, the aetiology of skin warts became more clearly understood but, perhaps because the disease was regarded as unimportant, its epidemiology received little attention. There was a tacit agreement that warts were contagious and caused by a virus, although the nature of the infecting unit transmitted (viral genome, virus particle, or infected cell) was unknown. While direct contact was thought to be the route of infection in some cases (for example, hand warts), the existence of inanimate vectors was convincingly shown in several studies. In one, an outbreak of hand warts among women in a cardboard box factory was traced to the practice of sharing a pot of warm glue into which all the workers put their hands. When each had an individual pot of glue no new cases occurred, and the shared glue pot had probably been a vector for the infection.[15] In another study, Lyell noted that plantar warts in a school were ten times more common in children who did gymnastics and danced barefoot than in those at the same school who were shod for these activities; here, the vector was thought to be the floor of the gymnasium.[16]

The epidemiology of genital warts was always contentious: was the disease sexually transmitted or not? The London surgeon Astley Cooper had no doubt; in 1835 he wrote:

> Warts are a local disease, yet when I say local I must observe that they frequently secrete a matter which is able to produce a similar disease in others. A gentleman in Sussex was called to a lady in labor; he felt something in the vagina, and found it to be a crop of warts. In conversation with the husband he told him that his lady had a number of warts. The gentleman stated that at the time he was married he had a wart on the penis and that he had no doubt but that he had communicated them to his wife.[17]

Nonetheless, by the end of the century genital warts were not generally regarded as being of "venereal" origin; they were held to be caused by chronic irritation. After the discovery of the presumed viral identity of genital and skin warts, this opinion had to be modified. It was now maintained that, since many patients with genital warts had common skin warts, they were due to the accidental transfer of virus from one site to the other. Sexual transmission of warts was thought to be very unusual; in a review of the literature in 1921, Heller could find only 11 cases where this had occurred.[18] These ideas were challenged in 1954 when Barrett et al. observed the frequent occurrence of penile warts in U.S. servicemen returning from the Far East who had intercourse with local girls. Moreover, many of the wives of these men developed vulval warts in turn. The authors proposed that genital warts should be regarded as a venereal disease.[19] This suggestion was regarded as outrageous, and 94% of a group of dermatovenereologists who were asked said that it was wrong.[20] For several years the idea of sexual transmission was quietly dropped, and belief in the "unitary" hypothesis—comforting because there was no implication of premarital sex or marital infidelity—was maintained. But later studies showed that Barrett and his colleagues were correct; the prevalence of skin warts had been overestimated, and in most patients with genital warts the disease had been acquired sexually.

In the ancient world, it had been generally believed that there was a connection between anal warts and sodomy, but this idea was forgotten. In the 18th century Hunter taught that they were a manifestation of syphilis. By the end of the 19th century, although there were occasional case reports of anal warts in homosexual men, for the most part the disease was attributed to poor personal hygiene, irritation from discharges, and other nonspecific factors. Male homosexuality was an emotive subject in those days, and the matter received scant attention until the decriminalization of most homosexual practices in the 1960s made epidemiological studies possible. The ancient association between anal warts and anal coitus was then confirmed.

III. SUBCLINICAL HPV INFECTION

Although by the middle of the 19th century surgeons were familiar with penile, anal, and vulval warts, cervical condylomas were not described until the 20th century. This may have been partly because of infrequent speculum examinations, but in 1921 it was stated that cervical condylomas were "one of the rarest of gynecological disorders,"[21] and as recently as 1952 Marsh, in a review of the world literature, could find only eight cases.[22] It is difficult to explain these observations because today cervical condylomas are found in 5–10% of women with vulval warts. Until 1976, exophytic condylomas were regarded as the only expression of HPV infection. In that year, "flat warts" of the cervix were described, invisible to the naked eye but identifiable by colposcopy after the application of acetic acid. These lesions were linked with cellular changes which included koilocytosis and dyskeratosis.[23] The term "koilocytotic atypia" had been introduced by Koss and Durfee 20 years earlier[24] to describe a series of cytological changes which initially had been thought to be a sign of dysplasia, not HPV infection. The discovery of subclinical HPV infection of the cervix was a most important event which opened up an entirely new concept of genital HPV infection which is still being explored. In the mid-1980s, subclinical infections of the external genitalia were also identified, but the epidemiology and significance of these lesions is at present unknown.

IV. TREATMENT

The treatment of skin warts by doctors in earlier times seems to have consisted of their simple excision or destruction. The Greek physician Galen (129–199 A.D.) is said to have known a "dexterous fellow" in Rome who could loosen myrmeciae by sucking them with his lips; when they protruded he would "suddenly divide them and snap them off with his fore teeth."[25] Warts and folklore have always been closely associated, and through the ages many patients with warts have preferred a bewildering variety of wart cures and charms to the painful and often ineffective treatment offered by the medical profession.[26]

The treatment of anogenital warts has also been problematic. In ancient Greece, Hippocrates advised the removal of anal thymia, if they were soft and friable, by pinching them off with the fingers. In Rome, patients with anal warts did not receive much sympathy; according to Dionysius (6th century A.D.):

The surgeons spared neither iron nor fire and were not moved by pity for the patients, because they had brought their trouble on themselves by their unnatural conduct.[27]

In the 18th century, Bell wrote that genital warts could be removed by a knife, scissors, or ligature, but "few patients will submit to the use of the scalpel for the extirpation of numerous warts." Nevertheless, this remained the favored treatment. Although cocaine became available as a local aesthetic in the mid-19th century, it was not always used, one surgeon maintaining that it was preferable "simply to cut them off without any anesthetic whatsoever." A new treatment of the application of podophyllin was introduced by Kaplan, a U.S. Army surgeon, in 1942.[28] It proved to be effective and has been widely (perhaps too widely) used ever since, with surgical extirpation reserved for recalcitrant or very extensive lesions. In recent years, the discovery of subclinical lesions has presented a fresh set of problems. Treatment seems to be remarkably ineffective, and there is no agreement on how, or indeed whether, they should be treated. Since Kaplan's work 50 years ago, there have been few real advances in therapy for anogenital warts, and a permanent cure is as elusive as ever.

V.   CONCLUSION

We have traced HPV infection from ancient times until today. It is clear that there have been two parallel epidemics, of diseases caused by different genotypes, with different epidemiology and clinical features. The first epidemic is of skin warts, associated with HPV 1–4, and spread by casual contact and probably by fomites; the second is of anogenital warts, associated with HPV 6 and 11, and spread for the most part by sexual contact. There is a little overlap between these two epidemics in that HPV 1–4 can sometimes affect the genitals, although HPV 6 and 11 only very rarely infect the nongenital skin. There is, in addition, a third epidemic, of infection by the so-called high risk genotypes, HPV 16, 18, and some others. This overlaps with the second epidemic. Knowledge about this third parallel epidemic is slowly accumulating at present; when its history comes to be written it will make interesting reading.

REFERENCES

1. Bafverstedt, B., Condylomata acuminata past and present, *Acta Derm. Venereol.*, 47, 376, 1967.
2. Anonymous, Peculiar sign, from *Ann. Soc. Méd. Roulers*, in *Lancet*, 2, 250, 1849.
3. Payne, J. F., On the contagiousness of common warts, *Br. J. Dermatol.*, 3, 185, 1891.
4. Gémy, quoted by Frei, E., Zur frage der aetiologischen Beziehung der Warzen und spitzen Kondylome, *Schweiz. Med. Wochenschr.*, 5, 215, 1924.
5. Variot, G., Un cas d'inoculation experimentale des verrues de l'enfant a l'homme, *J. Clin. Thérap. Infant.*, 2, 529, 1894.
6. Licht, C. de F., Om Vonters Smitsomhed, *Ugeskr. Laeg.*, 5 Raekke, 1, 368, 1894.
7. Ciuffo, G., Innesto positivo con filtrato di verruca volgare, *G. Ital. Mal. Ven. Pelle*, 48, 12, 1907.
8. Oriel, J. D., Natural history of genital warts, *Br. J. Vener. Dis.*, 47, 1, 1971.
9. Strauss, M. J., Shaw, E. W., Bunting, H., Melnick, J. L., "Crystalline" virus-like particles from skin papillomas characterised by intranuclear inclusion bodies, *Proc. Soc. Exp. Biol. Med.*, 72, 46, 1949.
10. Lipschütz, B., Zur Kenntnis der Ätiologie und der strukturellen Architektonic der Warze (Verruca vulgaris), *Arch. Dermatol. Syph.*, 148, 201, 1924.
11. Almeida, J. D., Howatson, A. F., Williams, M. G., Electron microscope study of human warts: sites sof virus production and nature of the inclusion bodies, *J. Inv. Dermatol.*, 38, 337, 1962.
12. Dunn, A. E. G., Ogilvie, M. M., Intranuclear virus particles in human genital wart tissue: observations on the ultrastructure of the epidermal layer, *J. Ultrastr. Res.*, 22, 282, 1968.
13. Almeida, J. D., Oriel, J. D., Stannard, L., Characterisation of the virus found in human genital warts, *Microbios*, 3, 225, 1969.
14. Gissmann, L., Pfister, H., zur Hausen, H., Human papillomaviruses. Characterisation of four different isolates, *Virology*, 76, 569, 1977.

15. McLaughlin, A. I. G., Edington, J. W., Infective warts in workers using bone-glue, *Lancet*, 2, 685, 1937.

16. Lyell, A., Warts (letter), *Br. Med. J.*, 2, 349, 1955.

17. Cooper, A., *Lectures on the Principals and Practice of Surgery*, 8th ed., Cox and Portwine, London, 1837, 497.

18. Heller, J., Zur Frage der Kontagiostität der spitzen Kondyloma, *Dermatol. Z.*, 34, 342, 1921.

19. Barrett, T. J., Silbar, J. D., McGinley, J. P., Genital warts - a venereal disease, *J. Am. Med. Assoc.*, 154, 333, 1954.

20. Ronchese, F., Genital warts: a venereal disease (letter), *J. Am. Med. Assoc.*, 154, 1198, 1954.

21. Wharton, L. R., Rare tumours of the cervix of the uterus of inflammatory origin — condyloma and granyuloma, *Surg. Gynecol. Obstet.*, 33, 145, 1921.

22. Marsh, M. R., Papilloma of the cervix, *Am. J. Obstet. Gynecol.*, 64, 281, 1952.

23. Meisels, A., Fortin, R., Roy, M., Condylomatious lesions of the cervix II Cytologic, colposcopic and histopathologic study, *Acta Cytol.*, 21, 379, 1977.

24. Koss, L. G., Durfee, G. R., Unusual patterns of squamous epithelium of the cervix: cytologic and pathologic study of koilocytotic atypia, *Ann. N.Y. Acad. Sci.*, 63, 1245, 1956.

25. Galen, quoted Lyell, A., Management of warts, *Br. Med. J.*, 2, 1576, 1966.

26. Burns, D. A., "Warts and all" — the history and folklore of warts: a review. *J. R. Soc. Med.*, 85, 37, 1992.

27. Dionysius, quoted Hyde, C. E., Condyloma acuminatum in the anal region in the male, *N.Y. Med. J.*, 106, 1125, 1917.

28. Kaplan, I. W., Condylomata acuminata, *New Orleans Med. Surg. J.*, 94, 388, 1942.

II. Virology and Basic Biology

2

Molecular Biology of HPV and Mechanisms of Keratinocyte Transformation

Pawel G. Fuchs and Herbert Pfister

CONTENTS

I. BIOLOGICAL PROPERTIES OF HUMAN PAPILLOMAVIRUSES

Human papillomaviruses (HPV) are small DNA viruses that multiply in the nuclei of differentiated keratinocytes and induce squamous epithelial tumors of the skin or mucosa. The virions are nonenveloped cubic particles of 55–60 nm, which encapsulate a single copy of the double-stranded genome in the form of a protein-complexed minichromosome.[1,2] The capsid proteins carry type-specific and genus-specific antigenic determinants.[3] To establish the viral DNA in the human epidermis, the virions probably have to infect cells of the basal layer. It may take weeks before tumors develop and up to 90% of the infections will have no clinical consequences.[4] Warts, papillomas, or dysplasias arise when virus-encoded proteins stimulate cellular proliferation and interfere with the proper differentiation of epithelial cells. Differentiating keratinocytes become increasingly permissive for HPV, which is reflected by the onset of vegetative viral DNA replication in prickle cells and by the synthesis of structural proteins, starting in the granular layer. Mature virus particles are spread throughout the cell nuclei in the stratum granulosum and appear embedded in keratin in the stratum corneum.

HPV induced papillomas or acanthomas may develop into carcinomas mainly in three conditions: the skin disease epidermodysplasia verruciformis (EV), dysplasias of the cervix uteri, and laryngeal papillomas of adults.[5,6] Carcinomas are not an early consequence of HPV infection but occur on the basis of long-persisting lesions with "latency periods" of many years.[7] No mature HPV particles are produced in carcinoma cells but persistence of viral DNA and ongoing expression of viral early genes could be demonstrated in carcinomas of EV patients and in anogenital cancer (see below). Due to the preferential association with malignant tumors, specific HPV types are regarded as representatives with a high carcinogenic potential as opposed to low risk viruses that prevail in predominantly benign proliferations.[4,6]

II.   GENOME ORGANIZATION

The HPV genome is a circular DNA molecule of 7500–8000 base pairs. A large number of HPV types have been sequenced in their entirety or at least partially.[8] Their organization turned out to be remarkably similar. All putative protein-encoding sequences (open reading frames, ORFs) are located on one DNA strand and occupy comparable positions relative to each other. Three representative genomes are shown in Figure 1. The individual ORFs are classified as "early" (E) or "late" (L) in analogy with other DNA viruses where this designation denotes the expression schedule in the viral life cycle. The expression in nonproductive, bovine papilloma virus 1 (BPV1) transformed cells defined the "early" segment of papillomavirus DNA, and a detailed genetic analysis indeed identified typical "early genes," whose products are involved in viral DNA replication, transcription control, and cellular transformation.[9] Only E4 seems to be predominantly expressed late in the viral life cycle, possibly playing a role in the collapse of the cytokeratin matrix and in virus release as shown for HPV16 E4.[10] The "late" ORFs encode the major viral capsid protein (L1) and a minor capsid component (L2) of uncertain localization.[11] ORFs L1 and E6 are consistently separated by a 400–1000 base pair noncoding DNA segment that contains the origin of viral DNA replication and numerous transcription control signals (see below). This segment is variably referred to as noncoding region (NCR), long control region, or upper regulatory region.

There are two noteworthy differences in the genome organization of HPV types belonging to various phylogenetic subgroups.[1,8] The noncoding DNA segment of EV-associated HPVs has roughly only half the length of the noncoding region of all other HPVs (Figure 1) and there is some evidence for transcriptional control elements integrated into flanking coding sequences.[12] The ORF E5 is located between ORFs E2 and L2 in genital HPVs like HPV 16[13] (Figure 1) and in more distantly related cutaneous HPVs like HPV2.[14] In contrast, there is little space between E2 and L2 in HPV1[15] and the coding part of E5 completely overlaps L2 (Figure 1). The ORF E5 of HPV1 is located downstream of a polyadenylation site at the beginning of L2 (see below) and therefore is not part of the early transcription unit. The amino acid sequence and the hydrophobicity profile of the putative HPV1 E5 protein show no similarity to E5 of HPV16-related viruses so it is questionable if the E5 ORFs of these viruses really represent homologous genes. There is no comparable ORF E5 in EV-associated HPVs like HPV8[12,16] (Figure 1).

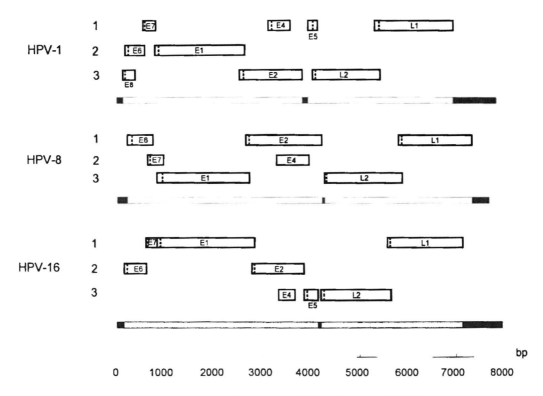

FIGURE 1   Genome organization of human papillomaviruses (HPV) 1, 8, and 16.[1,12,13,15] The circular genomes are linearized for convenience of alignment. Open reading frames are indicated by open boxes. Dotted lines within the frames represent the first methionine codon, which could serve as a start point of translation. Stippled areas of the genome bars represent coding sequences and black regions stand for noncoding regions. The scale is in base pairs (bp).

III.   GENE EXPRESSION

A.   Promoters and Transcripts

The early genome region of papillomaviruses is transcribed into multiple, differentially spliced, and partially overlapping RNA species, most of which share a common 3' end defined by a polyadenylation signal at the beginning of L2.[17-19] In the high-risk genital HPV types 16 and 18, one early promoter was identified in front of the E6 coding sequence[20,21] whereas the low-risk types 6 and 11 possess an additional E7-specific promoter within the E6 ORF.[22] A similar constellation of two independent E6- and E7-promoters has been reported for the EV-associated, skin-specific HPV types 5 and 8.[23,24]

The extensive analysis of BPV1 transcription suggests that there will be more promoter elements in the HPV genomes. At least 6 early promoters have been described for BPV1, only three of which map to the viral NCR.[17] Over 95% of all transcripts seen in HPV1-induced plantar warts had 5' ends in ORF E7[18], pointing to a strong nearby promoter, and the 5' ends of the most abundant, spliced E1^E4 mRNAs of HPV11 and HPV31 were mapped to a homologous site.[25,26] The HPV31 transcripts were shown to be induced following stratification of persistently infected cells in raft cultures. In spite of the abundance of the transcripts, the corresponding promoter is still poorly defined. The existence of an intragenic promoter in front of ORF E1 was furthermore suggested by cDNA and primer extension analysis of HPV16 transcripts.[27] A study on HPV18 revealed 3 novel promoters localized within the ORFs E1, E2, and L2, respectively, indicating that HPVs may actually show similar promoter plurality as BPV1.[28]

sites seems to be a constant feature (Figure 3). A genetic dissection revealed a modular structure of the enhancer by identifying several subunits which display limited enhancing activity on their own and synergistically contribute to the overall enhancement of transcription.[66,67] The enhancers in the central NCR are keratinocyte-specific[51,52,54] and may therefore constitute a basis for the epithelial cell tropism of the genital HPVs.

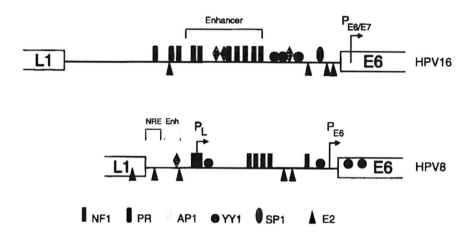

FIGURE 3 Schematic representation of the distribution of binding sites for the transcription factors NF1, AP1, SP1, YY1, the progesterone receptor (PR), and the viral E2 protein in the noncoding regions of the HPV16 and HPV8 genomes between open reading frames L1 and E6. The positions of enhancer (Enh) and negative regulatory elements (NRE) are indicated by brackets, the location of the E6 (P_{E6}) and the late (P_L) promoter by arrows. For details and references, see text.

The molecular mechanism directing the tissue specificity of the HPV-enhancers is still poorly understood. Data emerging during the last years suggest that the phenomenon depends rather on the balance of different ubiquitous transcription factors than on an "all-or-none" scenario where viral regulatory sequences would interact with one or more factor(s) present exclusively in epithelial cells. Among the candidates which might contribute to keratinocyte-specificity are jun B, AP1 proteins, members of the NF1 family, as well as TEF 1 and its cofactor.[57,58,60,66,69] Noteworthy is an apparently truly keratinocyte-specific factor KRF-1 that binds to the enhancer of HPV18.[70] Its general significance is questionable, however, because no KRF-1 binding sites could be identified in other genital HPV enhancers.

Progesterone and glucocorticoid response elements are consistent features of the NCRs of genital HPVs (Figure 3). They may reside within the central enhancer or in flanking regions and confer hormone inducibility to viral gene expression.[52,64] The genital HPVs may thus take advantage from temporarily increased progesterone concentrations during pregnancy and ovulation cycle. It is remarkable in this context that progesterone or progestins from oral contraceptives substantially enhanced transformation of rodent cells by HPV16 *in vitro*.[71] Dexamethasone also increased the transformation of HPV16 immortalized keratinocytes by the Ha-ras oncogene.[72]

Another group of constitutive enhancer elements has been found within the 5′ flank of HPV-NCRs. Such elements were identified for HPV11,[73,74] HPV18,[75] and HPV8 (Figure 3).[76] A similarly localized element has also been reported for BPV1.[77] Interestingly, these regulatory elements do not show the epithelial cell-specificity, characteristic for the central NCR enhancers. Whereas the HPV8 enhancer could be shown to be indispensable for the activity of the viral late promoter,[30,76] the target promoters of the other 5′-NCR enhancers remain unknown.

There is mounting evidence that the regulation of HPV transcription includes both positively acting enhancers and negatively regulating elements. Already, early functional dissections of NCRs suggested that these sequences were composed of intermingled domains mediating opposite regulatory effects.[78,79] Transcriptional silencers (*cis*-elements down-regulating the virus-specific transcription) have recently been uncovered in the NCRs of HPV8, 16, and 18. Silencers of the early promoter of HPV16 and 18 reside within the E6-proximal part of the NCRs, and their activity depends on the interaction with the ubiquitous multifunctional cellular protein YY1 (Figure 3).[80,81] Other negative elements depend on effects mediated by the epidermal growth factor,[82] retinoic acid receptor,[83] and the nuclear factor for the interleukin 6 expression (NF-IL6).[84]

A 38 bp sequence upstream of the late promoter of HPV8 downregulates its activity in an orientation-independent way (Figure 3).[85] This silencer element was shown to bind one cellular factor but three mutants have been identified which no longer bind protein but still repress transcription, indicating that protein-DNA interaction may not be relevant for its silencer function.

2. Viral Transcription Factors

E2 ORFs of papillomaviruses encode multifunctional DNA-binding phosphoproteins acting as transcriptional modulators and replication factors.[86,87] The E2 proteins consist of conserved N- and C-terminal domains of about 220 and 95 amino acid residues, respectively, joined by a variable sequence. The N-terminal part of E2 is responsible for transcriptional transactivation by the full-length protein. Another most interesting feature of the N-terminal E2-domain is its ability to mediate formation of DNA-loops *in vitro* between two DNA-bound E2 dimers.[88] This may allow E2 to bring together distantly located regulatory elements. The C-terminal sequences of the protein confer DNA-binding and dimerization capacities (Figure 4). The central, poorly conserved sequences have frequently been described as a hinge region, since due to their theoretically possible random coil structure they may serve as a flexible joint between the N- and C-termini of the E2 molecule. The hinge region appears to be relevant for the replicative functions of E2.[89]

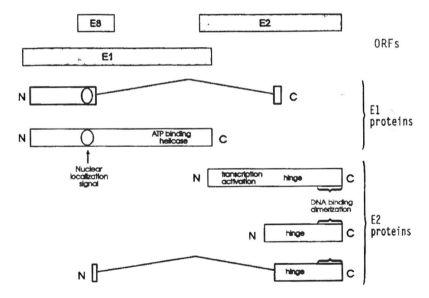

FIGURE 4 Schematic representation of E1 and E2 proteins of bovine papillomavirus 1. The proteins as translated from the open reading frames (ORFs, shown on top as shaded bars) are indicated by open boxes. The amino- and carboxy-termini are labeled by N and C. Functional domains are marked.

The E2 protein interacts as a dimer-molecule with its palindromic DNA target sites ACC(N)$_6$GGT or ACC(N)$_6$GTT.[90-93] These motifs occur several times in the genomes of all papillomaviruses and most of them are localized within the NCRs. The distribution of E2 binding sites within the NCRs is rather conserved among papillomaviruses of one phylogenetic branch but differs considerably between members of different lineages. This is most apparent in the HPVs specific for the mucosa vs. EV-associated viruses (Figure 3).[94]

Interaction of the E2 proteins with their target sequences may result in a variety of regulatory effects. Activation of transcription is an exclusive property of the full-length proteins. Already a single E2-binding palindrome in *cis* to a target promoter may mediate a weak stimulation in the presence of the E2 transactivator. Two E2-sites constitute a strong E2-dependent transcriptional enhancer that can stimulate promoters over a large distance.[96-98] The strong synergy of two E2 binding sites is partially due to the cooperative binding of E2 to adjacent palindromes.[99] On top of this, two DNA-bound dimers are required for cooperation with cellular factors such as USF and SP1 that may potentiate the stimulatory effect of E2.[97,100-102] Especially interesting seems to be the role of SP1, which can form a complex with full-length E2 and was shown to enhance the affinity of E2 to weak binding sites.[102] The specific targets of E2-activation are not yet clearly identified, but it seems possible that they include the components of the transcription-initiation complex.[103]

Although E2 was originally characterized as an activator of transcription, more recent studies showed that E2 proteins frequently inhibit gene expression.[86,87] Different mechanisms of E2-mediated repression have been revealed. Two N-terminally truncated E2 proteins are expressed by BPV1 that retain the ability to bind DNA but cannot stimulate transcription due to the lack of an activator domain (Figure 4). In fact, they act inhibitory when occupying the E2 target sites on DNA or inactivating the full-length E2 by forming inactive heterodimers. Negatively acting N-terminally truncated E2 proteins may also exist in HPV11 and HPV16 infected cells.[27,33,104,105] Another example presents the regulation of the BPV1 promoter P_{7185} which is subject to E2-repression due to the interference of E2 with binding of an essential promoter factor.[77,106] In this case, both the full length and repressor E2 forms may exert an inhibitory effect.

Among HPVs, the transcription-modulation by E2 has been studied primarily with the genital types 11, 16, and 18. Both positive and negative effects of E2 on the activity of the viral oncogene promoter have been observed, depending on slightly different experimental conditions with regard to E2-expression vectors and host cells. The E2-repression apparently depends on two E2 binding sites immediately preceding the TATA box of the early promoter and flanked at the 5'-side by a SP1 recognition motif. The inhibitory effect of E2 seems to be due to the hindrance of the assembly of the transcription preinitiation complex at the TATA box[103,107,108] and/or to the displacement of the stimulatory SP1 factor by E2-binding to the distal E2-site (Figure 3).[109-111] Both these binding sites are required for the repression of the HPV16 promoter,[108,111] whereas only the promoter-proximal site turned out to be necessary for E2-repression of HPV18.[112] The negative modulation of oncogene expression also occurs with the low-risk HPV11.[113] HPV16 E2 was shown to trans-activate the early promoter in rodent cells[114] and moderately stimulated viral gene expression in normal and immortalized keratinocytes.[115]

In HPV8, E2 clearly stimulates the late promoter.[30] A mutational analysis revealed that this is a net result of both positive and negative effects mediated by individual E2 binding sites.[116] Mainly high-affinity sites P0 and P1 and to a smaller extent medium- and low-affinity sites P3 and P4 serve to transactivate the promoter, whereas the low affinity site P2 is able to downmodulate E2-transactivation, finally repressing basal promoter activity at high E2 concentrations.[117] The negative regulation may depend on displacement of the TBP factor from the TATA-box by E2 protein as well as its interference with promoter-activating cellular factors which interact with the P2 sequence. The high conservation of the P2 sequence in the vicinity of the late promoter cap site of EV-associated HPVs, HPV1, CRPV, and BPV1 may suggest that an interplay of E2 and cellular factors at this sequence element is more generally important for the expression of structural proteins.

An HPV18 DNA sequence in the L1-proximal part of the LCR, which stimulates transcription, is dependent on the viral E6 gene product for function.[55] The mechanism remains to be established.

IV. REPLICATION

Two modes of viral DNA replication can be distinguished: (1) a "maintenance" replication during persistent infection that guarantees a constant copy number of viral genomes per cell, and (2) the vegetative replication representing an outburst of viral DNA synthesis in differentiated keratinocytes. The general model for the first strategy is replication of BPV 1 in transformed fibroblasts which is assumed to mimic HPV DNA replication in basal cells of the epidermis and in cultured keratinocytes.[118] Nothing is known so far at the molecular level about the switch to vegetative replication.

The full-length E1 and E2 proteins are necessary and sufficient *in trans* to drive BPV 1 DNA replication both *in vivo* and *in vitro*.[119-121] These factors cooperate with a *cis*-active element which apparently displays properties of an origin of replication (ori) and is localized within the viral NCR in close proximity to the early E6 promoter.[120]

E1 is the largest and most conserved ORF of papillomaviruses. In BPV1 it encodes at least two phosphorylated polypeptides: a small 23 kDa protein derived from the 5'-segment of E1 (recently shown to be nonessential for stable BPV1 replication[122]), and the 68 kDa full-length E1 phospho-protein (Figure 4).[123,124] In line with its role in replication, E1 is a nuclear protein.[124] Transport of E1 into the nucleus depends on a nuclear localization signal within the N-terminal part of the protein whose inactivation affects both the cellular localization and the ability of BPV1 to repli-cate.[125] The BPV1 E1 possesses a number of intrinsic activities characteristic for multifunctional replication factors, e.g., DNA helicase activity, DNA-dependent ATP-binding, and ATPase activity and an origin-specific ability to unwind the supercoiled DNA.[124,126]

In view of the absolute requirement of the replication process for both E1 and E2, the most interesting property of E1 is its ability to enter a stable physical complex with E2.[127] The sequence-specific binding of E1 to the viral origin of replication may be significantly enhanced by E2.[120,121,127-129] Ori mutants severely disabled in E1 binding still retained the capacity to bind considerable amounts of the E1/E2 complex which suggests the existence of a compensative E2-dependent mechanism.[130] The exact role of E2-binding site(s) remains unclear. Deletion of the ori proximal E2-binding site from the minimal BPV1-ori renders it inactive, but replication may be rescued by offering another E2-binding site(s), even at a distant position to the crippled ori-core. On the other hand, removal of the 3'-half of the ori-proximal palindrome does not affect replication although no E2 binding can be detected at the mutated site.[121,129] Mutational analysis revealed that the replication rates of BPV1 DNA roughly parallel the affinity of ori sequences to E1 or the E1/E2-complex.[130]

The *cis*-sequences active as minimal ori and target site of the E1 protein could be narrowed down to about 60 base pairs. They encompass an AT-rich stretch of nucleotides in their 5'-moiety, an inverted repeat, and a part of the neighboring E2-binding site.[121,129] This general outline is similar to the structures of origins of simple eucaryotic genomes.[131]

Studies with HPV1, 6b, 7, 11, 16, and 18 showed that the *cis*- and *trans*-requirements of the HPVs for transient replication were principally the same as those of BPV1.[132-135] Formation of the E1/E2 complex could be demonstrated for the HPV11-specific proteins which recognized the ori-containing DNA fragment in an E2-dependent manner.[136] In line with the initial observation for BPV1, the N-terminally shortened "repressor" forms of E2 did not support viral replication and rather acted inhibitory.[120,133] The ori-region of HPV11 could be mapped to an 80 base pair segment overlapping the early E6 promoter and displaying most of the characteristic features defined for the BPV1 minimal ori.[133] However, in some contrast to BPV 1, the ori-elements of HPV11 and 18 seem to depend on the presence of at least one complete E2-binding site.[133,135]

The replication of papillomavirus DNA, as measured by the transient assays, is obviously not cell type-specific.[120,132,134] The extreme host-and species-specificity observed for HPV infections therefore seems to be at least primarily due to the cellular control at the level of viral gene expression.

The intimate interconnection of replication and transcription control is remarkable. Not only is replication dependent on the transcription factor E2 but the *bona fide* replication protein E1 also appears involved in the repression of the BPV1 E6 promoter.[137] Although the exact mechanism of repression is still unclear, the E1 effect seemed to correlate with binding of the E1/E2 complex to the ori and not with the process of replication itself.

V.   TRANSFORMATION

Three viral proteins, namely E6, E7, and E5, revealed oncogenic activity in various transformation assays. The relative importance of the individual proteins is quite variable among different papillomaviruses. The transforming activity of a given virus can usually be put down to a cooperation of at least two oncoproteins. It is most interesting to note a correlation between some biochemical activities of the oncoproteins and the carcinogenic potential of the respective viruses suggesting that these functions are indeed relevant to tumorigenesis. The E6, E7, and E5 proteins could all be shown to interact with cellular proteins which on their part are involved in cell cycle control.

A.   The E7 Oncoprotein

The E7 proteins of HPV16 and HPV18 were studied in most detail. On their own, they are able to transform and immortalize rodent cells[138,139] and show weak immortalizing activity in primary human keratinocytes particularly when overexpressed under the control of a strong promoter.[140,141] In the context of the HPV genome, a cooperation of E7 and E6 genes is typically necessary to immortalize keratinocytes from the cervical mucosa and to alter their differentiation pattern.[142,143] The HPV6 E7 gene was about 10 times less efficient than HPV16 or HPV18 E7 when assaying induction of anchorage-independent growth in rodent fibroblasts.[144] In cooperation with an activated ras oncogene, HPV6 and HPV11 E7 transformed baby rat kidney cells with low efficiency but the transformed cells were highly tumorigenic in immunocompetent animals.[145] HPV6 E7 has no immortalizing activity in human epithelial cells on its own but can cooperate with HPV16 E6 in immortalization and stimulation of cell proliferation.[146]

The E7 genes of the cutaneous skin cancer-associated HPV types 8 and 47 failed to induce any detectable transformation of rodent cells,[147,148] in contrast to the E7 genes of genital papillomaviruses. In collaboration with the activated H-ras gene, however, HPV5 and 8 E7 gave rise to transformed cell lines.[149] The E7 gene of the plantar wart-specific HPV1 fully transformed the mouse fibroblast line C127.[150] In the case of cutaneous HPVs, the degree of morphological transformation by E7 genes therefore appears not correlated to the risk of malignant conversion of the lesions induced by the corresponding HPVs.

The E7 gene product is a multifunctional small phosphoprotein with about 100 amino acids (Figure 5) that appears bound to the nuclear matrix of the host cell.[151,152] No phosphorylation was detectable in the case of HPV8 E7.[23] The aminoterminal 40 amino acids show significant homology to oncoproteins of other DNA tumor viruses, namely to E1A of adenoviruses and large T of simian virus 40.[153] Analysis of mutants in the HPV16 E7 gene and of E7 peptides indicated that amino acids 1–40 are required for cellular transformation and stimulation of host DNA synthesis whereas amino acids 20–40 of E7 are critical for its ability to activate transcription from the adenovirus E2 promoter.[154-158] Amino acids 20–30 are responsible for the interaction with a number of cellular proteins (see below). The serines at position 31 and 32 serve as substrate for the cellular casein kinase II. The precise role of phosphorylation in transformation and transcription-activation is not yet clearly established.[155,158,159] Amino acids 40–98 contain two copies of a Cys-X-X-Cys sequence motif, which are involved in the zinc binding property of E7 (Figure 5).[160] This carboxy terminal portion of E7 is mainly responsible for the intracellular stability of the polypeptide,[158] but it may also contribute to transcription activation.[156,161,162]

An extremely interesting function of E7 is the ability to form complexes with several cellular proteins involved in cell cycle control. The first factor identified was the product of the retinoblastoma tumor suppressor gene, pRB.[163,164] The phosphorylated form of E7 binds preferentially to the underphosphorylated pRB, which exists in G_0 and G_1 of the cell cycle and is considered to be the active form restricting cell proliferation.[165,166] The underphosphorylated pRB binds and inhibits the transcription factor E2F.[167] The E7 protein in turn can dissociate the E2F-pRb complex,[161,162,168,169] and the released transcription factor may activate expression of cell cycle-regulated genes such as c-myc, thymidine kinase, and DNA polymerase α, required for DNA synthesis.[167] This function of E7 is appropriate to induce an S-phase environment to permit viral DNA amplification. Only in

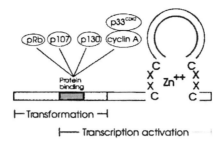

FIGURE 5 Structure and functional domains of the E7 oncoprotein. The zinc finger-like area is drawn schematically. The protein binding domain is responsible for complex formation with cellular proteins pRB, p107, p130, and the cyclin A-p33^{CDK2} complex.

the case of undue activity in basal cells of the epidermis may the function contribute to carcinogenesis analogous to mutations of the Rb gene. It is noteworthy that the E2F-pRb complex is absent in cervical carcinoma cell lines that express E7.[168]

The E7 protein was further shown to block pRb binding to DNA.[170] As pRb mutants defective in DNA-binding have lost the ability to inhibit cell growth, it was suggested that this E7 activity contributes to the inactivation of pRb.

The complex formation of viral oncoproteins and pRb may also partially explain the resistance of HPV transformed keratinocytes to transforming growth factor-ß (TGF-ß) mediated growth arrest in G1.[171] Addition of TGF-ß in mid to late G1 prevents phosphorylation of pRb.[172] TGF-ß therefore appears to function at least in part in the growth-inhibitory pathway dependent on the underphosphorylated state of pRb and this pathway is blocked in HPV transformed keratinocytes "downstream" of TGF-ß by the E7-pRb interaction. However, mutational analysis of E1A showed that binding to pRb, p107, and cyclin A elicited only partial resistance to TGF-ß growth inhibition.[173] This may indicate that additional functions are required to render cells insensitive to TGF-ß. E1A mutants binding to p300 could complement mutants interacting only with pRb to induce full resistance to TGF-ß, but there is no evidence for complex formation of E7 and p300.

Mutations within the E7 gene which prevent the E7-pRb interaction destroy many of the transforming and immortalizing activities in rodent cells.[155,174] This supports the functional significance of the pRb association. It is furthermore very interesting to note that the E7 proteins of low risk genital HPV types 6 and 11 bind to pRb with much lower affinity than the E7 proteins of HPV16 and 18,[164,165] and are less rapidly phosphorylated by casein kinase II[155] but transactivate the adenovirus E2 promoter with an efficiency similar to that of HPV16.[145,175] Studies with chimeric HPV6 and HPV16 proteins have shown that these differences are determined by the amino-terminal sequences whereas the carboxy-terminal regions are functionally equivalent.[175] A single amino acid difference at position 22 between the pRb binding sites of HPV16 and HPV6 turned out to be principally responsible for the reduced pRb binding affinity of HPV6 E7 and its low capacity to cooperate with an activated ras oncogene in transformation of baby rat kidney cells.[176,177] This may not explain, however, the weak immortalizing activity of the HPV6 E7 gene in human epithelial cells[146] because HPV16 E7 mutants which do not bind pRb are still able to immortalize primary human keratinocytes.[174]

There are various E7 mutants that retain pRb-binding activity and have lost transforming activity.[154,155,157,158] This indicates that complex formation with pRb may be important but not sufficient for cellular transformation.

More recent studies have demonstrated an interaction of E7 from HPV types 1, 6, 11, 16, 18, and 33 with p107, p130, cyclin A, and the cyclin-associated kinase p33^{CDK2}.[178-181] The E7/p107 interaction is cell cycle dependent, being maximal in the S and G$_2$ phase.[181] The same set of cellular proteins is bound by the homologous sequences in adenovirus E1A. However, p107 is required for E1A-cyclinA complex formation whereas HPV 16 E7 appears to interact directly with cyclin A.[179] Addition of E7 protein to cell extracts did not dissociate E2F from cyclin A, in contrast to adenovirus

E1A.[169] The E7-associated kinase activity was only 2–3% of the total cyclin A-associated kinase in HPV16 DNA containing cervical carcinoma cells.[179] The detection of E7-associated kinase activity correlated with the presence of cells in the G_2/M phase of the cell cycle where cyclin A is synthesized.[179-180] It is obvious from these data that HPV16 E7 is targeting a number of key players involved in the regulation of the cell cycle. This is intriguing by itself but further studies are needed to reveal all physical consequences of these interactions and their role in oncogenesis.

B. The E6 Oncoprotein

The E6 proteins of the genital high risk HPV types 16 and 18 are generally regarded as auxiliary oncoproteins. In rodent cells, E6 shows quite significant effects. It induces only subtle morphological changes in monolayer cell lines[182] but immortalizes primary cells,[183,184] leads to anchorage-independent growth of NIH3T3 and rat1 cells,[35,185] and even to tumorigenicity of ψ2 cells in nude mice.[186] In the human system, however, transforming ability could only be demonstrated with mammary epithelial cells.[187,188] In keratinocytes of the genital mucosa, which represents the authentic target tissue of HPV16 or 18, E6 revealed no activity on its own but cooperated with E7 in immortalization.[140,142,143] HPV16 E6 did not influence the degree of HPV16-E7 induced dysplastic changes of genital keratinocytes in the raft culture system.[146] The E6 genes of low risk genital HPVs do not have any appreciable cell-transforming activities,[144] but some low degree of cooperativity could be reported for HPV6-E6 and HPV16-E7.[146]

In contrast to HPVs infecting the genital mucosa, E6 seems to be the dominant oncogene of Ev-associated viruses. In rodent cell lines, E6 of HPV5, 8, 14, 21, 25, and 47 was shown to be sufficient to induce anchorage-independent growth and morphological transformation, whereas none of these effects could be reported for the E7 proteins of HPV8 and 47.[147,148,182,189] It should be noted that similar to E7 oncoproteins of genital HPVs, the cell transforming potential of EV-specific E6 proteins reflects the *in vivo* association of the corresponding virus types with cancer.[189]

The E6 proteins are small polypeptides with about 150 amino acids that contain four Cys-X-X-Cys motifs with the potential to form two zink finger-like domains. The spacing of the Cys-X-X-Cys motifs in both domains is exactly 29 amino acids like in the E7 oncoprotein.[94] E6 protein could indeed be shown to bind zinc.[190] Integrity of the cys-repeats is essential for stability and most of the biological properties of the polypeptide.[191,192] E6 proteins can interact with DNA in a sequence unspecific manner.[190,193,194] In line with this activity, HPV18 E6 could be detected in the nucleus but also in the non-nuclear membranes.[194]

The proteins of HPV 16 and 18 were shown to enter complexes with p53,[195] a multifunctional regulatory protein with properties of an anti-oncogene.[196] HPV E6 targets the p53 molecules in degradation via the ubiquitin-dependent proteolytic pathway,[197] suggesting that E6 can eliminate the negative growth regulator p53 and thereby push the cells towards uncontrolled proliferation. The reduced half life of p53 and low protein levels in some HPV-carrying cells support this hypothesis.[198-200] Formation of a stable complex between E6 and p53 and degradation of p53 require an additional factor, designated E6-associated protein (E6-AP).[201,202] E6-AP directly interacts with E6 also in the absence of p53 and stimulates the simultaneous association of both proteins with p53.

In contrast to the high risk HPV types 16 and 18, E6 proteins encoded by the low risk types 6 and 11 bind p53 with much lower affinity and do not mediate degradation.[195,197,203] No E6-p53 complexes could be demonstrated for the Ev-associated HPVs 5 and 8, as well as BPV1 and CRPV.[150,204-206]

The degradation of p53 induced by HPV16 E6 apparently represents an important step in the immortalization of human keratinocytes because dominant negative p53 mutants could be shown to substitute for E6 in this regard.[207] However, E6 has additional oncogenic activities mainly revealed by transformation of rodent cells which are independent of the p53 pathway. This is exemplified by E6 proteins of BPV1, CRPV, and HPVs 5 and 8, which have oncogenic properties although they do not complex p53[147,150,204-206] and even NIH 3T3 cell transformation by HPV16 E6 cannot be substituted by p53 mutants.[207]

A study by Keen et al.[205] disclosed at least five additional proteins (212, 182, 81, 75, and 33 kDa) interacting with E6 proteins of HPV16 and 18. E6 of HPV6 and 11 could bind (on average very weakly) different subsets of these proteins. All tested E6 proteins were found to bind a cellular kinase which could phosphorylate exogenous histone H1 and phosphorylate p182 as a part of the E6-associated protein complex. This activity was not due to p53-associated p33[cdc2] since it occurred also when extracts from p53-deficient cells were used. The kinase was not observed when testing the E6 proteins of HPV5 and 8, further substantiating biological differences between the E6-peptides of cutaneous and genital HPVs.

The yeast two-hybrid approach to E6-associated proteins recently revealed a new factor in HeLa cells (E6BP), specifically interacting with the E6 proteins of the high-risk genital HPVs.[208] Interestingly, E6BP represents a potential calcium-binding polypeptide. Since calcium ions and calcium-binding proteins are involved in cellular signaling and cell differentiation, this finding seems to expand the potential of E6 to interfere with the cellular growth control.

Consequences in terms of transformation might also be expected from the transactivation of heterologous promoters by E6.[35,191,207,209] Again there seem to be two possible mechanisms. Binding of E6 to p53 turned out to be sufficient to abrogate p53-mediated repression of multiple promoters.[200] On the other hand, transactivation of the adenovirus E2 promoter by E6 could not be mimicked by p53 mutants.[207] Rather, E6 represents a transactivating protein on its own which could replace the activating N-terminal domain of E2 to confer E2-binding site-dependent stimulation of promoters by E6-E2 fusion proteins.[191] The importance of the latter mechanism for oncogenesis is questionable because low risk and high risk genital HPVs did not differ in this activity.[35]

C.   The E5 Oncoprotein

The ORFs E5 of several animal papillomaviruses and genital HPVs encode highly hydrophobic polypeptides with a molecular mass of 8–10 kDa. E5 is a major oncogene of BPV1 and other fibropapilloma-inducing animal papillomaviruses.[9] The E5 protein displays two structurally distinct domains: an amino-terminal region with features of a typical transmembrane peptide and a short hydrophilic C-terminal sequence responsible for homodimer-formation.[210,211] The cell-transforming activity of BPV1-E5 was traced back to its interference with the cellular signal transduction pathways. Expression of E5 results in a prolonged half-life of the epidermal growth factor receptor (EGFR) and its retarded internalization,[212,213] as well as in a direct stimulation of the endogenous ß-type receptor for the platelet-derived growth factor (PDGFR).[214] Both events, which are independent of the natural growth factor ligand, are believed to expose the cell to a continous mitogenic stimulus.

The BPV-E5 protein was found to associate with the 16 kDa membrane-integral subunit of an ATPase which occurs in vacuoles, lysosomes, endosomes, and Golgi-vesicles, and constitutes a part of the cellular proton pump involved in the acidification of intracellular compartments.[215,216] The interaction depends on the hydrophobic domain of the E5 protein and its importance has been pinpointed by the observation that several mutations within this region simultanously hit the E5-ability to complex with p16 and to transform murine fibroblasts.[217] Most interestingly, it could be shown that p16 mediates *in vivo* formation of a ternary complex of E5-ATPase-PDGFR, thus establishing for the first time a physical link between a viral oncoprotein and the metabolism of a growth factor receptor.[218]

Another cellular factor which associates with E5 is the 120 kDa adaptin-like protein.[219] Adaptins are involved in recognition of receptors and targeting them to endocytosis and degradation. Engagement of adaptin(s) by E5 could result in maintenence of the activated receptors on the cell surface. This model may explain the ATPase-independent effect of E5 on the EGFR. Taken together, BPV1-E5 seems to disable a part of the normal cellular signaling circuits via its direct or indirect interactions with the functions of at least two growth factor receptors.

The HPV-encoded E5 proteins show very little sequence homology both with BPV1-E5 and among themselves. They are highly hydrophobic but, in contrast to BPV1-E5, seem to contain three putative transmembrane domains[220] and are not able to form dimers.[221] HPV6-E5 on its own transforms mouse cells.[222] The E5 protein of HPV16, although possessing rather little cell-transforming activity per se was shown to induce anchorage-independent growth (and eventually tumorigenicity in nude mice) upon stimulation of the E5-expressing mouse fibroblasts with EGF.[221,223,224] Since the E5-transformed cells revealed at the same time an elevated c-*fos* expression, it has been concluded that E5 enhances the ligand-dependent signal transduction into the nucleus.[224] These findings suggest that HPV-E5 oncoproteins use similar transformation strategies as BPV1-E5. More recent data could indeed substantiate this hypothesis. Both HPV6 and 16-E5 proteins are similarly localized in the cell as the BPV1 E5 protein and may as well form complexes with the p16-component of the vacuolar ATPase.[221] E5 of HPV6 was shown to associate with PDGFR and EGFR whereas no such interactions could be found for the HPV16-E5.[221,226]

HPV 16 E5 transformed mouse keratinocytes to tumorigenicity,[226] and showed mitogenic activity in human foreskin keratinocytes which was subject to a synergistic effect of EGF.[227] As compared to controls, the E5-expressing human cells showed an increased number of endogenous EGF receptors per cell. The normal EGFR response to its ligand in such cells is changed in that the receptors become hyperphosphorylated, their degradation is inhibited, and there is an increased recycling of the receptors to the cell surface. These effects may at least partially be due to an E5-induced block in acidification of the endosomes, which is probably related to the interaction of E5 with the p16-subunit of the vacuolar H^+-ATPase.[228]

An intriguing, albeit still unclear aspect of the E5 biology results from the recent demonstration of a possible cellular counterpart of the viral E5-sequence in the mouse genome.[229] Most interestingly, expression of this gene increases in animals and cell cultures treated with carcinogens.

D.　The E2 Protein

There is preliminary evidence that the E2 proteins, in addition to being involved in transcription control and replication, may also play a role in virus-induced cell transformation. Expression of HPV8 E2 in rodent fibroblasts led to anchorage-independent growth and reduced serum requirement of the cells.[230] HPV8 E2 furthermore allowed colony formation in soft agar when transfected into the spontaneously immortalized human skin keratinocyte line HaCaT, which in addition acquired an altered fibroblastoid morphology.[231] It seems possible that the cell-transforming activity presents a more general property of E2 proteins since E2 of BPV1 and HPV16 were also suggested to be involved in immortalization.[232,233]

VI.　MOLECULAR EVENTS ASSOCIATED WITH MALIGNANT CONVERSION

Carcinomas usually develop only after HPV induced lesions persist for several months or even years, which indicates that additional events are mandatory to trigger malignant conversion.[6,7] This is in line with the finding that HPV-immortalized keratinocytes are initially benign and become malignant only after numerous passages *in vitro*.[234,235] Tumor progression is enhanced by chemical or physical mutagens, which are likely to affect both viral and cellular functions and will thereby disturb the balanced persistent infection.[6,7] Several lines of evidence indicate that tumor progression is accompanied by an increase in viral oncogene expression, which continues in the malignant tumors.

A.　Physical State of Viral DNA

The integration of HPV16 or HPV18 DNA into the cellular DNA of many genital cancers, which is in contrast to the extrachromosomal persistence in benign lesions,[236-238] has attracted much attention as a potentially important event in tumor progression. HPV DNA integration is difficult to demonstrate in the presence of a vast excess of episomal viral DNA, but is likely to occur already in dysplastic lesions of increased severity. Using a cloned virus-cell DNA junction sequence from a bowenoid papule derived cell line as a probe, it was indeed possible to show that integration had taken place in the premalignant lesion that predominantly contained viral episomes.[239] Restriction enzyme cleavage of cancer DNAs with integrated viral sequences leads to tumor-specific patterns due to different junction fragments, which indicates that there is no consistent recombination site.[240] However, lymph node metastases of one patient usually show the same restriction enzyme cleavage pattern of viral DNA as the primary tumor, suggesting that integration had occurred prior to the events leading to the monoclonal spread of the carcinoma.[240,241]

Integration of HPV DNA may occur on different chromosomes such as 3, 8, 12, 13, or 20 in the vicinity of fragile sites, oncogenes, and chromosome breakpoints that are also characteristic of hematologic malignancies and solid tumors.[242-244] Viral sequences were found both in repetitive and single copy cellular DNA.[236] The repeatedly observed integration in the general vicinity of the cellular protooncogene *myc* may be noteworthy because *myc* appears rearranged and/or expressed at elevated levels in these cases.[243,245]

A detailed analysis of cervical cancer derived cell lines and several cancers showed that HPV DNA integration frequently occurs within the viral E1/E2 region,[246-251] thereby disrupting expression of these early genes. Engineered HPV16 DNAs with mutations in E1 and E2 revealed increased transformation efficiency *in vitro*,[252] which supports the notion that the naturally occurring inactivation may contribute to tumor progression. It has been suggested that the knock-out of the transcriptional modulator E2 would trigger uncontrolled expression of the oncogenes E6 and E7, and increased E6/E7 transcription was described in HPV18-immortalized human keratinocytes resulting from inactivation of E2.[253] However, the effect of E2 inactivation is not undisputed because Storey and colleagues[233] observed a lack of immortalizing activity of a HPV16 DNA with a mutation in the E2 gene. (See also Section III.C.2.)

Another remarkable consequence of integration is the formation of fusion transcripts of viral (E6-E7 genes) and cellular sequences[254,255] due to deletion of the viral splice acceptor site within E2 and the use of a nearby cellular splice acceptor. In one case, flanking cellular sequences downstream from the HPV16 genes E6 and E7 were shown to enhance gene expression, thus leading to transforming activity of the virus-cell DNA hybrid when tested with NIH 3T3 mouse fibroblasts.[256] The cell-derived 3'-termini of the mRNAs may affect the half life of the E6-E7 transcripts, which is indeed rather long, for example in HeLa cells,[257] and the increased steady-state levels of mRNA could account for increased amounts of viral oncoproteins.

Expression of integrated HPV DNA is furthermore obviously affected by the general cellular surroundings. Mapping of the nucleosomal organization around integrated HPV18 DNA in HeLa cells showed nuclease-hypersensitive sites as indicators of transcriptionally active areas in the viral control region and the 5' cellular flank.[258] HPV18 DNA in different cervical cancer derived cell lines showed a different response to steroid hormones, presumably depending on the chromosomal integration site.[259]

Whereas HPV18 DNA appears integrated in most of the cancers, a substantial proportion of HPV16 positive tumors and one cancer-derived cell line revealed only episomal viral DNA within the limits of detectability by Southern blot hybridization.[238,241,260-262] This suggests that integration is not absolutely required for tumor progression. A deregulation of viral oncogene expression, which was discussed as a possible consequence of viral DNA integration, may alternatively occur due to deletions in the viral control region, described for episomal HPV16 molecules from cervical and vulvar carcinomas.[263,264] Duplications, insertions, and point mutations within the transcriptional control region were also repeatedly observed in cancers associated with HPV6 and HPV11 DNAs.[265,268]

A more detailed analysis of a shortened control region of episomal HPV16 DNA from a cancer metastasis showed that two binding sites for the cellular transcriptional repressor YY1 were removed by a 106 bp deletion, resulting in a five- to six-fold increased promoter activity.[80] Expanding on this, deletions and point mutations of YY1 binding sites were identified in four out of five additional cervical cancers with exclusively episomal HPV16 DNAs. The expression of reporter genes under the control of three mutated LCRs was 3.8–6.0-fold higher than under the control of HPV16 wild-type LCR.[269] This suggests that deletion or mutation of target sequences for the cellular repressor

YY1 represents a repeatedly used strategy of HPV16 to escape from cellular control and to increase its transcription rate.

In contrast to cervical cancers, integration of the viral DNA into the cellular genome is a very rare event in EV-associated skin carcinomas. HPV14 was found once to be integrated into the cellular DNA, which may represent an unusual route for malignant conversion involving a weakly oncogenic EV virus.[270] In another case HPV5 DNA was not integrated in the primary cancer of the patient but only in a metastasis, which may be related to progressing malignancy.[271] Monomeric viral plasmids usually persist in high copy numbers accompanied by oligomeric molecules and genomes with deletions or duplications.[271-274] It is interesting to note that the deletions may extend into the transcription control region[274] affecting the L1 proximal silencer element.[30,85] It remains to be established if these deletions change the expression of viral oncogenes and contribute to malignant conversion.

B.   Viral Transcription in Precancerous Lesions and Carcinomas

In high-grade squamous intraepithelial lesions, transcription of the E6/E7 region is derepressed and *in situ* hybridization signals appear evenly distributed throughout the undifferentiated epithelium.[37,38,43] Viral transcription patterns in general and expression of the oncogenes E6 and E7 in particular are similar in precancerous lesions and in invasive carcinomas,[33,37,38,42] indicating that deregulation is an early event in tumor progression. Probes that were designed to detect unspliced transcripts of the E6/E7 region with a coding potential for a full length E6 protein generated no signals in genital cancers.[42] This demonstrates that the overall low levels of E6 mRNA[22] reflect low expression in every cell. The observed increase in E6/E7 transcripts is therefore due to higher levels of mRNAs with a coding potential for E7. The most abundant viral RNAs in HPV16 associated high-grade lesions and cancers hybridize to probes starting within the E7 gene.[42] They are likely to represent the spliced E1^E4 mRNA,[27] which is supported by comparable strong signals obtained with a probe specific for the second exon. In some cancers the second exon is missing, which may be a consequence of viral DNA integration accompanied by disruption of the early transcription unit and generation of viral-cellular fusion transcripts. Due to the abundance of mRNAs starting within E7, the levels of true E7 transcripts are lower than anticipated from earlier studies using E6/E7-specific probes for the *in situ* hybridization. In two HPV 6 associated cancers, no E6 mRNA could be detected. The E7 mRNA was the major transcript.[275]

In HPV18 lesions, the early transcription unit appeared consistently disrupted near the boundary of the E1 and E2 open reading frames in contrast to HPV 16-associated carcinomas, where it usually seemed to be intact.[33,37,38,42,43] This is in line with the different tendency of both virus types to integrate into the host genome. In spite of an in principle intact early region of HPV 16, there is in most cases little or no evidence for mRNAs encoding a full length E2 protein,[33,38,42] which may point to a specific downregulation of this transcriptional repressor. Both an HPV6 positive cervical and urinary bladder cancer showed signals after hybridization with an E2-specific probe.[275] As the grade of neoplasia increases, the L2 and L1 transcripts tend to disappear although some L1-specific signals may be detectable even in invasive cancers.[37,38,42] It has been proposed that these L1 colinear transcripts arise from flanking cellular promoters upstream of integrated viral DNA,[38] which would indicate integration into an actively transcribed host gene.

There is some indication of viral antisense transcripts in a subgroup of genital cancers,[276,277] although their identity is still a bit controversial. *In situ* hybridization with sense RNA probes showed focal, nuclear, and RNase-sensitive signals and in one tumor each, the presence of antisense RNA was confirmed by RNase protection assays and cDNA cloning. The RNAs mapped across the whole genome including the noncoding region and are assumed to arise from cellular promoters flanking integrated viral DNA. Antisense RNA was never detected in premalignant lesions[277] and occurred preferentially in cancers with a high copy number of viral DNA. One may speculate about the clinical significance of antisense transcripts because experimentally induced antisense RNA was shown to modulate the growth of cervical cancer cells,[278] but initial observations did not reveal effects, for example, on metastatic spread.[276]

C. Role of Alterations in the Host Genome

Almost all carcinomas carry aneuploid cells indicating massive genetic alterations acquired during tumor progression. Chromosomal mutations may activate cellular proto-oncogenes and inactivate growth control or tumor suppressor genes, thereby playing a decisive role in malignant conversion. An amplification of the *myc* or *ras* oncogenes, or both, has been observed in the late stage of cervical carcinomas[279] and a 4–20-fold overexpression of the c-*myc* gene was noted with 35% of stage I or II tumors.[280] This more generally observed increase in *myc* expression is probably only partially due to an integration of viral DNA in the vicinity of the cellular gene. As tumorigenicity is recessive with respect to the normal phenotype, the inactivation or loss of growth control genes may be more important than activation of a dominant oncogene. Initial studies with cervical carcinoma cell lines and a limited number of tumors showed all HPV-positive cases to carry p53 and pRb wild type sequences whereas HPV-negative cases presented mutations.[198,281-284] It was consequently speculated that inactivation of both these tumor suppressor proteins is important in cervical carcinogenesis and may be achieved either by complex formation with the HPV oncoproteins or by somatic mutations in the cellular genes.[139] However, the analysis of more tumors indicated that almost all cervical cancers display wild type p53 genes irrespective of the HPV status.[285-288] Moreover, it has recently been shown that HPV-positive cell lines contain a transactivation competent and DNA damage-responsive p53 protein.[289] These results argue against a decisive role of p53 mutations in cervical carcinogenesis.

A tumor suppressor gene encoded on chromosome 11 seems to be particularly important in preventing cervical cancer because the tumorigenic phenotype of HeLa and SiHa cells could be suppressed by introducing a normal chromosome 11.[290,291]

With regard to a role of the virus in malignant conversion, it is most remarkable that viral activities may induce chromosome abnormalities. Changes in ploidy have been observed as a consequence of high risk HPV infection in immortalized human epithelial cells *in vitro*.[235,292,293] Expression of the HPV16 E7 gene alone turned out to be sufficient to induce tetraploidy in human keratinocytes.[294] The follow-up of E7 gene-transfected mouse keratinocytes containing 100% tetraploid cells revealed a decrease in modal chromosome numbers reflecting a change from polyploidy to aneuploidy. The induction of polyploidy may result from duplicated DNA synthesis in the S-phase or dysfunction in chromosome segregation. With the known E7 protein functions in mind, it is tempting to speculate that cellular DNA replication is deregulated. A genetic instability can also be expected to result from E6 protein activities reducing the intracellular levels of p53. The p53 protein is normally known to be induced following DNA damage to arrest cells in the G_1-phase to provide sufficient time for DNA repair. A defect in this regard should increase the mutation rate particularly when cells are exposed to mutagens.[295]

An intriguing consequence of mutations in cellular genes appears to be elevated transcription of viral oncogenes. Zur Hausen postulated the existence of cellular interfering factors (CIF), which down regulate transcription of viral oncogenes thus preventing undue deregulation of cellular growth control.[7] In accordance with this model, the breakdown of intracellular surveillance by stepwise inactivation or loss of both alleles of the CIF genes is regarded as a crucial step in cancer development. A series of recent observations closely link the postulated control mechanism to the tumor suppressor function encoded on chromosome 11. A selective suppression of HPV18 transcription at the level of initiation was induced by the addition of the demethylating agent 5-azacytidin in nonmalignant hybrids of HeLa cells with either normal keratinocytes or fibroblasts. This occurred neither in parental HeLa cells nor in tumorigenic segregants, which have lost a normal chromosome 11.[296] Suppression of HPV expression was also induced *in vivo* in nontumorigenic HeLa x fibroblast hybrids 3 days after heterografting into nude mice.[297] Tumorigenic segregants, which lacked one normal chromosome 11, retained high levels of HPV expression. When an HPV18 transcriptional control region was introduced into SiHa cells, its constitutive activity was turned off right away after fusion with nontumorigenic human keratinocytes, whereas the endogenous HPV16 expression was not affected.[298] These data indicate that extrachromosomal HPV DNA is directly affected by the chromosome 11 related suppression mechanism, whereas further events have to be induced to allow repression of integrated viral sequences. This may be a complication specific for cell lines which depend on E6/E7 gene expression for *in vitro* growth and developed additional strategies to ensure expression.

HPV16 showed high early gene expression in human embryonic fibroblasts with a deletion in the short arm of chromosome 11 (from p 11.11 to p 15.1) in contrast to normal embryonic fibroblasts, and it is interesting that the del-11 cells were susceptible to transformation by HPV16, whereas the normal fibroblasts were resistant.[299] A more detailed analysis showed that the 55 kDa regulatory subunit PR55β of the protein phosphatase 2A is likely to be involved in the upregulation of viral transcription.[300] PR55β, which inhibits the phosphatase activity, is highly expressed in del-11 cells, and inhibition of the phosphatase by okadaic acid resulted in similar transactivation of the HPV16 control region in diploid cells. One may speculate that a protein encoded on the short arm of chromosome 11 normally downregulates the phosphatase inhibitor leading to dephosphorylation and directly or indirectly to activation/inactivation of negative/positive control factors of HPV transcription.

The presented list of possible events in the multistep scenario of tumor progression is certainly incomplete. However, evidence for genetic instability due to the activity of viral oncoproteins and a kind of "autocatalytic" increase in oncoprotein expression due to mutations in the viral and cellular genome identifies the virus as a major factor and driving force of progression.

ACKNOWLEDGMENTS

We thank Drs. T. Iftner and F. Stubenrauch for critical reading of the manuscript, S. Bethmann and R. Hott for excellent secretarial assistance, and R. Rippin for skillful art work. Unpublished work from our laboratory was supported by the Deutsche Forschungsgemeinschaft and the Dr. Mildred Scheel Stiftung for Cancer Research.

REFERENCES

1. Pfister, H. and Fuchs, P. G., Papillomaviruses: Particles, genome organization and proteins, in *Papillomaviruses and Human Disease*, Syrjänen, K., Gissmann, L. and Koss, L., Eds., Springer Verlag, Heidelberg, 1987, 1.
2. Pfister, H. and Fuchs, P. G., Anatomy, taxonomy and evolution of papillomaviruses, *Intervirology*, 37, 143, 1994.
3. Jenson, A. B., Rosenthal, J. D., Olson, C., Pass, F., Lancaster, W. D., and Shah, K., Immunologic relatedness of papillomaviruses from different species, *J. Natl. Cancer Inst.*, 64, 495, 1980.
4. Pfister, H., Human papillomaviruses and genital cancer, *Adv. Cancer Res.*, 48, 113, 1987.
5. zur Hausen, H., Human papillomaviruses and their possible role in squamous cell carcinomas, *Curr. Top. Microbiol. Immunol.*, 78, 1, 1977.
6. zur Hausen, H., Papillomaviruses as carcinomaviruses, *Adv. Viral Oncol.*, 8, 1, 1989.
7. zur Hausen, H., Intracellular surveillance of persisting viral infections, *Lancet*, 2, 489, 1986.
8. Delius, H. and Hofmann, B., Primer-directed sequencing of human papillomavirus types, in *Human Pathogenic Papillomaviruses*, zur Hausen, H., Ed., Springer Verlag, Berlin, 1994, 13.
9. DiMaio, D. and Neary, K., The genetics of bovine papillomavirus type 1, in *Papillomaviruses and Human Cancer*, Pfister, H., Ed., CRC Press, Boca Raton, 1990, 113.
10. Doorbar, J., Ely, S., McLean, C., and Crawford, L., Specific interaction between HPV 16 E1-E4 and cytokeratins results in collapse of the epithelial cell intermediate filament network, *Nature*, 352, 824, 1991.
11. Doorbar, J. and Gallimore, P., Identification of proteins encoded by the L1 and L2 open reading frames of human papillomavirus 1a, *J. Virol.*, 61, 2793, 1987.

12. Fuchs, P. G. and Pfister, H., Papillomaviruses in epidermodysplasia verruciformis, *Papillomavirus Report.*, 1, 1, 1990.
13. Seedorf, K., Kramer, G., Dürst, M., Suhai, S., and Roewekamp, W., Human papillomavirus type 16 DNA sequence, *Virology*, 145, 181, 1985.
14. Hirsch-Behnam, A., Delius, H., and de Villiers, E.-M., A comparative sequence analysis of two human papillomavirus (HPV) types 2a and 57, *Virus Res.*, 18, 81, 1990.
15. Danos, O., Engel, L. W., Chen, E. Y., Yaniv, M., and Howley, P. M., Comparative analysis of the human type 1a and bovine type 1 papillomavirus genomes, *J. Virol.*, 46, 557, 1983.
16. Fuchs, P. G., Iftner, T., Weninger, J., and Pfister, H., Epidermodysplasia verruciformis-associated human papillomavirus 8: genomic sequence and comparative analysis, *J. Virol.*, 58, 626, 1986.
17. Baker, C. C., Bovine papillomavirus type 1 transcription, in *Papillomaviruses and Human Cancer*, Pfister, H., Ed., CRC Press, Boca Raton, 1990, 91.
18. Chow, L. T., Reilly, S. S., Broker, T. R., and Taichman, L. B., Identification and mapping of human papillomavirus type 1 RNA transcripts recovered from plantar warts and infected epithelial cell cultures, *J. Virol.*, 61, 1913, 1987.
19. Chow, L. T., Nasseri, M., Wolinski, S. M., and Broker, T. R., Human papillomavirus types 6 and 11 mRNAs from genital condylomata acuminata, *J. Virol.*, 61, 2581, 1987.
20. Smotkin, D. and Wettstein, F. O., Transcription of human papillomavirus type 16 early genes in a cervical cancer and a cancer derived cell line and identification of the E7 protein, *Proc. Natl. Acad. Sci. U.S.A.*, 83, 4680, 1986.
21. Thierry, F., Heard, J. M., Dartmann, K., and Yaniv, M., Characterization of a transcriptional promoter of human papillomavirus 18 and modulation of its expression by simian virus 40 and adenovirus early antigens, *J. Virol.*, 61, 134, 1987.
22. Smotkin, D., Prokoph, H., and Wettstein, F. O., Oncogenic and nononcogenic human genital papillomaviruses generate the E7 mRNA by different mechanisms, *J. Virol.*, 63, 1441, 1989.
23. Iftner, T., Sagner, G., Pfister, H., and Wettstein, F. O., The E7 protein of human papillomavirus 8 is a nonphosphorylated protein of 17 kDa and can be generated by two different mechanisms, *Virology*, 179, 428, 1990.
24. Haller, K., Stubenrauch, F., and Pfister, H., Differentiation-dependent transcription of the epidermodysplasia verruciformis-associated human papillomavirus type 5 in benign lesions, *Virology*, 214, 245, 1995.
25. Nasseri, M., Hirochika, R., Broker, T. R., and Chow, L. T., A human papillomavirus type 11 transcript encoding an E1^E4 protein, *Virology*, 159, 433, 1987.
26. Hummel, M., Hudson, J. B., and Laimins L.A., Differentiation-induced and constitutive transcription of human papillomavirus type 31b in cell lines containing viral episomes, *J. Virol.*, 66, 6070, 1992.
27. Doorbar, J., Patron, A., Hartley, L., Crook, T., Stanley, M., and Crawford, L., Detection of novel splicing patterns in a HPV 16-containing keratinocyte cell line, *Virology*, 178, 254, 1990.
28. Karlen, S. and Beard, P., Identification and characterization of novel promoters in the genome of human papillomavirus type 18, *J. Virol.*, 67, 4296, 1993.
29. Palermo-Dilts, D. A., Broker, T. R., and Chow, L. T., Human papillomavirus type 1 produces redundant as well as polycistronic mRNAs in plantar warts, *J. Virol.*, 64, 3144, 1990.
30. Stubenrauch, F., Malejczyk, J., Fuchs, P. G., and Pfister, H., Late promoter of human papillomavirus type 8 and its regulation, *J. Virol.*, 66, 3485, 1992.
31. Rohlfs, M., Winkenbach, S., Meyer, S., Rupp, T., and Dürst, M., Viral transcription in human keratinocyte cell lines immortalized by human papillomavirus type-16, *Virology*, 183, 331, 1991.
32. Hummel, M., Lim, H. B., and Laimins, L. A., Human papillomavirus type 31b late gene expression is regulated through protein kinase C-mediated changes in RNA processing, *J. Virol.*, 69, 3381, 1995.
33. Sherman, L., Alloul, N., Golan, I., Dürst, M., and Baram, A., Expression and splicing patterns of human papillomavirus type-16 mRNAs in precancerous lesions and carcinomas of the cervix, in human keratinocytes immortalized by HPV 16 and in cell lines established from cervical cancers, *Int. J. Cancer*, 50, 356, 1992.
34. Sherman, L. and Alloul, N., Human papillomavirus type 16 expresses a variety of alternatively spliced mRNAs putatively encoding the E2 protein, *Virology*, 191, 953, 1992.
35. Sedman, A. S., Barbosa, M., Vass, W. C., Hubbert, N. L., Haas, J. A., Lowy, D. R., and Schiller, J. T., The full-length E6 protein of human papillomavirus 16 has transforming and transactivating activities and cooperates with E7 to immortalize keratinocytes in culture, *J. Virol.*, 64, 4860, 1991.

36. Beyer-Finkler, E., Stoler, M. H., Girardi, F., and Pfister, H., Cell differentiation-related gene expression of human papillomavirus 33, *Med. Microbiol. Immunol.*, 179, 185, 1990.

37. Dürst, M., Glitz, D., Schneider, A., and zur Hausen, H., Human papillomavirus type 16 (HPV 16) gene expression and DNA replication in cervical neoplasia: analysis by in situ hybridization, *Virology*, 189, 132, 1992.

38. Stoler, M. H., Rhodes, C. R., Whitbeck, A., Wolinsky, S. M., Chow, L. T., and Broker, T. R., Human papillomavirus type 16 and 18 gene expression in cervical neoplasias, *Hum. Pathol.*, 23, 117, 1992.

39. Stoler, M. H., Wolinsky, S. M., Whitbeck, A., Broker, T. R., and Chow, L. T., Differentiation-linked human papillomavirus types 6 and 11 transcription in genital condylomata revealed by in situ hybridization with message-specific RNA probes, *Virology*, 172, 331, 1989.

40. Iftner, T., Oft, M., Böhm, S., Wilczynski, S. P., and Pfister, H., Transcription of the E6 and E7 genes of human papillomavirus type 6 in anogenital condylomata is restricted to undifferentiated cell layers of the epithelium, *J. Virol.*, 66, 4639, 1992.

41. Dürst, M., Bosch, F. X., Glitz, D., Schneider, A., and zur Hausen, H., Inverse relationship between human papillomavirus (HPV) type 16 early gene expression and cell differentiation of nude mouse epithelial cysts and tumors induced by HPV-positive human cell lines, *J. Virol.*, 65, 796, 1991.

42. Böhm, S., Wilczynski, S. P., Pfister, H., and Iftner, T., The predominant mRNA class in HPV 16-infected anogenital neoplasia does not encode the E6 or the E7 protein, *Int. J. Cancer*, 55, 1, 1993.

43. Higgins, G. D., Uzelin, D. M., Phillips, G. E., McEvoy, P., Marin, R., and Burrell, C. J., Transcription patterns of human papillomavirus type 16 in genital intraepithelial neoplasia: evidence for promotor usage within the E7 open reading frame during epithelial differentiation, *J. Gen. Virol.*, 73, 2047, 1992.

44. Crum, C. P., Barber, S., Symbula, M., Snyder, K., Saleh, A. M., and Roche, J. K., Coexpression of the human papillomavirus type 16 E4 and L1 open reading frames in early cervical neoplasia, *Virology*, 178, 138, 1990.

45. Garcia-Carranca, A. Thierry, F., and Yaniv, M., Interplay of viral and cellular proteins along the long control region of human papillomavirus type 18, *J. Virol.*, 62, 4321, 1988.

46. Gloss, B., Chong, T., and Bernard, H.-U., Numerous nuclear proteins bind the long control region of human papillomavirus type 16: a subset of 6 of 23 DNase I-protected segments coincides with the location of the cell-type-specific enhancer, *J. Virol.*, 63, 1142, 1989.

47. May, M., Helbl, V., Pfister, H., and Fuchs, P. G., Unique topography of DNA-protein interactions in the noncoding region of epidermodysplasia verruciformis-associated human papillomaviruses, *J. Gen. Virol.*, 72, 2989, 1991.

48. Turek, P. L., The structure, function and regulation of papillomaviral genes in infection and cervical cancer, *Adv. Virol. Res.*, 44, 305, 1994.

49. Chin, M. T., Broker, T. R., and Chow, L. T., Identification of a novel constitutive enhancer element and an associated binding protein: implications for human papillomavirus type 11 enhancer regulation, *J.Virol.*, 63, 2967, 1989.

50. Dollard, S. C., Broker, T. R., and Chow, L. T., Regulation of the human papillomavirus type 11 E6 promoter by viral and host transcription factors in primary human keratinocytes, *J. Virol.*, 67, 1721, 1993.

51. Cripe, T. P., Haugen, T. H., Turk, J. P., Tabatabai, F., Schmid, P. G., III, Dürst, M., Gissmann, L., Roman, A., and Turek, L. P., Transcriptional regulation of the human papillomavirus-16 E6-E7 promoter by a keratinocyte-dependent enhancer, and by viral E2 trans-activator and repressor gene products: implication for cervical carcinogenesis, *EMBO J.*, 6, 3745, 1987.

52. Gloss, B., Bernard, H.-U., Seedorf, K., and Klock, G., The upstream regulatory region of the human papillomavirus-16 contains an E2 protein-independent enhancer which is specific for cervical carcinoma cells and regulated by glucocorticoid hormones, *EMBO J.*, 6, 3735, 1987.

53. Chong, T., Apt, D., Gloss, B., Isa, M., and Bernard, H.-U. The enhancer of human papillomaviruses type 16: binding sites for the ubiquitous transcription factors oct-1, NFA, TEF-2, NF1, and AP-1 participate in epithelial cell-specific transcription, *J. Virol.*, 65, 5933, 1991.

54. Swift, F. V., Bhat, K., Younghusband, H. B., and Hamada, H., Characterization of a cell type-specific enhancer found in the human papilloma virus type 18 genome, *EMBO J.*, 6, 1339, 1987.

55. Gius, D., Grossman, S., Bedell, M. A., and Laimins, L. A., Inducible and constitutive enhancer domains in the noncoding region of human papillomavirus type 18, *J. Virol.*, 62, 665, 1988.

56. Cripe, T. P., Alderborn, A., Anderson, R. D., Parkkinen, S., Bergman, P., Haugen, T. H., Petterson, U., and Turek, L. P., Transcriptional activation of the human papillomavirus-16 P97 promoter by an 88-nucleotide enhancer containing distinct cell-dependent and AP-1-responsive modules, *The New Biologist*, 2, 450, 1990.

57. Offord, E. A. and Beard, P., A member of the activator protein 1 family found in keratinocytes but not in fibroblasts required for transcription from a human papillomavirus type 18 promoter, *J. Virol.*, 64, 4792, 1990.

58. Thierry, F., Spyrou, G., Yaniv, M., and Howley, P. M., Two AP1 sites binding junB are essential for human papillomavirus type 18 transcription in keratinocytes, *J. Virol.*, 66, 3740, 1992.

59. Gloss, B., Yeo-Gloss, M., Meisterernst, M., Rogge, L., Winnacker, E. L., and Bernard, H.-U., Clusters of nuclear factor 1 binding sites identify enhancers of several papillomaviruses but alone are not sufficient for enhancer function, *Nucleic Acid Res.*, 17, 3519, 1989.

60. Apt, D., Chong, T., Liu, Y., and Bernard, H.-U., Nuclear factor I and epithelial cell-specific transcription of human papillomavirus type 16, *J. Virol.*, 67, 4455, 1993.

61. Royer, H.-D., Freyaldenhoven, M. P., Napierski, I., Spitkovsky, D. D., Bauknecht, T., and Dathan, N., Delineation of human papillomavirus type 18 enhancer binding proteins: the intracellular distribution of a novel octamer binding protein p92 is cell cycle regulated, *Nucleic Acid Res.*, 19, 2363, 1991.

62. Morris, P. J., Dent, C. L., Ring, C. J., and Latchman, D. S., The octamer binding site in the HPV 16 regulatory region produces opposite effects on gene expression in cervical and non-cervical cells, *Nucleic Acid Res.*, 21, 1019, 1993.

63. O'Connor, M. and Bernard, H.-U., Oct-1 activates the epithelial-specific enhancer of human papillomavirus type 16 via a synergistic interaction with NF1 at a conserved composite regulatory element, *Virology*, 207, 77, 1995.

64. Mittal, R., Pater, A., and Pater, M. M., Multiple human papillomavirus type 16 glucocorticoid response elements functional for transformation, transient expression, and DNA-protein interactions, *J. Virol.*, 67, 5656, 1993.

65. Cuthill, S., Sibbet, G. J., and Campo, M. S., Characterization of a nuclear factor, papillomavirus enhancer binding factor-1, that binds the long control region of human papillomavirus type 16 and contributes to enhancer activity, *Mol. Carcinog.*, 8, 96, 1993.

66. Ishiji, T., Lace, M. J., Pakkinen, S., Anderson, R. D., Haugen, T. H., Cripe, T. P., Xiao, J.-H., Davidson, I., Chambon, P., and Turek, L. P., Transcriptional enhancer factor (TEF)-1 and its cell-specific coactivator activate human papillomavirus-16 E6 and E7 oncogene transcription in keratinocytes and cervical carcinoma cells, *EMBO J.*, 11, 2271, 1992.

67. Chong, T., Chan, W. K., and Bernard, H.-U., Transcriptional activation of human papillomavirus 16 by nuclear factor I, AP1, steroid receptors and a possible novel transcription factor, PVF: a model for the composition of genital papillomavirus enhancers, *Nucleic Acid Res.*, 18, 465, 1990.

68. O'Connor, M., Chan, S.-Y., and Bernard, H.-U., Transcription factor binding sites in the long control region of genital HPVs, in *Human Papillomaviruses Database Compendium*, Halpern, A. and Myers, G., Eds., Los Alamos Laboratory, 1995.

69. Apt, D., Liu, Y., and Bernard, H.-U., Cloning and functional analysis of spliced isoforms of human nuclear factor 1-X: interference with transcriptional activation by NFl/CTF in a cell-type specific manner, *Nucleic Acids Res.*, 22, 3825, 1994.

70. Mack, D. H. and Laimins, L. A., A keratinocyte-specific transcription factor, KRF-1, interacts with AP-1 to activate expression of human papillomavirus type 18 in squamous epithelial cells, *Proc. Natl. Acad. Sci. U.S.A.*, 88, 9102, 1991.

71. Pater, A., Bayatpour, M., and Pater, M. M., Oncogenic transformation by a human papillomavirus 16 deoxyribonucleic acid in the presence of progesterone or progestins from oral contraceptives, *Am. J. Obstet. Gynecol.*, 162, 1099, 1990.

72. Dürst, M., Gallahan, D., Jay, G., and Rhin, J. S., Glucocorticoid-enhanced neoplastic transformation of human keratinocytes by human papillomavirus type 16 and an activated ras-oncogene, *Virology*, 173, 767, 1989.

73. Auborn, K. J., Galli, R. L., Dilorenzo, T. P., and Steinberg, B. M., Identification of DNA-protein interactions and enhancer activity at the 5'end of the upstream regulatory region in human papillomavirus type 1, *Virology*, 170, 123, 1989.

74. Auborn, K. J. and Steinberg, B. M., A key DNA-protein interaction determines the function of the 5'URR enhancer in human papillomavirus type 11, *Virology*, 181, 132, 1991.

75. Hoppe-Seyler, F. and Butz, K., A novel cis-stimulatory element maps to the 5'portion of the human papillomavirus type 18 upstream regulatory region and is functionally dependent on a sequence-aberrant Sp1 binding site, *J. Gen. Virol.*, 74, 281, 1993.

76. Horn, S., Pfister, H., and Fuchs, P. G., Constitutive transcriptional activator of epidermodysplasia verruciformis-associated human papillomavirus type 8, *Virology*, 196, 674, 1993.

77. Vande Pol, S. B. and Howley, P. M., A bovine papillomavirus constitutive enhancer is negatively regulated by the E2 repressor through competitive binding for a cellular factor, *J. Virol.*, 64, 5420, 1990.

78. Reh, H. and Pfister, H., Human papillomavirus type 8 contains cis-active positive and negative transcriptional control sequences, *J. Gen. Virol.*, 71, 2457, 1990.

79. Jackson, M. E. and Campo, M. S., Positive and negative E2-independent regulatory elements in the long control region of bovine papillomavirus type 4, *J. Gen. Virol.*, 72, 877, 1991.

80. May, M., Dong, X.-P., Beyer-Finkler, E., Stubenrauch, F., Fuchs, P. G., and Pfister, H., The E6-E7 promoter of extrachromosomal HPV16 DNA in cervical cancer escapes from cellular repression by mutation of target sequences for YY1, *EMBO J.*, 13, 1460, 1994.

81. Bauknecht, T., Angel, P., Royer, H.-D., and zur Hausen, H., Identification of a negative regulatory domain in the human papillomavirus type 18 promoter: interaction with the transcriptional repressor YY1, *EMBO J.*, 11, 4607, 1992.

82. Yasumoto, S., Taniguchi, A., and Sohma, K., Epidermal growth factor (EGF) elicits down-regulation of human papillomavirus type 16 (HPV-16) E6/E7 mRNA at the transcriptional level in an EGF-stimulated human keratinocyte cell line: functional role of EGF-responsive silencer in the HPV-16 long control region, *J. Virol.*, 65, 2000, 1991.

83. Bartsch, D., Boye, B., Baust, C., zur Hausen, H., and Schwarz, E., Retinoic acid-mediated repression of human papillomavirus 18 transcription and different ligand regulation of the retinoic acid receptor ß gene in non-tumorigenic and tumorigenic HeLa hybrid cells, *EMBO J.*, 11, 2283, 1992.

84. Kyo, S., Inoue, M., Nishio, Y., Nakanishi, K., Akira, S., Inoue, H., Yutsudo, M., Tanizawa, O., and Hakura, A., NF-IL6 represses early gene expression of human papillomavirus type 16 through binding to the noncoding region, *J. Virol.*, 67, 1058, 1993.

85. May, M., Grassmann, K., Pfister, H., and Fuchs, P. G., Transcriptional silencer of the human papillomavirus type 8 late promoter interacts alternatively with the viral transactivator E2 or with a cellular factor, *J. Virol.*, 68, 3612, 1994.

86. McBride, A., Romanczuk, H., and Howley, P. M., The papillomavirus E2 regulatory protein, *J. Biol. Chem.*, 266, 19411, 1991.

87. Ham, J., Dostatni, N., Gauthier, J.-M., and Yaniv, M., The papillomavirus E2 protein: a factor with many talents, *TIBS*, 16, 440, 1991.

88. Knight, J. D., Li, R., and Botchan, M., The activation domain of the papillomavirus E2 protein mediates association of DNA-bound dimers to form DNA loops, *Proc. Natl. Acad. Sci. U.S.A.*, 88, 3204, 1991.

89. Winokur, P. L. and McBride, A., Separation of the transcriptional activation and replication functions of the bovine papillomavirus-1 E2 protein, *EMBO J.*, 11, 4111, 1992.

90. Androphy, E., Lowy, D. R., and Schiller, J. T., Bovine papillomavirus E2 transactivating gene product binds to specific sites in papillomavirus DNA, *Nature*, 325, 70, 1987.

91. Li, R., Knight, J., Bream, G., Stenlund, A., and Botchan, M., Specific recognition nucleotides and their DNA context determine the affinity of E2 protein for 17 binding sites in the BPV1 genome, *Genes Dev.*, 3, 510, 1989.

92. Dostatni, N., Thierry, F., and Yaniv, M., A dimer of BPV-1 E2 containing a protease resistant core interacts with its DNA targets, *EMBO J.*, 7, 3807, 1988.

93. McBride, A., Schlegel, R., and Howley, P. M., E2 polypeptide encoded by the bovine papillomavirus type 1 form dimers through the common carboxyl-terminal domain: transactivation is mediated by the conserved amino-terminal domain, *Proc. Natl. Acad. Sci. U.S.A.*, 86, 510, 1989.

94. Iftner, T., Papillomavirus genomes: Sequence analysis related to functional aspects, in *Papillomaviruses and Human Disease*, Pfister, H., Ed., CRC Press, Boca Raton, 1990, 182.

95. Hawley-Nelson, P., Androphy, E. J., Lowy, D. R., and Schiller, J. T., The specific DNA recognition sequence of the bovine papillomavirus E2 protein is an E2-dependent enhancer, *EMBO J.*, 7, 525, 1988.

96. Thierry, F., Dostatni, N., Arnos, F., and Yaniv, M., Cooperative activation by bovine papillomavirus type 1 E2 can occur over a large distance, *Mol. Cell. Biol.*, 10, 4431, 1990.

97. Gauthier, J.-M., Dostatni, N., Luski, M., and Yaniv, M., Two DNA-bound E2 dimers are required for strong transcriptional activation and for cooperation with cellular factors in most cells, *The New Biologist*, 3, 1, 1991.

98. Lambert, P. F., Dostatni, N., McBride, A. A., and Yaniv, M., Functional analysis of the papillomavirus E2 transactivator in *Saccharomyces cerevisiae*, *Genes Dev.*, 3, 38, 1989.

99. Monini, P., Grossman, S. R., Pepinsky, B., Androphy, E. J., and Laimins, L. A., Cooperative binding of the E2 protein of bovine papillomavirus to adjacent E2-responsive sequences, *J. Virol.*, 65, 2124, 1991.

100. Ham, J., Dostatni, N., Arnos, F., and Yaniv, M., Several different upstream promoter elements can potentiate transactivation by the BPV-1 E2 protein, *EMBO J.*, 10, 2931, 1991.

101. Spalholz, B. A., Vande Pol, S. B., and Howley, P. M., Characterization of the cis elements involved in basal and E2-transactivated expression of the bovine papillomavirus P_{2443} promoter, *J. Virol.*, 65, 743, 1991.

102. Li, R., Knight, J. D., Jackson, S. P., Tijan, R., and Botchan, M., Interaction between Sp1 and the BPV enhancer E2 protein mediates synergistic activation of transcription, *Cell*, 65, 493, 1991.

103. Dostatni, N., Lambert, P. F., Sousa, R., Ham, J., Howley, P. M., and Yaniv, M., The functional BPV-1 E2 trans-activating protein can act as a repressor by preventing formation of the initiation complex, *Genes Dev.*, 5, 1657, 1991.

104. Chin, M. T., Hirochika, R., Hirochika, H., Broker, T. R., and Chow, L. T., Regulation of human papillomavirus type 11 enhancer and E6 promoter by activating and repressing proteins from the E2 open reading frame: functional and biochemical studies, *J. Virol.*, 62, 2994, 1988.

105. Chiang, C.-M., Broker, T. R., and Chow, L. T., An E1M^E2C fusion protein encoded by human papillomavirus type 11 is a sequence-specific transcription repressor, *J. Virol.*, 65, 3317, 1991.

106. Stenlund, A. and Botchan, M., The E2 transactivator can act as a repressor by interfering with a cellular transcription factor, *Genes Dev.*, 4, 123, 1990.

107. Thierry, F. and Howley, P. M., Functional analysis of E2-mediated repression of the HPV18 P_{105} promoter, *The New Biologist*, 3, 90, 1991.

108. Romanczuk, N., Thierry, F., and Howley, P. M., Mutational analysis of cis elements involved in E2 modulation of human papillomavirus type 16 P_{97} and type 18 P_{105} promoters, *J. Virol.*, 64, 2849, 1990.

109. Gloss, B. and Bernard, H.-U., The E6/E7 promoter of human papillomavirus type 16 is activated in the absence of E2 protein by sequence-aberrant Sp1 distal element, *J. Virol.*, 64, 5577, 1990.

110. Tan, S.-H., Gloss, B., and Bernard, H.-U., During negative regulation of the human papillomavirus-16 E6 promoter, the viral E2 protein can displace Sp1 from a proximal promoter element, *Nucleic Acid Res.*, 20, 251, 1992.

111. Tan, S.-H., Leong, L. E.-C., Walker, P. A., and Bernard, H.-U. The human papillomavirus type 16 E2 transcription factor binds with low cooperativity to two flanking sites and represses the E6 promoter through displacement of Sp1 and TFIID, *J. Virol.*, 68, 6411, 1994.

112. Demeret, C., Yaniv, M., and Thierry, F., The E2 transcriptional repressor can compensate for SP1 activation of the human papillomavirus type 18 early promoter, *J. Virol.*, 68, 7075, 1994.

113. Dong, G., Broker, T. R., and Chow, L. T., Human papillomavirus type 11 E2 proteins repress the homologous E6 promoter by interfering with the binding of host transcription factors to adjacent elements, *J. Virol.*, 68, 1115, 1994.

114. Lees, E., Osborn, K., Banks, L., and Crawford, L., Transformation of primary BRK cells by human papillomavirus type 16 and Ej-ras is increased by overexpression of the viral E2 protein, *J. Gen. Virol.*, 71, 183, 1990.

115. Bouvard, V., Storey, A., Pim, D., and Banks, L., Characterization of the human papillomavirus E2 protein: evidence of trans-activation and trans-repression in cervical keratinocytes, *EMBO J.*, 22, 5451, 1994.

116. Stubenrauch, F. and Pfister, H., Low-affinity E2-binding site mediates downmodulation of E2 trans-activation of the human papillomavirus type 8 late promoter, *J. Virol.*, 68, 6959, 1994.

117. Stubenrauch, F., Leigh, I. M., and Pfister, H. E2 represses the late gene promoter of human papillomavirus type 8 at high concentrations by interfering with cellular factors, *J. Virol.*, 70, 119, 1996.

118. LaPorta, R. F. and Taichman, L. B., Human papilloma viral DNA replicates as a stable episome in cultured epidermal keratinocytes, *Proc. Natl. Acad. Sci. U.S.A.*, 79, 3393, 1982.

119. Ustav, M. and Stenlund, A., Transient replication of BPV-1 requires two viral polypeptides encoded by the E1 and E2 open reading frames, *EMBO J.*, 10, 449, 1991.

120. Ustav, M., Ustav, E., Szymanski, P., and Stenlund, A., Identification of the origin of replication of bovine papillomavirus and characterization of the viral origin recognition factor E1, *EMBO J.*, 10, 4321, 1991.

121. Yang, L., Li, R., Mohr, I. J., Clark, R., and Botchan, M. R., Activation of BPV-1 replication *in vitro* by the transcription factor E2, *Nature*, 353, 628, 1991.

122. Hubert, W. G. and Lambert, P. F., The 23-kilodalton E1 phosphoprotein of bovine papillomavirus type 1 is nonessential for stable plasmid replication in murine C127 cells, *J. Virol.*, 67, 2932, 1993.

123. Thorner, L., Bucay, N., Choe, J., and Botchan, M., The product of the bovine papillomavirus type 1 modulator gene (M) is a phosphoprotein, *J. Virol.*, 62, 2474, 1988.

124. Sun, S., Thorner, L., Lentz, M., MacPherson, P., and Botchan, M., Identification of a 68-kilodalton nuclear ATP-binding phosphoprotein encoded by bovine papillomavirus type 1, *J. Virol.*, 64, 5093, 1990.

125. Lentz, M. R., Pak, D., Mohr, I., and Botchan, M. R., The E1 replication protein of bovine papillomavirus type 1 contains an extended nuclear localization signal that includes a p34^{cdc2} phosphorylation site, *J. Virol.*, 67, 1414, 1993.

126. Seo, Y.-S., Müller, F., Lusky, M., and Hurwitz, J., Bovine papillomavirus (BPV)-encoded E1 protein contains multiple activities required for BPV DNA replication, *Proc. Natl. Acad. Sci. U.S.A.*, 90, 702, 1993.

127. Mohr, I. J., Clark, R., Sun, S., Androphy, E. J., MacPherson, P., and Botchan, M. R., Targeting the E1 replication protein to the papillomavirus origin of replication by complex formation with the E2 transactivator, *Science*, 250, 1694, 1990.

128. Seo, Y.-S., Müller, F., Lusky, M., Gibbs, E., Kim, H.-E., Phillips, B., and Hurwitz, J., Bovine papillomavirus (BPV)-encoded E2 protein enhances binding of E1 protein to the BPV1 replication origin, *Proc. Natl. Acad. Sci. U.S.A.*, 90, 2865, 1993.

129. Ustav, E., Ustav, M., Szymanski, P., and Stenlund, A., The bovine papillomavirus origin of replication requires a binding site for the E2 transcriptional activator, *Proc. Natl. Acad. Sci. U.S.A.*, 90, 898, 1993.

130. Spalholz, B. A., McBride, A. A., Sarafi, T., and Quintero, J., Binding of bovine papillomavirus E1 to the origin is not sufficient for DNA replication, *Virology*, 193, 201, 1993.

131. DePamphilis, M. L., Eukaryotic DNA replication: Anatomy of an origin, *Annu. Rev. Biochem.*, 62, 29, 1993.

132. Chiang, C.-M., Ustav, M., Stenlund, A., Ho, T. F., Broker, T. R., and Chow, L. T., Viral E1 and E2 proteins support replication of homologous and heterologous papillomavirus origins, *Proc. Natl. Acad. Sci. U.S.A.*, 89, 5799, 1992.

133. Chiang, C.-M., Dong, G., Broker, T. R., and Chow, L. T., Control of human papillomavirus type 11 origin of replication by the E2 family of transcription regulatory proteins, *J. Virol.*, 66, 5224, 1992.

134. Del Vecchio, A. M., Romanczuk, H., Howley, P. M., and Baker, C. C., Transient replication of human papillomavirus DNAs, *J. Virol.*, 66, 5949, 1992.

135. Remm, M., Brain, R., and Jenkins, J. R., The E2 binding sites determine the efficiency of replication for the origin of human papillomavirus type 18, *Nucleic Acid Res.*, 20, 6015, 1992.

136. Bream, G. L., Ohmstede, C.-A., and Phelps, W. C., Characterization of human papillomavirus type 11 E1 and E2 proteins expressed in insect cells, *J. Virol.*, 67, 2655, 1993.

137. Sandler, A. B., Vande Pol, S. B., and Spalholz, B. A., Repression of bovine papillomavirus type 1 transcription by the E1 replication protein, *J. Virol.*, 67, 5079, 1993.

138. Vousden, K. H., Human papillomavirus transforming genes, *Seminars in Virology*, 2, 307, 1991.

139. Münger, K., Scheffner, M., Huibregtse, J. M., and Howley, P. M., Interactions of HPV E6 and E7 oncoproteins with tumour suppressor gene products, *Cancer Surveys*, 12, 197, 1992.

140. Hudson, J. B., Bedell, M. A., McCance, D. J., and Laimins, L. A., Immortalization and altered differentiation of human keratinocytes *in vitro* by the E6 and E7 open reading frames of human papillomavirus type 18, *J. Virol.*, 64, 519, 1990.

141. Halbert, C. L., Demers, G. W., and Galloway, D. A., The E7 gene of human papillomavirus type 16 is sufficient for immortalization of human epithelial cells, *J. Virol.*, 65, 473, 1991.

142. Hawley-Nelson, P., Vousden, K. H., Hubbert, N. L., Lowy, D. R., and Schiller, J. T., HPV16 E6 and E7 proteins cooperate to immortalize primary human foreskin keratinocytes, *EMBO J.*, 8, 3905, 1989.

143. Münger, K., Phelps, W. C., Bubb, V., Howley, P. M., and Schlegel, R., The E6 and E7 genes of the human papillomavirus type 16 together are necessary and sufficient for transformation of primary human keratinocytes, *J. Virol.*, 63, 4417, 1989.

144. Barbosa, M. S., Vass, W. C., Lowy, D. R., and Schiller, J. T., *In vitro* biological activities of the E6 and E7 genes vary among human papillomaviruses of different oncogenic potential, *J. Virol.*, 65, 292, 1991.

145. Storey, A., Osborn, K., and Crawford, L., Co-transformation by human papillomavirus types 6 and 11, *J. Gen. Virol.*, 71, 165, 1990.

146. Halbert, C. L., Demers, G. W., and Galloway, D. A., The E6 and E7 genes of human papillomavirus type 6 have weak immortalizing activity in human epithelial cells, *J. Virol.*, 66, 2125, 1992.

147. Iftner, T., Bierfelder, S., Csapo, Z., and Pfister, H., Involvement of human papillomavirus type 8 E6 and E7 genes in transformation and replication, *J. Virol.*, 62, 3655, 1988.

148. Kiyono, T., Nagashima, K., and Ishibashi, M., The primary structure of the major viral RNA in a rat cell line transfected with type 47 human papillomavirus DNA and the transforming activity of its cDNA and E6 gene, *Virology*, 173, 551, 1989.

149. Yamashita, T., Segawa, K., Fujinaga, Y., Nishikawa, T., and Fujinaga, K., Biological and biochemical activity of E7 genes of the cutaneous human papillomavirus type 5 and 8, *Oncogene*, 8, 2433, 1993.

150. Schmitt, A., Harry, J. B., Rapp, B., Wettstein, F. O., and Iftner, T. Comparison of the properties of the E6 and E7 genes of low- and high-risk cutaneous papillomaviruses reveals strongly transforming and high Rb-binding activity for the E7 protein of the low-risk human papillomavirus type 1, *J. Virol.*, 68, 7051, 1994.

151. Smotkin, D. and Wettstein, F. O., The major human papillomavirus protein in cervical cancers is a cytoplsmic phosphoprotein, *J. Virol.*, 61, 1686, 1987.

152. Greenfield, I., Nickerson, J., Penman, S., and Stanley, M., Human papillomavirus 16 E7 protein is associated with the nuclear matrix, *Proc. Natl. Acad. Sci. U.S.A.*, 88, 11217, 1991.

153. Phelps, W. C., Yee, C. L., Münger, K., and Howley, P. M., The human papillomavirus type 16 E7 gene encodes transactivation and transformation functions similar to adenovirus E1a, *Cell*, 53, 539.

154. Banks, L., Edmonds, C., and Vousden, K. H., Ability of the HPV16 E7 protein to bind RB and induce DNA synthesis is not sufficient for efficient transforming activity in NIH3T3 cells, *Oncogene*, 5, 1383, 1990.

155. Barbosa, M. S., Edmonds, C., Fisher, C., Schiller, J. T., Lowy, D. R., and Vousden, K. H., The region of the HPV E7 oncoprotein homologous to adenovirus E1a and SV40 large T antigen contains separate domains for Rb binding and casein kinase II phosphorylation, *EMBO J.*, 9, 153, 1990.

156. Rawls, J. A., Pusztai, R., and Green, M., Chemical synthesis of human papillomavirus type 16 E7 oncoprotein: autonomous protein domains for induction of cellular DNA synthesis and for *trans* activation, *J. Virol.*, 64, 6129, 1990.

157. Watanabe, S., Kanda, T., Sato, H., Furuno, A., and Yoshiike, K., Mutational analysis of human papillomavirus type 16 E7 functions, *J. Virol.*, 64, 207, 1990.

158. Phelps, W. C., Münger, K., Yee, C. L., Barnes, J. A., and Howley, P. M., Structure-function analysis of the human papillomavirus type 16 E7 oncoprotein, *J. Virol.*, 66, 2418, 1992.

159. Firzlaff, J. M., Lüscher, B., and Eisenman, R. N., Negative charge at the casein kinase II phosphorylation site is important for transformation but not for Rb protein binding by the E7 protein of human papillomavirus type 16, *Proc. Natl. Acad. Sci. U.S.A.*, 88, 5187, 1991.

160. McIntyre, M. C., Frattini, M. G., Grossman, S. R., and Laimins, L. A., Human papillomavirus type 18 E7 protein requires intact Cys-X-X-Cys motifs for zink binding, dimerization and transformation but not for Rb binding, *J. Virol.*, 67, 3142, 1993.

161. Wu, E. W., Clemens, K. E., Heck, R. V., and Münger, K., The human papillomavirus E7 oncoprotein and the cellular transcription factor E2F bind to separate sites on the retinoblastoma tumor suppressor protein, *J. Virol.*, 67, 2402, 1993.

162. Huang, P. S., Patrick, D. R., Edwards, G., Goodhart, P. J., Huber, H. E., Miles, L., Garsky, V. M., Oliff, A., and Heimbrook, D. C., Protein domains governing interactions between E2F, the retinoblastoma gene product, and human papillomavirus type 16 E7 protein, *Mol. Cell. Biol.*, 13, 953, 1993.

163. Dyson, N., Howley, P. M., Münger, K., and Harlow, E., The human papillomavirus 16 E7 oncoprotein is able to bind to the retinoblastoma gene product, *Science*, 243, 934, 1989.

164. Münger, K., Werness, B. A., Dyson, N., Phelps, W. C., Harlow, E., and Howley, P. M., Complex formation of human papillomavirus E7 proteins with the retinoblastoma tumor suppressor gene product, *EMBO J.*, 8, 4099, 1989.

165. Gage, J. R., Meyers, C., and Wettstein, F. O., The E7 proteins of the nononcogenic human papillomavirus type 6b (HPV-6b) and of the onocgenic HPV-16 differ in retinoblastoma protein binding and other properties, *J. Virol.*, 64, 723, 1990.

166. Imai, Y., Matsushima, Y., Sugimura, T., and Terada, M., Purification and characterization of human papillomavirus type 16 E7 protein with preferential binding capacity to the underphosphorylated form of retinoblastoma gene product, *J. Virol.*, 65, 4966, 1991.

167. Nevins, J. R., E2F: a link between the Rb tumor suppressor protein and viral oncoproteins, *Science*, 258, 424, 1992.

168. Chellappan, S., Kraus, V. B., Kroger, B., Münger, K., Howley, P. M., Phelps, W. C., and Nevins, J. R., Adenovirus E1A, simian virus 40 tumor antigen, and human papillomavirus E7 protein share the capacity to disrupt the interaction between transcription factor E2F and the retinoblastoma gene product, *Proc. Natl. Acad. Sci. U.S.A.*, 89, 4549, 1992.

169. Pagano, M., Dürst, M., Joswig, S., Draetta, G., and Jansen-Dürr, P., Binding of the human E2F transcription factor to the retinoblastoma protein but not to cyclin A is abolished in HPV-16-immortalized cells, *Oncogene*, 7, 1681, 1992.

170. Stirdivant, S. M., Huber, H. E., Patrick, D. R., Defeo-Jones, D., McAvoy, E. M., Garsky, V. M., Oliff, A., and Heimbrook, D. C., Human papillomavirus type 16 E7 protein inhibits DNA binding by the retinoblastoma gene product, *Mol. Cell. Biol.*, 12, 1905, 1992.

171. Pietenpol, J. A., Stein, R. W., Moran, E., Yaciuk, P., Schlegel, R., Lyons, R. M., Pittelkow, M. R., Münger, K., Howley, P. M., and Moses, H. L., TGF-ß1 inhibition of c-myc transcription and growth in keratinocytes is abrogated by viral transforming proteins with pRB binding domains, *Cell*, 61, 777, 1990.

172. Laiho, M., DeCaprio, J. A., Ludlow, J. W., Livingston, D. M., and Massagué, J., Growth inhibition by TGF-ß linked to suppression of retinoblastoma protein phosphorylation, *Cell*, 62, 175, 1990.

173. Missero, C., Filvaroff, E., and Dotto, G. P., Induction of transforming growth factor ß₁ resistance by the E1A oncogene requires binding to a specific set of cellular proteins, *Proc. Natl. Acad. Sci. U.S.A.*, 88, 3489, 1991.

174. Jewers, R. J., Hildebrandt, P., Ludlow, J. W., Kell, B., and McCance, D. J., Regions of human papillomavirus type 16 E7 oncoprotein required for immortalization of human keratinocytes, *J. Virol.*, 66, 1329, 1992.

175. Münger, K, Yee, C. L., Phelps, W. C., Pietenpol, J. A., Moses, H. L., and Howley, P. M, Biochemical and biological differences between E7 oncoproteins of the high and low risk HPV types are determined by aminoterminal sequences, *J. Virol.*, 65, 3943, 1991.

176. Heck, D. V., Yee, C. L., Howley, P. M., and Münger, K., Efficiency of binding the retinoblastoma protein correlates with the transforming capacity of the E7 oncoproteins of the human papillomavirus, *Proc. Natl. Acad. Sci., U.S.A.*, 89, 4442, 1992.

177. Sang, B-H. and Barbosa M., Single amino acid substitutions in "low-risk" human papillomavirus (HPV) type 6 E7 protein enhance features characteristic of the "high-risk" HPV E7 oncoproteins, *Proc. Natl. Acad. Sci. U.S.A.*, 89, 8063, 1992.

178. Dyson, N., Guida, P., Münger, K., and Harlow, E., Homologous sequences in adenovirs E1A and human papillomavirus E7 proteins mediate interaction with the same set of cellular proteins, *J. Virol.*, 66, 6893, 1992.

179. Tommasino, M., Adamczewski, J. P., Carlotti, F., Barth, C. F., Manetti, R., Contorni, M., Cavalieri, F., Hunt, T., and Crawford, L., HPV 16 E7 protein associates with the protein kinase p33^{CDK2} and cyclin A, *Oncogene*, 8, 195, 1993.

180. Davies, R., Hicks, R., Crook, T., Morris, J., and Vousden, K., Human papillomavirus type 16 E7 associates with a histone H1 kinase and with p107 through sequences necessary for transformation, *J. Virol.*, 67, 2521, 1993.

181. Ciccolini, F., Di Pasquale, G., Carlotti, F, Crawford, L., and Tomassino, M., Functional studies of E7 proteins from different HPV types, *Oncogene*, 9, 2633, 1994.

182. Hiraiwa, A., Kiyono, T., Segawa, K., Utsumi, K. R., Ohashi, M., and Ishibashi, M., Comparative study on E6 and E7 genes of some cutaneous and genital papillomaviruses of human origin for their ability to transform 3Y1 cells, *Virology*, 192, 102, 1993.

183. Kanda, T. Watanabe, S., and Yoshiike, K., Immortalization of primary rat cells by human papillomavirus type 16 subgenomic DNA fragments controled by the SV40 promoter, *Virology*, 165, 321, 1988.

184. Storey, A. and Banks, L., Human papillomavirus type 16 E6 gene cooperates with EJ-ras to immortalize primary mouse cells, *Oncogene*, 8, 919, 1983.

185. Bedell, M. A., Jones, K. H., Grossman, S. R., and Laimins L. A., Identification of human papillomavirus type 18 transforming genes in immortalized and primary cells, *J. Virol.*, 63, 1247, 1989.

186. Yutsudo, M., Okamoto, Y., and Hakura, A., Functional dissociation of transforming genes of human papillomavirus 16, *Virology*, 166, 594, 1988.

187. Band, V., Zajchowski, D., Kulesa, V., and Sager, R., Human papillomavirus DNAs immortalize normal epithelial cells and reduce their growth factor requirements. *Proc. Natl. Acad. Sci. U.S.A.*, 87, 463, 1990.

188. Shay, J. W., Wright, W. E., Brasǐskyte, D., and van der Haegen, B. A., E6 of human papillomavirus type 16 can overcome the M1 stage of immortalization in human mammary cells but not in human fibroblasts, *Oncogene*, 8, 1407, 1993.

189. Kiyono, T., Hiraiwa, A., and Ishibashi, M., Differences in transforming activity and coded amino acid sequence among E6 genes of several papillomaviruses associated with epidermodysplasia verruciformis,*Virology*, 186, 628, 1992.

190. Barbosa, M. S., Lowy, D. R., and Schiller, J. T., Papillomavirus polypeptides E6 and E7 are zinc-binding proteins, *J. Virol.*, 63, 1404, 1989.

191. Lamberti, C., Morrissey, L. C., Grossman, R., and Androphy, E. J., Transcriptional activation by the papillomavirus E6 zinc finger oncoproteins, *EMBO J.*, 9, 1907, 1990.

192. Kanda, T., Watanabe, S., Zanma, S., Sato, H., Furuno, A., and Yoshiika, K., Human papillomavirus type 16 E6 proteins with glycine substitution for cysteine in the metal-binding motif, *Virology*, 185, 536, 1991.

193. Mallon, R. G., Wojciechowicz, D., and Defendi, V., DNA-binding activity of papillomavirus proteins, *J. Virol.*, 61, 1655, 1987.

194. Grossman, S. R., Mora, R., and Laimins, L. A., Intracellular localization and DNA-binding properties of human papillomavirus type 18 protein expressed with a baculovirus vector, *J. Virol.*, 63, 366, 1989.

195. Werness, B. A., Levine, A. J., and Howley, P. M., Association of human papillomavirus types 16 and 18 E6 proteins with p53, *Science*, 248, 76, 1990.

196. Levine, A. J., Momand, J., and Finlay, C. A., The p53 tumor suppressor gene, *Nature*, 351, 453, 1991.

197. Scheffner, M., Werness, B. A., Huibregtse, J. M., Levine, A. J., and Howley, P. M., The E6 oncoprotein encoded by human papillomavirus types 16 and 18 promotes degradation of p53, *Cell*, 63, 1129, 1990.

198. Scheffner, M., Münger, K., Byrne, J. C., and Howley, P. M., The state of the p53 and retinoblastoma genes in human cervical carcinoma cell lines, *Proc. Natl. Acad. Sci. U.S.A.*, 88, 5523, 1991.

199. Hubbert, N., Sedman, S. A., and Schiller J. T., Human papillomavirus type 16 increases degradation rate of p53 in human keratinocytes, *J. Virol.*, 66, 6237, 1992.

200. Lechner, M. S., Mach, D. H., Finicle, A. B., Crook, T., Vousden, K. H., and Laimins, L. A., Human papillomavirus E6 proteins bind p53 *in vivo* and abrogate p53-mediated repression of transcription, *EMBO J.*, 11, 3045, 1992.

201. Huibregtse, J. M., Scheffner, M., and Howley, P. M., Cloning and expression of the cDNA for E6-AP, a protein that mediates the interaction of the human papillomavirus E6 oncoprotein with p53, *Mol. Cell. Biol.*, 13, 775, 1993.

202. Huibregtse, J. M., Scheffner, M., and Howley, P. M., A cellular protein mediates association of p53 with the E6 oncoprotein of human papillomavirus types 16 and 18, *EMBO J.*, 10, 4129, 1991.

203. Crook, T., Tidy, J. A., and Vousden, K. H., Degradation of p53 can be targeted by HPV E6 sequences distinct from those required for p53 binding and transactivation, *Cell*, 67, 547, 1991.

204. Steger, G. and Pfister, H., *In vitro* expressed HPV8 E6 protein does not bind p53, *Arch. Virol.*, 125, 355, 1992.

205. Keen, N., Elston, R., and Crawford, L., Interaction of the E6 protein of human papillomavirus with cellular proteins, *Oncogene*, 9, 1493, 1994.

206. Kiyono, T., Hiraiwa, A., Ishii, S., Takahashi, T., and Ishibashi, M. Inhibition of p53-mediated transactivation by E6 of type 1, but not type 5, 8, or 47 human papillomavirus of cutaneous origin, *J. Virol.*, 68, 4656, 1994.

207. Sedman, S. A., Hubbert, N. L., Vass, W. C., Lowy, D. R., and Schiller, J. T., Mutant p53 can substitute for human papillomavirus type 16EG in immortalization of human keratinocytes but does not have E6-associated trans-activation or transforming activity, *J. Virol.*, 66, 4201, 1992.

208. Chen, J. J., Reid, C. E., Band, V., and Androphy, E. J., Interaction of papillomavirus E6 oncoproteins with a putative calcium-binding protein, *Science*, 269, 529, 1995.

209. Desaintes, C., Hallez, S., Van Alphen, P., and Burny, A., Transcriptional activation of several promoters by the E6 protein of human papillomavirus type 16, *J. Virol.*, 66, 325, 1992.

210. Schlegel, R. and Wade-Glass, M., E5 transforming polypeptide of bovine papillomavirus, *Cancer Cells*, 5, 87, 1987.

211. Horwitz, B. H., Burkhardt, A., Schlegel, R., and DiMaio, D., 44-amino acid E5 transforming protein of bovine papillomavirus requires a hydrophobic core and specific carboxy-terminal amino acids, *Mol. Cell. Biol.*, 8, 4071, 1988.

212. Martin, P., Vass, W. C., Schiller, J. T., Lowy D. R., and Velu, T. J., The bovine papillomavirus E5 transforming protein can stimulate the transforming activity of EGF and and CSF-1 receptors, *Cell*, 59, 21, 1989.

213. Waters, C. M., Overholser, K. A., Sorkin, A., and Carpenter, G., Analysis of the influence of the E5 transforming protein on kinetic parameters of epidermal growth factor binding and metabolism, *J. Cell. Physiol.*, 152, 253, 1992.

214. Petti, L., Nilson, L. A., and DiMaio, D., Activation of the platelet-derived growth factor receptor by the bovine papillomavirus E5 transforming protein, *EMBO J.*, 10, 845, 1991.

215. Goldstein, D. J. and Schlegel, R., The E5 oncoprotein of bovine papillomavirus binds to a 16 KD cellular protein, *EMBO J.*, 9, 137, 1990.

216. Goldstein, D. J., Finbow, M. E., Andresson, T., McLean, P., Smith, K., Bubb, V., and Schlegel, R., Bovine papillomavirus E5 oncoprotein binds to the 16 K component of vacuolar H^+-ATPases, *Nature*, 352, 347, 1991.

217. Goldstein, D. J., Kulke, R., DiMaio, D., and Schlegel, R., A glutamine residue in the membrane-associating domain of the bovine papillomavirus type 1 E5 oncoprotein mediates its binding to a transmembrane component of the vacuolar H^+-ATPase, *J. Virol.*, 66, 405, 1992.

218. Goldstein, D. J., Andresson, T., Sparkowski, J. J., and Schlegel, R., The BPV-1 E5 protein, the 16 KDa membrane pore-forming protein and the PDGF receptor exist in a complex that is dependent on hydrophobic transmembrane interactions, *EMBO J.*, 11, 4851, 1992.

219. Cohen, B. D., Lowy, D. R., and Schiller, J. T., The conserved C-terminal domain of the bovine papillomavirus E5 oncoprotein can associate with an α-adaptin-like molecule: a possible link between growth factor receptors and viral transformation, *Mol. Cell. Biol.*, 13, 6462, 1993.

220. Bubb, V., McCance, D. J., and Schlegel, R., DNA sequence of the HPV-16 E5 ORF and the structure conservation of its encoded proteins, *Virology*, 163, 243, 1988.

221. Conrad, M., Bubb, V. J., and Schlegel, R., The HPV-6 and HPV-16 E5 proteins are membrane-associated proteins which associate with the 16 kD pore-forming protein, *J. Virol.*, 67, 6170, 1993.

222. Chen, S. L. and Mounts P., Transforming activity of E5a protein of human papillomavirus type 6 in NIH3T3 ans C127 cells, *J. Virol.*, 64, 3226, 1990.

223. Pim, D., Collins, M., and Banks, L., Human papillomavirus type 16 E5 gene stimulates the transforming activity of the epidermal growth factor receptor, *Oncogene*, 7, 27, 1992.

224. Leechanachai, P., Banks, L., Moreau, F., and Matlaschewski, G., The E5 gene from human papillomavirus type 16 is a oncogene which enhances growth factor-mediated signal transduction to the nucleus, *Oncogene*, 7, 19, 1992.

225. Conrad, M., Goldstein, D., Andresson, T., and Schlegel, R., The E5 protein of HPV-6, but not HPV-16, associates efficiently with cellular growth factor receptors, *Virology*, 200, 796, 1994.

226. Leptak, C., Ramon y Cajal, S., Kulke, R., Horwitz, B. H., Riese II, D. J., Dotto, G. P., and DiMaio, D., Tumorigenic transformation of murine keratinocytes by the E5 genes of bovine papillomavirus type 1 and human papillomavirus type 16, *J. Virol.*, 65, 7078, 1991.

227. Straight, S. W., Hinkle, P. M., Jewers, R. J., and McCance, D. J., The E5 oncoprotein of human papillomavirus type 16 transforms fibroblasts and effects the downregulation of the epidermal growth factor receptor in keratinocytes, *J. Virol.*, 67, 4521, 1993.

228. Straight, S. W., Herman, B., and McCance, D. J., The E5 oncoprotein of human papillomavirus type 16 inhibits the acidification of endosomes in human keratinocytes, *J. Virol.*, 69, 3185, 1995.

229. Kahn, T., Friesl, H., Copeland, N. G., Gilbert, D. J., Jenkins, N. A., Gissmann, L., Kramer, J., and zur Hausen, H., Molecular cloning, analysis and chromosomal localization of a mouse genomic sequence related to the human papillomavirus type 18 E5 region, *Mol. Carcinog.*, 6, 88, 1992.

230. Iftner, T., Fuchs, P. G., and Pfister, H., Two independently transforming functions of human papillomavirus 8, *Curr. Top. Microbiol. Immunol.*, 144, 167, 1989.

231. Fuchs, P. G., Horn, S., Iftner, T., May, M., Stubenrauch, F., and Pfister H., Molecular biology of epidermodysplasia verruciformis-associated human papillomaviruses, in *Virus Strategies*, Doerfler, W. and Böhm, P., Eds., Verlag Chemie, Weinheim, 1993, 517.

232. Cerni, C., Binetruy, B., Schiller, J. T., Lowy, D. R., Meneguzzi, G., and Cuzin, F., Successive steps in the process of immortalization identified by transfer of separate bovine papillomavirus genes into rat fibroblasts, *Proc. Natl. Acad. Sci. U.S.A.*, 86, 3266, 1989.

233. Storey, A., Greenfield, I., Banks, L., Pim, D., Crook, T., Crawford, L., and Stanley, M., Lack of immortalizing activity of a human papillomavirus type 16 variant with a mutation in the E2 gene isolated from normal human cervical keratinocytes, *Oncogene*, 7, 459, 1992.

234. Hurlin, P. J., Kaur, P., Smith, P. P., Perez-Reyes, N., Blanton, R. A., and McDougal, J. K., Progression of human papillomavirus type 18 immortalized keratinocytes to a malignant phenotype, *Proc. Natl. Acad. Sci. U.S.A.*, 88, 570, 1991.

235. Pecoraro, G., Lee, M., Morgan, D., and Defendi, V., Evolution of *in vitro* transformation and tumorigenesis of HPV16 and HPV18 immortalized primary cervical epithelial cells, *Am. J. Pathol.*, 138, 1, 1991.

236. Dürst, M., Kleinheinz, A., Hotz, M., and Gissmann, L., The physical state of human papillomavirus type 16 DNA in benign and malignant genital tumours, *J. gen. Virol.*, 66, 1515, 1985.

237. Lehn, H., Villa, L. L., Marziona, F., Hilgarth, M., Hillemans, H. G., and Sauer, G., Physical state and biological activity of human papillomavirus genomes in precancerous lesions of the female genital tract, *J. Gen. Virol.*, 69, 187, 1988.

238. Cullen, A. P., Reid, R., Campion, M., and Lörincz, A. T., Analysis of the physical state of different human papillomavirus DNAs in intraephitelial and invasive cervical neoplasm, *J. Virol.*, 65, 606, 1991.

239. Schneider-Maunoury, S., Croissant, O., and Orth, G., Integration of human papillomavirus type 16 DNA sequences: a possible early event in the progression of genital tumors, *J. Virol.*, 61, 3295, 1987.

240. Fuchs, P. G., Girardi, F., and Pfister, H., Human papillomavirus DNA in normal, acanthotic, preneoplastic and neoplastic epithelia of the cervix uteri, *Int. J. Cancer*, 41, 42, 1988.

241. Fuchs, P. G., Girardi, F., and Pfister, H., Human papillomavirus 16 DNA in cervical cancers and in lymph nodes of cervical cancer patients: a diagnostic marker for early metastases?, *Int. J. Cancer*, 43, 41, 1989.

242. Mincheva, A., Gissmann, L., and zur Hausen, H., Chromosomal integration sites of human papillomavirus DNA in three cervical cancer cell lines mapped by in situ hybridization, *Med. Microbiol. Immunol.*, 176, 245, 1987.

243. Dürst, M., Croce, C. M., Gissmann, L., Schwarz, E., and Huebner, K., Papillomavirus sequences integrate near cellular oncogenes in some cervical carcinomas, *Proc. Natl. Acad. Sci. U.S.A.*, 84, 1070, 1987.

244. Cannizarro, L. A., Dürst, M., Mendez, M. J., Hecht, B. K., and Hecht, F., Regional chromosome localization of human papillomavirus integration sites near fragile sites, oncogenes, and cancer chromosome breakpoints, *Cancer Genet. Cytogenet.*, 33, 93, 1988.

245. Couturier, J., Sastre-Garau, X., Schneider-Maunoury, S., Labib, A., and Orth, G., Integration of papillomavirus DNA near *myc* genes in genital carcinomas and its consequences for proto-oncogene expression, *J. Virol.*, 65, 4534, 1991.

246. Schwarz, E., Freese, U. K., Gissmann, L., Mayer, W., Roggenbuck, B., Stremlau, A., and zur Hausen, H., Structure and transcription of human papillomavirus sequences in cervical carcinoma cells, *Nature*, 314, 111, 1985.

247. Matsukura, T., Kanda, T., Furuno, A., Yoshikawa, H., Kawana, T., and Yoshiike, K., Cloning of monomeric human papillomavirus type 16 DNA integrated within cell DNA from a cervical carcinoma, *J. Virol.*, 58, 979, 1986.

248. Baker, C. C., Phelps, W. C., Lindgren, V., Braun, M. J., Gonda, M. A., and Howley, P. M., Structural and transcriptional analysis of human papillomavirus type 16 sequences in cervical carcinoma cell lines, *J. Virol.*, 61, 962, 1987.

249. El Awady, M. K., Kaplan, J. B., O'Brien, S. J., and Burk, R. D., Molecular analysis of integrated human papillomavirus 16 sequences in the cervical cancer cell line SiHa, *Virology,* 159, 389, 1987.

250. Choo, K. B., Pau, C. C., and Hau, S. H., Integration of human papillomavirus type 16 into cellular DNA of cervical carcinoma: preferential detection of the E2 gene and invariable retention of the long control region and the E6/E7 open reading frames, *Virology,* 161, 259, 1987.

251. Shirasawa, H., Tomita, Y., Sekiya, S., Takamizawa, H., and Bunsiti, S., Integration and transcription of human papillomavirus type 16 and 18 sequences in cell lines derived from cervical carcinomas, *J. Gen. Virol.,* 68, 583, 1987.

252. Romanczuk, H. and Howley, P. M., Disruption of either the E1 or the E2 regulatory gene of human papillomavirus type 16 increases viral immortalization capacity, *Proc. Natl. Acad. Sci. U.S.A.,* 89, 3159, 1992.

253. Sang, B.-C. and Barbosa, M. S., Increased E6/E7 transcription in HPV 18-immortalized human keratinocytes results from inactivation of E2 and additional cellular events, *Virology,* 189, 448, 1992.

254. Schneider-Gädicke, A. and Schwarz, E., Different human cervical carcinoma cell lines show similar transcription patterns of human papillomavirus type 18 early genes, *EMBO J.,* 5, 2285, 1986.

255. Smits, H. L., Cornelissen, M. T. E., Jebbink, M. F., Van den Tweel, J. G., Struyk, A. P. H. B., Briet, M., and ter Schegget, J., Human papillomavirus type 16 transcripts expressed from viral-cellular junctions and full-length viral copies in CaSki cells and in a cervical carcinoma, *Virology,* 182, 870, 1991.

256. Le, J.-Y. and Defendi, V., A viral cellular junction fragment form a human papillomavirus type 16-positive tumor is competent in transformation of NIH 3T3 cells, *J. Virol.,* 62, 4420, 1988.

257. Kleiner, E., Dietrich, W., and Pfister, H., Differential regulation of papilloma virus early gene expression in transformed fibroblasts and carcinoma cell lines, *EMBO J.,* 5, 1945, 1986.

258. Rösl, F., Westphal, E. M., and zur Hausen, H., Chromatin structure and transcriptional regulation of human papillomavirus type 18 DNA in HeLa cells, *Mol. Carcinog.,* 2, 72, 1989.

259. von Knebel Doeberitz, M., Bauknecht, T., Bartsch, D., and zur Hausen, H., Influence of chromosomal integration on glucocorticoid-regulated transcription of growth-stimulating papillomavirus genes E6 and E7 in cervical carcinoma cells, *Proc. Natl. Acad. Sci. U.S.A.,* 88, 1411, 1991.

260. Matsukura, T., Koi, S., and Sugase, M., Both episomal and integrated forms of human papillomavirus type 16 are involved in invasive cervical cancers, *Virology,* 172, 63, 1989.

261. Choo, K. B., Cheung, W.-F., Liew, L.-N., Lee, H.-H., and Han, S.-H., Presence of catenated human papillomavirus type 16 episomes in a cervical carcinoma cell line, *J. Virol.,* 63, 782, 1989.

262. Snijders, P. J. F., Meijer, C. J. L. M., van den Brule, A. J. C., Schrijnemakers, H. F. J., Snow, G. B., and Walboomers, J. M. M., Human papillomavirus (HPV) type 16 and 33 E6/E7 region transcripts in tonsillar carcinomas can originate from integrated and episomal HPV DNA, *J. Gen. Virol.,* 73, 2059, 1992.

263. Kennedy, I. M., Simpson, S., Macnab, J. C. M., and Clements, J. B., Human papillomavirus type 16 DNA from a vulvar carcinoma *in situ* is present as head-to-tail dimeric episomes with a deletion in the non-coding region, *J. Gen. Virol.,* 68, 451, 1987.

264. Girardi, F., Pickel, H., Beyer-Finkler, E., and Pfister, H. Specific rearrangements of human papillomavirus DNA provide molecular evidence for genetic heterogeneity of primary cervical cancers and lymph node metastases in two patients, *Gynecol. Oncol.,* 51, 281, 1993.

265. Rando, R. F., Groff, D. E., Chirikjian, J. G., and Lancaster, W. D., Isolation and characterization of a novel human papillomavirus type 6 from an invasive vulvar carcinoma, *J. Virol.,* 57, 3533, 1986.

266. Byrne, J., Tsao, M., Fraser, R. and Howley, P., Human papillomavirus-11 DNA in a patient with chronic laryngotracheobronchial papillomatosis and metastatic squamous-cell carcinoma of the lung, *N. Engl. J. Med.,* 317, 873, 1988.

267. DiLorenzo, T. P., Tamsen, A., Abramson, A. L., and Steinberg, B. M., Human papillomavirus type 6a DNA in the lung carcinoma of a patient with recurrent laryngeal papillomatosis is characterized by a partial duplication, *J. Gen. Virol.,* 73, 423, 1992.

268. McGlennen, R. C., Ghai, J., Ostrow, R. S., LaBresh, K., Schneider, J. F., and Faras, A. J., Cellular transformation by a unique isolate of human papillomavirus type 11, *Cancer Res.,* 52, 5872, 1992.

269. Dong, X.-P., Stubenrauch, F., Beyer-Finkler, E., and Pfister, H., Prevalence of deletions of YY1-binding sites in episomal HPV16 DNA from cervical cancers, *Int. J. Cancer,* 58, 803, 1994.

270. Orth, G., Epidermodysplasia varruciformis, in *The Papovaviridae,* Salzman, N. P. and Howley, P. M., Eds., Plenum Press, New York, 1987, 199.

271. Yabe Y., Tanimura Y., Sakai, A., Hitsumoto, T., and Nohara, N., Molecular characteristics and physical state of human papillomavirus DNA change with progressing malignancy: studies in a patient with epidermodysplasia verruciformis, *Int. J. Cancer*, 43, 1022, 1989.

272. Pfister, H., Gassenmaier, A., Nürnberger, F., and Stüttgen, G., Human papilloma virus 5-DNA of an Epidermodysplasia verruciformis patient infected with various human papillomavirus types, *Cancer Res.*, 43, 1436, 1983.

273. Ostrow R. S., Zachow, K. R., and Faras A. J., Molecular cloning and nucleotide sequence analysis of several naturally occuring HPV5 deletion mutant genomes, *Virology*, 158, 235, 1987.

274. Deaux, M.-C., Favre, M., and Orth, G., Genetic heterogeneity among human papillomaviruses (HPV) associated with epidermodysplasia verruciformis: evidence for multiple allelic forms of HPV5 and HPV8 genes, *Virology*, 184, 492, 1991.

275. Oft, M., Böhm, S., Wilczynski, S. P., and Iftner, T., Expression of the different viral mRNAs of human papillomavirus 6 in a squamous-cell carcinoma of the bladder and the cervix, *Int. J. Cancer*, 53, 924, 1993.

276. Higgins, G. D., Uzelin, D. M., Phillips, G. E., and Burrell, C. J., Presence and distribution of human papillomavirus sense and antisense RNA transcripts in genital cancers, *J. Gen. Virol.*, 72, 885, 1991.

277. Vormwald-Dogan, V., Fischer, B., Bludau, H., Freese, U. K., Gissmann, L., Glitz, D., Schwarz, E., and Dürst, M., Sense and antisense transcripts of human papillomavirus type 16 in cervical cancers, *J. Gen. Virol.*, 73, 1833, 1992.

278. von Knebel Doeberitz, M., Oltersdorf, T., Schwarz, E., and Gissmann, L., Correlation of modified human papillomavirus early gene expression with altered growth properties in C4-1 cervical carcinoma cells, *Cancer Res.*, 48, 3780, 1988.

279. Riou, G., Barrois, M., Tordjman, I., Dutroquay, V., and Orth, G., Présence de génomes de papillomavirus et amplification des oncogènes c-Ha-ras dans des cancers envahissants du col de l'utérus. *C.R. Acad. Sc. Paris*, 299, 575, 1984.

280. Riou, G., Barrois, M., Lê, M. G., George, M., Le Doussal, V., and Haie, C., C-myc proto-oncogene expression and prognosis in early carcinoma of the uterine cervix, *Lancet*, 2, 761, 1987.

281. Crook, T., Wrede, D., and Vousden, K. H., p53 point mutation in HPV negative human cervical carcinoma cell lines, *Oncogene*, 6, 873, 1991.

282. Yaginuma, Y. and Westphal, H., Analysis of the p53 gene in human uterine carcinoma cell lines, *Cancer Res.*, 51, 6506, 1991.

283. Wrede, D., Tidy, J.A., Crook, T., Lane, D., and Vousden, K. H., Expression of RB and p53 proteins in HPV-positive and HPV-negative cervical carcinoma cell lines, *Mol. Carcinog.*, 4, 171, 1991.

284. Crook, T., Wrede, D., Tidy J. A., Mason, W. P., Evans, D. J., and Vousden, K. H., Clonal p53 mutation in primary cervical cancer: association with human-papillomavirus-negative tumours, *Lancet*, 339, 1070, 1992.

285. Fujita, M., Inoue, M., Tanizawa, O., Iwamoto, S., and Enomoto, T., Alteration of the p53 gene in human primary cervical carcinoma with and without human papillomavirus infection, *Cancer Res.*, 52, 5323, 1992.

286. Chen, T. M., Chen, T. A., Hsieh, C. Y., Chang, D. Y., Chen, Y. H., and Defendi, V., The state of p53 in primary human cervical carcinomas and its effects in human papillomavirus-immortalized cervical cells, *Oncogene*, 8, 1551, 1993.

287. Choo, K. B. and Chong, K. Y., Absence of mutations in the p53 and the retinoblastoma susceptibility genes in primary cervical carcinomas, *Virology*, 193, 1042, 1993.

288. Park, D. J., Wilczynski, S. P., Paquette, R. L., Miller, C. W., and Koeffler, H. P., p53 mutations in HPV-negative carcinoma, *Oncogene*, 9, 205, 1994.

289. Butz, K., Shahabeddin, L., Geisen, C., Spitkowsky, D., Ullmann, A., and Hoppe-Seyler, F., Functional p53 protein in human papillomavirus-positive cancer cells, *Oncogene*, 10, 927, 1995.

290. Saxon, P. J., Srivatsan, E. S., and Stanbridge, E. J., Introduction of human chromosome 11 via microcell transfer controls tumorigenic expression of HeLa cells, *EMBO J.*, 5, 3461, 1986.

291. Koi, M., Morita, H., Yamada, H., Satoh, H., Barret, J. C., and Oshimura, M., Normal human chromosome 11 supresses tumorigenicity of human cervical tumor cell line SiHa, *Mol. Carcinogenesis*, 2, 12, 1989.

292. Dürst, M., Dzarlieva-Petrusevska, R. T., Boucamp, P., Fusenig, N. E., and Gissmann, L., Molecular and cytogenetic analysis of immortalized human primary keratinocytes obtained after transfection with human papillomavirus type 16 DNA, *Oncogene*, 1, 251, 1987.

293. Smith. P. P., Bryant, E. M., Kaur, P., and McDougall, J. K., Cytogenetic analysis of eight human papillomavirus immortalized human keratinocyte cell lines, *Int. J. Cancer*, 44, 1124, 1989.

294. Hashida, T. and Yasumoto, S., Induction of chromosome abnormalities in mouse and human epidermal keratinocytes by the human papillomavirus type 16 E7 oncogene, *J. Gen. Virol.*, 72, 1569, 1991.

295. Kessis, T. D., Slebos, R. J., Nelson, W. G., Kastan, M. B., Plunkett, B. S., Han, S. M., Lorincz, A. T., Hedrick, L., and Cho, K. R., Human papillomavirus 16 E6 expression disrupts the p53-mediated cellular response to DNA damage, *Proc. Natl. Acad. Sci. U.S.A.*, 90, 3988, 1993.

296. Rösl, F., Dürst, M., and zur Hausen, H., Selective suppression of human papillomavirus transcription in nontumorigenic cells by 5-azacytidine, *EMBO J.*, 7, 1321, 1988.

297. Bosch, F. X., Schwarz, E., Boukamp, P., Fusenig, N. E., Bartsch, D., and zur Hausen, H., Suppression *in vivo* of human papillomavirus type 18 E6-E7 gene expression in nontumorigenic HeLa x fibroblast hybrid cells, *J. Virol.*, 64, 4743, 1990.

298. Rösl, F., Achtstätter, T., Bauknecht, T., Futterman, G., Hutter, K. J., and zur Hausen, H., Extinction of the HPV18 upstream regulatory region in cervical carcinoma cells after fusion with non-tumorigenic human keratinocytes under non-selective conditions, *EMBO J.*, 10, 1337, 1991.

299. Smits, H. L., Raadsheer, E., Rood, I., Mehendale, S., Slater, R. M., van der Noordaa, J., and ter Schegget, J., Induction of anchorage-independent growth of human embryonic fibroblasts with a deletion in the short arm of chromosome 11 by human papillomavirus type 16 DNA, *J. Virol.*, 62, 4538, 1988.

300. Smits, P. H. M., Smits, H. L., Minnaar, R. P., Hemmings, B. A., Mayer-Jaekel, R. E., Schuurman, T., van der Noordaa, J., and ter Schegget, J., The 55kDa regulatory subunit of protein phosphatase 2A plays a role in the activation of the HPV16 long control region in human cells with a deletion in the short arm of chromosome 11, *EMBO J.*, 11, 4601, 1992.

3

The Nonhuman (Animal) Papillomaviruses: Host Range, Epitope Conservation, and Molecular Diversity

John P. Sundberg, Marc Van Ranst, Robert D. Burk, and A. Bennett Jenson

CONTENTS

I.   INTRODUCTION

"Many writers have imagined that the epidemic diseases which affect the human race are peculiar to our species, and have no influence on the inferior animals; and they have been not less decided in the opinion that the diseases of other animals are not communicable to man."[1] This statement introduced the most thorough historical dissertation on smallpox and its relationship to similar diseases in animals that led to Edward Jenner's development of vaccination.[2] These erroneous concepts are still held today by many clinicians and researchers, which severely limits their ability to take advantage of the nonhuman (so called "animal") papillomaviruses and the diseases they cause to use as animal models for the variety of serious human diseases that this genus of virus causes.

Papillomaviruses (PVs) infect a broad host range of vertebrate species; however, most that have been identified and characterized infect mammals (Table 1). Several avian PVs have been isolated and their DNAs cloned (Table 2). Reptiles and amphibians develop lesions suggestive of PV infections. With the exception of the Bolivian side necked turtle,[3] no lower vertebrate PVs have yet been convincingly identified (Table 2). Other agents, including poxviruses,[4-6] herpesviruses,[7-9] adenoviruses,[10] rhabdoviruses,[11] retroviruses,[9] anaerobic bacteria,[12,13] chemical carcinogens,[14] etc., will induce papillomatous lesions, and this becomes increasingly more prevalent in lower vertebrates and invertebrates.

0-8493-7356-5/97/$0.00+$.50
© 1997 by CRC Press, Inc.

TABLE 1 Phylogenetic Relationship of Mammalian Hosts Infected With Papillomaviruses, Based on Linnean Classification of Mammals[66] and the Proposed Nomenclature for Nonhuman Papillomaviruses[34]

Order/family/species (common name)	Published abbreviation	Proposed abbreviation	Lesion	Anatomical site	Carcinoma in host	Ref.
Marsupialia						
Didelphidae						
Didelphis virginiana (Virginian opossum)	none	DvPV[a]	Papilloma	Skin	unknown	67
Edentata						
Dasypodidae						
Chaetophractus villosus (hairy armadillo)	none	CvPV[a]	Papilloma	Skin	unknown	53
Primates						
Cercopithecidae						
Macaca mulatta (rhesus macaque)	RhPV	RhPV[b]	Squamous cell carcinoma	Genital	yes	33, 64
Colobus guereza (Eastern black and white colobus)	CgPV–1	CgPV–1	Papilloma	Genital	unknown	40, 65
Colobus guereza (Eastern black and white colobus)	CgPV–2	CgPV–2	Papilloma	Skin	unknown	33
Pongidae						
Pan paniscus (pygmy chimpanzee)	PpPV/PCPV	PpPV	Papilloma	Oral cavity	unknown	36–38
Pan troglodytes (chimpanzee)	PtPV	PtPV	Papilloma	Oral cavity	unknown	Favre, unpublished
Hominidae						
Homo sapiens (man)	HPV	HPV1–70 or more[c]				
Carnivora						
Canidae						
Canis familiaris (domestic dog)	COPV	COPV[c] COPV[d]	Papilloma Papilloma	Oral cavity Skin	yes yes	68–70 71, 72

Species		Virus	Lesion	Site	Malignant potential	Reference
Canis familiaris (domestic dog)	none	CfPV[d]	Papilloma	Genital	possibly	19
Canis latrans (coyote)	COPV	COPV[c]	Papilloma	Oral cavity	possibly	23, 73
Canis lupus (wolf)	none	COPV[ad]	Papilloma	Oral cavity	unknown	73
Ursidae						
Ursus arctos (Zodiac bear)	none	UaPV[a]	Papilloma	Genital	unknown	74
Procyonidae						
Procyon lotor (common raccoon)	none	RaPV[a]	Papilloma	Skin	unknown	77
Felidae						
Felis domesticus (domestic cat)	FdPV	FdPV	Papilloma	Skin	unknown	42, 44
Felis concolor (puma, cougar, Florida panther)	FcPV	FcPV	Papilloma	Oral cavity	unknown	Horner and Sundberg, unpublished
Felis rufus (bobcat)	FrPV	FrPV	Papilloma	Oral cavity	unknown	Horner and Sundberg, unpublished
Panthera leo (lion)	PlPV	PlPV	Papilloma	Oral cavity	unknown	41
Panthera uncia (snow leopard)	PuPV-1[d]	PuPV-1[d]	Papilloma	Oral cavity	unknown	Montali and Sundberg, unpublished
Panthera uncia (snow leopard)	PuPV-2[d]	PuPV-2[d]	Papilloma	Skin	unknown	Rowland and Sundberg, unpublished
Neofelis nebulosa (clouded leopard)	NnPV	NnPV	Papilloma	Oral cavity	unknown	Montali and Sundberg, unpublished
Cetacea						
Physeteridae						
Physeter catodon (sperm whale)	none	PcPV[a]	Papilloma	Genital	unknown	79

TABLE 1   Phylogenetic Relationship of Mammalian Hosts Infected With Papillomaviruses, Based on Linnean Classification of Mammals[66] and the Proposed Nomenclature for Nonhuman Papillomaviruses[34] (continued)

Order/family/species (common name)	Published abbreviation	Proposed abbreviation	Lesion	Anatomical site	Carcinoma in host	Ref.
Proboscidea						
Elephantidae						
Elaphas maximus (Indian elephant)	none	EmPV[A]	Papilloma	Oral cavity	unknown	76
Perissodactyla						
Equidae						
Equus caballus (domestic horse)	EQPV-1	EcPV-1	Papilloma	Skin	no	77
Equus caballus (domestic horse)	EQPV-2	EcPV-2	Papilloma	Genital	yes	77
Artiodactyla						
Cervidae						
Cervus elaphus (red deer, wapiti)	none	CePV-1[ad]	Fibropap.	Skin	unknown	78
Cervus elaphus (red deer, wapiti)	none	CePV-2[ad]	Papilloma	Skin	unknown	Favre, unpublished
Alces alces (Euopean elk, North American moose)	EEPV	AaPV	Fibroma	Skin	unknown	79-81
Rangifer tarandus (reindeer, caribou)	RDPV	RtPV	Fibropap.	Skin	unknown	82
Odocoileus hemionus (mule deer)	none	OhPV	Fibropap.	Skin	unknown	83
Odocoileus virginianus (white-tailed deer)	DPV	OvPV	Fibroma	Skin	unknown	83, 84
Giraffidae						
Giraffa camelopardalis (giraffe)	none	GcPV*	Papilloma	Skin	unknown	85
Antilocapridae						
Antilocapra americana (pronghorn antelope)	none	PrPV*+	Fibropap.	Skin	unknown	86

Bovidae					
Aepyceros melampus (impala)	none	AmPV[a]	Papilloma	Skin	unknown	85
Ovis aries (domestic sheep)	none	OaPV	Papilloma	Skin	possibly	87–91
Bos taurus (domestic cattle)	BPV-1	BPV-1[c]	Fibropap.	Skin	no	92, 93
Bos taurus (domestic cattle)	BPV-2	BPV-2[c]	Fibropap.	Skin, Genital	no	92
Bos taurus (domestic cattle)	BPV-3	BPV-3[c]	Papilloma	Skin	no	94
Bos taurus (domestic cattle)	BPV-4	BPV-4[c]	Papilloma	Esophagus	yes	95
Bos taurus (domestic cattle)	BPV-5	BPV-5[c]	Fibropap.	Teat skin	no	96
Bos taurus (domestic cattle)	BPV-6	BPV-6[c]	Papilloma	Teat skin	no	97
Capricornis crispus (Japanese serow)	none	CcPV	Papilloma	Skin	unknown	98
Rodentia					
Castoridae					
Castor canadensis (American beaver)	none	BePV[a]	Papilloma	Skin of feet	no	99
Murinae					
Micromys minutus (harvest mouse)	MmPV	MmPV	Papilloma	Skin	yes	30–32, 100
Mastomys (Praomys) natalensis (multimammate rat)	MnPV	MnPV	Papilloma	Skin	questionable	24, 100, 101

TABLE 1 Phylogenetic Relationship of Mammalian Hosts Infected With Papillomaviruses, Based on Linnean Classification of Mammals[66] and the Proposed Nomenclature for Nonhuman Papillomaviruses[34] (continued)

Order/family/species (common name)	Published abbreviation	Proposed abbreviation	Lesion	Anatomical site	Carcinoma in host	Ref.
Lagamorpha						
Leporidae						
Sylvilagus floridanus (Eastern cottontail rabbit)	CRPV	CRPV[c]	Papilloma	Skin	yes	106–109
Oryctolagus cuniculus (common rabbit)	ROPV	OcPV	Papilloma	Oral cavity	no	60

[a] No molecular work done to confirm initial observations.

[b] Genus and species abbreviation previously used, first two letters of common name used as an alternative.

[c] Long term usage of symbol precludes reason to change.

[d] Insufficient molecular work completed to determine if this is a separate species.

TABLE 2   Papillomavirus Infections in Nonmammalian Hosts

Host	Published abbreviation	Proposed abbreviation	Lesion	Anatomic site	Reference
Birds					
Fringilla coelebs (Chaffinch)	FPV	FcPV	Papilloma	Skin	110, 111
Fringilla monifringilla (Brambling)	none	FmPV[a]	Papilloma	Skin	112
Psittacus erithacus timneh (African grey parrot)	PePV	PePV	Papilloma	Skin	114, 115
Reptiles					
Platemys platycephala (Bolivian side necked turtle)	none	BoPV[b]	Epidermal hyperplasia	Skin	3

[a] No molecular work done to confirm initial observations.

[b] Genus and species abbreviation previously used; first two letters of common name used as an alternative.

The nonhuman PVs induce a variety of lesions with morphological features similar to those induced in humans. The cytopathic effect, in which there is both cell proliferation and lysis, follow common patterns regardless of the host species infected. Because of these underlying features, the nonhuman PVs are extremely valuable as models to understand the mechanisms underlying human PV infections and how the diseases induced can be prevented or treated.

This chapter will provide an extensive list of host species known to be infected by PVs. Also covered will be current concepts on epitope conservation between species and the phylogenetic evolution of PVs.

II.   PATHOLOGY OF PAPILLOMAVIRUS INDUCED LESIONS

All papillomaviruses induce proliferation of cells resulting in tumor formation. Only differentiated stratified squamous epithelial cells undergo a lytic process as the viruses complete their life cycles. Each virus produces very specific lesions but all follow fundamentally similar patterns of cellular proliferation and lysis.

Papillomaviruses are remarkably stable in the environment. Natural inoculation by rubbing on communally used posts or other animals probably forces desiccated cornified cells filled with millions of virions into wounds on susceptible hosts. The virus-packed cornified cells undergo dissolution and viruses invade surrounding cells. Target cells probably have surface receptors for normal cytokines by which the virus attaches and enters the cell such as an epidermal growth factor receptor for vaccinia.[15] The receptors for PVs are still undetermined. The primary target cells of PVs are basal cells of stratified squamous epithelia.[16] Transformation results in tumor formation. In some species, notably the ruminants (Artiodactyla), fibroblasts appear to be the primary target cells with overlying squamous cells being secondary.[17] This latter observation has been difficult to prove, however, sensitive *in situ* hybridization techniques may resolve this question.

These cell proliferation processes result in formation of three benign tumor types: papillomas (epidermal proliferation on thin fibrovascular stalks), fibropapillomas (epidermal proliferation on prominent fibrovascular structures forming a verrucous pattern), or fibromas (primarily fibroblasts and dense irregular collagenous connective tissue). Details of the lesions that occur in various species are published elsewhere.[18,19]

Epidermal degenerative changes, the second effect of PV infection, are usually limited to the cells in the stratum granulosum of the benign tumors but may include those in the upper stratum spinosum. The cytoplasm of these cells swells and stains poorly; large and/or abnormal keratohyalin granules become prominent; and nuclei may contain amphophilic inclusions of various sizes. The inclusions contain large crystalline arrays of virions when viewed by transmission electron microscopy. These infected cornified cells are sloughed into the environment as part of the normal exfoliation process, thus completing the life cycle of the virus.

Progression of PV induced tumors to malignancy (primarily squamous cell carcinomas) is discussed elsewhere in this book and in other reviews.[20] Regression of lesions is the result of the combined effects of the cellular and humoral immune system. Antibody titers can be detected following experimental inoculation and before regression of tumors. This is associated with a rise in viral genome copy number in tumors.[17,21] Perivascular lymphocytic infiltrates in the dermis immediately preclude tumor regression, indicating the role of the cellular immune system.[17] Simultaneous regression of coexisting, sometimes widely separated, benign warts or papillomas occur if these lesions are caused by the same PV type, suggesting that cell mediated immunity is responsible for spontaneous regression of PV induced lesions and that such immunity is PV type-specific.

The utilization of inbred laboratory mice in a variety of experiments in progress around the world will lead to a more thorough understanding of the pathogenesis of PV infections and the way mammals deal with it.

III. HOST RANGE AND NOMENCLATURE

At least 50 mammalian species have been confirmed to be infected by PVs (Table 1). Of these, 24 different PVs species have had their DNA cloned and characterized to various degrees. Three species of birds have had their respective PVs characterized (Table 2).

Nomenclature and symbols for the nonhuman PVs have been neglected because of the small number of viruses known. However, over the last 20 years, numerous novel nonhuman PVs have been identified by routine diagnostic methods such as electron microscopy and immunohistochemistry (Figure 1). Paralleling their discovery, many have been characterized to various degrees using modern molecular technology (Figure 1). As a result of the large number currently known, the nomenclature needs to be reevaluated using existing and proposed standards.

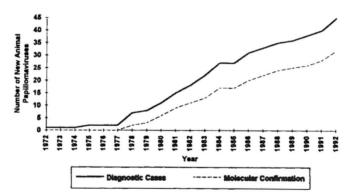

FIGURE 1   Over the past 20 years, initially few case reports identified new hosts for papillomaviruses. Following the molecular identification of BPV-1 and BPV-2 in 1978,[92] there has been a steady increase in the discovery of new nonhuman papillomaviruses and their molecular characterization.

The nomenclature of nonhuman papillomaviruses has been confusing and controversial. Several papillomaviruses have been studied for a long time and their designations are well known and should not be changed. These are limited to those that infect cattle (BPVs), cottontail rabbits (CRPV), and humans (HPVs). Eponyms should not be used. Since Richard Shope published the first report on the cottontail rabbit papillomavirus,[22] CRPV is often referred to as the Shope papillomavirus. His name is also associated with another unrelated virus, the Shope fibroma virus, which is a pox virus.[5] These designations are occasionally used interchangeably in review articles. A special case that falls into this group is the canine oral PV, designated COPV. In addition to having been in common use for many years, COPV has recently been found to infect two closely related canine species, domestic dogs and free-living coyotes.[23]

Muller and Gissmann[24] set a precedent in 1978 for naming PVs infecting uncommon hosts with their work on the multimammate rat (*Mastomys natalensis*) PV. They named the virus after the scientific name of the host species using the first letter of the genus (which is capitalized) followed by the first letter of the species (lower case) and then followed by PV (capitalized). In their case, the virus was designated MnPV. A year later, Coggins and zur Hausen[25] proposed use of the first two letters of the common name of the host species in a similar manner. Their original example was for the hamster papillomavirus, HaPV, which has subsequently been determined not to be a papillomavirus.[26-29] Based on these papers, we propose unifying the nonhuman PV nomenclature by using the scientific name of the host for the viral designation. If this is already taken in a prior publication, then the common name abbreviation should be used. An example would be the European harvest mouse (*Micromys minutus*) PV[30-32] and the rhesus macaque (*Macaca mulatta*) PV.[33] Since the mouse virus was reported first, it is designated MmPV. The nonhuman primate virus is designated RhPV, based on its common name.

Once molecular criteria have been met that differentiate two distinct PVs that infect a single host species (less than 50% homologous),[25,34] the viruses are numbered sequentially in the chronological order they are identified. For the nonhuman PVs, this has been limited to those infecting cattle, horses, and colobus monkeys (Table 1).

The use of a revised nomenclature system[34] would standardize the taxonomy of the nonhuman papillomaviruses. To this end, Tables 1 and 2 list the various designations used with adjustments to the standardized nomenclature system. The standardized nomenclature is then used in all subsequent tables and figures in this chapter.

IV. SPECIES SPECIFICITY

Although our knowledge is limited, most PVs appear to be species specific or at least restricted to infection between closely related animals within the same genus or family. The few known exceptions are listed in Table 3. These observations have two important implications: infection of humans when handling nonhuman primate PVs and importation and spread of foreign animal diseases related to endangered species programs.

TABLE 3   Papillomaviruses that Infect More Than One Species

Natural host	Virus	Experimental host	Reference
Domestic Cattle	BPV-1, 2	Horse	115
		Hamster	116,117
		Pica	118
		Mice	119,120
Cottontail Rabbit	CRPV	Domestic Rabbit	45
Domestic Rabbit	OcPV	Cottontail Rabbit	121
		Hamster	122
White-tailed deer	OvPV	Hamster	116
European elk	AaPV	Hamster	81
Domestic sheep	OaPV	Hamster	87
Coyote	COPV	Domestic Dog	23
Human	HPV-?	Baboon (?)	47

As more nonhuman primate papillomaviruses are identified and worked with,[34] particularly those phylogenetically closely related to humans such as chimpanzees,[36-38] it is possible that the nonhuman PVs will prove to be infectious and potentially tumorigenic in humans. A parallel example is herpes B virus infection in macaques.[39] In the natural host, herpes B virus infection causes only minor vesicles on oral mucous membranes. Infection of human caretakers may be fatal. The PVs isolated from nonhuman primates, although different, are very similar to HPVs at the molecular level.[36,37,40]

Endangered species programs work by bringing multiple individuals of a rare species into confinement to expand the population and increase the gene pool. This also establishes an ideal opportunity for spread of infectious diseases that can undermine an entire program. This situation arose in a captive breeding program involving the pygmy chimpanzee (*Pan paniscus*), an endangered ape closely related to humans. Pygmy chimpanzees were brought into a zoo for breeding purposes and were found, upon arrival, to be affected with PV positive oral papillomatosis. These animals were maintained in quarantine and could not be used for breeding purposes.[36]

Another potential problem recently occurred with endangered Asian lions. In their natural environment, India, a group of lions were found to have PV positive focal oral hyperplasia and papillomas.[41] Importation of the Asian lions into captive breeding programs has caused concerns about introduction of potential disease problems in domestic cats or wild felids on exhibit. Papillomatosis is a very rare disease in domestic cats. A PV infecting domestic cats has just recently been identified.[42-44]

Papillomavirus associated squamous cell carcinomas have perplexed scientists since the observation was first made where the cottontail rabbit cutaneous papillomavirus would induce squamous cell carcinomas when injected into domestic rabbits.[45] A biological observation that warrants follow-up is that many of the PVs that infect more than one species appear to be oncogenic in at least one of their hosts.[20,46] Bovine PV types 1 and 2 are associated with benign fibropapillomas in domestic cattle, disfiguring but basically benign sarcoids in horses, and fibrosarcomas in rodents.[46] Human PVs have proven to be very species specific, although most transmission studies utilized phylogenetically unrelated hosts. However, tissue extracts from a human papilloma were used successfully to induce lesions in a *Papio papio*, a nonhuman primate,[47] suggesting that primate PVs are able to infect closely related species, at least within the same order.

V.   ANTIBODY STUDIES

Papovaviridae is a family of viruses that includes two genera: papillomavirus and polyomavirus. These two genera have many differences[48] and probably should be reclassified into two distinct families. Neither the genomic DNA nor viral structural and nonstructural proteins are conserved between the papillomaviruses and polyomaviruses.[48-50] Group specific antibodies cross react within each genus, but not between them.

A large number of monoclonal and polyclonal antibodies have been generated to study the papillomaviruses. Their derivation and value is often misunderstood by users not familiar with the experiments that led to their development. Epitopes, antigenic determinants recognized by the paratopes of antibodies, fall into two broad categories: those that depend on tertiary protein structure and are conformational (species-specific) and those that depend on the primary structure of proteins and are linear (genus-specific). The protein determines the antigenic sites whereas the antibodies define the epitopes contained within these sites.

Each PV has major (L1) and minor (L2) structural viral proteins. The L1 protein, which comprises 95% of the mass of the virion, has a molecular mass of approximately 54 kD, whereas the L2 protein has the same approximate weight but migrates aberrantly in SDS-gels at around 77 kD. Although the nucleotide sequences encoding the L1 protein are highly conserved among all PVs, the corresponding conserved amino acid sequences, recognized as PV cross-reactive linear epitopes, have a cryptic location within the intact viral particles. The intact L1 protein, which is responsible for the structure of the capsomeres, expresses linear and discontinuous capsid surface epitopes that are type-specific. The conformational epitopes are the major target of neutralizing antibodies[51] and can be mimicked by conformationally correct L1 expressed alone. This finding has provided the basis for a preventive recombinant vaccine that has been used effectively in a dog model.[52,53] On the other hand, L2 proteins are poorly conserved, but type-specific and minimally cross-reactive epitopes appear to be internal to the capsid. The role of

L2 in viral assembly is unknown, but it may determine the site of genome encapsidation, since it is translocated to nucleoli, where native viral capsids are initially assembled when examined by electron microscopy.

Bovine papillomavirus type 1 (BPV-1) is the prototype PV. At least 17 distinct linear epitopes are encoded by the BPV-1 L1 gene. Most of these are conserved to various degrees among mammalian and avian PVs.[54,55] Polyclonal antibodies are produced by disrupting BPV-1 with sodium dodecyl sulfate, exposing internal, conserved structural antigens, which are then injected with adjuvents into rabbits to generate a multitude of cross reactive antibody populations. This type of preparation is available commercially (DAKO Corp., Carpinteria, CA) and is routinely used to screen tissue sections for evidence of productive infections. A number of monoclonal antibodies have also been produced against disrupted BPV-1 virions, and the linear epitopes defined by some of these monoclonal antibodies have been mapped to the exact location on the L1 gene product by the multipin synthesis system of Geysen et al.[56] Most of these epitopes are internal to the capsid, but they are reactive with monoclonal antibodies in productive infections, presumably because of an abundance of native linearized L1 protein synthesized in these lesions. Antibodies that recognize L2 proteins are not useful for detection or typing of PV in productive infections because of the relative small amounts of this structural protein available.

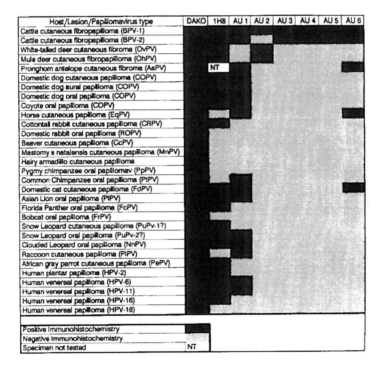

FIGURE 2   Rabbit polyclonal antibodies directed against epitopes of BPV-1 L1 and L2 gene products (DAKO) or mouse monoclonal antibodies directed against specific BPV-1 L1 epitopes (1H8, AU1-6) can be used in immuno-histochemical studies to identify epitope conservation between divergent papillomaviruses. The authors thank Drs. E. Amtmann and J. Kreider for blocks containing MnPV and CRPV, respectively.

Monoclonal antibodies against BPV-1 are specific for the papillomaviridae genus. However, other tissues and organisms may contain some of the antigenic determinants, which is one reason why precisely characterized monoclonal antibodies are important for detecting and typing productive infections. These antibodies can be used in a panel to evaluate and partially type papillomas by immunohistochemistry in tissue sections. The pattern of positive/negative staining can be compared to a table and the virus partially typed, or at least separated within a host species (Figure 2). This can be useful for specimens for which no frozen tissues are available for careful molecular studies. In harsh field conditions, such as the deserts of Saudi Arabia, specimen collection methods may be less than optimal for molecular studies, yet virus can be typed from fixed tissues by immunohistochemistry using these antibodies.[57]

VI.   HOST-VIRUS COEVOLUTION

The relatively small double-stranded DNA genomes of the papillomaviruses have been readily amenable to cloning and sequencing. All human and nonhuman papillomaviruses cloned to date have the same overall open reading frame organization. Although there is considerable variation between different virus types on the nucleotide and amino acid levels, the papillomavirus genomes manifest a very rigid "backbone structure," i.e., a framework of amino acids that are either identical or functionally conserved in all mammalian and avian PVs (Van Ranst et al., unpublished). As an example, Figure 3 (caption below) shows an amino acid alignment of E1 sequences of different human and nonhuman papillomaviruses. If one assumes that evolution tends to conserve structures that are critical for protein function, then a better delineation of this conserved framework, through sequencing of a wide range of human and nonhuman papillomaviruses, will contribute to provide a better understanding of the relationship between structure and function of the diverse viral proteins.

Molecular homology between nonhuman PV genomes has been useful for investigating anatomic site specificity and the phylogenetic relationship between the viruses and their hosts. This became evident with the use of reverse Southern blot technology under conditions of low stringency for entire genomes (Figure 4). Clusters of high cross hybridization correlate well to similarities in the categories listed above.[58]

If all mammalian and avian species are infected by multiple host species-specific PV types (as is the case of humans, colobus monkeys, horses, and cattle), the spectrum of PVs may well exceed 10^5–10^6 different types.[59] This enormous diversity of PVs most probably did not arise in the recent past, as papillomavirus types are relatively stable, slowly evolving genetic entities. Papillomaviruses do not encode their own DNA polymerase. Instead, they borrow the hardware of the host cell for replication of their viral genome. Although PVs undergo many replication cycles in a relatively short time span, they benefit from the high fidelity, proof reading capacity, and post-replication DNA repair mechanisms of the host DNA polymerase. This unquestionably contributes to the stability of the HPV genome, in contrast to retroviruses and RNA riboviruses which replicate their genomes through a more error-prone reverse transcriptase or RNA polymerase. Recombination between different PVs has not been substantiated, suggesting that they evolve either by the slow accumulation of point mutations and/or other nonstochastic mechanisms yet to be resolved that result in fixation of specific genome types. The slow rate of the mutation events is exemplified by the finding that a Swedish BPV-1 variant showed more than 99.9% DNA sequence similarity to a BPV-1 genome isolated in Wisconsin (U.S.) 30 years earlier.[60] The world-wide distribution in various mammalian and avian hosts of such a wide diversity of genetically stable host-restricted virus types that require close physical contact with virus-loaded exfoliated cells for transmission (i.e., not airborne), implies that papillomaviruses are ancient viruses that may have coevolved with their host species throughout vertebrate evolution.[61]

In order to test the coevolution hypothesis, two requirements have to be met consecutively. First, the viruses from evolutionarily related host species should themselves be phylogenetically closely

FIGURE 3   Amino acid alignment of a highly conserved region in the carboxyterminus of the E1 protein of 12 papillomaviruses (FcPV: chaffinch cutaneous PV;[111] COPV: canine oral PV;[70] CRPV: cottontail rabbit cutaneous PV;[106] HPV-1: human cutaneous PV;[123] HPV-5: human cutaneous PV;[124] HPV-13: human oral PV;[38] PpPV: pygmy chimpanzee oral PV;[38] RhPV: rhesus monkey venereal PV;[64] BPV-1, BPV-2: cattle cutaneous PV [Groff et al., unpublished;[93] OvPV: white-tailed deer cutaneous PV;[84] AaPV: European elk cutaneous PV.[80] Identical amino acids are marked with an asterisk (*), functionally conserved residues are marked with a pound sign (#).

```
          •   ••          •          •              •      ••    ••          •
FcPV    WKKILVFLTFQHINFKEFISILCMWLKGRPKKSCITIAGVPDS
COPV    WKEVVKFLRHQGIEFILFLADFKRFLRGRPKKNCLVFWGPPNT
CRPV    WKVVVHFLRHQRVEFIPFMVKLKAFLRGTPKKNCMVFYGPPNS
HPV  1  WKEIVRFLRFQEVEFISFMIAFKDLLCGKPKKNCLLIFGPPNT
HPV  5  WSDIVKFIRYQNINFIVFLTALKEFLHSVPKKNCILIYGPPNS
HPV 13  WKPIVQFLRHQNIEFIPFLSKLKLWLHGTPKKNCIAIVGPPDT
PpPV 1  WKPIVQFLRHQNIEFISFLSKLKLWLQGTPKKNCIAIVGPPDT
RhPV 1  WRPIVQFLRYQGVEFIAFLAALKLFLKGIPKKNCIVLFGPPNT
BPV  1  WKSILTFFNYQNIELITFINALKLWLKGIPKKNCLAFIGPPNT
BPV  2  WKSILTFFNYQNIELITFINALKLWLNGIPKKNCLAFIGPPKT
OvPV    WLSIMNLLKYHGIEHIQFVNALKPWLKGIPKYNCITIVGPPNS
AaPV    WLSIMNLLKFQGIEPINFVNALKPWLKGTPKHNCIAIVGPPNS


          •••        ••  •      •  •      ••    •        •   •••      •  •  ••  •  ••  •
FcPV    GKSMFAYSLIKFLNGSVLSFANSKSHFWLQPLTECKAALIDDV
COPV    GKSMFCMSLLSFLHGVVISYVNSKSHFWLQPLTEGKMGLLDDA
CRPV    GKSYFCMSLIRLLAGRVLSFANSRSHFWLQPLADAKLALVDDA
HPV  1  GKSMFCTSLLKLLGGKVISYCNSKSQFWLQPLADAKIGLLDDA
HPV  5  GKSSFAMSLIRVLKGRVLSFVNSKSQFWLQPLSECKIALLDDV
HPV 13  GKSCFCMSLIKFLGGTVISYVNSSSHFWLQPLCNAKVALLDDA
PpPV 1  GKSMFCMSLIKFLGGTVISYVNSSSHFWLQPLCNTKVALLDDA
RhPV 1  GKSYFGMSLIHFLQGSIISYVNSNSHFWLQPLADAKVAMLDDA
BPV  1  GKSMLCNSLIHFLGGSVLSFANHKSHFWLASLADTRAALCDDA
BPV  2  GKSMLCNSLIHFLGGSVLSFANHKSHFWLASLADARAALVDDA
OvPV    GKSLLCNSLIAFLGGKVLTFANHHSHFWLAPLADCRVALIDDA
AaPV    GKSLLCNTLMSFLGGKVLTFANHSSHFWLAPLTDCRVALIDDA


          •    ••        •  ••••  •••    ••• •  ••        •  ••••••••
FcPV    TLPCWDYVDTFLRNALDGNAICIDCKHRAPVQTKCPPLLLTSN
COPV    TRPCWLYIDTYLRNALDGNTFSVDCKHKAPLQLKCPPLLITTN
CRPV    TSACWDFIDTYLRNALDGNPISVDLKHKAPIEIKCPPLLITTN
HPV  1  TKPCWDYMDIYMRNALDGNTICIDLKHRAPQQIKCPPLLITSN
HPV  5  TDPCWIYMDTYLRNGLDGHYVSLDCKYRAPTQMKFPPLLLTSN
HPV 13  TQSCWVYMDTYMRNLLDGNPMSIDRKHKSLALIKCPPLLVTSN
PpPV 1  THSCWGYMDTYMRNLLDGNPMSIDRKHKSLALIKCPPLLVTSN
RhPV 1  TPQCWSYIDNYLRNALDGNPISVDRKHKNLVQMKCPPLLITSN
BPV  1  THACWRYFDTYLRNALDGYPVSIDRKHKAAVQIKAPPLLLTSN
BPV  2  THACWRYFDTYLRNALDGYPVSIDRKHKAAVQIKAPPLLVTSN
OvPV    TTACWRYFDTHLRNVLDGYPFGIDRKHNTAVQMKAPPLLVTSN
AaPV    THACWRYFDTYLRNVLDGYPVCIDRKHKSAVQLKAPPLLLTSN
```

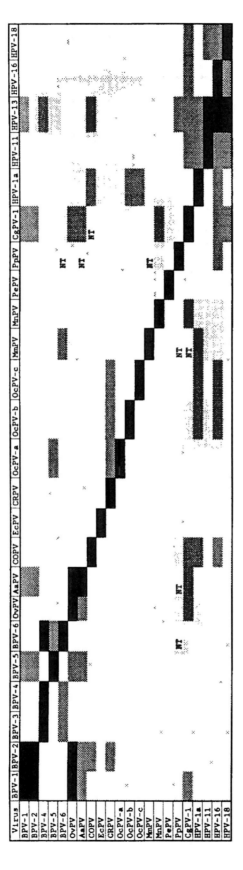

FIGURE 4 Low stringency reverse Southern blots reveals relative degrees of homology between entire papillomavirus genomes.[36,40,56,114] Black indicates a strong positive signal. Decreasing gray tones indicate decreasing signal strength. White indicates no signal. NT indicates where cross homologies were not tested.

related. More and more evidence is accumulating that this is the case for papillomaviruses. For example, PVs from host species belonging to the order of the Artiodactyla (even-toed ungulates) are phylogenetically related. Figure 5 shows the close phylogenetic relationship of cattle (*Bos taurus*) PV type 1 (BPV-1), BPV-2, European elk (*Alces alces*) PV, Reindeer (*Rangifer tarandus*) PV, and American white-tailed deer (*Odocoileus virginianus*) PV.[61] The PVs isolated from the Bovidae and Cervidae form monophyletic groups. Another example of the phylogenetic relationship of PVs from related species is in the Lagomorphae, where the mucosal rabbit oral PV (OcPV) from domestic rabbits and the cutaneous cottontail rabbit PV (CRPV) show more nucleotide similarity to each other than to other cloned cutaneous or mucosal papillomaviruses (Tachezy et al., unpublished).[62]

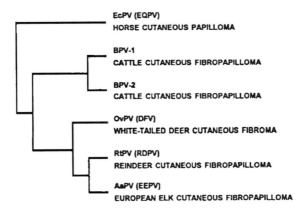

FIGURE 5   Phylogenetic relatedness of five different papillomaviruses from even–toed ungulate (artiodactyla) host species, based on an amino acid alignment of the E6 genes using the "Phylogenetic Analysis Using Parsimony" software (PAUP 3.0).[125] The domestic horse cutaneous PV (EcPV-1) was used as an outgroup (Kaplan et al., unpublished).[77]

The second and more important requirement to support a coevolution hypothesis is to demonstrate that PVs coevolved and cospeciated in synchrony with their hosts. This latter point can be argued when the branching pattern of the evolutionary tree derived from the viruses is concordant with the branching pattern of the host species tree. This is more difficult to substantiate since the phylogeny of the mammals is still heavily debated.[63] Only within the primates, where a large amount of comparative morphometric, biochemical, and molecular biological data are available, are the evolutionary relationships somewhat better defined and can the divergence times of the different primates be approximated with a reasonable degree of confidence. Primatologists concur that *Pan troglodytes* (common chimpanzee) and *P. paniscus* (pygmy chimpanzee) are the two species that are most closely related to humans.[64] The two chimpanzee species diverged from each other approximately 2.5 million years (Myr) ago, whereas the human branch and the ancestor of the two chimpanzee species diverged approximately 4.7 Myr ago.[65] Papillomaviruses characterized in these three species; *P. paniscus* PV (PpPV), *P. troglodytes* PV (PtPV), and HPV-13 are all associated with oral focal epithelial hyperplasia (FEH) in their respective hosts, and are extremely similar on the nucleotide level (Favre et al., unpublished).[36-38] The PpPV and PtPV are phylogenetically more closely related to each other than to their human PV counterparts. It appears that the phylogenetic relationship between the three FEH-related viruses is concordant with the evolutionary relationship between their hosts, supporting the notion that the hominoid PVs have coevolved with their hosts (Van Ranst et al., unpublished). The cercopithecoids (old world primates) and the human branch were estimated to have diverged about 40 Myr ago. Nonhuman primate PVs have been identified in two cercopithecidae, the black-and-white Abyssinian colobus (*Colobus guereza*, CgPV-1, and CgPV-2), and the rhesus macaque (*M. mulatta*, RhPV-1).[33,40,66,67] When included in a phylogenetic tree with HPVs, these nonhuman primate PVs are found among the human PVs, and their position in the tree reflects their tropism for specific anatomical sites. The branching points between the non-human primate PVs and their hypothetical HPV counterparts in the PV phylogenetic tree mirror the phylogeny of their respective hosts (Figure 6). We hypothesize that most (if not all) current human papillomavirus types will have counterparts in the nonhuman primates. The cloning and sequencing of a larger number of primate and other animal papillomaviruses is likely to shed more light on the diversity and molecular evolution of these DNA tumor viruses and on more basic aspects of the poorly understood speciation process.

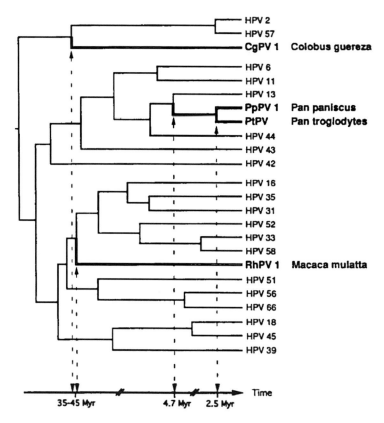

FIGURE 6 Phylogenetic tree generated from the alignment of the E6 genes of the nonhuman primate papillomaviruses (bold) and mucosal human papillomaviruses, using the UPGMA (Unweighted Pair Group Maximum Average) pairwise similarity matrix method.[126] HPV-1 was used as an outgroup (not shown). The time scale is not linear. The divergence time estimations of the primate host species[63,127] are indicated on the horizontal axis in million years (Myr.). Reprinted with permission of Cambridge University Press.[59]

REFERENCES

1. Baron, J., *The Life of Edward Jenner, M.D.*, Henry Colburn, London, 1838, 162.
2. Jenner, E., *An Inquiry into the Causes and Effects of the Variolae Vaccinae, a Disease Discovered in Some of the Western Counties of England, Particularly Gloucestershire, and Known by the Name of the Cow Pox*, Sampson Low, London, 1798.
3. Jacobson, E. R., Gaskin, J. M., Clubb, S., and Calderwood, M. B., Papilloma-like virus infection in Bolivian side-neck turtles, *J. Am. Vet. Med. Assoc.*, 181, 1325–1328, 1982.
4. McKenzie, R. A., Fay, F. R., and Prior, H. C., Poxvirus infection of the skin of an Eastern grey kangaroo, *Austr. Vet. J.*, 55, 188–190, 1979.
5. Tripathy, D. N., Hanson, L. E., and Crandell, R. A., Poxviruses of veterinary importance: diagnosis of infections. In *Comparative Diagnosis of Viral Diseases*, vol. III, Editors Kurstak, E., and Kurstak, C., Academic Press, New York, 1981, 267–346.

6. Papadimitriou, J. M. and Ashman, R. B., A poxvirus in a marsupial papilloma, *J. Gen. Virol.*, 16, 87–89, 1972.

7. Jacobson, E. R., Sundberg, J. P., Gaskin, J. M., Kollias, G. V., and O'Banion, M. K., Cutaneous papillomas associated with a herpes-like infection in a herd of captive African elephants, *J. Am. Vet. Med. Assoc.*, 189, 1075–1078, 1986.

8. Sano, T., Fukuda, H., and Furukawa, M., Herpesvirus cyprini: biological and oncogenic properties, *Fish Pathol.*, 20, 381–388, 1985.

9. Yamamoto, T., Kelly, R. K., and Nielsen, O., Epidermal hyperplasia of northern pike (*Esox lucius*) associated with herpesvirus and C-type particles, *Arch. Virol.*, 79, 255–272, 1983.

10. Bloch., B., Mellergaard S., and Nielsen, E., Adenovirus–like particles associated with epithelial hyperplasia in dab, *Limanda limanda* (L.), *J. Fish. Dis.*, 9, 281–285, 1986.

11. Ahne, W. and Thomsen, I., The existence of three different viral agents in a tumour bearing European eel (*Anguilla anguilla*), *Zbl. Vet. Med. B.*, 32, 228–235, 1985.

12. Read, D. H., Walker, R. L., Castro, A. E., Sundberg, J. P., and Thurmond, M. C., An invasive spirochaete associated with interdigital papillomatosis of dairy cattle, *Vet. Rec.*, 130, 59–60, 1992.

13. Wilson, D. G., Calderwood Mays, M. B., and Colahan, P. T., Equine canker: a prospective and retrospective study, *Vet. Surg.*, 14, 70, 1985.

14. Sundberg, J. P., Binder, R. L., Maurer, J. K., Newmann, E. A., and Cunniff, J. J., Absence of papillomavirus in skin tumors induced in SENCAR mice by a two–stage carcinogenesis protocol, *Carcinogenesis* 11, 341–344, 1990.

15. Eppstein, D. A., Marsh, Y. V., Schreiber, A. B., Newman, S. R., Todaro, G. J., and Nestor, J. J., Epidermal growth factor occupancy inhibits vaccinia virus infection, *Nature*, 318, 663–665, 1985.

16. Cheville, N. F. and Olson, C., Cytology of the canine oral papilloma, *Am. J. Pathol.*, 45, 849–872, 1964.

17. Sundberg, J. P., Chiodini, R. J., and Nielsen, S. W., Transmission of the white-tailed deer cutaneous fibroma, *Am. J. Vet. Res.*, 46, 1150–1154, 1985.

18. Sundberg, J. P., Animal models for papillomavirus research, *Contr. Oncol.*, 24, 11–38, 1987.

19. Sundberg, J. P., Papillomavirus infections in animals. in: Syrjanen, K., Gissmann, L., Koss, L. G., Eds., *Papillomaviruses and Human Disease*. Springer-Verlag, Heidelberg, 1987, 40–103.

20. Sundberg, J. P. and O'Banion, M. K., Animal papillomaviruses associated with malignant tumors, *Adv. Viral. Oncol.*, 8, 55–71, 1989.

21. O'Banion, M. K. and Sundberg, J. P., Papillomavirus genomes in experimentally induced fibromas in white-tailed deer, *Am. J. Vet. Res.*, 48, 1453–1455, 1987.

22. Shope, R. E. and Hurst, E. W., Infectious papillomatosis of rabbits, *J. Exp. Med.*, 58, 607–624, 1933.

23. Sundberg, J. P., Reszka, A., Williams, E., and Reichmann, M. E., An oral papillomavirus that infected one coyote and three dogs, *Vet. Pathol.*, 28, 87–88, 1991.

24. Muller, H. and Gissmann, L., *Mastomys natalensis* papillomavirus (MnPV), the causative agent of epithelial proliferations: characterization of the virus particle, *J. Gen. Virol.*, 41, 315–323, 1978.

25. Coggin, J. R. and zur Hausen, H., Workshop on papillomaviruses and cancer, *Cancer Res.*, 39, 545–546, 1979.

26. Scherneck, S., Vogel, F., Nguyen, H. L., and Feunteun, J., Sequence homology between polyoma virus, simian virus 40, and a papilloma-producing virus from a Syrian hamster: evidences for highly conserved sequences, *Virology*, 137, 41–48, 1984.

27. Delmas, V., Bastien C., Scherneck, S., and Feunteun, J., A new member of the polyomavirus family: the hamster papovavirus. Complete nucleotide sequence and transformation properties, *EMBO J.*, 4, 1279–1286, 1985.

28. Vogel, F., Scherneck, S., and Rohde, K., Characterization of the DNA of the hamster papovavirus. III. Mapping of the inverted repeated DNA sequences within the viral genome, *Biomed. Biochim. Acta*, 45, 887–895, 1986.

29. Vogel, F., Zimmermann, W., Krause, H., and Scherneck, S., Characterization of the DNA of the hamster papovavirus: I. Genom length and molecular cloning, *Arch. Geschwulstforschung*, 54, 433–442, 1984.

30. Sundberg, J. P., O'Banion, M. K., Shima, A., and Reichmann, M. E., Papillomas and carcinomas associated with a papillomavirus in European harvest mice (*Micromys minutus*), *Vet. Pathol.*, 25, 356–361, 1988.

31. Sundberg, J. P., O'Banion, M. K., and Reichmann, M. E., Mouse papillomavirus: Pathology and characterization of the virus, *Cancer Cells*, 5, 373–379, 1987.

32. O'Banion, M. K., Reichmann, M. E., and Sundberg, J. P., Cloning and characterization of a papillomavirus associated with papillomas and carcinomas in the European harvest mouse (*Micromys minutus*), *J. Virol.*, 62, 226–233, 1988.

33. Kloster, B. E., Manias, D. A., Ostrow, R. S., Shaver, M. K., McPherson S. W., Rangen, S. R. S., and Faras, A. J., Molecular cloning and characterization of the DNA of two papillomaviruses from monkeys, *Virology*, 166, 30–40, 1988.

34. Sundberg, J. P., Ghim, S.-J., Van Ranst, M., and Jenson, A. B., Nonhuman papillomaviruses: host range, pathology, epitope conservation, and new vaccine approaches, *Proc. First Congress Spontaneous Tumors in Animals* (in press).

35. Sundberg, J. P. and Reichmann, M. E., Papillomavirus infections. in: *Non-human Primates II. Monographs on Pathology of Laboratory Animals*, Jones, T. C., Mohr, U., and Hunt, R. D., Eds., Springer–Verlag, Heidelberg, 1993, 1–8.

36. Sundberg, J. P., Shima, A. L., and Adkison, D. L., Oral papillomavirus infection in a pygmy chimpanzee (*Pan paniscus*), *J. Vet. Lab. Invest.*, 4, 70–74, 1992.

37. Van Ranst, M., Fuse, A., Sobis, H., De Meurichy, W., Syrjanen, S. M., Billiau, A., and Opdenakker, G., A papillomavirus related to HPV type 13 in oral focal epithelial hyperplasia in the pygmy chimpanzee, *J. Oral. Pathol. Med.*, 20, 325–331, 1991.

38. Van Ranst, M., Fuse, A., Fiten, P., Beuken, E., Pfister, H., and Burk, R. D., Opdenakker, G., Human papillomavirus type 13 and pygmy chimpanzee papillomavirus type 1: comparison of the genome organizations, *Virology*, 190, 587–596, 1992.

39. Appleby, E. C., Graham-Jones, O., and Keeble, S. A., Primate diseases infectious to man, *Vet. Rec.*, 75, 81–86, 1963.

40. Reszka, A. A., Sundberg, J. P., and Reichmann, M. E., *In vitro* transformation and molecular characterization of colobus monkey venereal papillomavirus DNA, *Virology*, 181, 787–792, 1991.

41. Sundberg, J. P., Montali, R. J., Bush, M., Phillips, L. G., O'Brien, S. J., Jenson, A. B., Burk, R. D., and Van Ranst, M., Papillomavirus-associated focal oral hyperplasia in wild and captive Asian lions (*Panthera Leo Persica*), *J. Zoo Wildlife Med.*, 27, 61–70, 1996.

42. Carney, H. C., England, J. J., Hodgin, E. C., Whiteley, H. E., Adkison, D. L., and Sundberg, J. P., Papillomavirus infection of aged Persian cats, *J. Vet. Diag. Invest.*, 2, 294–299, 1990.

43. Egberink, H. F., Berrocal, A., Bax, H. A. D., van den Ingh, T. S. G. A. M., Walter, J. H., and Horzinek, M. C., Papillomavirus associated skin lesions in a cat seropositive for feline immunodeficiency virus, *Vet. Microbiol.*, 31, 117–125, 1992.

44. Van Ranst, M., Tachezy R., England, J., Sundberg, J. P., and Burk, R. D., Cloning and characterization of the domestic cat cutaneous papillomavirus, *Virology*, submitted.

45. Rous, P. and Beard, J. W., The progression to carcinoma of virus-induced rabbit papillomas (Shope), *J. Exp. Med.*, 62, 523–548, 1935.

46. Olson, C., Animal papillomaviruses. Historical perspectives. in: *The Papovaviridae*, vol. 2, *The Papillomaviruses*, Salzman, N. P. and Howley, P. M., Eds., Plenum Press, New York, 1987, 39–66.

47. Atanasiu, P., Transmission de la verrue commune au singe cynocephale (*Papio papio*), *Ann. Inst. Pasteur*, 74, 246–248, 1948.

48. Pfister, H., Papillomaviruses. General description, taxonomy, and classification. in: *The Papovaviridae*, vol. 2, *The Papillomaviruses*, Salzman, N. P. and Howley, P. M., Eds., Plenum Press, New York, 1987, 1–38.

49. Shah, K. H., Ozer, H. L., Ghazey, H. N., and Kelly, T. J., Common structural antigen of papovaviruses of the simian virus 40 - polyoma subgroup, *J. Virol.*, 21, 179–186, 1977.

50. Jenson, A. B., Rosenthal, J. R., Olson, C., Pass, F., Lancaster, W. D., and Shah, K., Immunological relatedness of papillomaviruses from different species, *J. Natl. Cancer Inst.*, 64, 495–500, 1980.

51. Ghim, S., Christensen, N. D., Kreider, J. W., and Jenson, A. B., Comparison of neutralization of BPV-1 infection of C127 cells and bovine fetal skin xenografts, *Int. J. Cancer*, 49, 285–289, 1991.

52. Bell, J., Sundberg, J. P., Ghim, S.-J., Newsome, J., Jenson, A. B., and Schelgel R., A formalin–inactivated vaccine protects against mucosal papillomavirus infection: a canine model, *Pathobiology*, 62, 194–198, 1994.

53. Ghim, S.-J., Suzich, J., Tamura, J., Bell, J. A., White, W., Newsome, J., Hill, F., Warrener, P., Sundberg, J., Jenson, A. B., and Schelgel, R., Formalin-inactivated oral papilloma extracts and recombinant L1 vaccines protect completely against mucosal papillomavirus infection: a canine model. *Vaccines 95*, Cold Spring Harbor Press, Cold Spring Harbor, NY, 1995, 375–379.

54. Sundberg, J. P., Junge, R. E., and Lancaster, W. D., Immunoperoxidase localization of papillomaviruses in hyperplastic and neoplastic epithelial lesions of animals, *Am. J. Vet. Res.*, 45, 1441–1446, 1984.

55. Lim, P. S., Jenson, A. B., Cowsert, L., Nakai, Y., Lim, L. Y., Jin, X. W., and Sundberg, J. P., Distribution and specific identification of papillomavirus major capsid protein epitopes by immunocytochemistry and epitope scanning of synthetic peptides, *J. Inf. Dis.*, 162, 1263–1269, 1990.

56. Geysen, H. M., Rodda, S. J., Mason, T. J., Tribbick, G., and Schoop, P. G. Strategies for epitope analysis using peptide synthesis, *J. Immunol. Methods*, 102, 259–274, 1987.

57. Elzein, E. T. A., Sundberg, J. P., Housawi, F. M., Gameel, A. A., Ramadan, R. O., and Hassanien, M. M., Genital bovine papillomavirus infection in Saudi Arabia, *J. Vet. Diag. Invest.*, 3, 36–38, 1991.

58. O'Banion, M. K., Sundberg, J. P., Reszka, A. A., and Reichmann, M. E., Cross-hybridization and relationships of various papillomavirus DNAs at different degrees of stringency, *Intervirology*, 28, 114–121, 1987.

59. Chan, S.-Y., Ho, L., Ong, C.-K., Chow, V., Drescher, B., Durst, M., ter Meulen, J., Villa, L., Luande, J., Mgaya, H. N., and Bernard, H.-U., Molecular variants of human papillomavirus type 16 from four continents suggest ancient pandemic spread of the virus and its coevolution with humankind, *J. Virology*, 66, 2057–2066, 1992.

60. Ahola, H., Stenlund, A., Moreno-Lopez, J., and Petterson, U., Sequences of bovine papillomavirus type 1 DNA; functional and evolutionary implications, *Nucleic Acids Res.*, 11, 2639–2650, 1983.

61. Van Ranst, M., Kaplan, J. B., Sundberg, J. P., and Burk, R. D., Molecular evolution of papillomaviruses. In *Coevolution of Viruses, Their Hosts and Vectors*, Garcia-Arenal, F. C., Calisher, C., and Gibbs, A. J., Eds., Cambridge University Press, Cambridge, 1995, 455–476.

62. O'Banion, M. K., Cialkowski, M. E., Reichmann, M. E., and Sundberg, J. P., Cloning and molecular characterization of an oral papillomavirus of domestic rabbits, *Virology*, 162, 221–231, 1988.

63. Novacek, M. J., Mammalian phylogeny: shaking the tree, *Nature*, 356, 121–125, 1992.

64. Begun, D. R., Miocene fossil Hominids and the chimp-human clade, *Science*, 257, 1929–1933, 1992.

65. Horai, S., Satta, Y., Hayasaka, K., Kondo, R., Inoue, T., Ishida, T., Hayashi, S., and Takahata, N., Man's place in Hominoidea revealed by mitochondrial DNA genealogy, *J. Mol. Evol.*, 35, 32–43, 1992.

66. Ostrow, R. S., Labresh, K. V., and Faras, A. J., Characterization of the complete RhPV–1 genomic sequence and an integration locus from a metastatic tumor, *Virology*, 181, 424–429, 1991.

67. O'Banion, M. K., Sundberg, J. P., Shima, A. L., and Reichmann, M. E., Venereal papilloma and papillomavirus in a colobus monkey (*Colobus guereza*), *Intervirology*, 28, 232–237, 1987.

68. Corbet, G. B. and Hill, J. E., *A World List of Mammalian Species*, British Museum Comstock Publ., London, 1980, 1–226.

69. Koller, L. D., Cutaneous papillomas on an opossum, *J. Natl. Cancer Inst.*, 49, 309–313, 1972.

70. Prister, H. and Meszaros, J., Partial characterization of canine oral papillomavirus, *Virology*, 104, 243–246, 1980.

71. Sundberg, J. P., O'Banion, M. K., Schmidt–Didier, E., and Reichmann, M. E., Cloning and characterization of a canine oral papillomavirus, *Am. J. Vet. Res.*, 47, 1142–1144, 1986.

72. Delius, H., Van Ranst, M., Jenson, A. B., zur Hausen, H., and Sundberg, J. P., Canine oral papillomavirus genomic sequence, *Virology*, 204, 447–452, 1994.

73. Watrach, A. M., The ultrastructure of canine cutaneous papilloma, *Cancer Res.*, 29, 2079–2084, 1969.

74. Sundberg, J. P., Smith, E. K., Herron, A. J., Jenson, A. B., Burk, R. D., and Van Ranst, M., Involvement of canine oral papillomavirus in generalized oral and cutaneous verrucosis in a Chinese shar pei dog. *Vet. Pathol.*, 31, 183–187, 1994.

75. Samuel, W. M., Chalmers, G. A., and Gunson, J. R., Oral papillomatosis in coyotes (*Canis latrans*) and wolves (*Canis lupus*) of Alberta, *J. Wildl. Dis.*, 14, 165–169, 1978.

76. Craft, C., Braun, L., and Strandberg, J., The use of immunohistochemical techniques in the diagnosis of virally-induced tumors, *Proc. Ann. Meet. Am. Coll. Vet. Pathol.*, 31, 102, 1980.

77. Hamir, A. N., Moser, G., Jenson, A. B., Sundberg, J. P., Hanlon, C., and Rupprecht, C. E., Papillomavirus infection in a raccoon (*Procyon lotor*), *J. Vet. Lab. Invest.*, 7, 549–551, 1995.

78. Sundberg, J. P., Montali, R., Bush, M., Van Ranst, M., Scott, D. W., Miller, W. H., Rowland, P. H., Homer, B. L., Roelke, M. E., England, J. J., and Jenson, A. B., Feline papillomaviruses: host range, molecular diversity, and epitope conservation, *Vet. Pathol.*, 31, 616, 1994.

79. Lambertsen, R. H., Kohn, B. A., Sundberg, J. P., and Buergelt, C. D., Genital papillomatosis in sperm whale bulls, *J. Wildl. Dis.*, 23, 361–367, 1987.

80. Sundberg, J. P., Russell, W., and Lancaster, W. D., Papillomatosis in Indian elephants, *Elaphus maximus*, *J. Am. Vet. Med. Assoc.*, 179, 1247–1248, 1981.

81. O'Banion, M. K., Reichmann, M. E., and Sundberg, J. P., Cloning and characterization of an equine cutaneous papillomavirus, *Virology*, 152, 100–109, 1986.

82. Moar, M. H. and Jarrett, W. F. H., A cutaneous fibropapilloma from a red deer (*Cervus elaphus*) associated with a papillomavirus, *Intervirology*, 24, 108–118, 1985.

83. Moreno-Lopez, J., Morner, T., and Pettersson, U., Papillomavirus DNA associated with pulmonary fibromatosis in European Elks, *J. Virol.*, 57, 1173–1176, 1986.

84. Moreno-Lopez, J., Pettersson, U., Dinter, Z., and Philipson, L., Characterization of a papilloma virus from the European Elk (EEPV), *Virology*, 112, 589–595, 1981.

85. Stenlund, A., Moreno-Lopez, J., Ahola, H., and Pettersson, U., European elk papillomavirus: characterization of the genome, induction of tumors in animals, and transformation *in vitro*, *J. Gen. Virol.*, 48, 370–376, 1983.

86. Moreno-Lopez, J., Ahola, H., Eriksson, A., Bergman, P., and Pettersson, U., Reindeer papillomavirus transforming properties correlate with a highly conserved E5 region, *J. Virol.*, 61, 3394–3400, 1987.

87. Lancaster, W. D. and Sundberg, J. P., Characterization of papillomaviruses isolated from cutaneous fibromas of white-tailed deer and mule deer, *Virology*, 123, 212–216, 1982.

88. Groff, D. E. and Lancaster, W. D., Molecular cloning and nucleotide sequence of deer papillomavirus, *J. Virol.*, 56, 85–91, 1983.

89. Karstad, L. and Kaminjolo, J. S., Skin papillomas in an impala (*Aepyceros melampus*) and a giraffe (*Giraffa camelopardalis*), *J. Wildl. Dis.*, 14, 309–313, 1978.

90. Sundberg, J. P., Williams, E., Thorne, E. T., and Lancaster, W. D., Cutaneous fibropapilloma in a pronghorn antelope, *J. Am. Vet. Med. Assoc.*, 183, 1333–1334, 1983.

91. Gibbs, E. P. J., Smale, C. J., and Lawman, M. J. P., Warts in sheep, *J. Comp. Pathol.*, 85, 327–334, 1975.

92. Hayward, M., Meischke, R., Baird, P., and Gissmann, L., Filiform squamous papillomas in sheep (OSP)-clinical features, histology, immunohistochemistry, transmission experiments, and analysis of papillomavirus DNA, *Proc. Internatl. Papillomavirus Workshop*, 11, 178, 1992.

93. Trenfield, K., Spradbrow, P. B., and Vanselow, B. A., Detection of papillomavirus DNA in precancerous lesions of the ears of sheep, *Vet. Microbiol.*, 25, 103–116, 1990.

94. Vanselow, B. A. and Spadbrow, P. B., Papillomaviruses, papillomas and squamous cell carcinomas in sheep, *Vet. Rec.*, 110, 561–562, 1982.

95. Vanselow, B. A. and Spadbrow, P. B., Squamous cell carcinoma of the vulva, hyperkeratosis and papillomaviruses in a ewe, *Aust. Vet. J.*, 60, 194–195, 1983.

96. Lancaster, W. D. and Olson, C., Demonstration of two distinct classes of bovine papillomaviruses, *Virology*, 89, 372–379, 1978.

97. Chen, E. Y., Howley, P. M., Levinson, A. D., and Seeburg, P. H., The primary structure and genetic organization of the bovine papillomavirus type 1 genome, *Nature*, 299, 529–534, 1982.

98. Pfister, H., Linz, U., Gissmann, L., Huchthausen, B., Hoffmann, D., and zur Hausen, H., Partial characterization of a new type of bovine papillomavirus, *Virology*, 96, 1–8, 1979.

99. Campo, M. S., Moar, M. H., Jarrett, W. F. H., and Laird, H. M., A new papillomavirus associated with alimentary cancer in cattle, *Nature*, 286, 180–182, 1980.

100. Campo, M. S., Moar, M. H., Laird, H. M., and Jarrett, W. F. H., Molecular heterogeneity and lesion site specificity of cutaneous bovine papillomaviruses, *Virology*, 113, 323–325, 1981.

101. Jarrett, W. F. H., Campo, M. S., O'Neil, B. W., Laird, H. M., and Coggins, L. W., A novel bovine papillomavirus (BPV-6) causing true epithelial papillomas of the mammary gland skin: a member of a proposed new BPV group, *Virology*, 136, 255–264, 1984.

102. Chihaya, Y., Oshima, K.-I., Miura, S., and Numakunai, S., Pathological study on cutaneous papillomatosis in a Japanese serow (*Capricornis crispus*), *Jap. J. Vet. Sci.*, 38, 327–338, 1976.

103. Carlson, B. L., Hill, D., and Nielsen, S. W., Cutaneous papillomatosis in a beaver, *J. Am. Vet. Med. Assoc.*, 183, 1283–1284, 1983.

104. Van Ranst, M., Tachezy, R., Pruss, J., and Burk, R. D., Primary structure of the E6 protein of *Micromys minutus* papillomavirus and *Mastomys natalensis* papillomavirus, *Nucleic. Acids Res.*, 20, 2889, 1992.

105. Amtmann, E., Volm, M., and Wayss, K., Tumour induction in the rodent *Mastomys natalensis* by activation of endogenous papilloma virus genomes, *Nature*, 308, 291–292, 1984.

106. Kahn, T., Friesl, H., Copeland, N. G., Gilbert, D. J., Jenkins, N. A., Gissmann, L., Kramer, J., and zur Hausen, H., Molecular cloning, analysis, and chromosomal localization of a mouse genomic sequence related to the human papillomavirus type 18 E5 region, *Mol. Carcinogenesis*, 6, 88–99, 1992.

107. Reeve, V. E., Greenoak, G. E., Canfield, P. J., Boehm-Wilcox, C., Tilbrook, P. A., Kulski, J. K., and Gallagher, C. H., Enhancement of u.v.-induced skin carcinogenesis in the hairless mouse by inoculation with cell-free extracts of skin tumours, *Immunol. Cell Biol.*, 67, 421–427, 1989.

108. Tilbrook, P. A., Greenoak, G. E., Reeve, V. E., Canfield, P. J., Gissmann, L., Gallagher, C. H., and Kulski, J. K., Identification of papillomaviral DNA sequences in hairless mouse tumours induced by ultraviolet irradiation, *J. Gen. Virol.*, 70, 1005–1009, 1989.

109. Sundberg, J. P., Inherited mouse mutations: Animal models and biomedical tools, *Lab. Animals*, 20, 40–49, 1991.

110. Giri, I., Danos, O., and Yaniv, M., Genomic structure of the cottontail rabbit (Shope) papillomavirus, *Proc. Natl. Acad. Sci. U.S.A.*, 82, 1580–1584, 1985.

111. Murphy, M. F., Potter, H. L., Abraham, J. M., Morgan, D. M., and Meinke, W. J., Analysis of a restriction endonuclease map for a rabbit papillomavirus DNA, *Curr. Microbiol.*, 5, 349–352, 1981.

112. Nasseri, M. and Wettstein, F. O., Differences exist between viral transcripts in cottontail rabbit papillomavirus-induced benign and malignant tumors as well as non-virus-producing and virus-producing tumors, *J. Virol.*, 51, 706–712, 1984.

113. Watts, S. L., Ostrow, R. S., Phelps, W. C., Prince, J. T., and Faras, A. J., Free cottontail papillomavirus DNA persists in warts and carcinomas of infected rabbits and in cells in culture transformed with virus or viral DNA, *Virology*, 125, 127–138, 1983.

114. Osterhaus, A. D. M. E., Ellens, D. J., and Horzinek, M. C., Identification and characterization of a papillomavirus from birds (Fringillidae), *Intervirology*, 8, 351–359, 1977.

115. Moreno-Lopez, J., Ahola, H., Stenlund, A., Osterhaus, A., and Pettersson, U., Genome of an avian papillomavirus, *J. Virol.*, 51, 872–875, 1984.

116. Lina, P. H. C., van Noord, M. J., and de Groot, F. G., Detection of virus in squamous papillomas of the wild bird species *Fringilla coelebs*, *J. Natl. Cancer Inst.*, 50, 567–571, 1973.

117. Jacobson, E. R., Mladinich, C. R., Clubb, S., Sundberg, J. P., and Lancaster, W. D., Papilloma-like virus infection in an African Gray Parrot, *J. Am. Vet. Med. Assoc.*, 183, 1307–1308, 1983.

118. O'Banion, M. K., Jacoboson, E. R., and Sundberg, J. P., Molecular cloning and partial characterization of a parrot papillomavirus, *Intervirology*, 33, 91–96, 1992.

119. Segre, D., Olson, C., and Hoerlein, A. B., Neutralization of bovine papillomavirus with serums from cattle and horses with experimental papillomas, *Am. J. Vet. Res.*, 16, 517–520, 1955.

120. Koller, L. D. and Olson, C., Attempted transmission of warts from man, cattle, and horses, and of deer fibroma to selected hosts, *J. Invest. Dermatol.*, 58, 366–368, 1972.

121. Freidman, J. C., Levy, J. P., Lasneret, J., Thomas, M., Boiron, M., and Bernard, J., Induction de fibromes sous-cutanes chez le hamster dore par inoculation d'extraits acellulaires de papillomes bovins, *C. R. Seances Acad. Ser. III*, 257, 2328–2331, 1963.

122. Puget, A., Favre, M., and Orth, G., Induction de tumeurs fibroblastiques cutanees ou sous-cutanees chez l'Ochotone afghan (*Ochotono rufescens rufescens*) par inoculation du virus du papillome bovin, *C. R. Acad. Sci.*, 280, 2813–2816, 1975.

123. Freidman, J. C., Lasneret, J., Gibeaux, L., and Boiron, M., Developpement de fibromes proliferatifs chez la souris a l'aide d'extraits acellulares de papillomes bovins et leur transformation maligne greffes isologues, *Rev. Med. Vet.*, 141, 115–122, 1965.

124. Boiron, M., Levy, J. P., Thomas, M., Friedman, J. C., and Bernard, J. C., Some properties of bovine papilloma virus, *Nature*, 201, 423, 1964.

125. Parsons, R. J. and Kidd, J. G., A virus causing oral papillomatosis in rabbits, *Proc. Soc. Exp. Biol. Med.*, 35, 441–443, 1936.

126. Sundberg, J. P., Junge, R. E., and El Shazly, M. O., Oral papillomatosis in New Zealand white rabbits, *Am. J. Vet. Res.*, 46, 664–668, 1985.

127. Danos, O., Katinka, M., and Yaniv, M., Human papillomavirus 1a complete DNA sequence: a novel type of genome organization among Papovaviridae, *EMBO J.*, 1, 231–236, 1982.

128. Zachow, A. P., Rutherford, J. D., and Corbitt, G., Nucleotide sequence and genome organization of human papillomavirus type 5, *Virology*, 158, 251–254, 1987.

129. Swofford, D. L., PAUP: Phylogenetic Analysis Using Parsimony, Version 3.0. Computer program and documentation. Distributed by the Illinois Natural History Survey, Champaign, IL, U.S.

130. Sokal, R. and Sneath, P. H. A., *Principles of Numerical Taxonomy.* San Francisco: Freeman, 1963, 1–153.
131. Miyamoto, M. M., Koop, B. F., Slightom, J. L., Goodman, M., and Tennant, M. R., Molecular systematics of higher primates: Genealogical relations and classification, *Proc. Natl. Acad. Sci. U.S.A.,* 85, 7627–7631, 1988.

4

Classification of the Human Papillomaviruses Based on Their Molecular Evolutionary Relationship

Marc Van Ranst, Ruth Tachezy, Hajo Delius, and Robert D. Burk

CONTENTS

I. INTRODUCTION

Papillomaviruses (PVs) are ancient viruses that are likely to have originated early in vertebrate evolution and coevolved and cospeciated in synchrony with their host species.[1] Lack of evidence for inter-PV recombination suggests that the PVs are evolving, in part, through the slow accumulation of point mutations that escape the proofreading capacity and DNA repair mechanisms of the high fidelity host DNA polymerase. The use of the host replication enzymes accounts for the relative genetic stability of the PVs, illustrated by the high nucleotide sequence conservation between a bovine papillomavirus type 1 (BPV-1) genome isolated in Wisconsin (U.S.) which was only 0.01% different from a Swedish BPV-1 variant isolated 30 years later.[2]

Since the first study of human papillomavirus (HPV) DNA in 1965 and the molecular cloning of HPV-1 in 1980, more than 75 different HPV types have been isolated.[3,4] It is now appreciated that the HPVs are a large and diverse group of viruses and that anatomically distinct HPV-related diseases are caused by specific virus types.[5] Based on the detection of a large number of related HPV types present on "low-stringent" Southern blot hybridization experiments, and the detection and rapid sequencing of an even broader spectrum of HPV genotypes by consensus or general primer-mediated polymerase chain reaction methods, it is likely that the total number of different HPV types will be greater than 100.[6-8]

Significant clinical and epidemiological associations between the detection of specific HPV types and the occurrence of cervical intraepithelial neoplasia and cancer suggest that screening and typing of HPVs may potentially become clinically relevant. Current data suggest that identification of HPV types with oncogenic potential may serve to differentiate patients with a higher risk to develop cancer.[9-11] Thus, detection of "high risk" (oncogenic) HPV types early in the natural course of infection may serve to identify women with a higher risk to develop cervical cancer.

The lack of a uniform classification system for the existent and expanding number of HPV types has created confusion among physicians and virologists. Recently, viral taxonomy based on phylogenetic relationships has gained wider acceptance among virologists to replace the classic phenetic classifications.[12] As suggested by Pfister et al. (1986), a classification of the papillomavirus types should ideally be based on homologies between genes that are relevant for differences in the biology of the viruses.[13] To rationally group HPV DNA types, phylogenetic trees were constructed based on nucleotide and amino acid sequence alignments using parsimony and distance matrix algorithms. The resulting phylogenetic trees provide an organization of the HPVs into specific groups encompassing the known tissue specificity and oncogenic potential of each HPV type.[14,15] Such an HPV-classification system allows the clinician to assess the "theoretical" oncogenic potential of recently characterized or newly isolated viruses. A more accurate knowledge of the phylogenetic relationships of the HPVs will further the understanding of speciation models for DNA viruses, and will have implications for the conceptualization of general strategies for diagnostic HPV-detection and vaccine development.

II. DEFINITION OF AN HPV TYPE

Traditionally, HPVs have been typed according to their genotype (i.e., new papillomavirus isolates have been defined as independent types when they exhibited less than 50% cross-hybridization to previously typed HPVs by reassociation kinetics).[16] More recently, the definition of a new HPV type has been modified to include nucleotide sequence data in the E6, E7, and L1 region in order to distinguish better between closely related HPVs. The complete genome of novel HPV isolates should be cloned entirely, and have less than 90% nucleotide sequence identity with other papillomavirus types in these regions in order to be recognized as a new HPV type.

As more individual HPV genomes are cloned and sequenced, the academic definition of what constitutes a new HPV type or subtype may take secondary importance to the phylogenetic definition of an HPV species. The International Committee on Taxonomy of Viruses (ICTV), after a decade of fierce debate, currently defines a virus species as "a polythetic class of viruses that constitutes a replicating lineage and occupies a particular ecological niche."[17] This new species definition has so far not been applied to papillomaviruses. A phylogenetic classification of the various papillomaviruses may help to elucidate the relationship between HPV types and HPV species.

III. PHYLOGENETIC TREES

A. Maximum Parsimony Method

Maximum parsimony algorithms search for the minimum number of genetic events (nucleotide substitutions or amino acid changes) to infer the most parsimonious tree from a set of sequences. These algorithms allow us to deduce the best supported genealogical hypothesis from an aligned set of sequences. The phylogenetic trees were made with the software package PAUP 3.0 (Phylogenetic Analysis Using Parsimony), developed by D. Swofford, using the heuristic search option with random stepwise addition of sequences (100 replications, holding 5 trees at every step), and "nearest neighbor interchanges" branch swapping.[18]

B. Phylogenetic Analysis Based on the Alignment of E6 Sequences

Phylogenetic trees were constructed, using parsimony algorithms, based on the alignment of the E6 sequences of 49 HPV types. This region was chosen for analysis because it allowed an unambiguous alignment of all sequences. Although the primary E6 protein sequences are remarkably divergent, all sequenced papillomavirus E6 proteins contain four copies of a Cysteine-X-X-Cysteine motif spaced at regular and invariant intervals. A tetrahedral arrangement of the four cysteine sulfur ligands of two of these motifs cooperate in binding of a single zinc ion, forming a zinc-stabilized loop (zinc-finger). The evolutionary conserved arrangement of the zinc binding motifs suggests that they are functionally important features in the three-dimensional structure of the E6 protein. Superimposed on the generally conserved amino acid framework are residues that are conserved in groups of papillomaviruses that share a specific tropism and/or malignant potential. Finally, the remainder of the protein consists of amino acids that are more or less characteristic for each papillomavirus type. The presence of these particular amino acids may be correlated to specific biochemical properties of a given virus type or alternatively may be fortuitous, i.e., not critical for the protein function.

The branching pattern of the most parsimonious phylogenetic tree (Figure 1) served to cluster different HPVs into groups corresponding to their known tissue tropism and oncogenic potential. One branch contains HPV-types that are associated with cutaneous lesions, the other branch groups viruses that are mainly associated with lesions of mucosal origin.

C. Phylogenetic Analysis Based on a Compounded Multiple Open Reading Frame Alignment

To show that the phylogenetic trees obtained with the E6 alignment were not restricted to this specific region, but were characteristic of the molecular evolution of the whole papillomavirus genome, amino acid sequence alignments were constructed for all major open reading frames of 18 HPVs where the complete nucleotide sequence was available. A compilation was made consisting of 14 stretches of 20 amino acids or more that could be unambiguously aligned (i.e., without gaps). This allowed back-translation into 3249 nucleotides, which were used for the generation of phylogenetic trees with PAUP 3.0. The exact nucleotide positions of the aligned parts (using the sequenced HPV-6 genome as a reference) were E6 (135-520), E1 (1687-2700), E2 (2723-3136; 3221-3280), L2 (4516-4641; 4894-5001; 5302-5400), and L1 (5834-5935; 5963-6169; 6200-6301; 6329-6583; 6656-6808; 6851-7036; 7088-7186). Except for the position of HPV-2 and HPV-57, the most parsimonious PAUP-phylogenetic tree for 3249 bp of 18 HPVs resulted in the same overall topology as the tree for the 384 bp region in the E6 gene of 49 HPVs (Figure 2).

D. The "Cutaneous" Branch

The cutaneous branch consists of viruses that infect the skin. HPV types such as HPV-1/4/41/49/63/65 were all cloned from verrucae vulgares or verrucae plantares. The HPV types specifically associated with epidermodysplasia verruciformis (EV) have a common evolutionary

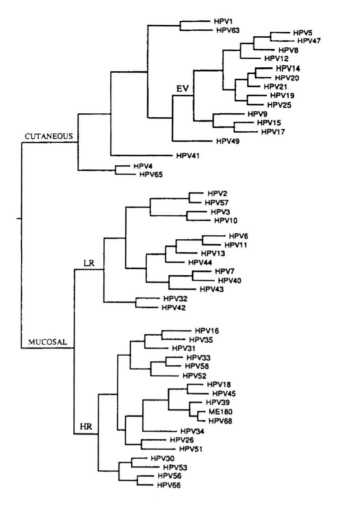

FIGURE 1 Phylogenetic tree constructed from the alignment of 384 nucleotides in the E6 genes of 49 human papillomavirus types using PAUP 3.0.

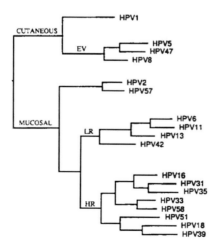

FIGURE 2 Phylogenetic tree constructed from the alignment of 3249 nucleotides in the E6, E1, E2, L2, and L1 genes of 18 human papillomavirus types using PAUP 3.0.

origin. There is a subgroup with HPV-5/8/12/47, a subgroup with HPV-14/19/20/21/25, and a subgroup with HPV-9/15/17. PVs in the first subgroup carry a significant risk for malignant degeneration, whereas viruses in the second and third subgroup are seldom found in malignant EV-lesions.

Given the relative rarity of epidermodysplasia verruciformis, it is a biological curiosity that more then 20 EV-specific HPV types were isolated from patients with this disease. Besides the unusually wide spectrum of EV-specific HPV types, the coding sequence divergence between different isolates of EV-types has been shown to be higher (3 to 10%), than the sequence divergence between different variants of mucosal HPV types (less than 1%).[19] The difference between an HPV type and a variant of that HPV type seems less distinct in the EV-group. The molecular basis for the increased genetic variation in the EV-HPVs is presently unknown. The biological constraints that counteract the success of mutational events may be more flexible for EV-specific HPVs than for mucosal HPVs. This may be explained by the observation that EV-lesions are often infected with multiple EV-HPV types.[20] Thus, coinfecting EV-specific HPVs or other cutaneous HPVs (such as HPV-3) may provide *trans*acting viral proteins that would allow the persistence of other episomal EV-HPV genomes with a biologically slightly inferior fitness. Ultraviolet light irradiation may also contribute to a higher mutation rate for EV-HPVs in the sun-exposed areas of the skin when compared to HPVs with a tropism for UV-inaccessible mucosal orogenital epithelia. An alternative hypothesis is that EV-HPV types utilize a subset of eukaryotic DNA polymerases with a lower fidelity or inferior DNA-proofreading or -repair mechanisms. Therefore, a mutation in a subset of the cellular DNA-processing enzymes, resulting in a lower fidelity of the viral replication process, may be hypothesized as a factor in the genetic basis of this disease. Finally, a (genetic?) defect in the cell-mediated immune response may lower the biological constraints against mutational events in EV-HPV types.

E.   The "Mucosal" Branch

The second major branch groups HPVs with a tropism to infect mucous membranes into a "low-risk" (LR) group and a "high-risk" (HR) group. On the 3249 bp-based tree (Figure 2), HPV-2 and HPV-57 occupied an intermediate position between the cutaneous and mucosal HPVs. Both viruses have been found in papillomas in the oral mucosa. However, they also appear to have retained the capacity to infect the skin and cause verruca vulgaris. The position of HPV-2 and HPV-57 was less stable in the E6 tree, where they were grouped with HPV-3 and HPV-10, two bona fide cutaneous viruses.

The rest of the HPVs in the "low-risk" (LR) group predominantly infect the genital and/or oral mucosae. This group comprises HPV-6/11/40/43/44/42, and is associated with benign genital condylomata and low grade cervical intraepithelial neoplasia (CIN). HPV-13 and HPV-32, involved in oral focal epithelial hyperplasia (Heck's disease), have also been identified in some genital lesions.[7,21] HPV-7, associated with cutaneous warts in meat handlers, lives up to its enigmatic status by being most closely related to genital types HPV-40 and HPV-43.

The HPVs in the second group (HR) were predominantly cloned from high grade CIN and invasive cervical cancer. One branch contains HPV-16/31/33/35/52/58. A second branch includes HPV-18/26/34/39/45/51/68/ME180, while a third group contains HPV-30/53/56/66.

IV.   CORRELATION WITH CLINICAL MANIFESTATIONS

Although further research on the correlation between the presence of different HPVs and their prognosis is warranted, HPV-typing may contribute to the identification and clinical management of high risk patients. With a rapidly growing number of HPV types being identified, an easily expandable classification system will allow the clinician to assign a potential oncogenic risk to recently characterized or new viruses. Our data indicate that phylogenetic analysis of HPV genomes can accurately classify distinct virus types into clinically relevant families. An advantage of this classification system is that it is derived solely from sequence data of the different papillomaviruses.

The correlation between the phylogenetic classification (i.e., "theoretical" oncogenicity) of HPVs and their clinical manifestations supports the notion that the different pathogenic consequences are determined, at least in part, by differences in the viral nucleotide sequences.

A.   Clinical Studies Support the Phylogenetic Division into "Low-Risk" and "High-Risk" Groups

Clinical studies conferring a relative risk estimate for the occurrence of a high grade intraepithelial lesion or invasive cervical cancer to different HPVs support the phylogenetic division of the mucogenital HPVs in a "low-risk" and a "high risk" group. In one recent multicenter study, viruses in the "low-risk" group were found in 20% of low grade CIN lesions, in 4% of high grade lesions, and never in invasive cancers. Viruses in the "high risk" group were found in 39% of low grade CIN, in 77% of high grade CIN, and in 91% of the cancers. HPV-16 was numerically the most important virus in the invasive cancers (47%).[9]

In the mucogenital "high-risk" group, there is a distinct phylogenetic branch for HPV-18/39/45/68/ME180. Clinical evidence is mounting to support a separate group with HPV-18 and HPV-45. These HPVs are detected in a disproportionately high percentage of adenocarcinomas and rapidly progressive invasive cervix cancers. Cancers containing HPV-18 occur in younger patients, and tend to have higher recurrence rates and a poorer prognosis than HPV-16-containing cancers.[9,22-24] The higher integration rate of HPV-18/45 DNA (in contrast to HPV-16/31/35) in invasive cervical cancer, may correlate with this more aggressive clinical behavior.[25]

B.   *In Vitro* Studies Confirm the Phylogenetic Division into "Low-Risk" And "High-Risk" Groups

The phylogenetic separation of the mucogenital group in "low-risk" and "high risk" HPVs correlates with experimental findings that the *in vitro* biological activities of the early genes vary among HPVs with different oncogenic capacity. The HPV types most commonly found in cervical carcinomas (HPV-16/18/31/33/51) were shown to have an increased *in vitro* potential over HPV-6 and -11 to immortalize and transform primary human foreskin or cervical epithelial cells.[26-31] The inactivation of the cell-encoded tumor suppressor protein p53 is thought to be an important step in the development of a variety of human tumors, including cervical cancer.[33,34] The E6 proteins of both "low risk" and "high-risk" mucogenital papillomaviruses were shown to associate *in vitro* with p53. However, only the E6 proteins of the "high-risk" viruses increased p53 degradation via the ubiquitin-dependent protease system. Mutational analysis of the E6 gene revealed that the region responsible for p53 inactivation was conserved in HPVs of the "high-risk" group only.[35,36]

The phylogenetic tree based on the E6 nucleotide sequences groups the papillomaviruses associated with epidermodysplasia verruciformis into a distinct branch. In this branch, there is a cluster with HPV-5/8/12/47, a cluster with HPV-14/19/20/21/25, and a cluster with HPV-9/15/17. Clinical and experimental evidence tends to support such a grouping. More than 20 HPV types have been detected in benign EV lesions, but mainly HPV 5 and 8 were consistently found in EV-related malignancies.[19,37] In transformation assays in rodent cell lines, the E6 genes of HPV-5, HPV-8, and HPV-47 were found to have a more potent transforming activity than the E6 of HPV-14/20/21/25.[38-40]

C.   Mucosal Papillomaviruses Associated with Cutaneous Lesions

Papillomaviruses are predominantly epitheliotropic and are generally specific for either skin or mucosa. Exceptions to this strict cutaneous vs. mucosal classification are HPV-2 and HPV-57, which display an ambivalent tropism, being found in both cutaneous and oral verrucae.[41] In the phylogenetic tree based on the multiple open reading frame alignment (Figure 2), these two viruses occupy an intermediate position, between the cutaneous viruses and the mucosal viruses. Their position in the E6-phylogenetic tree (Figure 1) is less clear. Together with HPV-3 and HPV-10, both associated with cutaneous verruca plana, they appear to share a common root with the mucosal "low-risk" papillomaviruses. However, slightly less parsimonious trees place them in the same intermediate position as in the multiple ORF tree (data not shown). More sequence data is needed to definitively root this group.

Cutaneous papillomaviruses, associated with skin warts or epidermodysplasia verruciformis, are rarely if ever recovered from genital tract lesions, and papillomaviruses from the "low risk" or "high risk" mucogenital group are usually not found in cutaneous lesions.[42] A notable exception is the presence of HPV-16 in digital periungual squamous cell carcinomas.[43,44] Squamous cell neoplasms from cutaneous sites other than the finger have yet to reveal the presence of HPV-16 DNA.[45-47] Guitart et al. reported the detection of HPV-16 DNA in a squamous cell carcinoma of the finger and in a cervical neoplasm in the same patient.[48] These data might imply digital transmission of HPV-16 from a mucogenital lesion to the nail bed region.

HPV-26 was isolated from an immune deficient patient with generalized cutaneous verrucosis, and was thought to be a cutaneous PV.[49] However, this patient also suffered from widespread anogenital condylomata. HPV-26 is phylogenetically related to HPV-51, which is found in CIN lesions and cervical carcinomas. But because of its original association with a skin lesion, HPV-26 has not been included in most of the probe panels in HPV-studies of the genital mucosa. Based on its phylogenetic position, one would predict the presence of HPV-26 in mucosal lesions. Recently, the presence of HPV-26 in the genital tract has been confirmed.[50]

HPV-7, a virus commonly found in cutaneous warts of butchers and fish handlers is positioned in the phylogenetic tree in the mucosal "low risk" group, together with HPV-40 and HPV-43, two viruses recovered from benign and low malignant mucosal lesions. However, HPV-7 was also recovered from oral lesions in HIV-seropositive patients, illustrating its potential for mucosal tropism.[51,52] The reason why butchers have a higher prevalence of hand warts, and why HPV-7 is more frequently found in warts from butchers then from other professions remains obscure.

D.   "Low-Risk" Papillomaviruses in "High-Risk" Lesions

Infection by "low-risk" HPV types such as HPV-6 and-11 does not entirely exclude the possibility of developing a malignant lesion. Although primarily found in benign lesions, HPV-6 and HPV-11 have been detected in premalignant and malignant lesions such as Buschke-Löwenstein tumor, carcinoma of the vulva, and laryngeal carcinoma. However, duplications and insertions are often found in the upstream regulatory region (URR) of "low-risk" papillomaviruses when they are present in "high-risk" lesions, potentially conferring deregulated growth properties to viruses otherwise associated with benign nonaggressive tumors.

1.   Buschke-Löwenstein Tumor

HPV-6 and HPV-11 were shown to be present as episomal molecules in Buschke-Löwenstein tumor, a large and uncommon verrucous perianogenital tumor, which is clinically regarded as malignant because of its tendency for local expansion with displacement and invasion of adjacent structures. It is not known, however, to lead to local lymph node involvement or distant metastases, and it histologically resembles condyloma acuminata. It has therefore been suggested that the Buschke-Löwenstein tumor is an unusually aggressive benign lesion, rather than a true carcinoma.[53] One of the HPV-6 subtypes (HPV-6d) isolated from a Buschke-Löwenstein tumor was found to have a tandem duplication of 459 base pairs in the upstream regulatory region (URR).[54] This duplicated the start sites and putative promoter and control elements for transcription of the early genes. Such duplications have been found in less than 5% of the HPV-6 URR in condylomata acuminata.[55]

2.   Vulvar Carcinoma

Whereas invasive cervical carcinomas predominantly contain HPV-16/18 or related viruses, vulvar carcinomas often contain HPV-6/11. But about half of these cases also have HPV-16 and/or HPV-18 present in the same lesion.[56] Characterization of episomal HPV-6 DNA from an invasive squamous carcinoma of the vulva (HPV-6-T70) revealed a 24 bp duplication, a 58 bp insertion, and a 49 bp deletion in the URR. The duplications and insertions in the URR of HPV-6-T70 are stretches of alternating purines and pyrimidines, capable of forming transcription-enhancing Z-DNA structures.[57] Another HPV-6 subtype isolated from a verrucous carcinoma of the vulva (HPV 6vc) contained three inserts of 74, 15, and 19 bp in the URR, which was shown to display enhanced transcriptional activity.[58,59]

3. Laryngeal Carcinoma

HPV-6 and HPV-11 are associated with benign juvenile and adult laryngeal papillomatosis.[60,61] After a long latency period, squamous cell carcinomas can arise in preexisting laryngeal papillomas and spread throughout the upper respiratory tract. Most of the HPV positive carcinomas contain HPV-16.[62-64] There are case reports describing the malignant progression of laryngopharyngeal lesions containing HPV-6 or -11.[65,66] However, Morgan et al. found that HPV-6/11 DNA was only present in adjacent tissue and absent from the malignant lesion itself. HPV-6 DNA, isolated from a bronchial carcinoma of a patient with recurrent laryngeal papillomatosis had a complete duplication of the URR.[67] HPV-6 genomes in the benign lesions in the same patient did not have this duplication, suggesting that sequence rearrangements in the URR were necessary to confer malignant potential to "low risk" HPVs.[68] An HPV-11 construct containing such a URR-duplication was shown to cooperate with the *ras*-oncogene in the transformation of rat kidney cells, whereas the standard HPV-11 DNA could not.[69]

V. CONCLUSION

There is a good correlation between the "theoretical" oncogenicity of an HPV type as deduced from phylogenetic analyses using HPV nucleotide sequence data, and the "clinical" and "*in vitro*" oncogenicity as determined from clinical studies and transformation assays, respectively.

The continued isolation, cloning, and characterization of novel HPV types will be of importance to further elucidate the biological spectrum of human papillomaviruses, their origin, and their molecular evolution. Some of the yet uncharacterized HPVs may turn out to be clinically important. Sequencing and phylogenetic analysis will provide information on their potential clinical relevance. Use of the novel HPV isolates in probe panels will improve the detection rate of HPV in clinical specimens in the future.

Further epidemiological studies with the typing of a larger number of HPV isolates will be necessary to assign more accurate relative risk values to different phylogenetic HPV groups or HPV types. Together with a definitive phylogenetic tree based on the whole genome alignment of a larger number of HPV types, this may lead to a better understanding of the causal relationship between the presence of an HPV genome and the development of an HPV-associated lesion.

ACKNOWLEDGMENTS

We thank G. Opdenakker and D. L. Swofford for helpful discussions, and G. Orth, A. Lorincz, M. Goldsborough, M. Ishibashi, and T. Kiyono for providing E6 nucleotide sequences prior to publication. This work was supported in part by NIH grant 5P30CA13330. Marc Van Ranst was the recipient of grants from the Belgian American Educational Foundation, the D. Collen Research Foundation, and NFWO Smith-Kline Beecham.

REFERENCES

1. Van Ranst, M., Sundberg, J. P., and Burk, R. D., Molecular evolution of papillomaviruses, in *Molecular Evolution of Viruses*, Calisher, C., Garcia-Arenal, F. C., and Gibbs A. J., Eds., Cambridge University Press, Cambridge, 1995.
2. Ahola, H., Stenlund, A., Moreno-Lopez, J., and Petterson, U., Sequences of bovine papillomavirus type 1 DNA; functional and evolutionary implications, *Nucleic Acids Res.*, 11, 2639, 1983.
3. Crawford, L.V., and Crawford, E. M., A comparative study of polyoma and papilloma viruses, *Virology*, 21, 258, 1983.
4. Heilman, C. E., Law, M.-F., Israel, M. A., and Howley, P. M., Cloning of human papilloma virus genomic DNAs and analysis of homologous polynucleotide sequences, *J. Virol.*, 36, 395, 1980.
5. De Villiers, E.-M., Heterogeneity of the Human Papillomavirus Group, *J. Virol.*, 63, 4898, 1989.
6. Manos, M. M., Ting, Y., Wright, D. K., Lewis, A. J., Broker, T. R., and Wolinsky, S. M., The use of polymerase chain reaction amplification for the detection of genital human papillomaviruses, *Cancer Cells*, 7, 209, 1989.
7. Snijders, P. J. F., Van den Brule, A. J. C., Schrijnemakers, H. F. J., Snow, G., Meijer, C. J. L. M., and Walboomers, J. M. M., The use of general primers in the polymerase chain reaction permits the detection of a broad spectrum of human papillomavirus genotypes, *J. Gen. Virol.*, 71, 173, 1990.
8. Van Ranst, M. A., Tachezy, R., and Burk R. T., Human papillomavirus nucleotide sequences: What's in stock ?, *Papillomavirus Report*, 5, 65, 1994.
9. Lorincz, A. T., Reid, R., Jenson, A. B., Greenberg, M. D., Lancaster, W., and Kurman, R. J., Human papillomavirus infection of the cervix: relative risk associations of 15 common anogenital types, *Obstet. Gynecol.*, 79, 328, 1992.
10. Lungu, O., Wei Sun, X., Felix, J., Richart, R. M., Silverstein, S., and Wright, T. C., Relationship of human papillomavirus type to grade of cervical intraepithelial neoplasia, *J. Am. Med. Assoc.*, 267, 2493, 1992.
11. Bergeron, C., Barasso, R., Beaudenon, S., Flamant, P., Croissant, O., and Orth, G. O., Human papillomaviruses associated with cervical intraepithelial neoplasia, *Am. J. Surg. Pathol.*, 16, 641, 1992.
12. Kingsbury, D. W., Biological concepts in virus classification, *Intervirology*, 29, 242, 1988.
13. Pfister, H., Krubke, J., Dietrich, W., Iftner, T., and Fuchs, P.G., Classification of the papillomaviruses: mapping the genome, in *Papillomaviruses: CIBA Foundation Symposium 120*, Evered, D. and Clark, S., Eds., John Wiley & Sons, New York, 1986, 3.
14. Van Ranst, M., Kaplan, J. B., and Burk, R. D., Phylogenetic classification of human papillomaviruses: correlation with clinical manifestations, *J. Gen. Virol.*, 73, 2653, 1992.
15. Chan, S.-Y., Bernard, H.-U., Ong, C.-K., Chan, S.-P., Hofmann, B., and Delius, H., Phylogenetic analysis of 48 papillomavirus types and 28 subtypes and variants: a showcase for the molecular evolution of DNA viruses, *J. Virol.*, 66, 5714, 1992.
16. Coggin, J. R. and zur Hausen, H., Workshop on papillomaviruses and cancer, *Cancer Res.*, 39, 545, 1979.
17. Van Regenmortel, M. H. V., Virus species, a much overlooked but essential concept in virus classification, *Intervirology*, 31, 241, 1990.
18. Swofford, D. L., PAUP: *Phylogenetic Analysis Using Parsimony*, Version 3.0, Computer program and documentation, Illinois Natural History Survey, Champaign, Illinois, 1991.
19. Deau, M.-C., Favre, M., and Orth, G., Genetic heterogeneity among human papillomaviruses associated with epidermodysplasia verruciformis: evidence for multiple allelic forms of HPV5 and HPV8 E6 genes, *Virology*, 184, 492, 1991.
20. Obalek, S., Favre, M., Szymanczyk, J., Misiewicz, J., Jablonska, S., and Orth, G., Human papillomavirus (HPV) types specific of epidermodysplasia verruciformis detected in warts induced by HPV3 or HPV3-related types in immunosuppressed patients, *J. Inv. Dermatol.*, 98, 336-941, 1992.
21. Rolighed, J., Sorensen, I. M., Jacobson, N. O., and Lindeberg, H., The presence of HPV types 6/11,13,16 and 33 in bowenoid papulosis in an HIV-positive male, demonstrated by DNA *in situ* hybridization, *Acta Patholog. Microbiol. Immunol. Scand.*, 99, 583, 1991.

22. Barnes, W., Delgado, G., Kurman, R. J., Petrilli, E. S., Smith, D. M., Ahmed, S., Lorincz, A. T., Temple, G. F., Jenson, A. B., and Lancaster, W. D., Possible prognostic significance of human papillomavirus type in cervical cancer, *Gynecol. Oncol.*, 29, 267, 1988.

23. Kurman, R. J., Schiffman, M. H., Lancaster, W. D., Reid, R., Jenson, A. B., Temple, G. F., and Lorincz, A. T., Analysis of individual human papillomavirus types in cervical neoplasia: a possible role for type 18 in rapid progression, *Am. J. Obst. Gynecol.*, 159, 293, 1988.

24. Franquemont, D. W., Ward, B. E., Anderson, W. A., and Crum, C. P., Prediction of "high-risk" cervical papillomavirus infection by biopsy morphology, *Am. J. Clin. Pathol.*, 92, 577, 1989.

25. Cullen, A. P., Reid, R., Campion, M., and Lorincz, A. T., Analysis of the physical state of different papillomavirus DNAs in intraepithelial and invasive cervical neoplasm, *J. Virol.*, 65, 606, 1991.

26. Schlegel, R., Phelps, W. C., Zhang, Y.-L., and Barbosa, M., Quantitative keratinocyte assay detects two biological activities of human papillomavirus DNA and identifies viral types associated with cervical carcinoma, *EMBO J.*, 7, 3181, 1988.

27. Storey, A., Pim, D., Murray, A., Osborn, K., Banks, L., and Crawford, L., Comparison of the *in vitro* transforming activities of human papillomavirus types, *EMBO J.*, 7, 1815, 1988.

28. Pecoraro, G., Morgan, D., and Defendi, V., Differential effects of human papillomavirus type 6, 16, and 18 DNAs on immortalization and transformation of human cervical epithelial cells, *Proc. Nat. Acad. Sci. U.S.A.*, 86, 563, 1989.

29. Woodworth, C. D., Doniger, J., and DiPaolo, J. A., Immortalization of human foreskin keratinocytes by various human papillomavirus DNAs corresponds to their association with cervical carcinoma, *J. Virol.*, 63, 159, 1989.

30. Vousden, K. H., Human papillomavirus oncoproteins, *Sem. Cancer Biol.*, 1, 415, 1990.

31. Barbosa, M. S., Vass, W. C., Lowy, D. R., and Schiller, J. T., *In vitro* biological activities of the E6 and E7 genes vary among human papillomaviruses of different oncogenic potential, *J. Virol.*, 65, 292, 1991.

32. Lungu, O., Crum, C. P., and Silverstein, S., Biologic properties and nucleotide sequence analysis of human papillomavirus type 51, *J. Virol.*, 65, 4216, 1991.

33. Crook, T., Wrede, D., and Vousden, K. H., p53 point mutation in HPV negative human cervical carcinoma cell lines, *Oncogene*, 6, 873, 1991.

34. Levine, A. J., Momand, J., and Finlay, C. A., The p53 tumor suppressor gene, *Nature*, 351, 453, 1991.

35. Scheffner, M., Werness, B. A., Huibregtse, J. M., Levine, A. J., and Howley, P. M., The E6 oncoprotein encoded by human papillomavirus types 16 and 18 promotes the degradation of p53, *Cell*, 63, 1129, 1990.

36. Crook, T., Tidy, J. A., and Vousden, K. H., Degradation of p53 can be targeted by HPV E6 sequences distinct from those required for p53 binding and trans-activation, *Cell*, 67, 547, 1991.

37. Orth, G., Epidermodysplasia verruciformis: a model for understanding the oncogenicity of human papillomaviruses, in *Papillomaviruses. CIBA Foundation Symposium 120*, D. Evered, D. and Clark, S., Eds., John Wiley & Sons, New York, 1986, 157.

38. Iftner, T., Bierfelder, S., Csapo, Z., and Pfister, H., Involvement of human papillomavirus type 8 genes E6 and E7 in transformation and replication, *J. Virol.*, 62, 3655, 1988.

39. Kiyono, T., Hiraiwa, A., and Ishibashi, M., Differences in transforming activity and coded amino acid sequence among E6 genes of several papillomaviruses associated with epidermodysplasia verruciformis, *Virology*, 186, 628, 1992.

40. Hiraiwa, A., Kiyono, T., Segawa, K., Utsumi, K. R., Ohasi, M., and Ishibashi, M., Comparative study on E6 and E7 genes of some cutaneous and genital papillomaviruses of human origin for their ability to transform 3Y1 cells, *Virology*, 192, 102, 1993.

41. Hirsch-Behnam, A., Delius, A., and de Villiers, E.-M., A comparative sequence analysis of two human papillomaviruses types 2a and 57, *Virus Res.*, 18, 81, 1990.

42. Grussendorf-Conen E.-I., Papillomavirus-induced tumors of the skin: cutaneous warts and epidermodysplasia verruciformis, in *Papillomaviruses and Human Disease*, Syrjanen, K., Gissmann, L., and Koss, L. G., Eds., Springer Verlag, Berlin, 1987, 158.

43. Moy, R. L., Eliezri, Y. D., Nuovo, G. J., Zitelli, J. A., Bennett, R. G., and Silverstein, S., Human papillomavirus type 16 DNA in periungual squamous cell carcinomas, *J. Am. Med. Assoc.*, 261, 2669, 1989.

44. Ostrow, R. S., Shaver, K., Turnquist, S., Viksnins, A., Bender, M., Vance, C., Kaye, V., and Faras, A. J., Human papillomavirus-16 DNA in a cutaneous invasive cancer. *Arch. Dermatol.*, 125, 666, 1989.

45. Eliezri, Y. D., Silverstein, S. J. and Nuovo, G. J., Occurrence of human papillomavirus type 16 DNA in cutaneous squamous and basal cell neoplasms, *J. Am. Acad. Dermatol.*, 23, 836, 1990.

46. Kawashima, M., Favre, M., Obalek, S., Jablonska, S., and Orth, G., Premalignant lesions and cancers of the skin in the general population: evaluation of the role of human papillomaviruses, *J. Inv. Dermatol.*, 95, 537, 1990.

47. Dyall-Smith, D., Trowell, H., Mark, A., and Dyall-Smith, M., Cutaneous squamous cell carcinomas and papillomaviruses in renal transplant recipients: a clinical and molecular biological study, *J. Dermatol. Sci.*, 2, 139, 1991.

48. Guitart, J., Bergfeld, W. F., Tuthill, R. J., Tubbs, R. R., Zienowicz, R.,and Fleegler, E. J., Squamous cell carcinoma of the nail bed : a clinico-pathological study of 12 cases, *Br. J. Dermatol.*, 123, 215, 1990.

49. Ostrow, R. S., Zachow, K. R., Thompson, O., and Faras, A. J., Molecular cloning and characterization of a unique type of human papillomavirus from an immune deficient patient, *J. Inv. Dermatol.*, 82, 362, 1984.

50. Gravitt, P. and Yi-Zhang, T., personal communication.

51. Greenspan, D., de Villiers, E.-M., Greenspan, J. S., De Souza, Y. G., and zur Hausen, H., Unusual HPV types in oral warts in association with HPV infection, *J. Oral Pathol. Med.*, 17, 482, 1988.

52. Syrjanen, S. M., Von Krogh, G., Kellokoski, J. and Syrjanen, K., Two different human papillomavirus types associated with oral mucosal lesions in an HIV seropositive man, *J. Oral Pathol. Med.*, 18, 366, 1989.

53. Dawson, D. F., Duckworth, J. K., Bernhardt, H., and Young, J. M., Giant condyloma and verrucous carcinoma of the genital area, *Arch. Pathol.*, 79, 225, 1965.

54. Boshart, M. and zur Hausen, H., Human papillomaviruses in Buschke-Lowenstein tumors: Physical state of the DNA and identification of a tandem duplication in the noncoding region of a human papillomavirus 6 subtype, *J. Virol.*, 58, 963, 1986.

55. Rubben, A., Beaudenon, S., Favre, M., Schmitz, W., Spelten, B., and Grussendorf-Conen, E.-I., Rearrangements of the upstream regulatory region of human papillomavirus type 6 can be found in both Buschke-Lowenstein tumors and in condylomata acuminata, *J. Gen. Virol.*, 73, 3147, 1992.

56. Sutton, G. P., Steh, F. B., Ehrlich, C. E., and Roman A., Human papillomavirus deoxyribonucleic acid in lesions of the female genital tract: evidence for type 6/11 in squamous carcinoma of the vulva, *Obstet. Gynecol.*, 70, 564, 1987.

57. Kasher, M. S. and Roman, A., Characterization of human papillomavirus type 6b DNA isolated from an invasive squamous carcinoma of the vulva, *Virology*, 165, 225, 1988.

58. Rando, R. F., Groff, D. E., Chirikjian, J. G., and Lancaster, W. D., Isolation and characterization of a novel human papillomavirus type 6 DNA from an invasive vulvar carcinoma, *J. Virol.*, 57, 353, 1986.

59. Rando, R. F., Lancaster, W. D., Han, P., and Lopez, C., The noncoding region of HPV-6vc contains two distinct transcriptional enhancing elements, *Virology*, 155, 545, 1986.

60. Terry, R. M., Lewis, F. A., Griffiths, S., Wells, M., and Bird, C. C., Demonstration of human papillomavirus types 6 and 11 in juvenile laryngeal papillomatosis by in situ DNA hybridization, *J. Pathol.*, 153, 245, 1987.

61. Mounts, P., Shah, K., and Kashima, H., Viral etiology of juvenile and adult-onset squamous papilloma of the larynx, *Proc. Nat. Acad. Sci. U.S.A.*, 79, 5425, 1982.

62. Hoshikawa, T., Nakajima, T., Uhara, H., Gotoh, M., Shimosato, Y., Tsutsumi, K., Ono, I., and Ebihara, S., Detection of human papillomavirus DNA in laryngeal squamous cell carcinomas by polymerase chain reaction, *Laryngoscope*, 100, 647, 1990.

63. Perez-Ayala, M., Ruiz-Cabello, F., Esteban, F, Concha, A., Redondo, M., Oliva, M. R., Cabrera, T., and Garrido, F., Presence of HPV 16 sequences in laryngeal carcinomas, *Int. J. Cancer*, 46, 8, 1990.

64. McCullough, D. W. and McNicol, P. J., Laryngeal carcinoma associated with human papillomavirus type 16, *J. Otolaryngol.*, 20, 97, 1991.

65. Zarod, A. P., Rutherford, J. D., and Corbitt, G., Malignant progression of laryngeal papilloma associated with human papillomavirus type 6 (HPV 6) DNA, *J. Clin. Pathol.*, 41, 280, 1988.

66. Lindeberg, H., Syrjanen, S., Karja, J., and Syrjanen K., Human papillomavirus type 11 DNA in squamous cell carcinomas and pre-existing multiple laryngeal papillomas, *Acta Otolaryngologica*, 107, 141, 1989.

67. Morgan, D. W., Abdullah, V., Quiney, R., and Myint, S., Human papilloma virus and carcinoma of the laryngopharynx, *J. Laryngol. Otol.*, 105, 288, 1991.

68. DiLorenzo, T. P., Tamsen, A., Abramson, A. L., and Steinberg, B. M., Human papillomavirus type 6a DNA in the lung carcinoma of a patient with recurrent laryngeal papillomatosis is characterized by a partial duplication, *J. Gen. Virol.*, 73, 423, 1992.

69. Rosen, M. and Auborn, K., Duplication of the upstream regulatory sequences increases the transformation potential of human papillomavirus type 11, *Virology*, 185, 484, 1991.

III. Epidemiology and Modes of Transmission

5

Epidemiology and Modes of Transmission

David A. Shoultz, Laura A. Koutsky, and Denise A. Galloway

CONTENTS

I. INTRODUCTION

Genital human papillomavirus (HPV) infections are common among young, sexually active individuals. Even among low risk populations where the prevalence of other sexually transmitted infections such as *Treponema pallidum*, *Neisseria gonnorrhoeae*, *Chlamydia trachomatis*, herpes simplex virus, or *Trichomonas vaginalis*, is less than 5% the prevalence of HPV infections is higher, ranging from 10 to 50%. One reason why HPV is more prevalent than other sexually transmitted diseases (STDs) is that HPV infection of the genital tract rarely causes visible signs or symptoms; thus, individuals do not know whether they or their partners are infectious. Because the virus is not cleared by currently available therapies, an important STD control activity that involves diagnosis and treatment of index cases and treatment of exposed partners cannot be used to reduce HPV transmission. Also, individuals may be infected by multiple types of HPV. It is not yet known whether cross protective immunity develops.

This chapter reviews findings that have broadened our knowledge of the epidemiology of genital HPV infections. The prevalence and incidence of genital HPV infections among female and male populations is discussed and recent findings on possible modes of nongenital transmission are presented. Additional reviews of the epidemiology of HPV infections can be found in the literature.[1-10]

II. HPV INFECTIONS OF WOMEN

Age and sexual behavior are two factors that clearly influence detection rates of genital HPV among different populations. As with other sexually transmitted infections, prevalence estimates for genital HPV infection are highest for sexually active young adults between 18 and 25 years of age. Based on data from several clinical surveys of genital warts, an annual prevalence of 1% for males and females between the ages of 15 and 49 years has been estimated.[2,11]

The annual incidence of genital warts among women was estimated to be 106 per 100,000 for the female population of Rochester, Minnesota, U.S., during the late 1970s.[12] The results of this study also showed that the age- and gender-adjusted incidence of genital warts in this community increased eight-fold between the early 1950s and the late 1970s from 13 per 100,000 to 106 per 100,000. This time period corresponds to years when rates for other sexually transmitted diseases were increasing dramatically in Europe and North America.[13] Additional studies show a 4.5-fold increase in the number of first office visits for condyloma in the United States between 1966 and 1984,[14] and a 2.5-fold increase in the incidence of condyloma for males and females in the United Kingdom between 1971 and 1982.[13] Data collected from STD clinics in New Zealand demonstrate an increase in the incidence of genital warts since 1977. During the period from 1988 to 1993, genital HPV infection was the most commonly detected STD, with 18% of new patients attending STD clinics receiving this diagnosis in 1993.[15]

In most clinical populations, the prevalence of HPV infection detected cytologically on Pap smears ranges between <1 and 3%.[11,16,17] Among women attending sexually transmitted disease clinics, 8 to 13% of Pap smears show signs of HPV infection.[18-20] Unlike the data for genital warts, there is no clear evidence supporting an increase over the last three decades in prevalence of cytologically detected cervical HPV infection. There may have been an increase in prevalence but the available data do not lend themselves to time-trend analysis. During the last 30 years there have been major changes in the classification of Pap smear abnormalities (particularly after the link between HPV and CIN was first suggested in 1976).[21,22] Also, until relatively recently, Pap screening was not routinely performed on young sexually active women between the ages of 15 and 25 years.

When DNA or RNA hybridization techniques are used to test cellular specimens obtained from genital or anal sites, additional subclinical HPV infections may be detected. The choice and performance of a particular hybridization method (Southern blot, filter *in situ*, dot blot, and PCR-based methods) used in epidemiological studies greatly influences how many infected individuals will be identified.

At present, specimen processing, hybridizing, and probing techniques vary considerably from laboratory to laboratory. Considerable interlaboratory variation in performance of Southern blots was demonstrated by Brandsma et al.[23] Interlaboratory agreement varied between 66 and 97% for HPV positively and between 77 and 96% for HPV type specificity among specimens considered to contain HPV. A similar interlaboratory comparison study of PCR results showed 83% agreement for HPV positivity among samples found satisfactory in both laboratories and 88% agreement for HPV type specificity.[24] A recent multilaboratory comparison of the reliability of HPV DNA detection by Hybrid Capture®, yielded rates of agreement ranging from 87 to 94%, with kappa values of 0.61 to 0.83.[25]

Surveys using a PCR-based method for HPV DNA detection have demonstrated prevalence estimates of up to 100% among gynecologic populations. The detection rates with PCR vary according to the protocol that is used. An important source of variation in results may be due to differences in the HPV type-specific probes that are used and whether, and which, consensus or generic primers are used.[26] For example, a probe specific for one HPV type will yield fewer positive results than will an assay employing general primers and a consensus probe allowing the identification of several HPV types. Lavage samples from 321 women with cervical lesions and 88 women with no history of cervical neoplasia were analyzed by Southern blot and two PCR systems both amplifying a product in the L1 region. For the 36 samples that were positive by Southern blot, PCR showed a sensitivity of 50% (18 of 36) for one set of primers and 100% (36 to 36) for the other set of primers. The overall HPV prevalence rates were 15% (18 of 120) and 47% (56 of 120) for the two sets of primers, respectively, compared with 30% (36 of 120) for Southern blot. However, 29% (16 of 56) of the HPV positives detected by the second set of primers were called nonclassified HPV types, the biologic meaning of which is not yet known.[27]

Results from recent studies using PCR-based methods to detect HPV DNA in genital tract specimens from sexually active women with negative Pap smears show prevalence estimates that range from 5 to 48%.[28-39] These studies include women from Europe, Africa, Latin America, North America, and Asia. Although different PCR methods and different HPV DNA probes were used in these studies, the following important conclusions can be drawn from the results.

1. Younger rather than older women are more likely to have HPV DNA detected.
2. HPV DNA is rarely detected in genital tract specimens of women who report no previous coitus.
3. Geographic differences in HPV prevalence estimates are not readily apparent.
4. Oncogenic types of HPV, particularly HPV 16, are the most common types detected in these studies of women with negative Pap smears.
5. Most genital HPV infections are only transiently detectable in sexually active young women, with the majority no longer being detectable after 1 to 2 years.[40]

Studies designed to evaluate risk factors for acquisition of HPV infection may be best performed among women who are initiating sexual activity. In general, these will be younger populations. Risk factor studies that include sexually active women of different ages are difficult to interpret because the HPV infections detected are a heterogeneous mixture of newly acquired, persisting, and recurrent infections.

A study conducted by Moscicki et al.[41] enrolled 661 nonpregnant sexually active females aged 13 to 19 who were attending one of three family planning clinics. HPV was the most prevalent sexually transmitted organism in the study population, having been detected by dot blot hybridization in 15% of participants as compared with 10% for *C. trachomatis*, 3% for *N. gonorrhoeae*, and 4% for *T. vaginalis*. The majority of HPV types detected were "high risk" types 16 or 18 or "intermediate risk" types 31, 33, or 35, so designated based upon the frequency of association of those HPV types with invasive cervical cancer.[42] The strongest risk factor for detection of HPV was number of lifetime sexual partners, with 61% of HPV positive women having had greater than 3 sexual partners as compared with 36% of HPV negative women [odds ratio (OR) = 2.8, 95% CI = 1.8, 4.5]. A study by Fisher et al.[43] detected HPV by Southern transfer hybridization in 32% of 107 white, suburban, sexually active adolescents (mean age 18.5 years). The prevalence of HPV types 16, 18, 31, 45, or 56 was 16%. Report of a lifetime number of sexual partners greater than two and younger age at menarche were significantly associated with detection of HPV DNA. A study conducted among inner-city teenagers, with DNA hybridizations having been performed in the same laboratory as that used in the Fisher et al. study,[43] found an HPV prevalence rate of 38%.[44] Martinez et al.[45] reported that 13% of inner-city adolescent females were positive for HPV DNA using low-stringency Southern transfer hybridization.

HPV DNA was detected in 18% of the cervical samples collected from 483 women between the ages of 16 to 81 years (median = 34 years) attending HMO obstetrics/gynecology clinics in Portland, Oregon. Using a PCR-based amplification system, it was determined that 40% of the HPV positive specimens contained DNA from HPV types known to be cancer associated.[46] Hildesheim et al.[38] used a similar detection method and reported a somewhat higher prevalence (34%) of cervical HPV DNA from a study conducted among 404 low-income cytologically normal women in Washington, D.C. between the ages of 16 and 72 years (median = 26). Recent sexual behavior was determined to be a more important predictor of HPV infection than was cumulative lifetime number of sexual partners. Using the PCR-based method of Bauer et al.,[32] cervical HPV DNA was detected in 44% of 357 cytologically normal women (aged 18 to 47 years, median = 23) attending a student health center in New Mexico.[39]

In our study of 18 to 20 year old university students, HPV DNA was detected by a PCR-based method in cervical or vulvo-vaginal specimens obtained from 2 (3.6%) of 55 women reporting no prior sexual intercourse, 17.5% of 63 women reporting 1 partner, 36.9% of 84 women reporting 2 to 4 partners and 85.4% of 41 women reporting 5 to 24 partners. Also, the frequency of detecting multiple types of HPV DNA in genital tract specimens increased with numbers of sexual partners, from 0% of women reporting no partners to 29% of those reporting 5 to 24 partners (L. Koutsky, unpublished data). Results from studies of older women[33,47] show that the association between increased number of sexual partners and detection of HPV DNA diminishes with age, suggesting that viral production decreases over time in most women, and that the virus may be eliminated in at least some women.

Information included in the above studies indicates that, similar to women with cervical neoplasia,[48-50] women with normal Pap smears are more likely to have HPV 16 vs. other classified types of HPV DNA. However, results from studies using consensus (generic) primers indicate that unclassified HPV types are detected most often. How much of the "unclassified" HPV DNA that is detected represents different types vs. very low levels of known HPV types is not clear.

Recent studies of the molecular evolution of HPV 18 suggest that this virus originated and evolved with the first *Homo sapiens* in Africa.[51] Variants of HPV 16 and 18 (and most likely, other genital types of HPV) appear to have coevolved with all human ethnic groups.[51,52] Although the prevalence of HPV infection appears to be similar in different regions of the world, recent data suggest that there may be geographic or ethnic differences in the prevalence of different variants of HPV types.[53] By sequencing segments from 118 HPV 16 isolates obtained from various patient populations in four countries (Singapore, Brazil, Tanzania, and Germany), Chan and colleagues[54] found that the observed distribution of HPV 16 subtypes suggests that HPV 16 evolved separately for a long enough period in Africa and Eurasia to create two molecularly distinguishable variants. The investigators speculated that because representatives from both HPV 16 branches are present in Brazil, the variants were probably transferred via past colonial immigration. Similar ethnic differences in the distribution of HPV 16 variants were not observed in a small survey of HPV 16 samples obtained from ethnically different patient populations in Seattle, Washington, U.S.[55] Whether variants of oncogenic types of HPV are important in predicting increased risk for invasive cancer of the genital tract or anus remains to be determined.

Results from our studies and those of Manos and colleagues indicate that prevalence estimates of HPV infection detected by PCR increase with the number of genital sites tested. For example, approximately 20% to 33% more women will be found positive for HPV when the cervix and vulva or vagina are sampled as opposed to the cervix alone (N. Kiviat and L. Koutsky, unpublished data).

Although few archival specimens from women with negative cytologies have been tested for HPV DNA, several groups from diverse geographical regions (Great Britain, the United States, China, Africa, and Japan) have used *in situ* hybridization techniques to examine archival tissue specimens from women diagnosed with cervical intraepithelial neoplasia or invasive cervical cancer.[54-58] Results from these studies provide a consistent picture over the past 25 to 50 years of the association of specific types of HPV with cervical intraepithelial neoplasia and invasive cervical cancer. In each time period and geographical location, high risk types of HPV (HPV 16 and 18) were most frequently detected. Also, more recently discovered HPV types (HPV 42–45, 51, 52, and 56) were found in archival specimens obtained 25 years earlier.

Prevalence estimates may still vary between studies despite the fact that similar populations were examined and the same hybridization techniques were used. Differences in prevalence estimates may be due to the method of sampling (swabs, lavages, wooden spatulas, biopsy, self-inserted swabs, or tampons) and the sites sampled (cervix, vagina, vulva, penis, or anus). Preliminary results based on comparisons of yields from clinician-obtained vs. patient-obtained specimens have been promising, with agreement between the two methods estimated to be above 80%.[59,60] Use of cervicovaginal lavages appears to identify more HPV infections by Southern blot hybridization than use of cervical swab specimens.[61] The increased yield from the lavages is probably due to both the improved adequacy of the cervical cell sample and to inclusion of HPV infections from vaginal sites. The issue of which site or sites are samples is very important as the yield of cells and the percentage of HPV positive tests may vary between samples from the external and internal genitalia and anus. The prevalence of HPV infection in the male population is probably similar to that observed among females, but because penile swabs yield relatively fewer cells, it can be difficult to obtain adequate specimens.[62]

When comparing PCR with filter *in-situ* and dot-blot hybridization, van den Brule et al.[63] estimated the prevalence of HPV infection to be 6 times higher by PCR in a population of women attending a community-based Pap screening program (6 vs. 1%) and 4 times higher in a population of women attending a gynecological clinic (12 vs. 3%). In another study of young women attending a university, the detection rate for HPV types 6, 11, 16, 18, 31, 33, and 35 by PCR was 2.3 times higher (25.5 vs. 11%) than when a nonamplified method of HPV DNA detection was used on the same specimens.[32] Although PCR-based methods may be optimal in answering questions concerning incidence, prevalence, transmission, and natural history of HPV infections, use of less sensitive methods such as dot blot or hybrid capture may be better for use in programs aimed at early detection and treatment of women at risk for cervical cancer. Previous investigations have shown that when a semi-quantitative approach is used for detecting HPV DNA, women with high grade intraepithelial lesions or invasive cervical cancer have higher levels of oncogenic HPV types detected in cervical specimens than women without neoplasia.[64-66] Bavin and colleagues recently reported that detecting high levels of HPV 16 using a semi-quantitative PCR method was better than a qualitative (dichotomous) result at discriminating between those who had high grade cervical lesions vs. those with low grade lesions or normal histologic findings.[64]

The main drawback to the use of PCR is the potential for false-positive results produced through contamination with plasmid DNA, with the PCR product, or through sample-to-sample contamination which cannot be ruled out in spite of the use of positive and negative controls.[26,67-69] Contamination with plasmid DNA can be reduced by using anti-contamination primers. These primers flank the cloning side of the plasmid so that, in case of contamination, no PCR produce is produced under standard conditions.[62] Use of anti-contamination primers can only partly exclude false-positive results because contamination from PCR-product carryover or from other clinical specimens is still possible. The inherent complexities associated with the interpretation of results from PCR-based detection methods have been reviewed elsewhere.[67-69]

III.   HPV INFECTIONS OF MEN

In contrast to the quantity and variety of HPV research carried out in female populations, there have been relatively few studies of men. Reported sex differences in the occurrence of condylomata could be more a function of health care behavior then biology.[12,58,59] In the public STD clinic setting, the frequency of condylomata is about 4% to 70% higher among males than among females, whereas in private practice, the ratio appears to be slightly higher for females. In at least three studies,[14,70,71] condylomata were diagnosed more frequently in Caucasian men than in African American men. Whether this difference is related to racial differences in innate susceptibility, acquired immunity, behavior, the effects of skin color on detectability of condylomata, or other factors has not been determined. Cook et al.[72] found that the most common site of genital warts among both circumcised and uncircumcised men attending an STD clinic was the base of the penile shaft. However, when warts were detected on the distal portion of the penis (glans, meatus) the diagnosis was made much more frequently in noncircumcised compared with circumcised men (OR = 10.0 95% CI 3.9, 25.7).

Most of the studies that have used hybridization methods to detect genital HPV infection among men have examined men with HPV-associated lesions,[73-78] or men who were partners of women either with CIN, genital warts, or partners of women who were attending a gynecology referral clinic.[69,79-84] These latter studies have found that 50–80% of male partners had lesions with clinical or morphological features consistent with HPV infection. More recently, studies among male partners of women with evidence of HPV infection have found HPV DNA as detected by molecular hybridization methods in 33 to 85%.[85-90] For example, Hippeläinen et al.[91] studied a total of 318 Finnish men at high-risk of HPV infection, most of whom were sexual partners of HPV-infected women. At the first study visit, 65% of the men were determined to have lesions suggestive of HPV infection. Nearly half (55%) of these men had HPV detected by *in situ* hybridization (ISH) for types 6/11, 16/18, 31, 33, or 42. Importantly, most lesions regressed within 16 months, and the median time of regression did not vary significantly with treatment.

The lack of satisfactory sampling techniques makes it difficult to determine the prevalence of genital HPV infections among males in the general population. Penile scrapings yield limited material and thus are generally negative for HPV DNA when analyzed by Southern blot or other non-PCR-based hybridization methods.[92] The relative detectability of HPV in samples from the urethra, semen, and anus is unclear.

Grussendorf-Conen et al.[62] obtained penile smear samples from 530 men (primarily blood donors) who had no evidence of clinically detectable genital tract HPV infection. HPV DNA was detected by dot blot hybridization in 31 samples (5.8%). Younger men were more likely to be HPV positive, with HPV DNA detected in specimens obtained from 7.9% of men 15 to 35 years of age and 1.7% of men over age 35 years. Higher HPV prevalence rates (using PCR) were observed in the studies of Wikström et al. (86%)[93] and Baken et al. (62%)[90]

Kataoka et al.[94] studied 105 Swedish Army recruits between 18 and 23 years of age, and collected urethral smears from everyone and penile biopsy specimens from men with visible lesions for detection of HPV DNA using dot blot or Southern blot and PCR. The reported mean number of lifetime sexual partners was 1.4. Examination by penoscopy revealed that 36% of men had areas of aceto-whitening on genital tract epithelium. Eighteen (17.1%) men had HPV DNA detected by PCR from the urethral specimens, with 26% of men with aceto-white lesions having HPV detected compared with 12% of men with normal epithelium. Similarly, Hippeläinen et al.[95] enrolled 432 Finnish conscripts (mean age = 20 years) in a clinical study aimed at detecting HPV DNA (by PCR) or HPV-related symptoms among an otherwise healthy male population. HPV DNA was detected in 17%, and a total of 26% were considered to be HPV positive when the determination was based upon PCR and/or peniscopic findings. Other studies where urethral smears were obtained from men attending an STD clinic[96] or a urology clinic[97] found a similar prevalence of HPV, although men from the STD clinics were more likely to have HPV 16 detected than were men from the urology clinic.

To determine the prevalence of HPV DNA using urogenital samples, Green et al.[98] obtained semen samples from 104 patients attending an infertility clinic. Using PCR, 23 samples (22%) were positive for HPV 11, 35 (33%) were positive for HPV 16 with 15 (14%) positive for both HPV types 11 and 16 for a total HPV prevalence rate of 41%. None of the specimens were positive for HPV DNA by Southern transfer hybridization. The clinical significance of the relatively high HPV prevalence rate in the semen observed among men without clinically apparent genital warts in this study with respect to either transmission of HPV or subsequent clinical manifestations remains to be clarified. HPV was not detected in semen specimens when non-PCR-based methods were used in studies by Nieminen et al.[99] and Ostrow et al.,[100] although relatively few men were studied. Nonetheless, Kyo et al.[101] studied 53 married Japanese couples and examined cervical and seman samples for HPV 16 and 18 DNA using a PCR-based method. Twelve (23%) of the semen samples were positive for HPV types 16 or 18, and the majority of these men (75%) had wives whose cervical samples were also positive for HPV DNA. Nonetheless, it is difficult to distinguish the actual source of virus in studies such as this (i.e., semen vs. exfoliated urethral mucosal cells) making this area of study largely unresolved to date.

Mandal et al.[102] studied 105 men (median age of 26 years) who were attending an STD clinic. Men included in the study did not have macroscopic evidence of warts on clinical examination. Pooled specimens consisting of exfoliated cells from the distal urethra, penile shaft, glans penis, and anorectal junction were used for detection of HPV DNA using dot blot hybridization techniques. HPV DNA was detected in 21 (20%) of men, with 95% of the HPVs detected being HPV 16. Of these men, 15 (14%) regularly used condoms and 17 (16%) were circumcised, neither of which was associated with detection of HPV DNA.

Although there have been relatively few prevalence studies of genital HPV infection in men, studies to date suggest that rates of infection are similar for men and women. Also, as with women, the prevalence of genital HPV infection is highest among sexually active young adults, and HPV 16 is the most common type of HPV detected. It should also be noted that the detection of HPV DNA in anogenital specimens is more common among men with human immunodeficiency virus (HIV) infection, particularly those with lower levels of circulating CD4 lymphocytes. Kiviat et al.[103] conducted a cross-sectional study of 285 HIV seropositive and 204 HIV seronegative men attending an HIV screening clinic in Seattle, Washington, U.S. Detection of anal HPV DNA by Southern transfer hybridization (STH) was found in 55% of the seropositive and 23% of the seronegative men. Furthermore, the authors concluded that among the HIV-infected men, the detection of type-specific anal HPV DNA was significantly associated with more advanced immunosuppression.

IV. MODES OF TRANSMISSION

The predominant mode of transmission for the genital types of HPV appears to be via genital to genital contact. The fact that HPV infection is so prevalent among young sexually active populations suggests that transmission is relatively efficient. It is thought that moisture and abrasion of the epithelial surface enhance transmission.[2,11] There are no data that conclusively address the question of whether condoms provide an effective barrier for transmission of HPV.

Perinatal transmission also occurs but with an unknown frequency. Juvenile-onset recurrent respiratory papillomatosis (JO-RRP) is a rare benign tumor that appears to develop in infants who have been perinatally exposed to HPV 6, or more commonly, HPV 11. Adult-onset recurrent respiratory papillomatosis (AO-RRP) is also associatd with HPV, but whether it develops years to decades after perinatal exposure or after exposure to HPV as an adult through oral-genital contact is not known. Kashima et al.[104] performed a case-control study that included two separate case groups: patients with JO-RRP and patients with AO-RRP. Separate control groups were assembled for each case group. Results from this study showed that JO-RRP patients were more often born vaginally to a teenage mother, and were more likely to be the first born child than were their juvenile controls. AO-RRP cases reported more sexual partners and a higher frequency of oral sex than their adult controls. These findings suggest that the mode of transmission for JO-RRP and AO-RRP may be different.

In recent years, a number of investigators have reported detecting HPV DNA in oral buccal mucosal scrapes or nasopharyngeal aspirate samples of newborns and young children. Sedlacek et al.[105] tested by Southern blot hybridization 45 neonatal nasopharyngeal aspirates obtained in term. HPV DNA was found in 15 (33%) of 45 samples. Smith et al.[106] found that only 2 (2.8%) of 72 infants tested by a dot blot method for HPV DNA 24 to 72 hours after delivery had a positive oral-pharyngeal sample. In a similar but separate investigation, Smith et al.[107] tested the oral-pharyngeal swabs of 203 newborns using a nonamplified liquid hybridization assay and found that only 2 (1%) of the neonates had detectable HPV DNA. Perhaps significantly, while 24 (12%) of the maternal cervical samples were HPV DNA positive in the third trimester, none were positive at the time of labor and delivery. Fredericks et al.[108] collected and tested for HPV DNA by a PCR-based method, exfoliating cervical epithelial cells from 30 women 6 weeks postpartum. Buccal scrapes from their babies were collected at the same visit and processed in an identical fashion. HPV DNA of a similar type could be detected in buccal mucosal scrapes of 8 of 11 babies born to women with HPV DNA detected in cervical specimens. Only 1 of the 19 babies born to women negative for HPV DNA had a positive buccal scrape sample. Interestingly, other investigators were able to demonstrate the presence of HPV DNA in amniotic fluid using a two-step PCR process. Of the 35 women with abnormal Pap smears who were tested, 27 (77%) had amniotic fluid samples which were HPV positive.[109] Because the issue of perinatal transmission is important to pregnant women, and results from these studies are quite inconsistent, it is important to develop more precise estimates of the rates of perinatal transmission by studying larger cohorts of women and their babies, collecting samples at birth and six weeks post-partum, and by using a sensitive method for HPV DNA testing.

Tang et al.[110] reported detection of anal condylomata at birth in a neonate born to a woman with vulvar condylomata whose membranes had not ruptured earlier than 24 hours prior to delivery, suggesting that the neonate was infected *in utero*. Recent reports of detecting anogenital warts or HPV DNA in young children are difficult to interpret. Gutman and colleagues[111] collected vaginal wash samples from 15 index girls aged 11 years or younger who showed signs and symptoms of sexual abuse and from a separate group of similarly aged girls who had negative findings for sexual abuse. Using Southern and reverse blot methods, HPV 6, 11, or 16 DNA was detected in samples from five (33%) of the 15 index patients and none of the 17 controls.

Some of the anogenital warts in children that have been typed are nongenital types that may have been digitally transferred by auto-inoculation or by the hands of a caregiver.[7,112] As noted above, some (perhaps many) anogenital HPV infections in children are the result of sexual abuse. Although some investigators suggest that many of the anal genital HPV infections seen in children and sexually inexperienced adolescents are the result of perinatal transmission, the fact that HPV DNA is rarely found in anal or genital specimens obtained from newborns, and the fact that two recent studies show no correlation between the types of HPV DNA detected in children and their mothers is puzzling.[112-114]

V.   SUMMARY

Human papillomavirus infections are very common among sexually active adolescents and young adults, with infection by more than one type seen frequently among those with multiple sexual partners. Genital HPV infection appears to be the most common STD. Perhaps this is because HPV rarely produces symptoms or signs and is better suited to establishing genital tract infection than other sexually transmitted organisms such as *T. pallidum*, *N. gonorrhoeae*, HSV, *T. vaginalis*, and *C. trachomatis*. Furthermore, HPV types known to be etiologically associated with invasive cancer of the cervix, vagina, vulva, and penis constitute the majority of infections detected among men and women.

There remain many issues to be clarified in future studies. One area of interest is the identification of host factors related to HPV detectability, including age, genetic differences, immunosuppression (either acquired or induced), frequency of exposure to HPV (recent and total number of sexual partners, condom use), other potential factors such as smoking, contraception, presence of other genital tract infections, and the specific anatomic site sampled (cervix, vagina, vulva, anus). Studies that are designed to address risk factors for the acquisition, persistence, and progression of HPV infection and HPV associated intraepithelial lesions are important. Studies of both men and women should be undertaken. Comparisons between studies is often difficult due to the use of different HPV detection systems and variation in test performance.

The frequency with which HPV is transmitted perinatally is still unclear. HPV-associated recurrent respiratory papillomatosis appears to arise after perinatal transmission of HPV 11, or to a lesser degree, HPV 6. However, risk of transmission to an infant from a pregnant woman with clinical or DNA evidence of HPV 6 or 11 remains extremely low. Data from studies designed to determine the frequency of HPV DNA detection in nasopharyngeal, oral buccal mucosal, or anogenital specimens obtained from newborns or young children are inconsistent. Additional research in the area of perinatal transmission is needed.

One of the present goals of papillomavirus research is to develop more cost effective ways to prevent, detect, and treat cancer precursor lesions. Genital papillomaviruses have been grouped into "low risk," "intermediate risk," and "high risk" types based on frequency of association with invasive cervical cancer. We do not know whether the ability to detect and treat specific types of HPV infection will improve cancer control, primarily because little is known about the natural history of these infections.

Currently, a variety of commercial HPV DNA tests are available but we are only beginning to study and understand whether and how these tests might be used in cervical cancer control efforts. Until we understand more fully how often to obtain samples for HPV detection, and the factors influencing the likelihood of progression or regression, HPV detection methods will not be widely used outside of research settings. In the future, when perhaps better tests and sampling methods are available, HPV testing may be useful in predicting which patients are at greatest risk for lesion persistence or progression. Most importantly, careful study of the costs and benefits of incorporating HPV DNA testing into cervical cancer control programs is necessary before any changes are made to the relatively successful Pap screening programs that are now in place in many countries throughout the world.

REFERENCES

1. zur Hausen, H., de Villiers, E.-M., and Gissman, L., Papillomavirus infections and human genital cancer, *Gynecol. Oncol.*, 1981; 12(Suppl.):S124–S128.
2. Koutsky, L. A., Galloway, D. A., and Holmes, K. K., Epidemiology of genital human papillomavirus infection, *Epidemiol. Rev.*, 1988; 10:122–163.
3. Beutner, K. R., Becker, T. M., and Stone, K. M., Epidemiology of human papillomavirus infections, *Dermatol. Clin.*, 1991; 9:211–218.
4. Franco, E. L., Viral etiology of cervical cancer: A critique of the evidence, *Rev. Infect. Dis.*, 1991; 13:1195–1206.
5. von Krough, G., Genitoanal papillomavirus infection: diagnositic and therapeutic objectives in the light of current epidemiological observations, *Int. J. STD AIDS*, 1991; 2:391–404.
6. Schneider, A. and Koutsky, L. A., Natural history and epidemiological features of genital HPV infection. In: Munoz, N., Bosch, F. X., Shah, K. V., Meheus, A., Eds., *The Epidemiology of Human Papillomavirus and Cervical Cancer*, (IARC Scientific Publications No. 119), Lyon, International Agency for Research on Cancer, 1992, 25–52.
7. Moscicki, A.-B., Human papillomavirus infections, *Adv. Pediatr.*, 1992; 139:257–281.
8. Schneider, A., Pathogenesis of genital HPV infection, *Genitourin Med.*, 1993; 69:165–173.
9. Northfeld, D. W. and Palefsky, J. M., Human papillomavirus-associated anogenital neoplasia in persons with HIV infection, *AIDS Clin. Rev.*, 1992, pp. 241–2519.
10. Critchlow, C. W. and Koutsky, L. A., The epidemiology of human papillomavirus infection. In: Mindel, A., Ed., *Genital Warts: Human Papillomavirus Infection*, London, Edward Arnold, 1995.
11. Schiffman, M. H. and Burk, R. D., Human papillomavirus. In: Evans, A. S. and Kaslow, R., Eds., *Viral Infections of Humans*, 4th Edition, New York, Plenum Medical, 1995.
12. Chuang, T. Y., Perry, H. O., Kurland, L. T., and Ilstrup, D. M., Condyloma acuminatum in Rochester, Minnesota, 1950-1978. (Parts I and II), *Arch. Dermatol.*, 1984; 120:469–483.
13. Aral, S. O. and Holmes, K. K., Epidemiology of sexual behavior and sexually transmitted diseases. In: Holmes, K. K., Mardh, P.-A., Sparling, P. F., Wiesner, P. J., Cates, W., Lemon, S. M., and Stamm, W. E., Eds., *Sexually Transmitted Diseases*, Second Edition, New York, McGraw-Hill, 1990.
14. Becker, T. M., Stone, K. M., and Alexander, E. R., Genital human papilomavirus infection: a growing concern, *Obstet. Gynecol. Clin. N. Am.*, 1987; 14:389–96.
15. Lyttle, P. H., Surveillance report: disease trends at New Zealand sexually transmitted disease clinics 1977-1993, *Genitourin. Med.*, 1994; 70:329–35.
16. de Brux, J., Orth, G., Croissant, O., Cochard, B., and Ionesco, M., Condylomatous lesions of the cervix uteri: development in 2466 patients, *Bull. Cancer*, 1983; 70:410–422.
17. Meisels, A. and Morin, C., Flat condyloma of the cervix: two variants with different prognosis. In: Peto, R. and zur Hausen, H., Eds., *Viral Etiology of Cervical Cancer* (Banbury Report No. 21), Cold Spring Harbor, NY, CSH Press, 1986.
18. Drake, M., Medley, G., and Mitchell, H., Cytological detection of human papillomarus infection, *Obstet. Gynecol. Clin. North Am.*, 1987; 14:431–450.
19. Kiviat, N. B., Koutsky, L. A., Paavonen, J. A., Galloway, D. A., Critchlow, C. W., Beckmann, A. M., McDougall, J. K., Peterson, M. L., Stevens, C. E., Lipinski, C. M., and Holmes, K. K., Prevalence of genital papillomavirus infection among women attending a college student health clinic or an STD clinic, *J. Infec. Dis.*, 1989; 159:293–302.

20. Kiviat, N. B., Koutsky, L. A., Critchlow, C. W., Lorincz, A. T., Cullen, A. P., Browckway, J., and Holmes, K. K., Prevalence and cytologic manifestations of human papillomavirus (HPV) types 6, 11, 16, 18, 31, 33, 35, 42, 43, 44, 45, 51, 52, and 56 among 500 consecutive women, *Int. J. Gynecol. Pathol.*, 1992; 11:197–203.

21. Valente, P. T., Update on the Bethesda System for reporting cervical/vaginal diagnoses, *Cancer Treat Res.*, 1994; 70:15–28.

22. Kiviat, N. B., Critchlow, C. W., and Kurman, R. J., Reassessment of the morpholigical continuum of cervical intraepithelial lesions: does it reflect different stages in the progression to cervical carcinoma. In: Munoz, N., Bosch, F. X., Shah, K. V., and Meheus, A., Eds., *The Epidemiology of Human Papillomavirus and Cervical Cancer* (IARC Scientific Publications No. 119), Lyon, International Agency for Research on Cancer, 1992.

23. Brandsma, J., Burk, R. D., Lancaster, W. D., Pfister, H., and Schiffman, M. H., Interlaboratory variation as an explanation for varying prevalence estimates of human papillomavirus infection, *Int. J. Cancer*, 1989; 43:260–262.

24. Kuypers, J. M., Critchlow, C. W., Gravitt, P. E., Vernon, D. A., Sayer, J. B., Manos, M. M., and Kiviat, N. B., Comparison of dot filter hybridization, Southern transfer hybridization, and polymerase chain reaction amplification for diagnosis of anal human papillomavirus infection, *J. Clin. Microbiol.*, 1993; 31:1003–1006.

25. Schiffman, M. H., Kiviat, N. B., Burk, R. D., Shah, K. V., Daniel, R. W., Lewis, R., Kuypers, J., Manos, M. M., Scott, D. R., Sherman, M. E., Kurman, R. J., Stoler, M. H., Glass, A. G., Rush, B. B., Mielzynska, I., and Lorincz, A. T., Accuracy and interlaboratory reliability of human papillomavirus DNA testing by hybrid capture, *J. Clin. Microbiol.*, 1995; 33:545–50.

26. Gravitt, P. E. and Manos, M. M., Polymerase chain reaction-based methods for the detection of human papillomavirus DNA. In: Munoz, N., Bosch, F. X., Shah, K. V., and Meheus, A., Eds., *The Epidemiology of Human Papillomavirus and Cervical Cancer* (IARC Scientific Publications No. 119), Lyon, International Agency for Research on Cancer, pp. 121–133, 1992.

27. Schiffman, M. H., Bauer, H. M., Lorincz, A. T., Manos, M. M., Bryne, J. C., Glass, A. G., Cadell, D. M., and Howley, P. M., A comparison of Southern blot hybridization and polymerase chain reaction methods for the detection of human papillomavirus DNA, *J. Clin. Microbiol.*, 1991; 29:573–577.

28. Melkert, P. W. J., Hopman, E., van den Brule, A., Risse, E. K. J., van Diest, P. J., Bleker, O. P., Helmerhorst, T., Schipper, M. I., Meijer, C. J. L. M., and Walboomers, J. M. M., Prevalence of HPV in cytomorphologically normal cervical smears, as determined by the polymerase chain reaction, is age-dependent, *Int. J. Cancer*, 1993; 53:919–923.

29. Schiffman, M. H., Bauer, H. M., Hoover, R. N., Glass, A. G., Cadell, D. M., Rush, B. B., Scott, D. R., Sherman, M. E., Kurman, R. J., Wacholder, S., Stanton, C. K., and Manos, M. M., Epidemiologic evidence showing that human papillomavirus causes most cervical intraepithelial neoplasia, *J. Natl. Cancer Inst.*, 1993; 85:958–964.

30. Kjaer, S. K. de Villiers, E.-M., Çaglayan, H., Svare, E., Haugaard, B. J., Engholm, G., Christensen, R. B., Møller, K. A., Poll, P., Jensen, H., Vestergaard, B. F., Lynge, E., and Jensen, O. M., Human papillomavirus, *Herpes simplex* virus and other potential risk factors for cervical cancer in a high-risk area (Greenland) and a low-risk area (Denmark)- a second look, *Br. J. Cancer*, 1993; 67:830–837.

31. ter-Meulen, J., Eberhardt, H. C., Luande, J., Mgaya, H. N., Chang-Claude, J., Mtiro, H., Mhina, M., Kashaija, P., Ockert, S., Yu, X., Meinhardt, G., Gissmann, L., and Pawlita, M., Human papillomavirus (HPV) infection, HIV infection and cervical cancer in Tanzania, East Africa, *Int. J. Cancer*, 1992; 51:515–521.

32. Bauer, H. M., Ting, Y., Greer, C. E., Chambers, J. C., Tashiro, C. J., Chimera, J., Reingold, A., and Manos, M. M., Genital human papillomavirus infection in female university students as determined by a PCR-based method, *J. Am. Med. Assoc.*, 1991; 265:472–477.

33. Nishikawa, A., Fukushima, M., Shimada, M., Yamakawa, Y., Shimano, S., Kato, I., and Fujinaga, K., Relatively low prevalence of human papillomavirus 16, 18 and 33 DNA in the normal cervices of Japanese women shown by polymerase chain reaction, *J. Cancer Res.*, 1991; 82:532–326.

34. Czeglédy, J., Rogo, K. O., Evander, M., and Wadell, G., High-risk human papillomavirus types in cytologically normal cervical scrapes from Kenya, *Med. Microbiol. Immunol.*, 1992; 180:321–326.

35. Munoz, N., Bosch, R. X., de Sanjose, S., Tafur, L., Izarzugaza, I., Gili, M., Viladiu, P., Navarro, C., Martos, C., Ascunce, N., Gonzalez, L. C., Kaldor, J. M., Guerrero, E., Lorincz, A., Samtamaria, M., Alonso de Ruiz, P., Aristizabal, N., and Shah, K., The causal link between human papillomavirus and invasive cervical cancer: a population-based case-control study in Columbia and Spain, *Int. J. Cancer*, 1992; 52:743–749.

36. Pao, C. C., Lin, C.-Y., Maa, J.-S., Lai, C.-H., Wu, S.-Y., and Soong, Y.-K., Detection of human papillomavirus in cervicovaginal cells using polymerase chain reaction, *J. Infect. Dis.*, 1990; 161:113–115.

37. Agorastus, T., Bontis, J., Lambropoulos, A. F., Constantinidis, T. C., Nasioutziki, M., Tagou, C., and Katsouyiannopoulous, V., Epidemiology of human papillomavirus infection in Greek asymptomatic women, *Eur. J. Cancer Prev.*, 1995; 4:159–67.

38. Hildesheim, A., Gravitt, P., Schiffman, M. H., Kurman, R. J., Barnes, W., Jones, S., Tchabo, J. G., Brinton, L. A., Copeland, C., Epp, J., and Manos, M. M., Determinants of genital human papillomavirus infection in low-income women in Washington, D.C., *Sex Trans. Dis.*, 1993; 20:279–85.

39. Wheeler, C. M., Parmenter, C. A., Hunt, W. C., Becker, T. M., Greer, C. E., Hildesheim, A., and Manos, M. M., Determinants of genital human papillomavirus infection among cytologically normal women attending the University of New Mexico study health center, *Sex Trans. Dis.*, 1993; 20:286–9.

40. Evander, M., Edlund, K., Gustafsson, A., Jonsson, M., Karlsoon, R., Rylander, E., and Wadell, G., Human papillomavirus infectiton is transient in young women: a population-based cohort study, *J. Infect. Dis.*, 1995; 171:1026–30.

41. Moscicki, A.-B., Palefsky, J., Gonzales, J., and Schoolnik, G. K., Human papillomavirus infection in sexually active adolescent females: prevalence and risk factors, *Pediatr. Res.*, 1990; 28:507–513.

42. Lorincz, A. T., Reid, R., Jenson, A. B., Greenberg, M. D., Lancaster, W., and Kurman, R. J., Human papillomavirus infection of the cervix: Relative risk associations of fifteen common anogenital types, *Obstet. Gynecol.*, 1992; 79:328–337.

43. Fisher, M., Rosenfeld, W. D., and Burk, R. D., Cervicovaginal human papillomavirus infection in suburban adolescents and young adults, *J. Pediatr.*, 1991; 119:821–825.

44. Rosenfeld, W. D., Vermund, S. H., Wentz, S. H., and Burk, R. D., High prevalence rate of human papillomavirus infection and association with abnormal Papanicolaou smears in sexually active adolescents, *Am. J. Dis. Child.*, 1989; 143:1443–1447.

45. Martinez, J., Smith, R., Farmer, M., Resau, J., Alge, L., Daniel, L., Gupta, J., Shah, K., and Naghashfar, Z., High prevalence of genital tract papillomavirus infection in female adolescents, *Pediatrics*, 1988; 82:604–608.

46. Bauer, H. M., Hildesheim, A., Schiffman, M. H., Glass, A. G., Rush, B. B., Scott, D. R., Cadell, D. M., Kurman, R. J., and Manos, M. M., Determinants of genital human papillomavirus infection in low-risk women in Portland, Oregon, *Sex Trans. Dis.*, 1993; 20:274–8.

47. de Villiers, E.-M., Wagner, D., Schneider, A., Wesch, H., Munz, F., Miklaw, H., and zur Hausen, H., Human papillomavirus DNA in women without and with cytological abnormalities: results of a five-year follow-up study, *Gynecol. Oncol.*, 1992; 44:33–39.

48. Bergeron, C., Barrasso, R., Beaudenon, S., Flamant, P., Croissant, O., and Orth, G., Human papillomavirus associated with cervical intraepithelial neoplasia, *Am. J. Surg. Pathol.*, 1992: 16:641–649.

49. McCance, D. J., Campion, M. J., Clarkson, P. K., Chesters, P. M., Jenkins, D., and Singer, A., Prevalence of human papillomavirus type 16 DNA sequences in cervical intraepithelial neoplasia and invasive carcinoma of the cervix, *Br. J. Obstet. Gynaecol.*, 1985; 92:1101–1105.

50. Lorincz, A. T., Schiffman, M. H., Jaffurs, W. J., Marlow, J., Quinn, A. P., and Temple, G. F., Temporal associations of human papillomavirus infection with cervical cytologic abnormalities, *Am. J. Obstet. Gynecol.*, 1990; 162:645–651.

51. Ong, C.-K., Chan, S.-Y., Savaria, C. M., Fujninaga, K., Mavromara-Nazos, P., Labropoulou, V., Pfister, H., Tay, S.-K., ter Meulen, J., Villa, L. L., and Bernard, H.-U., Evolution of human papillomavirus type 18: an ancient phylogenetic root in Africa and intratype diversity reflect coevolution with human ethnic groups, *J. Virol.*, 1993; 67:6424–6431.

52. Ho, L., Chan, S.-Y., Burk, R. D., Das, B. C., Fujinaga, K., Icenogle, J. P., Kahn, T., Kiviat, N., Lancaster, W., Mavromara-Nazos, P., Labropoulou, V., Mitrani-Rosenbaum, S., Norrild, B., Radhakrishna, P. M., Stoerker, J., Syrjaenen, K., Syrjaenen, S., Tay, S.-K., Villa, L. L., Wheeler, C. M., Williamson, A.-L., and Bernard, H.-U., The genetic drift of human papillomavirus type 16 is a means of reconstructing prehistoric viral spread and the movement of ancient human populations, *J. Virol.,* 1993; 67:6413–6423.

53. Bosch, F. X., Manos, M. M., Munoz, N., Sherman, M., Jansen, A. M., Peto, J., Schiffman, M. H., Moreno, V., Kurman, R., and Shah, K. V., Prevalence of human papillomavirus in cervical cancer: a worldwide perspective, International Biological Study on Cervical Cancer Study Group, *J. Natl. Cancer Inst.,* 1995; 87:796–802.

54. Chan, S.-Y., Bernard, H.-U., Ong, C. K., Chan, S. P., Hofmann, B., and Delius, H., Phylogenetic analysis of 48 papillomavirus types and 28 subtypes and variants: a showcase for the molecular evolution of DNA viruses, *J. Virol.,* 1992; 66:5714–5725.

55. Xi, L. F., Demers, G. W., Koutsky, L. A., Kiviat, N. B., Kuypers, J., Watts, D. H., Holmes, K. K., and Galloway, D. A., Analysis of human papillomavirus type 16 variants indicates establishment of persistent infection, *J. Infect. Dis.,* 172:747–755.

56. Collins, J. E., Jenkins, D., and McCance, D. J., Detection of human papillomavirus DNA sequences by *in situ* DNA-DNA hybridization in cervical intraepithelial neoplasia and invasive carcinoma: a retrospective study, *J. Clin. Pathol.,* 1988; 41:289–295.

57. Nuovo, G. J., MacConnell, P., Forde, A., and Delvenne, P., Detection of human papillomavirus DNA in formalin-fixed tissues by *in situ* hybridization after amplification by polymerase chain reaction, *Am. J. Pathol.,* 1991; 139:847–854.

58. Anderson, S. M., Brooke, P. K., Van-Eyck, S. L., Noell, H., and Frable, W. J., Distribution of human papillomavirus types in genital lesions from two temporally distinct populations determined by *in situ* hybridization, *Hum. Pathol.,* 1993; 24:547–553.

59. Morrison, E. A., Goldberg, G. L., Hagan, R. J., Kadish, A. S., and Burk, R. D., Self-administered home cervicovaginal lavage: a novel tool for the clinical-epidemiologic investigation of genital human papillomavirus infections, *Am. J. Obstet. Gynecol.,* 1992; 167:104–107.

60. Moscicki, A.-B., Comparison between methods for human papillomavirus DNA testing: a model for self-testing in young women, *J. Infect. Dis.,* 1993; 167:723–725.

61. Burk, R. D., Kadish, A. S., Calderin, S., and Romney, S. L., Human papillomavirus infection of the cervix detected by cervicovaginal lavage and molecular hybridization: Correlation with biopsy results and Papanicolaou smear, *Am. J. Obstet. Gynecol.,* 1986; 154:982–989.

62. Grussendorf-Conen, E. I., de Villiers, E.-M., and Gissman, L., Human papillomavirus genomes in penile smears of healthy men [letter], *Lancet,* 1986; II:1092.

63. van den Brule, A. J., Claas, E. C., du Maine, M., Melchers, W. J., Helmerhorst, T., Quint, W. G., Lindeman, J., Meijer, C. J., and Walboomers, J. M., Use of anticontamination primers in the polymerase chain reaction for the detection of human papilloma virus genotypes in cervical scrapes and biopsies, *J. Med. Virol.,* 1989; 29:20–27.

64. Bavin, P. J., Giles, J. A., Deery, A., Crow, J., Griffiths, P. D., Emery, V. C., and Walker, P. G., Use of semi-quantitative PCR for human papillomavirus DNA type 16 to identify women with high grade cervical disease in a population presenting with a mildly dyskaryotic smear report, *Br. J. Cancer,* 1993; 67:602–605.

65. Cuzick, J., Singer, A., De Stavola, B. L., and Chomet, J., Case-control study of risks factors for cervical intraepithelial neoplasia in young women, *Eur. J. Cancer,* 1990; 26:684–690.

66. Reeves, W. C., Brinton, L. A., Garcia, M., Brenes, M. M., Herrero, R., Gaitan, E., Tenorio, P., De Britton, R. C., and Rawls, W. E., Human papillomavirus infection and cervical cancer in Latin America, *New Engl. J. Med.,* 1989; 320: 1437–1441.

67. Mullis, K., Faloona, F., Scharf, S., Saiki, R., Horn, G., and Erlich, H., Specific enzymatic amplification of DNA *in vitro*: the polymerase chain reaction. *Cold Spring Harb. Symp. Quant. Biol.,* 1986; 51:263–73.

68. Saiki, R. K., Gelfand, D. H., Stoffel, S., Scharf, S. J., Higuchi, R., Horn, G. T., Mullis, K. B., and Erlich, H. A., Primer-directed enzymatic amplification of DNA with a thermostable DNA polymerase, *Science,* 1988; 239:487–91.

69. Quinn, T. C., Recent advcances in diagnosis of sexually transmitted diseases, *Sex. Trans. Dis.,* 1994; 21:S19–27.

70. Oriel, J. D., Natural history of genital warts, *Br. J. Vener. Dis.*, 1971; 47:1–13.
71. Cook, L. S., Koutsky, L. A., and Holmes, K. K., Circumsion and sexually transmitted diseases, *Am. J. Public Health*, 1994; 84:197–201.
72. Cook, L. S., Koutsky, L. A., and Holmes, K. K., Clinical presentation of genital warts among circumcised and uncircumcised heterosexual men attending an urban STD clinic, *Genitourin. Med.*, 1993; 69:262–64.
73. Syrjänen, S. M., von Krogh, G., and Syrjänen, K. J., Detection of human papillomavirus DNA in anogenital condylomata in men using *in situ* DNA hybridisation applied to paraffin sections, *Genitourin. Med.*, 1987; 63:32–39.
74. Nuovo, G. J., Hochman, H. A., Eliezri, Y. D., Lastarria, D., Comite, S. L., and Silvers, D. N., Detection of human papillomavirus DNA in penile lesions histologically negative for condylomata. Analysis by *in situ* hybridization and the polymerase chain reaction, *Am. J. Surg. Pathol.*, 1990; 14:829–836.
75. Hillman, R. J., Botcherby, M., Ryait, B. K., Hanna, N., and Taylor-Robinson, D., Detection of human papillomavirus DNA in the urogenital tracts of men with anogenital warts, *Sex Transm. Dis.*, 1993; 20:21–27.
76. Rock, B., Shah, K. V., Farmer, E. R., A morpholigic, pathologic, and virologic study of anogenital warts in men, *Arch. Dermatol.*, 1992; 127:495–500.
77. Demeter, L. M., Stoler, M. H., Bonnez, W., Corey, L., Pappas, P., Strussenberg, J., and Reichman, R. C., Penile intraepithelial neoplasia: Clinical presentation and an analysis of the physical state of human papillomavirus DNA, *J. Infect. Dis.*, 1993; 168:38–46.
78. Langenberg, A., Cone, R. W., McDougall, J., Kiviat, N., and Corey, L., Dual infection with human papillomavirus in a population with overt genital condylomas, *J. Am. Acad. Dermatol.*, 1993; 28:434–442.
79. Levine, R. U., Crum, C. P., Herman, E., Silvers, D., Ferenczy, A., and Richart, R. M., Cervical papillomavirus infection and intraepithelial neoplasia: a study of the male sexual partners, *Obstetr. Gynecol.*, 1984; 64:16–20.
80. Sand, P., Bowen, L., Blischke, S., and Ostergard, D. R., Evaluation of male consorts of women with genital human papillomavirus infection, *Obstetr. Gynecol.*, 1986; 68:679–681.
81. Sedlacek, T. V., Cunnane, M., and Carpiniello, V., Colposcopy in the diagnosis of penile condyloma, *Am. J. Obstetr. Gynecol.*, 1986; 154:494–496.
82. Brasso, R., de Brux, J., Croissant, O., and Orth, G., High prevalence of papillomavirus-associated penile intraepithelial neoplasia in sexual partners of women with cervical intraepithelial neoplasia, *New Engl. J. Med.*, 1987; 317:916–923.
83. Krebs, H. B. and Schneider, V., Human papillomavirus-associated lesions of the penis: colposcopy, cytology and histology, *Obstetr. Gynecol.*, 1987; 70:299–304.
84. Cecchini, S., Cipparone, I., Confortini, M., Scuderi, A., Meini, L., and Piazzesi, G., Urethral cytology of cytobrush specimens: a new technique for detecting subclinical HPV infection in men, *Acta. Cytol.*, 1988; 32:314–317.
85. Campion, M. J., McCance, D. J., Mitchell, H. S., Jenkins, D., and Singer, A., Subclinical penile human papillomavirus infection and dysplasia in consorts of women with cervical neoplasia, *Genitourin. Med.*, 1988; 64:90–99.
86. Schneider, A., Kirchmayr, R., De Villiers, E.-M., and Gissman, L., Subclinical human papillomavirus infections in male sexual partners of female carriers, *J. Urol.*, 1988; 140:1431–1434.
87. Costa, S., Syrjänen, S., Vendra, C., Chang, F., Guida, G., Tervahauta, A., Hippeläinen, M., and Syrjänen, K., Detection of human papillomavirus infections in the male sexual partners of women attending an STD clinic in Bologna, *Int. J. STD AIDS*, 1992; 3:338–346.
88. Wikström, A., Hedblad, M.-A., Johansson, B., Kalantari, M., Syrjänen, Lindberg, M., and von Krogh, G., The acetic acid test in evaluation of subclinical genital papillomavirus infection: A comparative study on penoscopy, histopathology, virology and scanning electron microscopy findings, *Genitourin. Med.*, 1992; 68:90–99.
89. Mazzatenta, C., Andreassi, L., Biagioli, M., Ricci, S., and Ratti, G., Detection and typing of genital papillomaviruses in men with a single polymerase chain reaction and type-specific DNA probes, *J. Am. Acad. Dermatol.*, 1993; 28:704–710.
90. Baken, L. A., Koutsky, L. A., Kuypers, J., Kosorok, M. R., Lee, S. K., Kiviat, N. B., and Holmes, K. K., Genital human papillomavirus infection among male and female sex partners: prevalence and type-specific concordance, *J. Infect. Dis.*, 1995; 171:429–32.

91. Hippeläinen, M., Yliskoski, M., Saarikoski, S., Syrjänen, S., and Syrjänen, K., Genital human papillomavirus lesions of the male sexual partners: the diagnostic accuracy of peniscopy, *Genitoruin. Med.*, 1991; 67:291–296.

92. Barrasso, R., HPV-related genital lesions in men. In: Munoz, N., Bosch, F. X., Shah, K. V., and Meheus, A., Eds., *The Epidemiology of Human Papillomavirus and Cervical Cancer* (IARC Scientific Publications No. 119), Lyon, International Agency for Research on Cancer, 1992, 85–92.

93. Wikström, A., Lidbrink, P., Johansson, B., and von Krogh, G., Penile human papillomavirus carriage among men attending Swedish STD clinics, *Int. J. STD AIDS*, 1991; 12:105–109.

94. Kataoka, A., Claesson, U., Hansson, B. G., Eriksson, M., and Lindh, E., Human papillomavirus infection of the male diagnosed by Southern-blot hybridization and polymerase chain reaction: comparison between urethra samples and penile biopsy samples, *J. Med. Virol.*, 1991; 33:159–164.

95. Hippeläinen, M., Syrjänen, S., Hippeläinen, M., Koskela, H., Pulkkinen, J., Saarikoski, S., and Syrjänen, K., Prevalence and risk factors of genital human papillomavirus (HPV) infection in healthy males: a study on Finnish conscripts, *Sex. Trans. Dis.*, 1993; 20:321–8.

96. van Doornum, G. J. J., Hooykaas, C., Juffermans, L. H. J., van der Lans, S. M. G. A., van der Linden, M. M. D., Coutinho, R. A., and Quint, W. G. V., Prevalence of human papillomavirus infections among heterosexual men and women with multiple sexual partners, *J. Med. Virol.*, 1992; 37:13–21.

97. Omar, R., Choudhury, M., Fischer, J., and Ezpeleta, C., A "Pap" test for men? Male urethral smears as screening tool for detecting subclinical human papillomavirus infection, *Urology*, 1991; 37:110–115.

98. Green, J., Monteiro, E., Bolton, V. N., Sanders, P., and Gibson, P. E., Detection of human papillomavirus DNA by PCR in semen from patients with and without penile warts, *Genitourin. Med.*, 1991; 67:207–210.

99. Nieminen, P., Koskimies, A. I., and Paavonen, J., Human papillomavirus DNA is not transmitted by semen, *Int. J. STD AIDS*, 1991; 2:207–208.

100. Ostrow, R. S., Zachow, K. R., Nimura, M., Okagaki, T., Muller, S., Bender, M., and Faras, A. J., Detection of papillomavirus DNA in human semen, *Science*, 1986; 231:731–733.

101. Kyo, S., Inoue, M., Koyama, M., Fujita, M., Tanizawa, O., and Hakura, A., Detection of high-risk human papillomavirus in the cervix and semen of sex partners, *J. Infect. Dis.*, 1994; 170:682–5.

102. Mandal, D., Haye, K. R., Ray, T. K., Goorney, B. P., Stanbridge, C. M., and Corbitt, G., Prevalence of occult human papillomavirus infection, determined by cytology and DNA hybridization, in heterosexual men attending a genitourinary medicine clinic, *Int. J. STD AIDS*, 1991; 2:351–355.

103. Kiviat, N. B., Critchlow, C. W., Holmes, K. K., Kuypers, J., Sayer, J., Dunphy, C., Surawicz, C., Kirby, P., Wood, R., and Daling, J. R., Association of anal dysplasia and human papillomavirus with immunosuppression and HIV infection among homosexual men, *AIDS*, 1993; 7:43–9.

104. Kashima, H. K., Shah, F., Lyles, A., Glackin, R., Muhammad, N., Turner, L., Van Zandt, S., Whitt, S., and Shah, K., A comparison of risk factors in juvenile-onset and adult-onset recurrent respiratory papillomatosis, *Laryngoscope*, 1992; 102(1):9–13.

105. Sedlacek, T. V., Lindheim, S., Eder, C., Hasty, L., Woodland, M., Ludomirsky, A., and Rando, R. F., Mechanism for human papillomavirus transmission at birth, *Am. J. Obstetr. Gynecol.*, 1989; 161(1):55–59.

106. Smith, E. M., Johnson, S. R., Cripe, T. P., Pignatari, S., and Turek, L., Perinatal vertical transmission of human papillomavirus and subsequent development of respiratory tract papillomatosis, *Anns. of Otology, Rhinol. Laryngol.*, 1991; 100(6):479–483.

107. Smith, E. M., Johnson, S. R., Cripe, T. P., Perlman, S., McGuinnes, G., Jiang, D., Cripe, L., and Turek, L. P., Perinatal transmission and maternal risks of human papillomavirus infection, *Cancer Detect. Prev.*, 1995; 2995:196–205.

108. Fredericks, B. D., Balkin, A., Daniel, H. W., Schonrock, J., Ward, B., and Frazer, I. H., Transmission of human papillomaviruses from mother to child, *Aust. NZ J. Obstetr. Gynaecol.*, 1993; 33:30–2.

109. Armbruster-Moraes, E., Ioshimoto, L. M., Leao, E., Zugaib, M., Presence of human papillomavirus DNA in amniotic fluids of pregnant women with cervical lesions, *Gynecol. Oncol.*, 1994; 54:152–8.

110. Tang, C., Shermeta, D. W., and Wood, C., Congenital condylomata acuminata, *Am. J. Obstetr. Gynecol.*, 1978; 131:912–13.

111. Gutman, L. T., St. Claire, K., Herman-Giddens, M. E., Johnson, W. W., and Phelps, W. C., Evaluation of sexually abused and nonabused young girls for intravaginal human papillomavirus infection, *Am. J. Dis. Children*, 1992; 146(6):694–699.

112. Frasier, L. D., Human papillomavirus infections in children, *Pediatr. Ann.*, 1994; 23:354–60.

113. St. Louis, M. E., Icengole, J. P., Manzila, T., Kamenga, M., Ryder, R. W., Heyward, W. L., and Reeves, W. C., Genital types of papillomavirus in children of women with HIV-1 infection in Kinshasa, Zaire, *Int. J. Cancer*, 1993; 54:181–84.

114. Obalek, S., Misiewicz, J., Jablonska, S., Favre, M., and Orth, G., Childhood condyloma acuminatum: association with genital and cutaneous human papillomaviruses, *Ped. Dermatol.*, 1993; 10:101–106.

IV. Natural History and Association to Cancer

6

HPV Types in Human Disease

Ethel-Michele de Villiers

CONTENTS

I.   INTRODUCTION

As early as the beginning of this century, papillomas were successfully transmitted by cell-free extracts.[1] Soon thereafter, volunteers were subcutaneously inoculated with extracts from laryngeal and genital condylomas. The resulting papillomatous lesions resembled verrucae planae rather than the lesions with exophytic growth from which the extracts originated.[2] These experiments were, at that stage, already indicative of the pathogenic diversity induced by the papillomaviruses.

The human papillomavirus group presently consists of 77 different characterized types, with an additional 30 types already identified, but their complete DNA genomes not yet isolated. The present definition of a new HPV type is that it differs by more than 10% in the DNA sequence of its L1 open reading frame (ORF) to that of the closest related HPV type.

The human papillomaviruses have historically been grouped into the cutaneous types, i.e., those identified in lesions of the skin, and in the mucosal types, i.e., those identified in lesions of mucosal origin, mainly of the genital tract. The DNA genomes of almost all the HPV types have been sequenced during the last few years.[3,4] This lead to a phylogenetic analysis grouping the viruses into different subgroups[5] which, in some cases, does not correspond to the known biological associations. A classification based on DNA sequence only, would certainly present a biased view. The very diverse clinical entities in which these viruses are present will have to be taken into consideration.

The association of a papillomavirus infection to a number of diseases, such as the benign and malignant, mainly squamous cell proliferations of the mucosa of the genital tract, is well known. Not only has its role in the pathogenesis of such benign lesions been of interest, but the mechanism by which a number of HPV types induces malignant changes has been studied and reviewed extensively.[6,7]

The detection of papillomavirus infections in other disease entities has been hampered, in some instances, by the limitations of the detection methods available, and in others, by lack of interest. The mere presence of HPV DNA in benign or malignant lesions does not prove the etiological role of these viruses in the induction of these diseases, but it forms the foundation from which the mechanism of tumor induction can be studied. Probably the most interesting development recently in the detection of papillomavirus DNA sequences in different types of tumors has been the association of HPV DNA to various types of cystic tumors, e.g., epidermoid cysts of the skin,[8] cholesteatomas of the middle ear,[9] and odontogenic cysts.[10] Inverted papillomas of the sinuses[11] and nasal cavity[12] fall into this category as well. These will be discussed in more detail in the following sections.

II.   CUTANEOUS LESIONS

A large number of HPV types have been identified in, and isolated from, benign and malignant lesions of the skin.[13-17]

The HPV types associated primarily with skin lesions are frequently characterized by type-specific macro- and microscopic features. The various types of cutaneous warts can be classified according to the clinical morphology and the infecting HPV type. HPV 1, HPV 2, HPV 3, and HPV 4 each induce a distinct cytopathic effect.[18] This observation formed the foundation for the identification of HPV infection in other cutaneous lesions of which the etiology had previously been unknown.[19] HPV 4 infections are characterized by a homogenous type of inclusion body.[19] Lesions regularly presenting similar cytopathic features are epidermoid cysts. An analysis of a number of such palmoplantar cysts led to the identification and isolation of HPV 60 and HPV 65,[8,20,21] which are both related in their DNA sequences to HPV 4. The homogenous type of inclusion body was also indentifed in different types of pigmented lesions, including pigmented common warts, keratotic flat lesions, and cutaneous horns.[21] The identification of HPV 63 in multiple punctated keratotic lesions on the sole of the foot[21] was based on the same principal. An infection with this HPV type is typically associated with a filamentous type of inclusion body. Although the DNA sequence of HPV 63 is distantly related to that of HPV 1, the type of inclusion bodies induced by these two viruses differ extensively.[19] An HPV 1-induced lesion histologically presents a granular type of inclusion body[19] which is associated with the presence of the E4 protein of this virus.[22,23] The clinical features of the lesions induced by HPV 1 may differ, depending on the anatomical site of such a lesion, e.g., a digitate wart on the upper lip, cutaneous horn on the finger, and a common wart on the dorsum of the foot, in contrast to the classical palmoplantar lesions and lesions occurring on the lateral surfaces of the hands and feet.[24] They do, however, all display the same cytopathic effect, i.e., the granular type of inclusion body.

Epidermodysplasia verruciformis (EV) is an example of a multifactorial disease involving genetic, immunological, and extrinsic factors. Many different types of HPV are induced to cause greatly differing clinical features in these patients. The majority of these HPV types has, over the years, been thought to have infected only this population.[25] Certain lesions, containing the DNA of, e.g., HPV 5, 8, 14, 17, 20, or 47, could, primarily at sun-exposed sites, develop into squamous cell carcinomas.[25-27] Black-skinned patients with EV have a much lower incidence of skin cancer, but develop seborrhoic keratoses, harboring HPV 5 on the sun-exposed areas of the skin.[29]

The development of warts and nonmelanoma skin cancer in patients under immunosuppression has provided us with valuable information. The majority of renal allograft recipients (RARs) develop warts during the period of immunosuppressive therapy.[30] A large proportion of these lesions progress through dysplasia to carcinoma *in situ* or invasive carcinoma on sun-exposed sites.[31,32] Prior to the advent of the highly sensitive polymerase chain reaction (PCR) technique, the DNA of known HPV types were used to probe lesions for identical or related sequences. This lead to the identification of the common cutaneous types, e.g., HPV 2, 3, and 10 in the benign lesions[33] and in single cases, e.g., HPV 5,[34,35] which is usually only found in lesions from EV patients. These latter results could not be confirmed by applying PCR on a number of these same biopsies,[36] indicating a possible cross-hybridization between different HPV types in the method which was applied.

Analyses of similar lesions by using the PCR technique have been reported.[15-17,37] The primers used for amplifying the cellular DNA by Tieben et al.[37] and Berkhout et al.[17] had been designed to amplify the EV-specific group, as well as closely related HPV types. They detected EV-specific, as well as a few putative new HPV types, in benign and malignant lesions from RARs. The results from this laboratory, as well as our own results, revealed the definite presence of the EV-HPV types in the general population. A careful analysis of a large series of warts, pre- and malignant lesions of the skin, which we performed by applying a degenerate PCR technique, lead to the identification of 20 new HPV types, the majority of them related to the HPV 4, 48, 50, 60, and 65-group and the EV-group of HPVs.[15,16] This degenerate PCR method was designed to detect not only all known papillomavirus types, but any related sequences, i.e., putative new papillomaviruses. In a first round of amplification using a mixture of the degenerate primers, i.e., thereby losing in sensitivity and specificity, 62% of the benign proliferations and 56% of the malignant lesions contained HPV DNA. Sequencing of the products revealed a different spectrum of HPV types than the previous Southern blot analyses had resulted in. HPV 27 and HPV 57, both closely related to HPV 2, were detected in 14% of the samples, whereas HPV 2 itself was not present. The same applied for the group of HPV 3-related viruses. HPV 10, HPV 28, and HPV 77 were detected in 24% of the lesions, whereas HPV 3 itself was not detected.

In order to increase the sensitivity and specificity, each biopsy from the malignant lesions was again subjected to DNA amplification, using 16 individual primer combinations. The resulting products were cloned and sequenced.[16] Six HPV types belonging to the so-called "high risk"[38] mucosal group (HPV 16, 51, 54, 56, 61, and 69), were detected in these malignant cutaneous lesions, in contrast to HPV 41 and HPV 60 only, as cutaneous types. The detection of HPV 16 in single cutaneous lesions had been reported earlier. These included an epidermal naevus and a case of squamous cell carcinoma developing from an arsenic keratosis,[38] pre- and malignant lesions of the hand[40-45] and of the lip,[46] as well as HPV 35 in a bowenoid lesion of the finger.[47] These results all accentuate the misconception which existed previously, that is, the strict division by which specific HPV types can only infect specific types of tissue. In a similar investigation of nonmelanoma skin cancers from the nonimmunosuppressed population, the "mucosal" types HPV 6b, 32, 42, and 51 were detected. HPV 6b and HPV 42 are "low-risk" mucosal viruses. Here again, the results underline the notion that any HPV type can infect any cell, although the mechanism by which their genomes are activated to induce lesions in the different cell types may be subjected to specific cellular controlling genes. The detection of a number of EV-specific types in these lesions from the nonimmunosuppressed group, accentuates the general ability of these viruses to infect any population, with the subsequent restricted control of its functions by cellular genes of the host, probably forcing the viral genome into latency. Another observation resulting from the analyses of lesions from immunosuppressed vs. nonimmunosuppressed populations, is multiple infections within one lesion in the former group vs. only one virus type detectable in the latter. The mechanism by which the viral genes are activated here awaits further investigation.

Limited studies have been performed on the role of the papillomavirus genome in the induction of malignant cutaneous lesions. The E6 and E7 open reading frames (ORF) of the "high-risk" HPV types have been shown to be essential for immortalization and the maintenance of the malignant phenotype in the development of malignant genital tumors.[6] It is not clear whether these proteins of the papillomavirus types found in cutaneous lesions, act in a similar way. The mechanism by which they play a role in malignant conversion has not been clarified. *In vitro* studies on HPV types belonging to the EV group and which have been found in malignant lesions HPV 5, 8, and 47, have been reported. These studies have been performed mainly in rodent cells in which the E6 ORF alone seems to be sufficient to induce morphological transformation, whereas the E7 ORF cannot.[48-50] This is in contrast to the corresponding ORFs of HPV 1, which act in the same manner as the "high-risk" genital HPV types[51] and which has been detected in single malignant cutaneous lesions.[32,52]

Another HPV type which has been detected in a small number of squamous cell carcinomas of the skin, is HPV 41. Three of the four patients from whom these biopsies had been taken had received PUVA treatment over an extended period of time.[53] It is known that nonmelanoma skin cancers develop apparently only after modifications had been induced into cellular genes, occurring either as a hereditary event[54] and/or after prolonged exposure to external factors, e.g., UV-radiation or PUVA treatment.[55,56] The tumor suppressor gene, p53, is mutated in about 90% of nonmelanoma carcinomas of the skin. These mutations are typical for UV-radiation.[54,57] p53 plays, among others, an important role in the DNA repair process after exposure to UV-radiation or carcinogens and mutagens.[58] The DNA genome of the prototype HPV 41, isolated from disseminated warts, contains a frame-shift mutation in the E7 ORF. The E7 ORF of a second isolate from an arsenic keratosis lesion was intact.[59] We utilized the E6 and E7 ORFs of these two isolates to transfect the HaCaT cells, a spontaneously immortalized cutaneous keratinocyte cell line harboring a UV-induced mutation in its p53 gene.[60,61] The cell lines resulting after transfection, both induced tumors in nude mice after subcutaneous inoculation, in contrast to the parental nontransfected HaCat cells.[62] The cell line harboring the E6 and interrupted E7 ORFs produced large cystic tumors of highly proliferative cells, whereas the cell line containing the E6 and intact E7 ORFs produced small flat cysts giving the impression of ruptured cysts as evidenced by the formation of foreign body granulomas and the implantation of keratin rests. The mechanism by which this hyperproliferative growth is induced by the E6-interrupted E7 ORFs, is still unclear. It seems as if the E7 ORF may even exert an inhibitory effect on the function of the E6 ORF of this HPV type.

III. URETHRA

Several studies have reported the presence of HPV DNA in samples taken from the distal urethra and from urine. The results from these two types of samples were not always in concordance. HPV DNA was detected in 12/138 (8%) of urethra samples taken from presumably healthy military conscripts, whereas 8/138 (5%) had positive urine samples.[63] In a group of men with external genital condyloma, HPV DNA was present in 114/135 (84%) of these lesions, whereas only 14 (12.3%) had intraurethral condyloma.[64] A similar pattern was observed in female patients, where HPV DNA was present in 83% of the wart biopsies vs. 25% of urethral loop specimens.[65]

Reports on the presence of HPV DNA in carcinoma of the urethra are limited. Grußendorf-Conen et al.[66] detected HPV 6 DNA in such a lesion, and Wiener et al.[67] tested archival surgical specimens from 14 patients. They detected HPV 16 DNA in 4 (29%) of these samples, whereas none of the other 10 HPV types tested for was present. The clinical data revealed that the HPV positive tumors were located in the pendulous urethra, rather than in the bulbar urethra.

These results again point to the fact that, although the HPV infections may be widespread throughout the urogenital tract, certain types of tissues have a predilection for the replication of the papillomavirus genome in comparison to others.

IV. BLADDER

The observation of koilocytotic changes in the histology of bladder neoplasias has been indicative of the association of an HPV infection.[68] Attempts to identify HPV sequences in such lesions has, however, resulted in varying opinions. By using the most sensitive techniques, Knowles[69] could not detect one positive sample among biopsies from 100 transitional cell tumors, 6 carcinoma *in situ*, 2 adenocarcinoma, 1 squamous cell carcinoma, and 12 bladder cell lines, and Chang et al. (1994) did not find HPV DNA in 108 transitional cell tumors. In contrast, Furihata et al.[71] and LaRue et al.[72] found 28/90 (31%) and 28/71 (39%) of these tumors to contain HPV DNA. In a study on archival bladder carcinoma specimens, Maloney et al.[73] detected HPV 18 in 1/22 squamous cell carcinomas, but in 0/20 transitional carcinomas. The patient from which this HPV 18 containing biopsy was taken had been a renal transplant recipient. Similarly, in a study testing 75 transitional cell carcinomas, HPV 16 DNA was detected in 2 cases, and in both the patients had been immunosuppressed after undergoing renal and cardiac transplantation.[74]

We have examined a large series of malignant bladder tumors, as well as several cell lines, for the presence of known HPV types. Only one sample contained HPV-related sequences. Additional studies using degenerate primers in the PCR, are required to determine the possible etiological role of an infection with a yet unidentified HPV type in the development of carcinoma of the bladder.

V. COLON

The possible association of an HPV infection with the development of carcinoma of the colon could not be established to date. Shah et al.[75] examined 50 samples of colorectal carcinoma using the PCR technique. No HPV DNA could be detected in any of these biopsies. Koulos et al.[76] examined 7 colorectal adenocarcinomas and 3 adenomatous polyps of the colon and found all samples void of detectable HPV DNA. Schroyer et al.[77] could not detect HPV DNA in 22 colonic adenocarcinomas, but found such DNA in 5 (100%) of anorectal carcinomas tested. We could not detect any HPV DNA sequences in our series of colorectal tumors.

VI. BREAST

Normal ductal cells of the breast can be immortalized by the HPV 16 and HPV 18 E6 genes. The mechanism of this immortalization is different from that observed in genital keratinocytes[78] in which both the E6 and E7 genes are needed to induce this change. We, as others,[79,80] have failed to detect any HPV sequences in malignant tumors of the breast, although one group has reported the presence of HPV 16 DNA in 29% of carcinomas.[81]

VII. EYE

Papillomatous changes of the conjunctiva may develop, although this is a rare event. A few single cases of conjunctival papillomas containing HPV DNA, have been reported.[82] In a larger study,[83] the presence of HPV 6 and HPV 11 DNA was reported in 15 of 23 conjunctival papillomas. We could detect HPV 6/11 sequences in 14 of 20 papillomatous changes of the conjunctiva.[84]

Malignant changes of the conjunctiva is also a rare event. McDonnell et al.[85] detected HPV 16 DNA in 88% of samples in a series of 42 lesions ranging from mild dysplasia to infiltrating squamous cell carcinoma. Lauer et al.[86] found HPV 16 (4 of 5 samples) and HPV 18 (2 of 5 samples) in conjunctival intraepithelial neoplasias, and Oldrich et al.[87] and Tritten et al.[88] each reported patients with bilateral malignant tumors containing HPV DNA. We could demonstrate HPV 16 DNA in one case of squamous cell carcinoma of the conjunctiva.

VIII. LESIONS OF THE UPPER AERODIGESTIVE TRACT

A.   Oral Cavity

A number of HPV types commonly found in the lesions of the genital tract were originally identified and isolated from lesions of the upper respiratory tract. The first HPV 11 isolate originates from a laryngeal papilloma,[89] HPV 30 from a laryngeal carcinoma,[90] and HPV 57 from an inverted papilloma of the maxillary sinus.[11] The two HPV types isolated from oral lesions, i.e., focal epithelial hyperplasia, HPV 13 and HPV 32, have not been associated with lesions other than the oral cavity.[91]

Infection of the oral mucosa with HPV types usually associated with genital lesions is not surprising, although these infections most probably remain subclinical.[92] The majority of papillomatous lesions of the oral mucosa in the nonimmunosuppressed population contain HPV 6, HPV 11, or in single cases, HPV 2 DNA.[91,93] To our knowledge, all efforts to detect HPV DNA in florid oral papillomatosis have remained negative.

The lesions developing in patients under immunosuppression again gives us an indication of possible latent infections in the immunocompetent population. Patients infected with HIV frequently develop oral papillomas,[94] as well as facial skin lesions.[95] In these studies, HPV 7 DNA was detected in a large percentage of the lesions. This was surprising at the time, as HPV 7 had previously been isolated from, and associated with, cutaneous warts developing extensively on the hands of people handling meat,[96] and had otherwise only been identified in cutaneous lesions of immunosuppressed patients.[97] We recently reexamined the lesions originating from HIV infected patients by applying the polymerase chain reaction with different combinations of degenerate primers.[98] HPV DNA was detected in 67% (45/67) of the samples. HPV 7 (19%) and HPV 32 (22%) were the most predominant HPV types. Other known HPV types detected were HPV 2a, 6b, 13, 16, 18, 55, 59, and 69. Two new HPV types, HPV 72 and HPV 73, were isolated from oral warts with atypia. An interesting result was the presence of HPV 32 in 2/4 fibromas. Control samples, taken from normal oral mucosa, contained HPV 16 and HPV 18 in 2/7 samples tested.

Many investigations have been published[93] subsequent to the report of HPV 16 DNA in tongue carcinoma.[99] Cofactors, such as smoking and alcohol, have regularly been associated with the development of malignant oral lesions. HPV DNA was recently reported in 74% of oral cancers in Indian betel quid chewers,[100] although another study on betel-associated oral cancers from Papua, New Guinea could detect HPV DNA in only 2/30 samples (6.7%).[101] The clinical entity, proliferative verrucous leukoplakia, described as multifocal oral lesions frequently progressing to oral cancer in the absence of tobacco use, has also been shown to contain HPV DNA in the majority of lesions tested.[102] Another study also reported the presence of HPV DNA in oral cancers of a percentage of patients who had never smoked.[103]

Tongue carcinomas often contain HPV 16 DNA, although other HPV types such as HPV 2, HPV 6, HPV 33, and HPV-related types have been reported.[91,93,104,105]

The number of HPV negative tumors of the oral cavity, however, remains large, even though the histology is indicative of an infection by papillomaviruses.[106]

The origin of the odontogenic cysts is, similar to cholesteatomas, either developmental or inflammatory.[107] These are cysts lined with epithelium and located in the jaw. We recently examined odontogenic cysts for the presence of HPV DNA and detected such sequences in more than 50% of the 20 samples.[10]

B.   Nasal and Paranasal Sinuses

Evidence of papillomavirus DNA in papillomatous lesions and cancers of the nasal cavity and the paranasal sinuses has increased rapidly. Inverted papillomas frequently develop in this area and tend to progress to malignant tumors. These tumors subsequently lead to bone erosion, often resulting in the death of the patient. HPV 57 was isolated from such an inverted papilloma of the maxillary sinus.[11] This lesion recurred and the patient died after skull erosion. These inverted papillomas tend to follow the same clinical progression as seen in cholesteatomas of the middle ear. HPV 57 has subsequently been detected in a series of benign squamous papillomas, as well as inverted papillomas with and without carcinoma.[12] HPV 6 and HPV 11 are also often found in these lesions,[108] whereas the malignant lesions contain HPV 16 and HPV 18[108,109] and, in single cases, HPV 6 DNA.[110,111]

C. Tonsils

Tonsillar carcinoma is a rare disease. HPV DNA has been detected in 10/10 lesions examined by Snijders et al.[112] HPV 7, 16, 33, and an HPV-related DNA sequence were present. Two of 3 samples tested by Brachman et al.[113] contained HPV 16-related DNA sequences and 2 of 4 samples tested by Lewensohn-Fuchs et al.[114] contained HPV 16 DNA. HPV 6 was found in a single tonsillar carcinoma by Bercovich et al.,[115] and we detected HPV DNA in 3 of 5 of the lesions.[116]

D. Pharynx and Larynx

Laryngeal carcinomas have frequently received attention. It has not been possible to pinpoint a specific HPV type as being the most prevalent in either squamous cell carcinoma or verrucous carcinoma of the larynx. The detection of HPV DNA reported in different studies varies considerably from 0% (0/11),[117] 8% (3/40),[118] 10.5% (6/57),[119] 22.2% (8/36),[120] 24% (11/45),[121] and 45% (13/29),[122] to mention only a few. These data deserve clarification in additional studies. HPV DNA has also been detected in a few cases of carcinoma of the pharynx and hypopharynx.[123,124]

E. Ear

Cholesteatoma of the middle ear is a relatively common aural disorder which frequently results in hearing loss and other complications relating to bone resorption.[125] The accumulation of keratinizing squamous epithelium is characteristic and it is histopathologically defined as an epidermoid cyst.[126] In the majority of cases, cholesteatomas are acquired (vs. congenital), e.g., after perforation of the tympanic membrane, and is usually associated with an inflammatory reaction. Histologically, this aggressively growing, bone-destructing tumor shows papillary growth and koilocytosis, which are characteristics of papillomavirus-induced lesions. We examined a series of 45 biopsies from 42 patients with middle-ear cholesteatoma.[9] HPV DNA was detected in 36% (16/45). The PCR products hybridized under stringent conditions to HPV 11 DNA after HPV 11 had been confirmed by sequencing 3 of these products.

F. Lung

Benign and malignant tumors of the bronchi often develop in patients with a history of multiple laryngeal papillomas. Such patients who had been treated with irradiation have a 16-fold increased risk of a subsequent carcinoma in the respiratory system.[127] These carcinomas usually contain HPV DNA.[128-131]

Lung carcinomas developing in other patients have been tested extensively for the presence of papillomavirus DNA. Stremlau et al.[132] initially reported HPV 16-related DNA in an anaplastic tumor of the lung. Subsequent studies by other groups revealed controversial results.[93] We could not detect any HPV sequences in a series of 80 biopsies from lung cancers by using a degenerate PCR technique.[133] Similar results have been reported.[134,135] These results are in contrast to the clinical and histological data on the development of such tumors. Based on this information, an HPV etiology had been suggested for these tumors almost 20 years ago.[136] A reexamination of carcinomas of the lung, using a series of primer combinations in the PCR as has been performed on cutaneous lesions,[16] will probably solve this controversy.

G.   Esophagus

Squamous cell papilloma of the esophagus is apparently very rarely diagnosed. These lesions develop mainly as a result of mucosal damage. HPV DNA has been demonstrated in such lesions, i.e., HPV 16 DNA at an endoscopic injection sclerotherapy site[137] and HPV 6 DNA in 1/23 papillomas[138] developing in a group of patients presenting with hiatus hernia, gastroesophageal reflux, or esophagitis.[139] In another study, Poljak et al.[140] detected HPV 6 in 1/29 (3%) esophageal papillomas.

Esophageal carcinoma occurs very frequently in certain groups of people, e.g., in the high-incidence area of China. In a series of 85 tumors from China, HPV DNA was detected in 34 (40%) biopsies. The HPV types included HPV 6, 11, 16, 18, and 30.[141] Other groups report HPV DNA in 3/45 (7%) of lesions,[142] 5/12 (42%),[143] 24/71 (34%),[144] 24/40 (60%),[145] 25/48 (52%),[146] and 0/31 (0%).[147] These samples were taken from cases from different population groups, i.e., either with high or with low incidence rates. We have tested more than 100 samples obtained from different population groups, but have to date been unable to detect any HPV sequences. Togawa et al.[148] recently reported HPV 16 and HPV 18, as well as the isolation of an HPV 23-related DNA sequence amplified by PCR, in 22% (17/72) of the esophageal carcinomas tested. This putative new sequence was present in 14% of the carcinomas tested.[149] It will be of great importance to use this sequence in analyzing the samples included in the studies mentioned above. This may contribute to the clarification of an otherwise confusing field of research.

REFERENCES

1. Ciuffo, G., Innesto positivo con filtrada de verrucae volgare. *G. Ital. Mal. Venereol.*, 48, 12, 1907.
2. Waelsch, L., Übertragungsversuche mit spitzem Kondylom. *Arch. Dermat. Syph.*, 124, 625–646, 1917.
3. Delius, H., Hofmann, B., Primer-directed sequencing of human papillomavirus types. *Curr. Top. Microbiol. Immunol.*, 86, 13–31, 1994.
4. Delius, H., unpublished data, 1995.
5. Chan, S.-Y., Delius, H., Halpern, A. L., Bernard, H.-U. Analysis of genomic sequences of 95 papillomavirus types: Uniting typing, phylogeny, and taxonomy. *J. Virol.*, 69, 3074–3083, 1995.
6. zur Hausen, H., Molecular pathogenesis of cancer of the cervix and its causation by specific human papillomavirus types, *Curr. Top. Microbiol. Immunol.*, 186, 131–156.
7. zur Hausen, H., de Villiers, E.-M., Human papillomaviruses, *Ann. Rev. Mircobiol.*, 48, 427–447, 1994.
8. Egawa, K., Inaba, Y., Ono, T., Arao, T., "Cystic papilloma" in humans? Demonstration of human papillomavirus in plantar epidermoid cysts, *Arch. Dermatol.*, 126, 1599–1603, 1990.
9. Bergmann, K., Hoppe, F., He, Y., Helms, J., Müller-Hermelink, H.-K., Stremlau, A., de Villiers, E.-M., Human-papillomavirus DNA in cholesteatomas, *Int. J. Cancer*, 59, 463–466, 1994.
10. Neumann, T., Williams, D., de Villiers, E.-M., unpublished results, 1995.
11. de Villiers, E.-M., Hirsch-Behnam, A., von Knebel Doeberitz, C., Neumann, C., zur Hausen, H., Two newly identified human papillomavirus types (HPV 40 and 57) isolated from mucosal lesions, *Virology*, 171, 248–253, 1989.
12. Wu, T.-C., Trujillo, J. M., Kashima, H. K., Mounts, P., Association of human papillomavirus with nasal neoplasia, *Lancet*, 341, 522–524, 1993.
13. de Villiers, E.-M., Heterogeneity of the human papillomavirus group, *J. Virol.*, 63, 4898–4903, 1989.
14. de Villiers, E.-M., Human papillomavirus: An update, *Curr. Top. Microbiol. Immunol.*, 186, 1-12, 1994.
15. Shamanin, V., Glover, M., Rausch, C., Proby, C., Leigh, I. M., zur Hausen, H., de Villiers, E.-M., Specific types of human papillomavirus found in benign proliferations and carcinomas of the skin in immunosuppressed patients, *Cancer Res.*, 54, 4610–4613, 1994.
16. Shamanin, V., zur Hausen, H., Lavergne, D., Proby, C. M., Leigh, I. M., Neumann, C., Hamm, H., Goos, M., Haustein, U.-F., Jung, E. G., Plewig, G., Wolff, H., de Villiers, E.-M., HPV infections in nonmelanoma skin cancers from renal transplant recipients and nonimmunosuppressed patients, *J. Natl. Cancer Inst.*, 88, 802–811, 1996.

17. Berkhout, R. J. M., Tieben, L. M., Smits, H. L., Bouwes Bavinck, J. N., Vermeer, B. J., ter Schegget, J., Nested PCR approach for detection and typing of epidermodysplasia verruciformis-associated human papillomavirus types in cutaneous cancers from renal transplant recipients, *J. Clin. Microbiol.,* 33, 690–695, 1995.

18. Jablonska, S., Orth, G., Obalek, S., Croissant, O., Cutaneous warts. Clinical, histological and virological correlations, in *Clinics in Dermatology,* Jablonska, S., and Orth, G., Eds., Lippinkott, Philadelphia, 1985, vol. 3, 71–82.

19. Egawa, K., New types of human papillomaviruses and intracytoplasmic inclusion bodies: a classification of inclusion warts according to clinical features, histology and associated HPV types, *Br. J. Dermatol.,* 130, 158–166, 1994.

20. Matsukura, T., Iwasaki, T., Kawashima, M., Molecular cloning of a novel human papillomavirus (type 60) from a plantar cyst with characteristic pathological changes, *Virology,* 190, 561–564, 1992.

21. Egawa, K., Delius, H., Matsukura, T., Kawashima, M., de Villiers, E.-M., Two novel types of human papillomavirus, HPV 63 and HPV 65: comparisons of their clinical and histological features and DNA sequences to other HPV types. *Virology,* 94, 789–799, 1993.

22. Doorbar, J., Evans, H. S., Coneron, I., Crawford, L. V., Gallimore, P. H., Analysis of HPV-1 E4 gene expression using epitope-defined antibodies, *EMBO J.,* 7, 825–833, 1988.

23. Rogel-Gaillard, C., Breitburd, F., Orth, G., Human papillomavirus type 1 E4 proteins differing by their N-terminal ends have distinct cellular localizations when transiently expressed in vitro. *J. Virol.,* 66, 816–823, 1992.

24. Egawa, K., Inaba, Y., Yoshimura, K., Ono, T., Varied clinical morphology of HPV-1-induced warts, depending on anatomical factors, *Br. J. Dermatol.,* 128, 271-276, 1993.

25. Orth, G., Epidermodysplasia verruciformis: a model for understanding the oncogenicity of human papillomaviruses, in *Papillomaviruses,* Ciba Foundation Symp. 120, John Wiley & Sons, Chichester, 1986, 157–174.

26. Yutsudo, M., Shimake, T., Hakura, A., Human papillomavirus type 17 DNA in skin carcinoma tissue of a patient with epidermodysplasia verruciformis, *Virology,* 144, 295–298, 1985.

27. Kanda, R., Tanigaki, T., Kitano, Y., Yoshikawa, K., Yutsudo, M., Hakura, A., Types of human papillomavirus isolated from Japanese patients with epidermodysplasia verruciformis, *Br. J. Dermatol.,* 121, 463–469, 1989.

28. Kiyono, T., Adachi, A., Ishibashi, M., Genome organisation and taxonomic position of human papillomavirus type 47 inferred from its DNA sequence, *Virology,* 177, 401–405, 1990.

29. Jacyk, W. K., de Villiers, E-M., Epidermodysplasia verruciformis in Africans, *Int. J. Dermatol.,* 32, 806–810, 1993.

30. Penn, I., Post-transplant kidney cancers and skin cancers (including Kaposi's sarcoma), in *Cancer in Organ Transplant Recipients,* Schmähl, D., and Penn, I., Eds., Springer-Verlag, Berlin, 1991, 46–53.

31. Purdie, K. J., Sexton, C. J., Proby, C. M., Glover, M. T., Williams, A. T., Stables, J. N., Leigh, I. M., Malignant transformation of cutaneous lesions in renal allograft patients: a role for human papillomavirus? *Cancer Res.,* 53, 5328–5333, 1993.

32. Stark, L. A., Arends, M. J., McLaren, K. M., Benton, E. C., Shahidullah, H., Hunter, J. A. A., Bird, C. C., Prevalence of human papillomavirus DNA in cutaneous neoplasms from renal allograft recipients supports a possible viral role in tumor promotion, *Br. J. Cancer,* 69, 222–229, 1994.

33. Obalek, S., Favre, M., Szymanczyk, J., Misiwiecz, J., Jablonska, S., Orth, G., Human papillomavirus (HPV) types specific of epidermodysplasia veruciformis induced by HPV 3 or HPV 3-related types in immunosuppressed patients, *J. Invest. Dermatol.,* 98, 936–941, 1992.

34. Barr, B. B. B., Beriton, E. C., McLaren, K., Bunney, M. H., Smith, J. W., Blessing, K., Hunter, J. A. A., Human papillomavirus infection in skin cancer in renal allograft recipients, *Lancet,* i, 124–129, 1988.

35. Soler, C., Chardonnet, Y., Euvrard, S., Chignol, M. C., Thivolet, J., Evaluation of human papillomavirus type 5 on frozen sections of multiple lesions from transplant recipients with in situ hybridization and non-isotopic probes, *Dermatology,* 184, 248–253, 1992.

36. de Villiers, E.-M., Benton, E. C., unpublished data, 1995.

37. Tieben, L. M., Berkhout, R. J. M., Smits, H. L., Bouwes Bavinck, J. N., Vermeer, B. J., Bruijn, J. A., van der Woude, F. J., ter Schegget, J., Detection of epidermodysplasia verruciformis-like human papillomavirus types in malignant and premalignant skin lesions of renal transplant recipients. *Br. J. Dermatol.,* 131, 226–230, 1994.

38. zur Hausen, H., Human genital cancer: synergism between two virus infections or synergism between a virus infection and initiating events. *Lancet*, 2, 1370–1372, 1986.

39. de Villiers, E.-M., Implication of papillomaviruses in nongenital tumours, in *Herpes and Papillomaviruses*, de Palo, R., Rilke, F., and zur Hausen, H., Eds., Raven Press, New York, 1988, 65–70.

40. Kühnl-Petzold, C., Grösser, A., de Villiers, E.-M., HPV 16 assozierter bowenoid-verrucösser Tumor der palmaren Haut. *Akt. Dermatologica*, 14, 848–849, 1988.

41. Moy, R. L., Eliezri, Y. D., Nuovo, G. J., Zitelle, J. A., Bennett, B. G., Silverstein, S., Human papillomavirus type 16 DNA in periungual squamous cell carcinomas, *J. Am. Med. Assoc.*, 261, 2669–2673, 1989.

42. Ostrow, R. S., Shaver, M. K., Turnquist, S., Viksnins, A., Bender, M., Vance, C., Kaye, V., Faras, A. J., Human papillomavirus-16 DNA in a cutaneous invasive cancer, *Arch. Dermatol.*, 125, 666–669, 1989.

43. Eliezri, Y. D., Silverstein, S. J., Nuovo, G. J., Occurrence of human papillomavirus type 16 DNA in cutaneous squamous and basal cell neoplasms, *J. Am. Acad. Dermatol.*, 23, 836–842, 1990.

44. Moy, R. L., Quan, M. B., The presence of human papillomavirus type 16 in squamous cell carcinoma of the proximal finger and reconstruction with a bilobed transposition flap, *J. Dermatol. Surg. Oncol.*, 17, 171–175, 1991.

45. Grob, J. J., Zarour, H., Jacquemier, J., Hassoun, J., Bonerandi, J. J., Extra-genital HPV 16-related bowenoid papulosis, *Genitourin. Med.*, 67, 18–20, 1991.

46. Kawashima, M., Favre, M., Obalek, S., Jablonska, S., Orth, G., Premalignant lesions and cancers of the skin in the general population: evaluation of the role of human papillomaviruses. *J. Invest. Dermatol.*, 95, 537–542, 1990.

47. Rüdlinger, R., Grob, R., Yu, Y. X., Schnyder, U. W., Human papillomavirus-35-positive verruca with bowenoid dysplasia of the periungual area, *Arch. Dermatol.*, 125, 655–659, 1989.

48. Kiyono, T., Nagashima, K., Ishibashi, M., The primary structure of major viral RNA in a rat cell line transfected with type 47 human papillomavirus DNA and the transforming activity of its cDNA and E6 gene, *Virology*, 173, 473-478, 1989.

49. Hiraiwa, A., Kiyono, T., Segawa, K., Utsumi, K. R., Ohashi, M., Ishibashi, M., Comparative study on E6 and E7 genes of some cutaneous and genital papillomaviruses of human origin for their ability to transform 3Y1 cells, *Virology*, 192, 102–111, 1993.

50. Kiyono, T., Hiraiwa, A., Ishii, S., Takahashi, T., Ishibashi, M., Inhibition of p53-mediated transactivation by E6 of type 1, but not type 5, 8, or 47 human papillomavirus of cutaneous origin, *J. Virol.*, 68, 4656–4661, 1994.

51. Schmitt, A., Harry, J. B., Rapp, B., Wettstein, F. O., Iftner, T., Comparison of the properties of the E6 and E7 genes of low- and high-risk cutaneous papillomaviruses reveals strongly transforming and high Rb-binding activity for the E7 protein of the low-risk human papillomavirus type 1, *J. Virol.*, 68, 7051–7059, 1994.

52. Euvrard, S., Chardonnet, Y., Pouteil-Noble, C., Kanitakis, J., Chignol, M. C., Thivolet, J., Touraine, J. L., Association of skin malignancies with various and multiple carcinogenic and noncarcinogenic human papillomaviruses in renal transplant recipients, *Cancer*, 72, 2198–2206, 1993.

53. de Villiers, E.-M., Human papillomaviruses, in Schmähl, D., and Penn, I., Eds., *Cancer in Organ Transplant Recipients*, Springer-Verlag, Berlin Heidelberg, 1991, 106–112.

54. Rees, J., Genetic alterations in nonmelanoma skin cancer, *J. Invest. Dermatol.*, 103, 747–750, 1994.

55. Preston, D. S., Stern, R. S., Nonmelanoma cancers of the skin, *New Engl. J. Med.*, 327, 1649–1662, 1992.

56. Lever, L. R., Farr, P. M., Skin cancers or premalignant lesions occur in half of high-dose PUVA patients, *Br. J. Dermatol.*, 131, 215–219, 1994.

57. Zielger, A., Lefell, D. J., Kunals, S., Sharma, H. W., Gailani, M., Simon, J. A., Halperin, A. J., Baden, H. P., Shapiro, P. E., Bale, A. E., Brash, D. E., Mutation hotspots due to sunlight in the p53 gene of nonmelanoma skin cancers, *Proc. Natl. Acad. Sci. U.S.A.*, 90, 4216–4220, 1993.

58. Smith, M. L., Chen, I.-T., Zhan, Q., O'Connor, P. M., Fornace, A. J., Involvement of the p53 tumor suppressor in repair of U.V.-type DNA damage, *Oncogene*, 10, 1053–1059, 1995.

59. Hirt, L., Hirsch-Behnam, A., de Villiers, E.-M., Nucleotide sequence of human papillomavirus (HPV) type 41: an unusual HPV type without a typical E2 binding site consensus sequence. *Virus Res.*, 18, 179–190, 1990.

60. Boukamp, P., Petrussevska, D., Breitkreuz, D., Hornung, J., Markham, A., Fusenig, N., Normal keratinization in a spontaneously immortalized aneuploid human keratinocyte cell line, *J. Cell Biol.*, 106, 761–771, 1988.

61. Lehman, T.A., Modali, R., Boukamp, P., Stanek, J., Bennett, W. P., Welsh, J. A., Metcalf, R. A., Stampfer, M. R., Fusenig, N., Rogan, E. M., Redell, R., Harris, C. C., p53 mutations in human immortalized epithelial cell lines, *Carcinogenesis*, 14, 833–839, 1993.

62. Fischer, M., Frick, M., Beinlich, A., Mincheva, A., Lichter, P., de Villiers, E.-M., Non-tumorigenic human cutaneous keratinocytes (HaCaT) induce tumors after transfection with the E6 and an interrupted E7 ORFs of the cutaneous papillomavirus HPV 41 DNA, submitted.

63. Forslund, O., Hansson, B. G., Rymark, P., Bjerre, B., Human papillomavirus DNA in urine samples compared with that in simultaneously collected urethra and cervix samples, *J. Clin. Microbiol.*, 31, 1975–1979, 1993.

64. Fralick, R. A., Malek, R. S., Goellner, J. R., Hyland, K. M., Urethroscopy and urethral cytology in men with external condyloma, *Urology*, 43, 361–364, 1994.

65. Hillman, R. J., Ryait, B. K., Botcherby, M., Taylor-Robinson, D., Changes in HPV infection in patients with anogenital warts and their partners, *Genitourin. Med.*, 69, 450–456, 1993.

66. Grußendorf-Conen, E. I., Deutz, F. J., de Villiers, E.-M., Detection of human papillomavirus-6 in primary carcinoma of the urethra in men, *Cancer*, 60, 1832–1835, 1987.

67. Wiener, J. S., Liu, E. T., Walther, P. J., Oncogenic human papillomavirus type 16 is associated with squamous cell cancer of the male urethra, *Cancer Res.*, 52, 5018–5023, 1992.

68. Hartveit, F., Maehle, B. O., Thunold, S., Koilocytosis in neoplasia of the urinary bladder, *Br. J. Urol.*, 69, 46–48, 1992.

69. Knowles, M. A., Human papillomavirus sequences are not detectable by Southern blotting or general primer-mediated polymerase chain reaction in transitional cell tumours if the bladder, *Urol. Res.*, 20, 297–301, 1992.

70. Chang, F., Lipponen, P., Tervahauta, A., Syrjänen, S., Syrjänen, K., Transitional cell carcinoma of the bladder: Failure to demonstrate human papillomavirus deoxyribonucleic acid by in situ hybridization and polymerase chain reaction, *J. Urol.*, 152, 1429–1433, 1994.

71. Furihata, M., Inoue, K., Ohtsuki, Y., Hashimoto, H., Terao, N., Fujita, Y., High-risk human papillomavirus infections and overexpression of p53 protein as prognostic indicators in transitional cell carcinoma of the urinary bladder, *Cancer Res.*, 53, 4823–4827, 1993.

72. LaRue, H., Simoneau, M., Fradet, Y., Human papillomavirus in transitional cell carcinoma of the urinary bladder, *Clin. Cancer Res.*, 1, 435–440, 1995.

73. Maloney, K. E., Wiener, J. S., Walther, P. J., Oncogenic human papillomaviruses are rarely associated with squamous cell carcinoma of the bladder: evaluation by differential polymerase chain reaction, *J. Urol.*, 151, 360–364, 1994.

74. Noel, J. C., Thiry, L., Verhest, A., Deschepper, N., Peny, M. O., Sattar, A. A., Schulman, C. C., Haot, J., Transitional cell carcinoma of the bladder: evaluation of the role of human papillomaviruses, *Urology*, 44, 671–675, 1994.

75. Shah, K. V., Daniel, R. W., Simos, J. W., Vogelstein, B., Investigation of colon cancers for human papillomavirus genomic sequences by polymerase chain reaction. *J. Surg. Oncol.*, 51, 5–7, 1992.

76. Koulos, J., Symmans, F., Chumas, J., Nuovo, G., Human papillomavirus detection in adenocarcinoma of the anus, *Mod. Pathol.*, 4, 58–61, 1991.

77. Shroyer, K. R., Kim, J. G., Manos, M. M., Greer, C. E., Pearlman, N. W., Franklin, W. A., Papillomavirus found in anorectal squamous carcinoma, not in colon adenocarcinoma, *Arch. Surg.*, 127, 741–744, 1992.

78. Band, V., Zajchowski, D., Kulesa, V., Sager, R., Human papillomavirus DNAs immortalize normal human mammary epithelial cells and reduce their growth factor requirements, *Proc. Natl. Acad. Sci. U.S.A.*, 87, 463–467, 1990.

79. Bratthauer, G. L., Tavassoli, F. A., O'Leary, T. J., Etiology of breast carcinoma: no apparent role for papillomavirus types 6/11/16/18, *Pathol. Res. Pract.*, 188, 384–386, 1992.

80. Wrede, D., Lugman, Y. A., Coombes, R. C., Vousden, K. H., Absence of HPV 16 and 18 DNA in breast cancer, *Br. J. Cancer*, 65, 891–894, 1992.

81. Di Lonardo, A., Venuti, A., Marcante, M. L., Human papillomavirus in breast cancer, *Breast Cancer Res. Treat.*, 21, 95–100, 1992.

82. Shah, K. V., Papillomavirus infections of the repsiratory tract, the conjunctiva, and the oral cavity, in *Papillomaviruses and Human Cancer*, Pfister H., Ed., CRC Press, Boca Raton, Florida, 1990, 74–90.

83. McDonnell, P. J., McDonnell, J. M., Kessis, T., Green, W. R., Shah, K. V., Detection of human papillomavirus type 6/11 DNA in conjunctival papillomas by in situ hybridization with radioactive probes, *Human Pathol.*, 18, 1115, 1987.

84. de Villiers, E.-M., Strunck-Kortenbusch, B., Sundmacher, R., unpublished data, 1990.

85. McDonnell,J. M., McDonnell, P. J., Sun, Y. Y., Human papillomavirus DNA in tissues and ocular surface swabs of patients with conjunctival epithelial neoplasia, *Invest. Opthalmol. Vis. Sci.*, 33, 184–189, 1992.

86. Lauer, S. A., Malter, J. S., Meier, J. R., Human papillomavirus type 18 in conjunctival intraepithelial neoplasia, *Am J. Opthalmol.*,110, 23–27, 1990.

87. Oldrich, M. G., Jakobiec, F. A., Lancaster, W. D., Kenyon, K. R., Kelly, L. D., Kormehl, E. W., Steinert, R. F., Grove, A. S. Jr., Shore, J. W., Gregoire, L., A spectrum of bilateral squamous conjunctival tumors associated with human papillomavirus type 16, *Opthalmology*, 98, 628–635, 1991.

88. Tritten, J. J., Beati, D., Sahli, R., Uffer, S., Bilateral conjunctival and eyelid tumor associated with human papillomavirus in an immunocompetent man. *Klin. Monatsbl. Augenheilkd.*, 204, 453–455, 1994.

89. Gissmann, L., Diehl, V., Schultz-Coulon, H., zur Hausen, H., Molecular cloning and characterization of human papillomavirus DNA from a laryngeal papilloma, *J. Virol.*, 44, 393–400, 1982.

90. Kahn, T., Schwarz, E., zur Hausen, H., Molecular cloning and characterization of the DNA of the new human papillomavirus (HPV 30) from a laryngeal carcinoma, *Int. J. Cancer*, 37, 61–65, 1986.

91. de Villiers, E.-M., Papillomaviruses in cancers and papillomas of the aerodigestive tract, *Biomed. Pharmacother.*, 43, 31–36, 1989.

92. Kellokoski, J., Syrjänen, S., Syrjänen, K., Yliskoski, M., Oral mucosa changes in women with genital HPV infection, *J. Oral Pathol. Med.*, 19, 142–148, 1990.

93. Snijders, P. J. F., van den Brule, A. J. C., Meijer, C. J. L. M., Walboomers, J. M. M., Papillomaviruses and cancer of the upper digestive and respiratory tracts, *Curr. Top. Microbiol. Immunol.*, 186, 177–198, 1994.

94. Greenspan, D., de Villiers, E.-M., Greenspan, J. S., de Souza, Y. G., zur Hausen, H., Unusual HPV types in oral warts in association with HIV infection, *J. Oral. Pathol.*, 17, 482–487, 1988.

95. de Villiers, E.-M., Prevalence of HPV 7 papillomas in the oral mucosa and facial skin of patients with human immunodeficiency virus, *Arch. Dermatol.*, 125, 1590, 1989.

96. Orth, G., Jablonska, S., Favre, M., Croissant, O., Obalek, S., Jarzabek-Chorzelska, M., Jibard, N., Identification of papillomavirus in butcher's warts, *J. Invest. Dermatol.*, 76, 97–102, 1981.

97. de Villiers, E.-M., Neumann, C., Oltersdorf, T., Fierlbeck, G., zur Hausen, H., Butcher's wart virus (HPV 7) infections in non-butchers, *J. Invest. Dermatol.*, 87, 236–238, 1986.

98. Völter, C., He, Y., Delius, H., Roy-Burman, A., Greenspan, J. S., Greenspan, D., de Villiers, E-M., Novel HPV types present in oral papillomatous lesions from patients with HIV infection, *Int. J. Cancer*, 66, 453–456, 1996.

99. de Villiers, E.-M., Weidauer, H., Otto, H., zur Hausen, H., Papillomavirus DNA in human tongue carcinomas, *Int. J. Cancer*, 36, 575–578, 1985.

100. Balaram, P., Nalinakumari, K. R., Abraham, E., Balan, A., Hareendran, N. K., Bernard, H. U., Chan, S. Y., Human papillomaviruses in 91 oral cancers from Indian betel quid chewers - high prevalence and multiplicity of infections, *Int. J. Cancer*, 16, 450–454, 1995.

101. Thomas, S., Brennan, J., Martel, G., Frazer, I., Montesano, R., Sidransky, D., Hollstein, M., Mutations in the conserved regions of p53 are infrequent in betel-associated oral cancers from Papua New Guinea, *Cancer Res.*, 54, 3588–3593, 1994.

102. Palefsky, J.M., Silverman, S. Jr., Abdel-Salaam, M., Daniels, T. E., Greenspan, J. S., Association between proliferative verrucous leukoplakia and infection with human papillomavirus type 16, *J. Oral Pathol. Med.*, 24, 193–197, 1995.

103. Brandwein, M., Zeitlin, J., Nuovo, G. J., MacConnell, P., Bodian, C., Urken, M., Biller, H., HPV detection using "hot start" polymerase chain reaction in patients with oral cancer: a clinicopathological study of 64 patients, *Mod. Pathol.*, 7, 720–727, 1994.

104. Shindoh, M., Sawada, Y., Kohgo, T., Amamiya, A., Fujinaga, K., Detection of human papillomavirus DNA sequences in tongue squamous-cell carcinoma utilizing polymerase chain reaction method, *Int. J. Cancer*, 50, 167–171, 1992.

105. Kitasato, H., Delius, H., zur Hausen, H., Sorger, K., Rösl, F., de Villiers, E.-M., Sequence rearrangements in the upstream regulatory region of human papillomavirus type 6: are these involved in malignant transition?, *J. Gen. Virol.*, 75, 1157–1162, 1994.

106. Kashima, H. K., Kutcher, M., Kessis, T., Levin, L. S., de Villiers, E.-M., Shah, K. V., Human papillomavirus in squamous cell carcinoma, leukoplakia, lichen planus, and clinically normal epithelium of the oral cavitiy, *Ann. Otol. Rhinol. Laryngol.*, 99, 55–61, 1990.

107. Shear, M., Developmental odonotogenic cysts. An update, *J. Oral Pathol.*, 23,1–11, 1994.

108. Kashima, H. K., Kessis, T., Hruban, R. H., Wu, T. C., Zinreich, S. J., Shah, K. V., Human papillomavirus in sinonasal papillomas and squamous cell carcinoma, *Laryngoscope*, 102, 973–976, 1992.

109. Furuta, Y., Takasu, T., Asai, T., Shinohara, T., Sawa, H., Nagashima, K., Inuyama, Y., Detection of human papillomavirus DNA in carcinomas of the nasal cavities and paranasal sinuses by polymerase chain reaction, *Cancer*, 69, 353–357, 1992.

110. Judd, R., Zaki, S.R., Coffield, L. M., Evatt, B. L., Human papillomavirus type 6 detected by polymerase chain reaction in invasive sinonasal papillary squamous cell carcinoma, *Arch. Pathol. Lab. Med.*, 115, 1150–1153, 1991.

111. Buchwald, C., Franzmann, M. B., Jacobsen, G. K., Lindeberg, H., Human papillomavirus (HPV) in sinonasal papillomas: a study of 78 cases using in situ hybridization and polymerase chain reaction, *Laryngoscope*, 105, 66–71, 1995.

112. Snijders, P.J.F., Cromme, F. V., van den Brule, A. J. C., Schrijnemakers, H. F. J., Snow, G. B., Meijer, C. J. L. M., Walboomers, J. M. M., Prevalence and expression of human papillomavirus in tonsillar carcinomas, indicating a possible viral etiology, *Int. J. Cancer*, 51, 845–850, 1992.

113. Brachman, D. G., Graves, D., Vokes, E., Beckett, M., Haraf, D., Montag, A., Dunphy, E., Mick, R., Yandell, D., Weichselbaum, R. R., Occurrence of p53 gene deletions and human papillomavirus infection in human head and neck cancer, *Cancer Res.*, 52, 4832–4836, 1992.

114. Lewensohn-Fuchs, I., Munck-Wikland, E., Berke, Z., Magnusson, K. P., Pallesen, G., Auer, G., Lindholm, J., Linde, A., Aberg, B., Rubio, C., Kuylenstierna, R., Wiman, K. G., Dalianis, T., Involvement of aberrant p53 expression and human papillomavirus in carcinoma of the head, neck and esophagus, *Anticancer Res.*, 14, 1281–1286, 1994.

115. Bercovich, J. A., Centeno, C. R., Aguilar, O. G., Grinstein, S., Kahn. T., Presence and integration of human papillomavirus type 6 in a tonsillar carcinoma, *J. Gen. Virol.*, 72, 2569–2572, 1991.

116. de Villiers, E.-M., Weidauer, H., unpublished results, 1992.

117. Multhaupt, H. A., Fessler, J. N., Warhol, M. J., Detection of human papillomavirus in laryngeal lesions by in situ hybridization, *Human Pathol.*, 25, 1302–1305, 1994.

118. Brandwein, M. S., Nuovo, G. J., Biller, H., Analysis of prevalence of human papillomavirus in laryngeal carcinomas. Study of 40 cases using polymerase chain reaction and consensus primers. *Ann. Otol. Rhinol. Laryngol.*, 102, 309–313, 1993.

119. Fouret, P., Dabit, D., Sibony, M., Alili, D., Commo, F., Saint-Guily, J. L., Callard, P., Expression of p53 protein related to the presence of human papillomavirus infection in precancer lesions of the larynx, *Am. J. Pathol.*, 146, 599–604, 1995.

120. Salam, M. A., Rockett, J., Morris, A., General primer-mediated polymerase chain reaction for simultaneous detection and typing of human papillomavirus DNA in laryngeal squamous cell carcinomas, *Clin. Otolaryngol.*, 20, 84–88, 1995.

121. Shidara, K., Suzuki, T., Hara, F., Nakajima, T., Lack of synergistic association between human papillomavirus and ras gene point mutation in laryngeal carcinomas, *Laryngoscope*, 104, 1008–1012, 1994.

122. Fliss, D. M., Noble-Topham, S. E., McLachlin, M., Freeman, J. L., Noyek, A. M., van Nostrand, A. W., Hartwick, R. W., Laryngeal verrucous carcinoma: a clinicopathological study and detection of human papillomavirus using polymerase chain reaction, *Laryngoscope*, 104, 146–152, 1994.

123. Hoshikawa, T., Detection of human papillomavirus DNA in hypopharyngeal carcinoma, *Nippon Jibiinkoka Gakkai Kaiho*, 94, 1151–1157, 1994.

124. Ogura, H., Watanabe, S., Fukushima, K., Masuda, Y., Fujiwara, T., Yabe, Y., Presence of human papillomavirus type 18 DNA in a pharyngeal and a laryngeal carcinoma, *Jpn. J. Cancer Res.*, 82, 1184–1186, 1991.

125. Abramson, M., Moriyama, H., Huang, C. C., Pathogenic factors in bone resorption in cholesteatoma, *Acta Otolaryngol.*, 97, 437–442, 1984.

126. Broekaert, D., Pattin, C., Coucke, P., de Bersaques, J., Marquet, J., Keratinization of middle-ear cholesteatomas. I. A histochemical study of epidermal transglutaminase, *Europ. Arch. Otorhinolaryngol.*, 247, 312–317, 1990.

127. Lindeberg, H., Elbrond, O., Malignant tumours in patients with a history of multiple laryngeal papillomas: the significance of irradiation, *Clin. Otolaryngol.*, 16, 149–151, 1991.

128. Byrne, J. C., Tsao, M. S., Fraser, R. S., Howley, P. M., Human papillomavirus-11 DNA in a patient with chronic laryngotracheobronchial papillomatosis and metastatic squamous cell carcinoma of the lung, *N. Engl. J. Med.*, 317, 873, 1987.

129. DiLorenzo, T. P., Tamsen, A., Abramson, A. L., Steinberg, B. M., Human papillomavirus type 6a DNA in lung carcinoma of patient with recurrent laryngeal papillomatosis is characterized by a partial duplication, *J. Gen. Virol.*, 73, 423–428, 1992.

130. Simma, B., Burger, R., Uehlinger, J., Ghelfi, D., Hof, E., Dangel, P., Briner, J., Fanconi, S., Squamous cell carcinoma arising in a non-irradiated child with recurrent respiratory papillomatosis, *Eur. J. Pediatr.*, 152, 776–778, 1993.

131. Doyle, D. J., Henderson, L. A., LeJeune, F. E. Jr., Miller, R. H., Changes in human papillomavirus typing of recurrent respiratory papillomatosis progressing to malignant neoplasm, *Arch. Otolaryngol. Head Neck Surg.*, 120, 1273–1276, 1994.

132. Stremlau, A., Gissmann, L., Ikenberg, H., Stark, M., Bannasch, P., zur Hausen, H., Human papillomavirus type 16 related DNA in an anaplastic carcinoma of the lung, *Cancer*, 55, 1737–1740, 1985.

133. Shamanin, V., Delius, H., de Villiers, E.-M., Development of a broad spectrum PCR assay for papillomaviruses and its application in screening lung cancer biopsies, *J. Gen. Virol.*, 75, 1149–1156, 1994.

134. Szabo, I., Sepp, R., Nakamoto, K., Maeda, M., Sakamoto, H., Uda, H., Human papillomavirus not found in squamous cell lung carcinomas by polymerase chain reaction, *Cancer*, 73, 2740–2744, 1994.

135. Fong, K. M., Schonrock, J., Frazer, I. M., Zimmerman, P. V., Smith, P. J., Human papillomavirus not found in squamous cell lung carcinomas by polymerase chain reaction, *Cancer*, 75, 2400–2401, 1995.

136. zur Hausen, H., Condylomata acuminata and genital cancer, *Cancer Res.*, 36, 530, 1976.

137. Yamada, Y., Ninomiya, M., Kato, T., Nagaki, M., Kato, M., Hatakeyama, H., Moriwaki, H., Muto, Y., Human papillomavirus type 16-positive esophageal papilloma at an endoscopic injection sclerotherapy site, *Gastroenterology*, 108, 550–553, 1995.

138. Carr, N. J., Bratthauer, G. L., Kichy, J. H., Taubenberger, J. K., Monihan, J. M., Sobin, L. H., Squamous cell papillomas of the esophagus: a study of 23 lesions for human papillomavirus by in situ hybridization and the polymerase chain reaction, *Human Pathol.*, 25, 536–540, 1994a.

139. Carr, N. J., Monihan, J. M., Sobin, L. H., Squamous cell papilloma of the esophagus: a clinicopathologic and follow-up study of 25 cases, *Am. J. Gastroenterol.*, 89, 245–248, 1994b.

140. Poljak, M., Orlowska, J., Cerar, A., Human papillomavirus infection in esophageal squamous cell papillomas: a study of 29 lesions, *Anticancer Res.*, 15, 965–969, 1995.

141. Chang, F., Syrjänen, S., Shen, Q., Wang, L., Syrjänen, K., Screening for human papillomavirus infections in oesophageal squamous cell carcinomas by *in situ* hybridization, *Cancer*, 72, 2525–2530, 1993.

142. Toh, Y., Kuwano, H., Tanaka, S., Baba, K., Matsuda, H., Sugimachi, K., Mori, R., Detection of human papillomavirus DNA in esophageal carcinoma in Japan by polymerase chain reaction, *Cancer*, 70, 2234–2248, 1992.

143. Benamouzig, R., Pigot, F., Quiroga, G., Validire, P., Chaussade, S., Catalan, F., Couturier, D., Human papillomavirus infection in esophageal squamous-cell carcinoma in western countries, *Int. J. Cancer*, 50, 549–552, 1992.

144. Furihata, M., Ohtsuki, Y., Ogoshi, S., Takahashi, A., Tamiya, T., Ogata, T., Prognostic significance of human papillomavirus genomes (type-16, -18) and aberrant expression of p53 protein in esophageal cancer, *Int. J. Cancer*, 54, 226–230, 1993.

145. Chen, B., Yin, H., Dhurandhar, N., Detection of human papillomavirus DNA in esophageal squamous cell carcinomas by the polymerase chain reaction using general consensus primers, *Hum. Pathol.*, 25, 920–923, 1994.

146. Cooper, K., Taylor, L., Govind, S., Human papillomavirus DNA in oesophageal carcinomas in South Africa, *J. Pathol.*, 175, 273–277, 1995.

147. Akutsu, N., Shirasawa, H., Nakano, K., Tanzawa, H., Asano, T., Kobayashi, S., Isono, K., Simizu, B., Rare association of human papillomavirus DNA with oesophageal cancer in Japan, *J. Infect. Dis.*, 171, 425–428, 1995.

148. Togawa, T., Jaskiewicz, K., Takahashi, T., Meltzer, S. J., Rustgi, A. K., Human papillomavirus DNA sequences in esophagus squamous cell carcinoma, *Gastroenterol.*, 107, 128–136, 1994.

149. Togawa, K., Rustgi, A. K., A novel human papillomavirus sequence based on L1 general primers, *Virus Res.*, 36, 293–297, 1994.

7

Warts and HPV-Related Squamous Cell Tumors of the Skin

Elke-Ingrid Grussendorf-Conen

CONTENTS

I. INTRODUCTION

Human papillomaviruses (HPV) affect mucosae and skin of immunocompetent as well as that of immunosuppressed patients. They produce epithelial proliferation with different patterns of growth depending on the site and HPV type. It is assumed that infectious virus particles penetrate through breaks in the epithelium or epidermis and enter one or more basal cells. Nevertheless, it takes months before warts develop and up to 90% of the HPV infections will have no clinical consequences at

0-8493-7356-5/97/$0.00+$.50
© 1997 by CRC Press, Inc.

all. The viral DNA seems to persist extrachromosomally, but nothing is known about transcription and translation in the state of clinically silent latency.

The viral replication cycle appears to be linked to the differentiation process of the epithelium, and there is evidence that HPV can modify keratinocyte maturation.[1] Virus-encoded proteins stimulate cellular proliferation and interfere with the proper differentiation of the epithelial cells. Increased cell supply from the basal layer and the delayed terminal differentiation finally lead to hyperplasia of the spinous layer and the beginning of wart growth.

Following replication, viral DNA is sufficiently abundant within nuclei in intermediate and superficial cell layers. The amount of viruses produced correlates to some extent with the type of lesion (plantar> common wart> anogenital wart) and the age of the lesion (new>old).[2]

The striking feature of different human papillomavirus types is the preference of infection for squamous epithelia at specific sites (Table 1). Although such site specificity is not fully understood, it may be explained by attachment of viral capsid proteins to specific surface receptors on epithelial cells.[3,4] Alternatively, there may be close linkage of the site-specific epithelial differentiation program with permissiveness for viral replication, perhaps through cellular regulatory proteins binding to viral DNA at transcription control sequences.

TABLE 1   HPV Type Grouping Based on Site of Infection and on DNA-Sequence Homology

Site	Group (overall DNA-sequence homology determined by cross-hybridization 1-40%)	HPV Type
Skin	A	[1]
	B	[2,3,10,27–29,57]
	C	[4]
	F	[7]
	I	[26]
	O	[41]
	Q	[48[a]]
Skin of EV	D	[5[b],8[b],9,12,14,15, 17,19,20–25, 36–38,46,47,49]
	R	[50]
Anogenital and oral mucosa	E	[6,11,13,44,55]
	G	[16[b],31[a]]
	H	[18[b],32,42,45]
	J	[30[a],53]
	K	[33[a],52]
	M	[35[a]]
	N	[39[a]]
	P	[43]
	S	[54]
	T	[56]

[a] HPV types suggested to have malignant potential or cloned from a cancer.

[b] HPV types strongly associated with malignant tumors.

Source: Modified from Classification by Pfister[3] and Arends et al.[4]

II. INCIDENCE OF CUTANEOUS WARTS

Although it is well known since ancient times that cutaneous warts are common, there is a surprising lack of new epidemiologic information. Their frequency in the general European and American population is estimated to be 7 to 10%.[5] Recently, a Russian epidemiologic study estimated the population incidence of viral warts to be 12.94% in and surrounding Tomsk.[6] The analysis is based on a total of 30,518 patients. In Great Britain, 10 to 25% of new patients who present themselves at dermatologic clinics do so for treatment of warts.[7] In 1987, Stern and co-workers[8] calculated that approximately 8% of office visits to dermatologists were for warts but only half of the patients with warts were seen by dermatologists. The remainder of these patients were cared for by general or family practitioners, internists, and pediatricians. In a general survey of skin diseases among 2180 adults, 3.5% were found to have warts.[8] "Verruca vulgaris" was the fifth most common diagnosis in a university pediatric dermatologic clinic, and was noted in nearly 5% of patients.[9]

Warts are rare before the age of five, with their incidence increasing as children become older, reaching a maximum between the ages of 10 and 14 years, declining rapidly until 20 years old, than gradually increasing after 25 years. In a well-designed study published in 1989, Steele and co-workers[10] analysed 826 patients with cutaneous warts. The age distribution was from 2-81 years, with children being the most frequently affected. The median age at presentation was 11 years. Of the patients 30% were between 10 and 14 years, and 65% were between 5 and 20 years of age. Only 16% of these patients were over 35 years of age. In general, the age distribution differs somewhat in patients with verrucae vulgares and those with plantar warts, suggesting different modes of acquisition.[11,12]

III. INCIDENCE OF CUTANEOUS WARTS IN IMMUNOCOMPROMISED PATIENTS

Manifestations of nongenital HPV infection in the immunocompromised population have been well studied.[13,14] To date, the best-documented immunocompromised population consists of renal allograft recipients. Reported incidences of common warts range from 24-48%.[15] With each year of immunosuppression, there is an increase in the number of warts. Dyall-Smith and co-workers[16] studied a total of 198 renal transplant recipients for warts. They discovered that of the patients transplanted for more than 5 years, 92% were found to have warts and 65% had more than five warts each. These immunocompromised patients were infected by the same HPV types as seen in immunocompetent patients. It is not known whether immunocompromised patients develop verrucae vulgares because of an increased susceptibility to HPV infection or because of latent infection. That this population suffers reactivation of other latent viral infections is well known, and HPV is clearly capable of establishing latent infection. Thus, reactivity may be the most plausible explanation of these observations. A lack of effective immune response with partial inhibition of activation markers expressed by keratinocytes could be found in papillomavirus infected skin lesions from transplant recipients,[17] indicating the importance of host factors.

IV. CLASSIFICATION

The traditional classification of cutaneous warts is based on clinical appearance and location. It includes the following clinical types: verruca vulgaris or common wart, deep hyperkeratotic palmoplantar wart or myrmecia, superficial mosaic type palmoplantar wart, verruca plana or flat wart, and intermediate wart.

V.   CLINICAL MANIFESTATION

A.   Verrucae Vulgares (Common Warts)

Common warts begin as little, flat or dome-shaped, firm, skin-colored papules. With increasing elevation, their surface becomes rough, irregular, and hyperkeratotic. Their size varies from a few millimeters to more than 1 cm, and their color changes to gray or brownish. They may occur singly or in clusters and are sometimes confluent and hypertrophic, especially in periungual location. They may appear anywhere on the skin, including the thin epithelia of the anal and genital regions and the vermillion of the lips, but they are most commonly localised on the dorsal aspects of the fingers and hands. On the soles, common warts usually appear as *mosaic warts*.[18] They are painless, only slightly raised above the skin level, multiple, and often so closely set that they may impinge one against the other and form a coherent plate of warts. There may be only one large plaque, but it is common to find several small warts of the same structure in its neighborhood. *Endophytic* common warts also appear characteristically in palmar and plantar localizations. They are usually multiple, painless, and have a slightly raised hyperkeratotic surface. Sometimes they are surrounded by a horny wall which defines the size of the lesion. If they are small, they may resemble keratosis punctata.[19]

On the face, head, neck and in flexures, verrucae vulgares can become elongated and papillomatous. Depending on their clinical characteristics and size, they are often referred to as *filiform, digitate, or multidigitate warts*. Hyperproliferative, papillomatous common warts with a cauliflowerlike, vegetating appearance have been found on the hands of butchers.[20,21]

B.   Myrmecia

The prototype of myrmecia is the single, painful palmoplantar wart deeply set in the skin. It is usually associated with considerable tenderness and may show swelling and redness. When it occurs multiply, the individual lesions do not coalesce. Myrmecia do not only occur on the palm and soles, but also on the lateral aspects of the fingers and toes, under the nails, on the pulp of the digits and, rarely, on the face, scalp, and body. Usually the deep palmoplantar wart is covered with a thick callus. When this horny plate is removed, the wart tissue appears soft and crumbly and shows a white opaque color. This sort of wart occurs frequently in children between 5 and 15 years of age.

C.   Verrucae Planae (Plane Warts, Flat Warts)

Verrucae planae are slightly elevated, small, skin-colored papules. They always appear as multiple, irregularly disseminated or grouped lesions sometimes in linear distribution. The forehead and the dorsal aspects of the hands are most commonly affected; rarely do they occur on the forearms and lower extremities.

D.   Intermediate Warts

The term *intermediate warts* was applied by Jablonska et al. in 1985[19] to lesions that cannot be classified as common or plane warts, as they combine clinical features of both. If they are hyperkeratotic, raised, and coalescent, these papillomas differ from common warts by a flatter surface. Typical flat warts are often found between the raised ones. The clinical recognition of intermediate warts and their differentiation from young common warts may be impossible. The histology is of diagnostic significance.

VI.   CUTANEOUS WARTS AND INFECTING HPV TYPE

Disclosure of the plurality of HPV types associated with skin warts raises the problem of the relation of clinical morphology to distinct types of HPV. This was first suggested by the characterizing of distinct HPV from different types of lesions: HPV 1 from deep plantar warts, HPV 2 from common hand warts, and HPV 3 from plane warts. At present, more than 70 types of HPV are recognized, with several subtypes for many of them. Some HPV types are especially associated with cutaneous warts and a great number of them are associated with skin warts in epidermodysplasia verruciformis (see Table 1). A great number of different HPV types pertain to only a limited variety of clinically and histologically different sorts of warts as mentioned above. Table 2 shows how the HPV types are related to clinically defined warts:

TABLE 2   The Relationship Between Clinically
           Defined Warts and HPV Types

Myrmecia:	HPV 1
Common warts:	HPV 2,4,7,26–29,49,57
Plane warts:	HPV 3,10,28

HPV 1 is characterized through its enormous virus production which leads to highly characteristic histologic features.[22] It is associated with deep plantar warts, such as myrmecia, and only rarely with other common warts. The HPV 1 induced wart has a dome-shaped clinical appearance with a central depression. Nevertheless, the clinical morphology of HPV 1 warts varies, depending on their localization. Lesions on the face, for example, can have the clinical features of digitate or filiforme warts.[23]

According to their DNA sequence homology, some of the HPV types show a close relationship to each other as HPV 2, 27, 29, and 57. HPV 2 and its subtypes are the prototypes of common warts.[24] The HPV 2 related type 57 can also be found in genital lesions.[25] Plane warts and intermediate warts are commonly associated with the related HPV types HPV 3, 10, and 28.[26] HPV 4 induces small multiple warts and endophytic warts. With HPV 4, related are HPV 60 and 65. Recently these types have been associated with pigmented warts.[27] Another group of related HPV types are HPV 7 and HPV 40. HPV 7 was first detected in butcher's warts[28,29] and later was found in other skin warts and in oral warts in HIV-infected people.[30,31] The HPV 7 related HPV 40 could be demonstrated in genital warts and bowenoid lesions.[25] Originally, HPV 41 was isolated from facial skin warts of a child. Later on, it was detected in some cases of actinic keratosis and in skin cancer.[32]

VII. REGRESSION AND IMMUNOLOGY

Skin warts usually regress spontaneously. It is generally stated that 35% of patients lose their warts within 2–6 months,[33,34] 63% within 1 year, and 67% within 2 years. However, there are a number of people who have had warts for decades. The mechanism of wart regression has been the subject of much speculation and research. The spontaneous disappearance, frequently observed simultaneously for multiple warts, may indicate that wart rejection is due to humoral and/or cell-mediated immune reactions toward the wart cells. Numerous studies have been done by different groups of investigators on the humoral or cellular immunity to HPVs using various techniques.[35] HPV-specific antibodies seem to have rather less significance in the regression of warts, while there is considerable evidence that cell-mediated immunity plays the major role in the control of HPV infection.[36] The incidence of warts increases during immunosuppressive treatment and in persons with cell-mediated immune deficiency. On the other hand, regression of warts has been reported after inflammation or treatment with dinitrochlorobenzene and with a variety of immune adjuvants. Tagami and colleagues[37] reported as early as 1974 the occurrence of mononuclear cell infiltration in the dermis and epidermis of regressing flat warts. This was confirmed by Berman and Winkelman,[38] who have shown similar changes in resolving common warts. *In situ* investigation of the cellular immune response is another approach provided by the use of monoclonal antibodies directed against surface antigens of T cells, B cells, and Langerhans cells. It has been demonstrated that Langerhans cells in the epidermis play an important role as antigen carriers, elicitors, and targets of immunological reactions. In skin warts, Langerhans cells are markedly reduced in number, suggesting a decrease of immunological surveillance which might induce tolerance to HPV.[36,39] Involution of common warts, myrmecia, and plane warts is associated with a mononuclear cell infiltration, exocytosis, and degenerative epidermal changes, indicating that regression represents a cell-mediated immune rejection of the warts.

A.   Clinical Signs of Regression

A deep plantar wart in regression is dark or almost black and becomes painful. The edges sometimes peel slightly. The superficial part of the wart is dry. In advanced regression, the whole wart is dry and friable.[40] Common warts, however, usually shrink silently. Itching sometimes precedes resolution. They involute individually, in part probably due to an immune response of the host, but nearly always due either to simple occlusion of blood vessels in the tumor tissue or to changes in the keratinocytes which are not favorable to the propagation of HPV.

Flat warts in normal people present a dramatic, systemic, regression phenomenon based on the development of a cellular immune response of the host against HPV-transformed cells.[41] Before involution, the warts suddenly begin to exacerbate. They become reddened and swell up, causing intense pruritus. In severe cases, extensive vesiculation may appear on the top of the warts. After 2–7 weeks, when the inflammation subsides with associated scaling and crusting, generally all warts have disappeared.

VIII. RELATION BETWEEN HPV INFECTION AND CUTANEOUS CANCER

A.   Association of HPV with Malignancies in the Immunocompetent Population

In contrast to the frequent detection of genomes of specific HPV in a high proportion of genital cancers, there is less information on their association with the malignant tumors of the skin in the general population. However, the presence of specific HPV genomes in cancers and premalignant lesions of patients with epidermodysplasia verruciformis (EV), a rare, lifelong disease, indicates that at least some HPV types present a high-risk factor for the development of skin carcinomas. Thus, EV was the first model of viral cutaneous oncogenesis in humans.

In the general population, the association of premalignant lesions and cancers of the skin with HPV appears to be very weak. Kawashima and co-workers[42] studied 314 biopsies obtained from 227 patients to evaluate the role of HPV in the development of skin malignancies. Their results suggest that the known HPV types play only a minor role in skin carcinogenesis. Nevertheless, DNA of HPV 2, 16, 34, 35, or 41 have been identified in a few cases of extragenital Bowen's disease and squamous cell skin tumors[32,43-47] (Table 3). Remarkable is a strong association between the genital HPV type 16 and squamous cell neoplasmas from the finger[51-53] (Table 4). From this location, 7 of 11 tumors contained HPV 16 DNA and two more contained HPV 16-related sequences, whereas 16 cutaneous carcinomas from other sites showed no such association.[54] The authors stress that a direct inoculation of the periungual region with virus from genital lesions may have occurred. Possibly, the anatomical peculiarity of the nail fold and the nail bed favour infection with mucosal HPV types. This problem deserves further investigation.

1.   Bowen's Disease

Although the etiology of Bowen's disease is unknown, a viral involvement has long been proposed based on clinical observation and electron-microscopic findings.[55] Association of Bowen's disease with HPV has been reported in several cases. In 1984, Pfister and Haneke[44] described HPV 2 in cutaneous Bowen's disease. Kawashima et al.[56] described HPV 34 in a lesion of Bowen's disease of the skin in 1986, and in 1989 Rüdlinger et al.[47] observed a periungual HPV 35-positive bowenoid lesion. Remarkable, however, is the frequent association of Bowen's disease with HPV 16. Kettler et al.[46] detected six cases with HPV 16 or HPV 16 related DNA out of 26 cases. As digitally

TABLE 3 HPV-DNA in Cutaneous Premalignant Lesions and in Skin Cancers of the General Population

Diagnosis	Number of cases tested	Number of cases with HPV	HPV-type	Ref. (year)
Actinic keratosis				
	3	1	41	32 (1988)
	50	1	41	63 (1990)
	51	3	36	
			2x untyped	42 (1990)
Kerato-acanthoma				
	5	2	25-related	64 (1986)
	6	1	9,37	65 (1986)
	8	8	16-related	67 (1989)
	13	1	25	66 (1990)
	32	0	—	42 (1990)
	31	0	—	68 (1992)
Basal cell carcinoma				
	52	1	20	42 (1990)
	16	3	16	69 (1991)
Bowen's disease				
	5	2	16	43 (1983)
	1	1	2	44 (1984)
	1	1	16	58 (1988)
	11	5	16 2x 3x untyped	61 (1991)
	26	6	16 4x 16-related 2x	46 (1990)
	81	2	34	42 (1990)
Squamous cell carcinoma				
	10	2	41	32 (1988)
	1	1	11	71 (1989)
	61	1	5 and 16-related	42 (1990)
	1	1	11,18	72 (1991)
	21	4	16	69 (1991)
	10	1	16	70 (1992)
	1	1	5	73 (1992)
	1	1	33	74 (1992)

localized, HPV 16 was found in 7 of 11 tumors, this suggested a genital-digital route of transmission.[54]

Recently,[57] a case report was presented of a patient with multiple Bowen's lesions of three fingers in which HPV 16 was detected utilizing PCR. Grussendorf-Conen[58] found HPV 16 DNA in bowenoid papulosis on the neck (1988). Grob et al.[59] could also demonstrate HPV 16 in a case of bowenoid papulosis on the face by *in situ* hybridization. The detection of genus-specific antigens of papillomaviruses in 28 out of 144 cases (19.4%) of cutaneous Bowen's disease, in contrast to the low detection rate of viral DNA in these lesions,[60] supports the possibility that the relevant HPV types are not yet characterized and persisting viral DNA is not detected due to its lack of cross-hybridization with presently available probes. Guerin-Reverchon and co-workers[61] detected HPV-DNA in 5 of 11 samples of cutaneous Bowen's disease, using *in situ* hybridization with biotinylated probes of HPV 1, 2, 5, 6, 11, 16, and 18, under stringent and/or

TABLE 4   HPV-DNA in Bowen's Disease and Skin Carcinomas of the Fingers

Diagnosis	Number of cases tested	Number of cases with HPV	HPV-type	Ref.(year)
Bowen's disease				
	1	1	35	47 (1989)
	11	7	16	54 (1990)
	1	1	16	57 (1993)
Squamous cell carcinoma				
	10	6	16	75 (1988)
	1	1	16	52 (1989)
	12	1	16	53 (1990)
	12	7	16 5x	76 (1991)
			2x untyped	
Total number:				
	48	24		

nonstringent conditions. HPV 16 was found in two cases associated, however, either with HPV 2 or HPV 18. Three additional lesions reacted only under nonstringent conditions; HPV could not be typed with the probes used. This, too, points to a possible association of cutaneous Bowen's disease with possibly not yet detected HPV types.

2.   Actinic Keratosis

The incidence of HPV-positive cases in actinic keratosis is actually low. Kawashima and colleagues[42] reported 51 specimens from 40 patients in which only 3 specimens from 2 patients were found to be HPV positive. HPV 36 was characterized from an actinic keratosis by Kawashima et al. in 1986.[62] In one of three patients with actinic keratosis, Grimmel et al. detected HPV 41. Out of 50 cases with actinic keratosis tested by *in situ* hybridization, 1 case proved to be HPV 41-positive.[63]

3.   Kerato-Acanthoma

Pfister et al.[64] found HPV-DNA related to HPV 19 and 25 in two of five cases of kerato-acanthoma, and Scheurlen et al.[65] characterized HPV 9 and HPV 37 in one of six cases. HPV 25 DNA was detected in one of 13 kerato-acanthomas in Australian patients.[66] Magee et al.[67] reported the detection of HPV 16 related DNA in 8 kerato-acanthomas by DNA hybridization. Six of the eight tumors occurred in immunosuppressed renal transplant patients. Kawashima et al.[42] tested 32 specimens of 29 patients with kerato-acanthomas and none proved to be positive. Hopfl and co-workers[68] reported 31 kerato-acanthomas which were consistently negative for HPV using *in situ* hybridization.

4.   Basal Cell and Squamous Cell Carcinoma

Kawashima et al.[42] tested 52 basal cell carcinomas from 35 patients and found HPV 20 in only one case. Only one case containing HPV-DNA could be detected by the same authors out of 61 specimens of squamous cell carcinomas. Other authors have found HPV 16 DNA in cutaneous squamous cell carcinomas in an increasing number of nonimmunosuppressed persons. A total number of 37 nonmelanoma skin cancers was analyzed by Pierceall et al.[69] for the presence of HPV sequences using PCR with primers designed to amplify DNA encoding the E6-E7 region of different genital HPV types. HPV 16 sequences were detected in 4 of 21 squamous cell carcinomas and 3 of 16 basal cell carcinomas. The presence of HPV 16 in the seven skin tumors was confirmed by dot blot hybridization of PCR-amplified material to ^{32}P-labeled HPV 16. Pfister's group[70] tested 10 cases of squamous cell cancer and found 1 specimen positive for HPV 16. Out of 25 patients with squamous cell carcinoma of the lip, HPV 16 was found in one case.[42] In 1989, Knobler et al.[71] reported a case of verrucous carcinoma of the lower leg to be positive for HPV 11. Garven et al.[72] detected HPV 11 and HPV 18 in a verrucous carcinoma of the leg by *in situ* hybridization. Noel et al.[45] demonstrated HPV 2 in a verrucous carcinoma of the foot by the PCR. HPV 41 could be shown in two of ten squamous cell carcinomas.[32] HPV 5 DNA was detected in one squamous cell carcinoma of a nonimmunosuppressed patient. This tumor also reacted with an HPV 16 probe.[73] In 1992, a case of Bowen's carcinoma of the nipple was reported, containing HPV 6 DNA.[74]

In analogy to the frequent occurrence of HPV 16 in digitally located Bowen's disease, Moy et al.[75] found that six of ten periungual squamous cell carcinomas contained HPV 16 DNA. Gordon and Palusci[52] reported HPV 16 in periungual carcinoma, as did Guitart et al.,[53] when they reviewed 12 cases of squamous cell carcinoma of the nail bed. Ashinoff et al.[76] found HPV DNA in 7 of 12 patients with squamous cell carcinoma of the finger and the nail bed, none of whom were originally diagnosed as having a malignant lesion. Five of the seven periungual lesions were found to contain HPV 16. These data confirm the association between HPV and squamous cell carcinoma of the periungual region and suggest that biopsies should be performed on chronic, solitary finger lesions in adults before therapy is initiated.

B.   Cutaneous Malignancies in Immunosuppressed Patients

In renal transplant recipients, squamous cell skin cancers are about 30–40 times as frequent as in the normal population, in contrast to basal cell carcinomas which are only 3–4 times as frequent.[77] The incidence of skin carcinomas appears to increase with the time after transplantation, from 8% at 1 year after allograft to 17% after 4 years.[78] In another series, malignancies appeared in 3% of the patients within the first year of immunosuppression, and the incidence increased up to 44% after 9 years, with a characteristic shifting of the ratio of basal cell to squamous cell carcinomas from 4:1 to 1:1.[79] Dyall-Smith et al.[80] calculated the probability of developing squamous cell carcinoma to be 25% after 9.5 years, rising to 50% after 20.6 years. The squamous cell carcinomas may have an aggressive course with a 5 to 8% metastasis rate,[81] and they are often preceded by warts and actinic keratoses. Studying 64 biopsies of 20 renal transplant patients, Euvrard and co-workers[81] differentiated 12 precancerous actinic keratoses, 2 Bowen's disease lesions, 11 kerato-acanthomas, 2 basal cell carcinomas, and 24 squamous cell carcinomas. HPV-DNA was detected in 4 of the precancerous keratoses, in 1 Bowen's disease, in 7 kerato-acanthomas, and in 13 squamous cell carcinomas (Table 5). HPV 16 or 18 was found in lesions from sun-exposed areas, but HPV 1 or 2 could also be found in 4 squamous cell carcinomas. The authors point out that oncogenic and benign HPV types may play an important role in the development of squamous cell carcinoma along with other cocarcinogenic factors, significant factors being UV exposure and immunosuppressive treatment. The presence of warts in graft recipients must lead to a dermatologic surveillance for early detection and treatment of warts, precancerous actinic keratosis, and squamous cell carcinomas. Patients should be advised to avoid sun exposure as soon as they have received their graft.

Interesting in this context is the finding of HPV 11 in multiple squamous cell carcinomas in a patient with subacute cutaneous lupus erythematosus who was treated with azathioprine and pred-nisone.[82]

As renal transplant recipients and EV-patients share a defect in immunological responses with occurrence of skin cancers on sun exposed areas, one could hypothetize that EV-specific HPV types play a role in skin carcinogenesis of iatrogenic immunosuppressed people, too. Thus, HPV 5 or HPV 5-related HPV, HPV 8, and other EV-specific HPVs have been detected in a small number of skin carcinomas of the immunosuppressed.[14,83,84]

Cancers, both squamous and basal cell carcinomas, develop mostly in sun-exposed areas.[78,79,81,85] However, Soler and colleagues[73] studied 92 lesions of transplant recipients, including 27 malignant skin tumors of transplant recipients, without being able to find HPV 5 DNA in any single case. Taking into account the high incidence of skin cancers in immunosuppressed people, however, the prevalence of EV-specific HPV types is extremely low. This indicates that immunosuppression is

TABLE 5   HPV-DNA in Malignant Skin Tumors of Immunosuppressed Patients

Diagnosis	Number of cases tested	Number of cases with HPV	HPV-type	Ref.(year)
Basal cell carcinoma				
	2	2	2	50 (1988)
	2	0	—	81 (1993)
Squamous cell carcinoma				
	1	1	5	83 (1983)
	1	1	2,4	86 (1987)
	4	3	5,8	84 (1989)
	1	1	48	48 (1989)
	188	0	—	80 (1991)
	1	1	1	49 (1991)
	1	1	11	82 (1992)
	24	13	1,2,16,18	81 (1993)

only one, and obviously a minor factor, determing the susceptibility of EV-specific HPV. Compared with the high incidence of HPV-containing plane and common warts, the incidence of skin carcinomas harboring HPV-DNA is in transplant recipients as low as in the general population.

REFERENCES

1. Brescia RJ, Jenson AB, Lancaster WD, et al: The role of human papillomaviruses in the pathogenesis and histologic classification of precancerous lesions of the cervix. *Hum Pathol* 17:552–559, 1986.
2. Cobb MW: Human papillomavirus infection. *J Am Acad Dermatol* 22:547–566, 1990.
3. Pfister H: General introduction to papillomaviruses. In: Pfister H (Ed.): *Papillomaviruses and Human Cancer.* CRC Press Boca Raton, Florida, 1990, 2–9.
4. Arends MJ, Wyllie AH, Bird CC: Papillomavirus and human cancer. *Hum Pathol* 21:686–698, 1990.
5. Laurent R, Kienzler JL: Epidemiology of HPV infections. *Clin Dermatol* 3:56–70, 1985.
6. Beliaeva TL: The population incidence of warts. *Vestn Dermatol Venerol* 2:55–58, 1990.
7. Nagington J, Rook A, Highet AS: Virus and related infections. In: Rook A, Wilkinson DS, Ebling FJG, Eds. *Textbook of Dermatology.* Oxford: Blackwell, 1986: pp 668–679.
8. Stern RS, Johnson ML, DeLozier J: Utilization of physician services for dermatologic complaints. *Arch Dermatol* 113:1062–1066, 1987.
9. Schachner L, Ling NS, Press S: A statistical analysis of a pediatric dermatology clinic. *Pediatr Dermatol* 1:157-164, 1983.
10. Steele K, Irwin WG, Merrett JD: Warts in general practice. *Ir Med J* 82:122–124, 1989.
11. Barr A, Coles RB: Plantar warts: a statistical survey. *Trans St Johns Hosp Derm Soc* 52:226, 1966.
12. Barr A, Coles RB: Warts on the hands: a statistical survey. *Trans Hosp Derm Soc* 55:69–73, 1969.
13. Gassenmeier A, Fuchs P, Schell H et al: Papillomavirus DNA in warts of immunosuppressed renal allograft recipients. *Arch Dermatol Res* 278: 219–223, 1986.
14. Rüdlinger R, Smith IW, Bunney MH, Hunter JAA: Human papillomavirus infections in a group of renal transplant recipients. *Br J Dermatol* 115:681, 1986.
15. Beutner KR, Becker TM, Stone KM: Epidemiology of human papillomavirus infections. *Derm Clin* 9:211–218, 1991.
16. Dyall-Smith D, Trowell H, Dyall-Smith ML: Benign human papillomavirus infection in renal transplant recipients. *Int J Dermatol* 30:785–789, 1991.
17. Viac J, Chardonnet Y, Euvrard S et al: Langerhans cells, inflammation markers and human papillomavirus infections in benign and malignant epithelial tumors from transplant recipients. *J Dermatol* 19:67–77, 1992.
18. Montgomery AH: Paper read before the West Side Clinical Society, March 1928. Cited in: Montgomery AH, Montgomery RM. *NY State J Med* 37: 1978, 1937.
19. Jablonska S, Orth G, Obalek S, Croissant O: Cutaneous warts: clinical, histologic, and virologic correlation. *Clin Dermatol* 3:71–82, 1985.

20. Orth G, Jablonska S, Favre M: Identification of papillomviruses in butcher's warts. *J Invest Dermatol* 76:97–102, 1981.
21. Jablonska S, Orth G, Glinski W: Morphology and immunology of human warts and familiar warts. In: Bachmann PA (Ed): *Leukemias, Lymphomas and Papillomas: Comparative Aspects*. Taylor and Francis, London 1981, pp 107–131.
22. Grußendorf, E-I: Lichtmikroskopische Untersuchungen an typisierten Viruswarzen (HPV 1 und HPV 4). *Arch Dermatol Res* 268:141–148, 1980.
23. Egawa K. Inaba Y, Yoshimura K, Ono T: Varied clinical morphology of HPV 1-induced warts, depending on anatomical factors. *Brit J Dermatol* 128:271–276, 1993.
24. Rübben A, Krones R, Schwetschenau B, Grussendorf-Conen EI: Common warts from immunocompetent patients show the same distribution of human papillomavirus types as common warts from immunocompromised patients. *Br J Dermatol* 128:264–170, 1993.
25. de Villiers EM, Hirsch-Behnan A, von Knebel Doeberitz C, Neumann C, zur Hausen H: Two newly identified human papillomavirus types (HPV 40 and 57) isolated from mucosal lesions. *Virology* 171:248–253, 1989.
26. Favre M, Obalek S, Jablonska S, Orth G: Human papillomavirus type 28 (HPV 28), an HPV-3-related type associated with skin warts. *J Virol* 63:4909, 1989.
27. Egawa K, Matsukura T, Kawashima M, de Villiers EM: A novel family of human papillomavirus (HPV 4,60 and 65) associated with black warts with specific intracytoplasmic inclusion bodies. In: *Proceedings of the Papillomavirus Workshop*. Seattle, U.S., July 1991. Fred Hutchinson Cancer Research Center.
28. Orth G, Jablonska S, Favre M, Croissant O, Obalek S, Jarzabek-Chorzelska M, Jibard N: Identification of papillomavirus in butchers' warts. *J Invest Dermatol* 76:97–102, 1981.
29. Oltersdorf T, Campo MS, Favre M, Dartmann K, Gissmann L: Molecular cloning and characterization of human papillomavirus type 7 DNA. *Virology* 149:247–250, 1986.
30. Greenspan D, de Villiers E-M, Greenspan JS, de Souza YG, zur Hausen H: Unusual HPV types in oral warts in association with HIV infection. *J Oral Pathol* 17:482–487, 1988.
31. de Villiers E-M: Prevalence of HPV 7 papillomas in the oral mucosa and facial skin of patients with human immunodeficiency virus. *Arch Dermatol* 125:1590, 1989.
32. Grimmel M, de Villiers E-M, Pawlita M, Neumann C, zur Hausen H: Characterization of a new human papillomavirus type (41) isolated from disseminated warts and the detection of closely related sequences in some squamous cell carcinomas. *Int J Cancer* 41:5–9, 1988.
33. Massing AM, Epstein WL: Natural history of warts. *Arch Dermatol* 87:306–310, 1963.
34. Bunney MH: *Viral Warts: Their Biology and Treatment*. Oxford University Press, Oxford 1982.
35. Tagami H, Oguchi M, Ofuji S: Immunological aspects of wart regression with special reference to regression phenomena of numerous flat warts: an experiment on tumor immunity in man by nature. *J Dermatol* 10:1–12, 1983.
36. Chardonnet Y, Viac J, Staquet MJ, Thivolet J: Cell-mediated immunity to human papillomavirus. *Clin Dermatol* 3: 156–164, 1985.
37. Tagami H, Ogino A, Takigawa M: Regression of plane warts following spontaneous inflammation. *Br J Dermatol* 90:147–154, 1974.
38. Berman A, Winkelman RK: Flat warts undergoing involution: histopathological findings. *Arch Dermatol* 113:1219–1221, 1977.
39. Grußendorf-Conen E-I: Langerhanszellen in HPV-induzierten Warzen. *Akt. Dermatol.* 13:224–225, 1987.
40. Rasmussen KA: Verrucae plantares: symptomatology and epidemiology. *Acta Derm Venereol* (Stockh) 38 (Suppl 39): 1–146, 1958.
41. Tagami H, Setsuya A, Masakuzu R (1985): Regression of flat warts and common warts. *Clin Dermatol* 3: 170–178, 1985.
42. Kawashima M, Favre M, Obalek S, Jablonska S, Orth G: Premalignant lesions and cancers of the skin in the general population: evaluation of the role of human papillomavirus. *J Invest Dermatol* 95:537–542, 1990.
43. Ikenberg, H, Gissmann L, Gross G, Grussendorf-Conen EI, zur Hausen H: Human papillomavirus type 16-related DNA in genital Bowen's disease and in Bowenoid papulosis. *Int J Cancer* 32:563–565, 1983.

44. Pfister H, Haneke E: Demonstration of human papillomavirus type 2 DNA in Bowen's disease. *Arch Dermatol Res* 276: 123–125, 1984.

45. Noel JC, Peny MO, Detremmerie O, Verhest A, Heenen M, Thiry G, de Dobbeleer G: Demonstration of huamn papillomavirus type 2 in a verrucous carcinoma of the foot. *Dermatology* 187:58–61, 1993.

46. Kettler AH, Rutledge M, Tschen JA, Buffone G: Detection of human papillomavirus in nongenital Bowen's disease by *in situ* DNA hybridization. *Arch Dermatol* 126:77–781, 1990.

47. Rüdlinger R, Grob R, Yu YX, Schnyder UW: Human papillomavirus-35-positive bowenoid papulosis of the anogenital area and concurrent human papillomavirus-35-positive verruca with bowenoid dysplasia of the periungual area. *Arch Dermatol* 125:655–659, 1989.

48. Müller M, Kelly G, Fiedler M, Gissmann L: Human papillomavirus type 48. *J Virol* 63:4907–4908, 1989.

49. Euvrard S, Chardonnet Y, Dureau G, Hermier C, Thivolet J: Human papillomavirus type 1-associated squamous cell carcinoma in a heart transplant recipient. *Arch Dermatol* 127:559–564, 1991.

50. Obalek S, Favre M, Jablonska S, Szymanczyk J, Orth G: Human papillomavirus type 2-associated basal cell carcinomas in two immunosuppressed patients. *Arch Dermatol* 124:930–934,1988.

51. Eliezri YD, Silverstein A, Moy RL: Human papillomavirus and digital sqamous cell carcinomas. *J Invest Dermatol* 90 (Abstr.) 556, 1988.

52. Gordon M, Papusci VJ: Human papillomavirus type 16 periungual carcinoma (Letter). *J Am Med Assoc* 262:3407–3408, 1989.

53. Guitart J, Bergfeld WF, Tuthill et al: Squamous cell carcinoma of the nail bed: a clinicopathological study of 12 cases. *Br J Dermatol* 123:215–222, 1990.

54. Eliezri YD, Silverstein SJ, Nuovo GJ: Occurrence of human papillomavirus type 16 DNA in cutaneous squamous and basal cell neoplasmas. *J Am Acad Dermatol* 23:836–842, 1990.

55. Kimura S, Hirai A, Harada R et al: So-called multicentric pigmented Bowen's disease. *Dermatologica* 157: 229–237, 1978.

56. Kawashima M, Jablonska S, Favre M, Obalek S, Croissant O, Orth G: Characterization of a new type of human papillomavirus found in a lesion of Bowen's disease of the skin. *J Virol* 57: 688–692, 1986.

57. Mcgrae JD et al: Multiple Bowen's disease of the fingers associated with human papillomavirus type 16. *Int J Dermatol* 32:104–107, 1993.

58. Grussendorf-Conen E-I: HPV-induzierte pigmentierte bowenoide Papulose am Hals. *Akt. Dermatol* 14:317–319, 1988.

59. Grob JJ, Zarour H, Jaquemier J et al: Extra-anogenital HPV 16-related bowenoid papulosis. *Genitourin Med* 67:18–20, 1991.

60. Grussendorf-Conen E-I, Giesen M: Papillomavirus Common Antigen in Bowen's Disease. *Dermatologica* 181:11–15, 1990.

61. Guerin-Reverchon I, Chardonnet Y, Viac J et al: Human papillomavirus infection and filaggrin expression in paraffin-embedded biopsy specimens of extragenital Bowen's disease and genital bowenoid papulosis. *J Cancer Res Clin Oncol* 116:295–300, 1990.

62. Kawashima M, Favre M, Jablonska S, Obalek S, Orth G: Characterization of a new type of human papillomavirus (HPV) related to HPV 5 from a case of actinic keratosis. *Virology* 154:389–394, 1986.

63. Grußendorf-Conen E-I, de Villiers E-M: Detection and localization of HPV-41 DNA in actinic keratosis by *in situ* hybridization. Papillomvirus workshop, Heidelberg 1990.

64. Pfister H, Gassenmeier A, Fuchs PG: Demonstration of human papillomavirus DNA in two keratoakanthomas. *Arch Dermatol Res* 218:243–246, 1986.

65. Scheurlen W, Gissmann L, Gross G, zur Hausen H: Molecular cloning of the two new HPV-types HPV 37 and HPV 38 from a keratoakanthoma and malignant melanoma. *Int J Cancer* 37:505, 1986.

66. Trowell HE, Dyall-Smith ML, Dyall-Smith DJ: Human papillomavirus associated with keratoakanthomas in Australian patients. (Letter). *Arch Dermatol* 126:1654, 1990.

67. Magee KL, Rapini RP, Duvic M, Adler-Storthz K: Human paillomavirus associated with keratoakanthoma. *Arch Dermatol* 125:1587–1589, 1989.

68. Hopfl RM, Schirr MM, Fritsch PO: Keratoakanthomas: human papillomavirus associated? (Letter) *Arch Dermatol* 128:563–564, 1992.

69. Pierceall WE, Goldberg LH, Ananthaswamy HN: Presence of human papilloma virus type 16 DNA sequences in human nonmelanoma skin cancers. *J Invest Dermatol* 97:880–884, 1991.

70. Pfister H: Human papillomaviruses and skin cancer. *Semin Cancer Biol* 3:263–271, 1992.

71. Knobler RM, Schneider S, Neumann RA et al: DNA dot-blot hybridization implicates human papillomavirus type 11 DNA in epithelioma cuniculatum. *J Med Virol* 29:33–37, 1989.

72. Garven TC, Thelmo WL, Victor J, Pertschuk L: Verrucous carcinoma of the leg positive for human papillomavirus DNA 11 and 18: A case report. *Hum Pathol* 22:1170–1173, 1991.

73. Soler C, Chardonnet Y, Euvrard S, Chignol MC, Thivolet J: Evaluation of human papillomavirus type 5 on frozen sections of multiple lesions from transplant recipients with *in situ* hybridization and non-isotopic probes. *Dermatology* 184:248–253, 1992.

74. Rübben A, Grußendorf-Conen E.-I.: HPV 16-verwandte DNA in einem Bowen-Karzinom der Mamille. *ZHautkr* 67:563–565, 1992.

75. Moy RL, Eliezri YD, Nuovo GJ et al: Human papillomavirus type 16 DNA in periungual squamous cell carcinomas. *J Am Med Assoc* 261:2669-2673, 1988.

76. Ashinoff R, Li JJ, Jacobson M et al: Detection of human papillomvirus DNA in squamous cell carcinoma of the nail bed and finger determined by polymerase chain reaction. *Arch Dermatol* 127:1813–1818, 1991.

77. Hoxtell EO, Mandel JS, Murray SS, Schuman LM, Goltz RW: Incidence of skin carcinoma after renal transplantation. *Arch Dermatol* 113:436–438.

78. Marshall V: Premalignant and malignant skin tumors in immunosuppressed patients. *Tranplantation* 17:272,1974.

79. Hardie JR, Strong RW, Hartley LCJ, Woodruff PWH, Clunie GJA: Skin cancer in caucasian renal allograft recipients living in a subtropical climate. *Surgery* 87:177, 1980.

80. Dyall-Smith D, Trowell H, Mark A, Dyall-Smith M: Cutaneous squamous cell carcinomas and papillomaviruses in renal transplant recipients: a clinical and molecular biologic study. *J Dermatol Sci* 2:139–146, 1991.

81. Euvrard S, Chardonnet Y, Pouteil-Noble CP, Kanitakis J, Thivolet J, Touraine JL: Skin malignancies and human papillomavirus in renal transplant recipients. *Transplant Proc* 25: 1392–1393, 1993.

82. Cohen LM, Tyring SK, Rady P, Callen JP: Human papillomavirus type 11 in multiple squamous cell carcinomas in a patient with subacute cutaneous lupus erythematosus. *J Am Acad Dermatol* 26:840–845, 1992.

83. Lutzner MA, Orth G, Dutronquay V, Ducasse MF, Kreis H, Crosnier J: Detection of human paillomavirus type 5 DNA in skin cancers of an immunosuppressed renal allograft recipient. *Lancet II*: 422–424,1983.

84. Barr BBB, McLaren K, Smith IW, Benton EC, Bunney MH, Blessing K, Hunter JAA: Human papillomavirus infection and skin cancer in renal allograft recipients. *Lancet I*: 124–128, 1989.

85. Boyle J, Briggs JD, MacKie RM, Junor BJR, Aitchison TC: Cancer, warts and sunshine in renal transplant patients. *Lancet I*: 702, 198.

86. Van der Leest RJ, Zachow KR, Ostrow RS, Bender M, Pass F, Faras AJ: Human papillomavirus. Heterogeneity in 36 renal transplant recipients. *Arch Dermatol* 123:354–357, 1987.

8

Epidermodysplasia Verruciformis as a Model for HPV-Related Oncogenesis

Slawomir Majewski, Stefania Jablonska, and Gerard Orth

CONTENTS

I.   INTRODUCTION

Epidermodysplasia verruciformis (EV) is a human skin disorder that provides strong evidence for a close relationship between infection with human papillomaviruses (HPVs) and cutaneous carcinogenesis.[1-3] EV is characterized by genetically determined unusual susceptibility to infection with EV HPVs resulting in the appearance in the early childhood of persisting warts and characteristic macular lesions.[4] The patients suffering from EV are unable to reject skin lesions, in spite of preserved nonspecific immunity to a variety of non EV HPV antigens. Benign lesions of EV are found associated with about 20 various HPVs.[3]

Most patients are infected with several (up to 10) various EV HPVs; however, in EV cancers two oncogenic HPVs (HPV5 and HPV8) predominate. The skin carcinomas that develop mainly in the sun-exposed area in adults have an unusual characteristic—in spite of invasive histology, they do not form metastases.[4,5] Recent molecular studies on the EV HPV genomes revealed the transforming potential of the E6 gene, and several genes were shown to be involved in regulation of viral DNA transcription in the process of tumor progression. Since EV-like lesions induced by EV HPVs were reported in single cases of heavily immunosuppressed patients, it was suggested that the abrogation of immune reactivity against EV HPV antigens could be responsible for persistence of cutaneous infection, and possibly for tumor progression and malignant conversion of EV skin lesions.

II.   EV SPECIFIC HPVs

A majority of characterized HPVs have been classified into groups according to their related genotypes, tissue tropism, and oncogenic potential.[6] A proportion of EV HPVs within the phylogenetic tree of papillomaviruses is quite remarkable.[7,8] There is a great diversity of EV HPVs: 21 are already characterized and cloned, and characterization of others referred to tentatively as EV HPV related is pending. EV HPVs could be preliminarily classified into subgroups of related genotypes based on DNA homology:

> Subgroup 1: HPV, 5, 8, 12, 19–21, 24, 25, 36, and 47
> Subgroup 2: HPV 9, 15, 17, 22, 23, 37, 38, and 49

More distantly related:

> HPV 48 and 50

Genetic heterogeneity of HPV5 and HPV8 and the presence of stable variants[9] suggests that the diversity of HPVs associated with EV is still greater. In spite of large spectrum EV HPVs in benign skin lesions of EV, the predominant HPVs in skin cancers of the patients are HPV5 and HPV8, and much more rarely HPV14, 17, 20, and 47.[3]

A high prevalence of novel EV HPV types differing from all other known EV HPVs was found in immunosuppressed population with the use of a very sensitive nested PCR enabling detection of HPV DNA at low copy numbers.[10,11] Thus it is to be presumed that EV-specific and EV HPV-related HPVs are in a latent form widespread in the general population all over the world. The role of these potentially novel EV HPV-related types in cutaneous oncogenesis in immunosuppressed population and in the general population is still poorly understood and remains to be demonstrated.

III. EPIDEMIOLOGY

A. EV HPVs in Immunosuppressed Population

In immunosuppressed patients appear all types of warts, induced by cutaneous HPVs. The frequency of HPV infection differs in various series, since the most important factor influencing the prevalence of cutaneous warts was found to be the duration of immunosuppression, i.e., graft survival time in allograft recipients. The prevalence is from about 35% for less than 5 years to over 80% for more than 5 years after grafting.[12,13]

In the previous studies of EV HPVs, mostly HPV5 and HPV8 were repeatedly found in allograft patients, both in single or disseminated lesions showing clinical similarity to EV,[12-22] and in plane, intermediate, or common-type warts.[17,23-25] With the use of PCR technique a low prevalence of HPV5 and HPV8 was detected in skin cancers of allograft patients.[26] However, PCR with the use of consensus primers proved to be not sensitive enough.[27] The most recent studies by PCR with the use of degenerate primers and subsequent sequencing of the amplified fragments enabled detection of EV HPVs in a proportion of allograft patients.[10,11] There was a high prevalence of EV-related HPV DNA sequences, distinct from the known EV HPVs or showing sequences related to EV HPVs.[11] EV-related HPVs were detected both in warts and in skin cancers. It should be stressed that a very high prevalence of EV-related HPVs was found in skin cancers (81%) in the series of Berkhout et al.,[11] and 56% of various skin malignancies were associated with different EV-related HPVs or HPVs responsible for warts in the general population.[10] One squamous cell carcinoma (SSC) contained HPV41. It is significant that in both studies a proportion of HPV-positive samples contained more than one HPV type. In the study by Shamanin et al.[10] EV-related HPVs were found to coexist with HPV3 or related HPV10 and HPV28, which were responsible for plane or intermediate warts in the general population.

The mere presence of EV HPVs does not appear to be sufficient for a full expression of EV phenotype, since EV HPV DNA was detected in typical cutaneous warts with no features of EV.[17,23,25] In our series of 100 immunosuppressed patients with warts, we found EV HPVs in 7 cases: HPV5, HPV20, and HPV23, always associated with HPV3 or related HPVs (HPV10 and HPV28), and responsible for plane or intermediate warts in the general population.[25] A novel HPV149, characterized in the immunosuppressed patients,[28] proved also to be EV specific HPV, like some other new not fully characterized types.[10] Absence of clinical and histological features of EV was probably due to still operative host cell restriction. Since EV HPVs were associated with HPVs responsible for flat or intermediate warts, it could be presumed that HPV3 or related HPVs provide the functions required in trans to allow episomal persistence of EV HPV genomes without expression of the EV gene. It should be stressed that EV patients found to be infected with HPV3 and EV HPVs had the lowest level of cell mediated immunity, comparable to that in allograft recipients.[29] EV HPVs are probably present in latent form by preserved host cell restriction. Their appearance in heavily immunosuppressed population is probably due to some rearrangement of cellular genome, with mutation of suppressor genes (e.g., p53), as shown for HPV16 E6,[30] and/or activation of cellular oncogenes, e.g., c-myc and Ha-ras, as shown for benign and malignant lesions associated with HPV.[31]

In summary, the immunosuppressed population is at risk to acquire EV HPV infection, which may be latent, and if activated, may play a role in the development of cutaneous cancers.

B. EV HPVs Associated with Tumors in the Immunosuppressed Population

The appearance of potentially oncogenic EV HPVs could be responsible for a great prevalence of malignancies in the immunosuppressed population.[22,32] Some new types of HPV were characterized from cancers of immunosuppressed persons: HPV 35 from Bowen's disease of the finger,[20] HPV 48 disclosed in one SCC,[37] HPV 37 and HPV 38 cloned from a case of keratoacantoma, and a case of malignant melanoma, respectively.[38] The prevalence of EV HPVs reported in malignancies in this population differs considerably. From rare or not, at all detection rates of HPV5 in squamous cell carcinomas[33-36] to 60% in a series of Barr,[22] and to 81% in a series of Berkhout et al.[11] This discrepancy appears to depend not only on the series studied, the graft survival time, the intensity of immunosuppression and the applied co-carcinogens, but also on the technique of detection. EV HPV DNA was detected significantly more frequently in patients with cancers, which suggests their possible role in the etiology of squamous cell carcinomas,[22] and possibly in other cutaneous malignancies.[10] Cancers were mainly or exclusively located in the sun-exposed areas, and UVB radiation was found to be an important co-cancerogen.[4]

The role of x-rays in evoking EV changes is best evidenced in a case of Hodgkin's disease, associated as a rule with deep immunosuppression in which developed typical EV lesions harboring EV HPVs.[21] These changes were exclusively limited to the skin subjected to irradiation and did not spread to other locations, including those characteristic of EV.

C. EV HPVs Associated with Tumors in the General Population

The association of cutaneous malignancies with EV HPVs in the general population appears to be weak. In a large series of 227 patients with malignant and premalignant skin lesions, HPV20 was disclosed only in one patient.[39] A new HPV36 was characterized originally from actinic keratoses of an immunocompetent patient, and later was found in several patients with EV, thus proved to be an EV HPV.[40] HPV34—slightly related to HPV16—was characterized from bowenoid papulosis of the finger.[41] A not entirely characterized EV-related HPV DNA was demonstrated in 2 keratoacanthomas.[42] The findings were not confirmed in a large series of patients with these tumors. However, cancers in an immunocompetent population, studied with the use of more sensitive techniques, were found to be positive mainly for HPV16.[43,44] With the use of newest techniques (nested PCR), about 70% of BCC and SCC in the general population was found to be associated with EV HPVs, some never found previously in immunosuppressed or in EV patients.[11] However, their role in the pathogenesis of cancers has to be established.

IV. GENETICS

EV is a multifactorial disease, but several data strongly suggest a genetic basis for the susceptibility to EV HPVs. A frequent familial occurrence of the disease, parental consanguinity, and high frequency (25%) of siblings with EV, as well as sex ratio (about 1), suggest that EV is an autosomal recessive disorder.[3,45] Another mode of EV inheritance, i.e., X-linked recessive, was described in a family in which only the males were affected.[46] However, a sex limitation to women was found in another family.[47] The existence of different recessive modes of EV transmission may suggest that abnormal susceptibility to EV HPVs depends on several genes localized on various chromosomes.[3] A role of genetic factor in EV is indirectly supported by appearance (in about 8% of cases) of mental retardation and other congenital abnormalities.[45] Neither chromosomal abnormalities[3,45] nor association with specific HLA-A,B,C alleles[48] were detected in EV patients. However, our recent studies on the polymorphism of class II MHC genes (DR-DQ), in a large series of 57 patients with EV from Europe, Africa, and America, suggest that specific halotypes are associated with EV (unpublished).

V. CLINICAL PRESENTATION

There are two main varieties of EV: the most common form associated with EV HPVs and a rare variety associated with HPV3, 10.[1,4,49] Sometimes a mixed infection with EV HPVs and HPV3 occurs.

A. EV Induced by EV HPVs

Cutaneous lesions are diverse: plane wart-like (Figure 1), and red, red-brownish, and brownish plaques (Figure 2). Achromic plaques with pigmented borders and red-brownish plaques on the trunk sometimes show a striking resemblance to pityriasis versicolor. The disseminated plane-wart like lesions, localized mainly on the hands, upper and lower limbs, and the face, are usually flatter, somewhat more reddish, and much more abundant than plane warts. Red and brownish plaques with irregular outlines and a slightly scaly surface are mainly distributed on the trunk, neck, and the proximal parts of the upper and lower extremities. Red single plaques localized exclusively on the trunk are not infrequently overlooked, and in these patients EV is recognized first after malignant tumors begin to appear on the face. In some patients, the lesions are widely disseminated, confluent, or almost generalized. In the form associated exclusively with EV HPV, other types of warts—common warts induced by HPV2 or HPV4—plantar and genital warts are very rare due to restrictive sensitivity to EV HPVs. The patients are, however, sometimes also infected with HPV3 and, in a majority of the cases, with several EV HPVs.

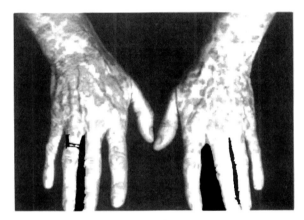

FIGURE 1 Very numerous, plane wart-like lesions on the dorsa of the hands and the forearms, more reddish and flatter than verruca plana in the general population, with some confluent, forming irregular plaques. The lesions were found to be associated with EV HPV5, 21, 23.

Oral mucosa and lymph nodes are not involved. There is also no visceral involvement and the general condition of the patients is satisfactory. Single cases were reported to be associated with mental retardation.[45]

B. EV Associated with HPV3

In this variety, the cutaneous changes are of plane wart type, widely disseminated over the trunk, face, and limbs (Figure 3), usually larger than plane warts, or plaque-like lesions. Follow-up of the patients with this variety of EV for over 30 years, we have seen in several of them superinfection with EV HPVs. Thus this life-long infection with HPV3 presents a risk factor for development of the major form of EV.

The mixed infection with EV HPVs and HPV3 is characterized by plane warts on the extremities, and red plaques and pityriasis versicolor-like lesions on the trunk and face.

C. The Course of the Disease

The course of the disease is extremely chronic and the infection is, as a rule, lifelong, starting at the age of 5–7 years. It is not clear why the lesions never appear in newborn and younger children.

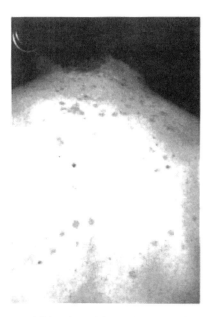

FIGURE 2 Characteristic red plaques—reddish or brownish macular lesions disseminated on the back. Red plaques were associated with EV HPV5 and 36.

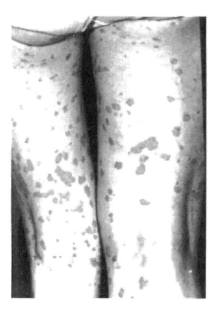

FIGURE 3 Plane wart-like lesions in EV found to be induced by HPV3. The lesions are more elevated than plane warts induced by EV HPVs, and in some areas they appear in linear arrangement (Koebner phenomenon). This patient had mixed infection with highly prevalent EV HPVs on the face and back, and HPV3 on the limbs.

It can be presumed that this is related with some changes in the immune system at this age. The cutaneous changes appear progressively, becoming widespread in some patients, or limited in others. Thus the patients differ considerably not only by clinical pattern, but also by the extent and activity of the disease. It should be stressed that the characteristic and invariable feature is persistence of changes throughout life. We have seen disappearance of lesions in some areas and/or flattening of plane warts, which became almost invisible, but there was never full regression of EV induced by EV HPVs. However, we have observed regression of generalized warts induced by HPV3 in a familial EV case. Contrary to the regression of plane warts in the general population, the lesions disappeared without any inflammatory reaction and not simultaneously.[50] The patient recovered completely and the depressed cell mediated immunity normalized.

VI. HISTOLOGIC AND ELECTRONMICROSCOPIC FEATURES

A. EV HPVs

The characteristic cytopathic effect consists of the presence of clear large dysplastic cells with finely granular cytoplasm and vacuolized nuclei, arranged in nests in the upper layers of the epidermis, not infrequently starting suprabasally and almost completely replacing the epidermis. The horny layer is loose, having a basket-weave like appearance, with prominent keratohyaline granules of various sizes and stainability over the dysplastic clear cells of the granular layer (Figure 4).

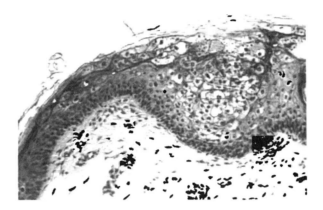

FIGURE 4 Histology of EV HPV5 associated red plaque. Characteristic hysplastic clear cells starting suprabasally, with overlying prominent keratohyaline granules in the upper parts of the epidermis. H + E, ×160.

The EV pattern is identical for diverse EV HPVs, and the extent of dysplastic changes depends only on the viral load and the activity of the disease.

B. HPV3-Associated EV

The histological pattern has all the characteristics of HPV3-induced plane warts in the general population. The characteristic feature is the "bird's eye" appearance due to vacualization around the pyknotic and a strongly stained nuclei, by well defined cell borders. The stratum corneum is in general loose with slight or no parakeratosis. Warts induced by HPV10 show frequently more pronounced papillomatosis and hyperkeratosis with more or less prominent parakeratosis. Thus, these warts have some features of verruca vulgaris but the cytopathic effect is not HPV3 type. Such warts, associated with HPV3 related viruses, are often referred to as intermediate verrucae, recognized clinically as common warts.

C. Electronmicroscopic Findings

The dysplastic cells have characteristic features: the cytoplasm is almost completely devoid of organelles except for ribosomes; the nucleoplasm is clear with chromatin pushed to the margins of the cell; the nucleoli are prominent; and viral particles, often in crystalline array, fill the nuclei of the superficial cells. The keratohyaline, not associated with tonofilaments, which are rarified, appear as isolated granules.

The electronmicroscopic features of HPV3-induced lesions have all the characteristics of plane warts in the general population: clarification around the nuclei with cytoplasmic organelles pushed to the periphery. There are no vacuoles in the nuclei and the chromatin is not marginated.

D.   Tumors in Patients with EV

Tumors arising from EV lesions may be benign papillomata (Figure 5) or seborrhoic ketatosis, and/or premalignant and malignant, i.e., actinic keratosis and squamous cell carcinomas (SCC). Papillomata develop both from HPV3- or EV HPV-associated lesions, and were reported as the main cutaneous finding in black patients.[51] Papillomata associated with EV HPVs may display the characteristic cytopathic effect.

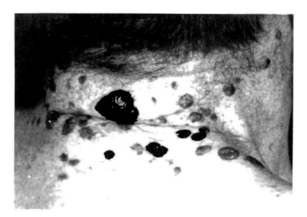

FIGURE 5   Numerous pigmented papillomata on the neck found to be associated with HPV8 and still unidentified HPVX.

Malignancies develop in one third to one half of the patients.[3] They start to appear in the fourth or fifth decades, are usually multiple, and arise as a rule from actinic keratoses localized mainly on the sun-exposed and/or traumatized parts of the body. The red or red-brownish plaques become hyperkeratotic, scaling, elevated, and, if very numerous, confluent, especially on the forehead (Figure 6). In contrast to a very rare malignant conversion of actinic keratosis in the general population, in EV patients this occurs gradually in numerous lesions.

The histology of premalignant lesions is characteristic of actinic keratosis with more numerous dyskeratotic cells and pronounced Bowen's atypia (Figure 7). The cytopathic effect disappears or is only slightly pronounced in some areas. The HPV DNA is often detected in a great amount. The premalignant lesions remain limited to the epidermis for several—usually more than 10—years. Early malignant conversion starts as an irregular downward proliferation of the epidermis displaying basaloid features.

The microinvasive growth occurs frequently in and around hair follicles. Invasive carcinomas are of SCC type with preserved Bowen's atypia: large dyskeratotic, pleomorphic, and multinucleated cells, with numerous atypical mitotic figures. Sometimes the invasive tumors are basaliomas. However, by studying serial sections, it is often possible to find, in some areas, multinucleated and dyskeratotic cells characteristic or Bowen's atypia.

EV tumors develop slowly, are mainly locally destructive, e.g., by periorbital localization, they do not destroy an eyeball. The metastatic potential is weak, if no co-carcinogens are applied, e.g., by x-ray irradiation.

The electronmicroscopy of EV tumors shows pronounced apoptosis, a most characteristic feature of Bowen's atypia. The apoptotic bodies, composed mainly of tonofilaments intermingled with traces of cytoplasmic organelles and/or remnants of nuclei, are engulfed by neighboring keratinocytes, and undergo gradual lysis. This phenomenon is probably responsible for a very slow progression of the tumors and noninvasive growth.

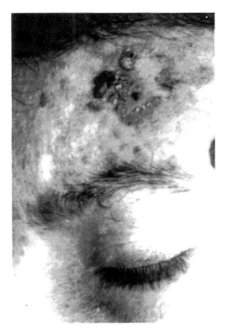

FIGURE 6   Microinvasive and invasive Bowen's carcinomas and disseminated premalignant lesions involving almost the entire forehead found to be associated with HPV5 and HPV9. This patient was infected with 10 EV HPVs and, additionally, with HPV3a.

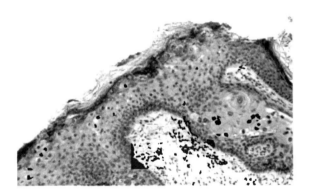

FIGURE 7   Actinic keratosis in EV with still pronounced cytopathic effect and downward proliferation of rete ridges displaying some early features of Bowen's atypia. H+E, ×120.

VII.   VIROLOGICAL ASPECTS

A.   Potentially Oncogenic EV HPVs

HPV 5, 8, and 47 have a "high oncogenic" potential and appear in more than 90% of EV skin carcinomas.[3,4] The E6 gene of "high oncogenic" HPVs was shown *in vitro* to have a higher transforming potential as compared to E6 of "low oncogenic" HPVs (HPV 14, 17, 20).[3] Characterization of molecular differences between "high oncogenic" and "low oncogenic" EV HPVs could be very helpful in understanding the process of viral cutaneous carcinogenesis in humans.

B.   Genetic Heterogeneity Among EV HPVs and the Role in Malignant Conversion

Molecular hybridization revealed in EV multiple DNA copies of EV HPV with no integration of viral sequences into the host genome.[3] Such integration was exceptionally described in EV cancers.[3,52] In spite of lack of EV HPV DNA integration, the role of EV HPVs in tumor progression is strongly supported by the detection of transcripts of the early region (E6 and E7) of the viral genome in the skin cancers.[3,9,53]

Using a rodent fibroblast and anchorage independence assay, it was shown that E6 genes of "high oncogenic" viruses (HPV 5, 8, and 47) encode proteins with higher transforming capability, compared to that of "low oncogenic" viruses.[54] In contrast to the anogenital types of HPVs, E7 of HPV8 and HPV47 did not induce transformation of cells.[55,56] However, unlike anogenital HPVs, E6 and E7 proteins of EV HPVs did not bind either p53 or pRB antioncogene proteins.[58] Immunostaining with a monoclonal anti-p53 antibody was found to be positive in over 90% of benign lesions of EV, whereas it was negative in all non-EV warts studied.[57] However, no p53 mutations were detected in exons 5–8 of the p53 gene in 4 analyzed lesions.[57] The authors concluded that the immunostaining was probably due to accumulation of wild type p53. They believe that over-expressed p53 protein might not be functional, or its suppressor function may be overcome by an unknown mechanism in EV leading to malignant transformation. Therefore, it was suggested that EV HPVs disturb the growth control of human keratinocytes by mechanisms that differ from those of the anogenital HPVs.[59] One of the possibilities is a derangement of function of E2-coded *trans*-activator of regulatory elements within the LCR (long control region) of HPV8.[60,61] It was shown that loss of E2 trans-activating function is associated with the loss of transforming function of this gene. In addition to the *trans*-acting factors, several *cis*-acting transcription control elements within the noncoding region (NCR) of the viral DNA have been identified.[62] The pattern of conserved sequences of NCR of EV HPVs differs substantially from that of other HPV types.[63,64]

Recently, a negatively acting oligonucleotide - SIL (for silence) was cloned from HPV8 sequences between 7384 and 7421, and was shown to act as a *cis*-acting element down-regulating the transcription.[59] Moreover, it was found that the SIL region contains the palindromic sequence P1 which binds the viral *trans*-activator protein E2. Therefore, it was suggested that viral factor (E2) can relieve repression by SIL leading to an elevated transcription of HPV8 genes in the process of malignant progression.[59] Recently, a constitutive transcriptional activator of HPV8 was identified which consists of M33 motif in the 3'-part of the NCR consistently followed by an API binding site.[65] This element showed properties of a constitutive enhancer capable also of stimulating the activity of thymidine kinase.

The question arises of whether modifications of the episomal viral genomes (for example due to UVB-induced mutations) could be involved in tumor progression in EV. It is known that in about half of the EV cancers there are deletions in EV HPV DNA,[3] including those affecting sequences homologous to the SIL.[9] The sequencing data of the regions flanking the deletions and the E6 genes of HPV5 and HPV8 did not support the involvement in EV of point mutations in tumor progression.[9]

It is to be stressed that oncogenic EV HPVs showed an unusual for HPVs genomic heterogeneity, even in the isolates from the same skin lesion of an EV patient suggesting that E6 genes code for different forms of E6 proteins.[9] These different allelic forms of transforming E6 gene could present different affinities for their target proteins or DNA sequences as well as other biological functions. It is possible that some EV HPV oncogene products can be involved not only in cell transformation, but also can serve as a source of specific antigens recognized by the host immune mechanisms.

VIII. IMMUNOLOGICAL ASPECTS

Tumor development and progression are multistep processes that involve complex interactions between the transformed cell, surrounding extracellular matrix, and cells of the immune system.[66,67] All these interactions constitute a basis for *immunosurveillance*, i.e., immune control of HPV infection and malignant progression. The role of immunosurveillance in EV is supported by a specific defect of cell-mediated immunity (CMI) against EV HPV-harboring kertatinocytes,[68,69] and by detection of EV HPVs in heavily immunosuppressed patients. In spite of the specific immune defect, a majority of EV patients also present variable abnormalities of nonspecific CMI, both local and systemic.[5] An intriguing possibility is that some of the derangement of CMI in EV patients are related to the long-lasting presence of EV HPVs and skin tumors. Recently, it was shown that the long-term presence of cancer, both in animals and in man, leads to alterations in T cell receptor-associated CD3 molecules, and to the abrogation of function of internal kinases (Lck and Fyn), resulting in depression of immune reactions.[70]

A.   Immunotolerance (Defect of Specific Immunity Against EV HPVs)

The nature of specific immune defect in EV patients is unknown, but it seems that abrogated immunosurveillance mechanisms against HPV infected/transformed keratinocytes is a result of genetically determined abnormalities of the process of presentation or recognition of EV HPV antigens.

It is well known that recognition of foreign antigens by T cells requires their presentation by glycoproteins encoded by genes within MHC.[71,72] MHC class I and class II molecules bind fragments of protein molecules (peptides) and present these fragments on the surface of antigen-presenting cells (APC) to CD8 and CD4 cell, respectively.[73,74] Class I molecules bind peptides derived from viruses, other intracellular pathogens, and endogenously synthesized proteins.[73] Class II molecules select peptides that are derived from proteins taken up by internalization, e.g., structural proteins of pathogenic microorganisms.[74] The particular immunogenic peptides are selected by MHC molecules depending on the affinity of different MHC alleles.[75] The optimal presentation of endo- and exogeneous antigens depends not only on HLA alleles but also on the other genes within MHC coding substances responsible for antigen degradation (proteasomes)[76] and peptide transportation (transporters),[77,78] and it is influenced by some other gene products, e.g., TNFα (tumor necrosis factor-alpha) (see below).

There is increasing evidence that specific immune responses to papillomaviruses are also genetically determined and depend on alleles of MHC. In a rabbit Shope papilloma-carcinoma complex, regression or malignant conversion of rabbit viral papillomas are linked to MHC class II genes.[79] In these studies, RFLP analysis of class II MHC in the rabbits revealed a strong linkage between papilloma regression and a DR EcoRI fragment, whereas malignant conversion of the lesions was associated with a DQ PvuII fragment. Further studies, based on sequencing the exon 2 encoding the DRα1 antigen binding domains of the different alleles, revealed that polymorphism thus characterized cannot account for the differences observed in wart regression. In contrast, the DQ allele associated with a higher risk of malignant conversion of skin papillomas encodes a highly divergent antigen binding domain which could account for deranged capacity to present viral or cellular antigens. Our most recent studies revealed similar negative and positive associations of specific class II MHC haplotypes in EV patients (unpublished).

The hypothesis of genetic immunosurveillance of HPV infection is further supported by the findings that a high risk of SCC of the cervix,[80] as well as the recurrent respiratory papillomatosis[81] is associated with some class II MHC alleles. Apple et al.[80] have shown that DRB1* 1501-DQB1* 0602 haplotypes were associated positively, while DR13 haplotype was associated negatively with HPV16 cervical cancers. Therefore, it is possible that particular MHC class II alleles, involved in viral antigen presentation, could condition the host immune reactions into immunity or immuno-tolerance, leading to regression or progression of the tumor.

In EV, a specific immunotolerance to EV HPVs manifests clinically as the inability of the patients to reject the HPV-induced skin lesions which then progress into skin cancers. Immunologically, this defect is reflected by the inability of natural cytotoxic cells to lyse EV HPV-harboring keratinocytes,[68] and by unresponsiveness of the patients' T lymphocytes to autologous HPV-infected epidermal cells.[69] One of the possibilities of the specific immunotolerance to EV HPVs could be due to derangement of HPV antigen processing within infected/transformed keratinocyte. Recently, some human cancers were found to be deficient in antigen processing capability.[82] However, nothing is known about proteasome-transporter genes of MHC in the control of HPV antigen presentation.

The most important and constant immune abnormality in EV is cutaneous anergy to locally applied DNCB and other contact sensitizers,[83,84] suggesting that the main immune defect is related to the local CMI reactions. This defect is most pronounced in EV patients with mixed infection with EV HPVs and HPV3. The abrogation of local CMI in EV suggests an important defect in the functions of antigen presenting cells (APC). However, recent studies did not disclose any significant differences in distribution of Langerhans cells (LC) in noninvolved skin of the patients with EV as compared with normal controls.[85] In the wart-like and benign red plaques, there was a decrease in LC number per unit of epidermal volume; however, this decrease was comparable to that in plane warts of non EV patients.[85] Also, a preserved *in vitro* function of LC from EV patients was reported,[69] suggesting that *in vivo* defect in APC function is due to some locally operating factors in the skin of EV patients. One of such factors seems to be UVB radiation, a main co-carcinogen in EV patients.

B.   Role of UVB in Generation of Specific Immune Defect in EV

The most characteristic feature of tumor progression in EV is its relation to sun exposure.[4] UVB is an important factor for both induction of local or systemic immunosuppression and probably for generation of specific derangement of the antigen processing and presentation. It was found that UVB impairs induction of contact hypersensitivity (CHS), as measured by the response to the locally applied DNCB.[86] This UVB-dependent immunological unresponsiveness seems to be genetically determined, both in animals and humans, and in man it presents a risk factor for skin cancer.[87]

One of the factors responsible for UVB-induced local immunotolerance could be urocanic acid (UCA) which is isomerized from *trans* to *cis* form upon UVB irradiation.[88] Cis UCA, when applied locally on the skin, suppresses the delayed type of hypersensitivity to herpes simplex antigens and to a variety of contact sensitizers[89,90] with simultaneous generation of specific T suppressor cells.[88] In our study, we found that the stratum corneum of the epidermis from sun-exposed areas in EV patients contains several-fold increased levels of the cis-isomer. Moreover, family members of EV patients showed an increased capability of isomerizing of UCA in the stratum corneum.

The mechanism of action of UCA is not known. Recent studies have suggested that TNFα could mediate the deleterious effect of UCA on the induction of CHS.[91] TNFα is a cytokine released within minutes after application of contact sensitizers or after UVB exposure,[92] and its amounts in EV epidermis were found to be increased both on the mRNA and protein levels.[93] The experimental data in the mouse have shown that local intradermal injection of recombinant TNFα into the sites painted with a hapten, impaired the induction of CHS in a similar way as observed after UVB exposure.[86] Recently it was shown that TNF can prevent LC from migration into the regional lymph nodes, thus affecting antigen presentation.[91] Since the production of TNFα is genetically determined,[94] it was suggested that susceptibility or resistance to the effects of UVB are dictated by polymorphic loci within MHC, including TNF genes.[81]

The important factor controlling the local action of TNFα is a TNFα receptor-inhibitor. The expression of a cell-associated TNFα receptor in EV is unknown. In contrast to the increased levels of soluble forms of TNFα receptors found in advanced malignancies,[95] or preliminary studies showed normal levels of circulating TNFα receptors in EV patients. It is tempting to speculate that increased levels of soluble TNFα receptors enable the autocrine action of endogeneous TNFα limiting proliferation of infected or transformed EV keratinocytes.

Another cytokine which could be of importance for generation of the immune defect in EV is TGF-β1 found to be overexpressed in both benign and premalignant EV skin lesions.[93] Moreover, we found by a dot-blot analysis presence of TGF-β1 in the supernatants of short-term culture of EV keratinocytes. TGFβ shows various immunosuppressive properties including inhibition of T cell proliferation, decrease of IL-1-dependent antigen presentation, and natural cytotoxicity.[96] TGFβ is also capable of enhancing TNFα gene transcription.[97] Thus, the local TGF-β1 activity in the skin of EV patients could be an additional immunosuppressive factor, enhancing a specific defect of host immune system toward EV HPV-infected keratinocytes.

T cells can be rendered anergic by antigen stimulation, also due to the local action of other cytokines, e.g., IL-4 and IL-10. These cytokines were not studied in EV; however, they were found to mediate susceptibility to infection by some pathogens via inhibition of Th1 cells leading to immunosuppression of CMI responses.[98] Of importance is that IL-4 is a main mediator of the induction of T cell tolerance due to administration of high doses of antigens.[99]

C. Role of Extracellular Matrix (ECM) in Tumor Progression in EV

Various cytokines and growth factors could affect tumor progression in EV through their effects on cell-ECM interactions. The highly characteristic feature of EV cancers is their low potential for invasive growth and metastasis formation.[4] Of special importance for ECM metabolism seems to be TGFβ found to be a strong inhibitor of several proteases involved in metastases (by inducing TIMP tissue inhibitors of metaloproteinases).[96] TGFβ also induces synthesis of ECM proteins and stimulates expression of integrins, i.e., cellular receptors for ECM components. Integrins play an essential role in tumor cell dissemination, both providing traction for cell migration on ECM and regulating deposition of such matrix.[100] These receptors are a family of glycoproteins consisting of two subunits (alpha and beta), and they have extracellular, transmembrane, and cytoplasmic domains.[100] Various abnormalities in integrin expression were described in different tumors depending on their origin.[101,102]

Recently, we have studied the expression of VLA-2 (collagen receptor), VLA-3 (multispecific receptor for collagen, fibronectin, and laminin), and VLA-6 (laminin receptor) in EV skin lesions as compared to that in benign and premalignant tumors in the general population. We found a simultaneous increase of VLA-2 and VLA-6 but not VLA-3 expression in EV lesions associated with EV HPVs (HPV5 and HPV8), but not with HPV3 (Majewski et al., in preparation). VLA-6 was also upregulated in benign actinic keratoses but not in basal cell carcinomas in the general population. It is conceivable that increased expression of VLA-6 could contribute to a low invasiveness of EV tumors. Recently it was found that in human papillomavirus-associated cervical neoplasms, in contrast to melanoma, a nonintegrin high affinity laminin receptor gene expression correlated with cell proliferation rather than invasion of tumors.[103] Also, we have found that *in vitro* expression of VLA-6 correlates with the proliferation rate of HPV16-harboring keratinocystes. Studies on the role of cell-ECM interactions and mechanisms of a low invasiveness of EV cancers could provide a new basis for therapy of HPV-associated tumors.

IX. MANAGEMENT

There is no specific therapy for EV, and no drug is effective against EV HPVs. The experimental therapies have been conducted with the use of interferons and retinoids.

A. Interferons

Application of IFNα in EV patients gave partial responses: slight clinical improvement and a marked decrease in the number of cells positive for HPV antigen.[104] However, within 1–3 months after cessation of therapy, all warts reappeared. Negative results were reported by other.[105,106] We have tried IFNα and β in various doses of $1–9 \times 10^6$ U/daily in 3 EV patients, with only slight and temporary improvement. Although systemic IFN proved to be in general ineffective in EV, the intralesional application appears to be a promising treatment for Bowen's carcinomas and basaliomas originating from EV lesions[107] as was found for basaliomas[108] and early carcinomas in the general population.[109] The treatment regimen is $1.5–3 \times 10^6$ U IFNα or IFNβ daily, 3 times weekly, for 3 weeks. In our EV patients, the results were not satisfactory.

B.   Retinoids

Orally administered etretinate or Isotretinoin were reported to have some temporary effect.[107] However, the reduction in size of the lesions was reversed after discontinuation of the therapy. We did not see beneficial effects in EV cases associated with EV HPVs. However, in one case of HPV3-induced EV, generalized plane warts regressed completely after 4 months of etretinate treatment combined with removal of single warts, which could induce immunostimulation by the wart-associated antigen. In another patient, we achieved a remarkable improvement; however, in 3 months after discontinuation of the treatment the warts reappeared.[110] Retinoids combined with IFN present a new promising combination for therapy of cutaneous tumours because of potentiation of anti-proliferative and immunostimulatory effects.[111] However, the results in EV patients were not satisfactory.

C.   Combined Therapy with 1.25-Dihydroxyvitamin D3 and Retinoids

This combination appears to be promising[112] since it was shown that *in vitro* there are synergistic antiangiogenic and antiproliferative effects for cell lines harboring HPV.[113,114] The results of this therapy in EV patients are still difficult to evaluate.

D.   Topical Therapy

The topical therapy with all trans-retinoic acid (0.05%–0.1%) or Isotretinoin (2%) applied alternately with 5% 5-fluorouracil proved effective exclusively for very early premalignant lesions.

E.   Prophylaxis

There are no effective measures to prevent EV HPV infection in the families of EV. In cases of EV induced by EV HPVs, the patients are at risk to develop cancers and since UVB is a most potent co-carcinogen, they should be protected against UVB from early infancy. The further measure of prevention is protection against chemical and mechanical irritations. For arising carcinomas, gamma irradiation is strongly contraindicated since its deleterious effect is comparable to that seen in patients with laryngeal papillomata. In EV, there are operative potent defense mechanisms limiting the growth of tumors and preventing metastases, and therefore the surgery could be less aggressive.

F.   Skin Grafting

By very numerous premalignant and malignant changes involving the entire forehead, we recommend removal of the frontal skin with its replacement by unexposed skin from the internal aspect of the arm. This method was applied in six patients, and we did not see any malignancies within the graft during up to 16 years of follow-up, although around it developed multiple Bowen's carcinomas. Nine years after grafting, single red plaques started to appear in the grafted skin, however with no tendency to malignant conversion. This method of preventing carcinomas provided an interesting model to study the development of benign changes in EV and their malignant conversion, which is a multistep process over more than 20–30 years.

REFERENCES

1. Orth, G., Jablonska, S., Breitburd, F., Favre, M., and Croissant, O., The human papillomaviruses, *Bull. Cancer* (Paris), 65, 151, 1978.
2. Orth, G., Jablonska, S., Jarzabek-Chorzelska, M., Rzesa, G., Obalek, S., Favre, M., and Croissant, O., Characteristics of the lesions and risk of malignant conversion as related to the type of the human papillomavirus involved in epidermodysplasia verruciformis, *Cancer Res.*, 39, 1074, 1979.

3. Orth, G., Epidermodysplasia verruciformis, In: Salzman, H. P., Howley, P. M., (Eds). *The Papovaviridae*. London, Plenum Press, 2, 101, 1987.

4. Jablonska, S., Epidermodysplasia verruciformis, In: Friedman, R. J., (Ed). *Skin Cancers*. W.B. Saunders, 101, 1991.

5. Majewski, S. and Jablonska, S., Epidermodysplasia verruciformis as a model of human papillomavirus-induced genetic cnacers: the role of local immunosurveillance, *Am. J. Med. Sci.*, 304, 174, 1992.

6. De Villiers, E. M., Human pathogenic papillomavirus types: an update. H. Zur Hausen (Ed). *Current Topics in Microbiology and Immunology*, Volume 186, Springer-Verlag, Berlin, Heidelberg, 1994, pp 1–12.

7. Chan, S. Y., Bernard, C. K., Ong, S. P., Chan, B., Hofmann, B., and Delius, H., Phylogenetic analysis of 48 papillomavirus types and 28 subtypes and variants: a showcase for the molecular evolution of DNA viruses, *J. Virol.*, 66, 5714, 1994.

8. Bernard, H. U., Chan, S. Y., and Delius, H., Evolution of papillomaviruses. H. Zur Hausen (Ed). *Current Topics in Microbiology and Immunology*, Volume 186, Springer-Verlag, Berlin, Heidelberg, 1994, pp 33–54.

9. Deau, M. C., Favre, M., and Orth, G., Genetic heterogeneity among papillomaviruses HPV associated with epidermodysplasia verruciformis: Evidence for multiplfe allelic forms of HPV5 and HPV8 E6 genes, *Virology*, 184, 492, 1991.

10. Shamanin, V., Glover, M., Rausch, C., Proby, C., Liegh, I. M., and Zur Hausaen, H., Specific types of human papillomaviruses found in benign proliferations and carcinomas of the skin in immunosuppressed patients, *Cancer Res.*, 54, 4610, 1994.

11. Berkhout, R. J. M., Tieben, L. M., Smits, H. L., Bouwes Bavinck, J. N., Vermeer, B. J., and Ter Schegget, J., Nested PCR approach for detection and typing of epidermodysplasia verruciformis-associated human papillomaviruses types in curtaneous cancers from renal transplant recipients, *J. Clin. Microbiol.*, 33, 690, 1995.

12. Rudlinger, R., Smith, J. W., Bunney, M. H., and Hunter, J. A. A., Human papillomaviruses infections in a group of renal transplant recipients, *Br. J. Dermatol.*, 115, 681, 1986.

13. Benton, E. C., McLaren, K., Barr, B. B., Blessing, K., Bunney, M. H., Rudlinger, R., Smith, I. W., and Hunter, J. A. A., Human papiloma virus infection and its relationship to skin cancer in a group of renal allograft recipients, Fritsch, P., Schuler, G., Hintner, H. (Eds): *Immunodeficiency* and *Curr. Probl. Dermatol.*, Basel, Karger, 18, 168, 1989.

14. Lutzner, M., Croissant, O., Ducasse, M. F., Kreis, H., Crosnier, J., and Orth, G., A potentially oncogenic human papillomavirus (HPV5) found in two renal allograft recipients, *J. Invest. Dermatol.*, 75, 353, 1980.

15. Goldes, J. A., Filippovitch, A. H., Neudorf, S. M., Bender, M. E., Ostrow, R. S., Faras, A., and Goltz, R. W., Epidermodysplasia verruficormis in a setting of common variable immunodeficiency, *Pediatr. Dermatol.*, 2, 136, 1984.

16. Pfister, H., Iftner, T., and Fuchs, P. G., Papillomaviruses from epidermodysplasia verruciformis patients and renal allograft recipients, In: *Papillomaviruses: Molecular and Clinical Aspects*. Howley, P. M., Broker, T. R. (Eds), A.R. Liss, New York, 85, 1985.

17. Gassenmaier, A., Fuchs, P., Schell, H., and Pfister, H., Papillomavirus DNA in warts of immunosuppressed renal allograft recipients, *Arch. Dermatol. Res.*, 278, 219, 1986.

18. Tanigaki, T., Kanda, R., and Sato, K., Epidermodysplasia verruciformis in a patient with systemic lupus erythematosus, *Arch. Dermatol. Res.*, 278, 247, 1986.

19. Rudlinger, R., Grob, R., Buchmann, P., Christen, D., and Steiner, R., Anogenital warts of the condyloma acuminatum type in HIV-positive patients, *Dermatologica*, 176, 277, 1988.

20. Rudlinger, R., Grob, R., Yu, Y. X., and Schnyder, U. W., Human papillomavirus-35-positive bowenoid papulosis of the anogenital area and concurrent human papillomavirus-35-positive verruca with bowenoid dysplasia of the periungual area, *Arch. Dermatol.*, 125, 655, 1989.

21. Gross, G., Ellinger, K., Roussaki, A., Fuchs, P. G., Peter, H. H., and Pfister, H., Epidermodysplasia verruciformis in a patient with Hodgkins disease: characterization of a new papillomavirus type and interferon treatment, *J. Invest. Dermatol.*, 91, 43, 1989.

22. Barr, B. B. B., Benton, B. C., McLoren, K., Bunney, M. H., Smith, I. W., Blessing, M. H., and Hunter, J. A. A., Human papillomavirus infection and skin cancer in renal allograft recipients, *Lancet*, 2, 124, 1989.

23. Van de Leest, R. J., Zachow, K. R., Ostrow, R. S., Bencler, M., Pass, F., and Faras, A. J., Human papillomavirus heterogeneity in 36 renal transplant recipients, *Arch. Dermatol.*, 123, 354, 1987.

24. Euvrard, S., Chardonnet, Y., Hermier, C., Viac, J., and Thivoler, J., Verrues et carcinomes epidermoides après transplantation renale, *Ann. Derm. Venereol.*, 166, 201, 1989.

25. Obalek, S., Favre, M., Szymanczyk, J., Misiewicz, J., Jablonska, S., and Orth, G., Human papillomavirus (HPV) types specific of epidermodysplasia verruciformis detected in warts induced by HPV3 or HPV3-related types in immunosuppressed patients, *J. Invest. Dermatol.*, 98, 936, 1992.

26. Stark, L. A., Arends, M. J., McLaren, K. M., Benton, E. C., Shahidullah, H., Hunter, J. A. A., and Bird, C. C., Prevalence of human papillomavirus DNA in cutaneous neoplasm from renal allograft recipients support a possible viral role in tumour promotion, *Br. J. Cancer*, 69, 222, 1994.

27. Tieben, L. M., ter Schegget, J., Minnaar, R. P., Bouwes Banvinck, J. N., Berkhout, R. J. M., Vermeer, B. J., Jebbink, M. F., and Smith, H. L., Detection of cutaneous and genital HPV types in clinical samples by PCR using consensus primers, *J. Virol. Methods*, 42, 265, 1993.

28. Favre, M., Obalek, S., Jablonska, S., and Orth, G., Human papillomavirus type 49: a type isolated from flat warts of renal transplant patients, *J. Virol.*, 63, 4909, 1989.

29. Majewski, S., Skopinska-Rozewska, E., Jablonska, S., Wasik, M., Misiewicz, J., and Orth, G., Partial defects of cell-mediated immunity in patients with epidermodysplasia verruciformis, *J. Am. Acad. Dermatol.*, 15, 966, 1986.

30. Hubbert, N. L., Sedman, S. A., and Schiller, J. T., Human papillomavirus type E6 increases the degradation rate of p53 in human keratinocytes, *J. Virol.*, 66, 6237, 1992.

31. Pelisson, J., Soler, C., Pechoux, C., Chignol, M. C., Viac, J., and Euverard, S., c-myc and c-Ha-ras cellular oncogenes and human papillomaviruses in benign and malignant cutaneous lesions, *J. Dermatol. Sci.*, 3, 56, 1992.

32. Bunney, M. H., Barr, B. B., McLoren, K., Smith, I. W., Benton, E. C., Anderton, I. L., and Hunter, J. A. A., Human papillomavirus type 5 and skin cancer in renal allograft recipients, *Lancet*, 2, 151, 1987.

33. Rudlinger, R. and Grob, R., Papillomavirus infection and skin cancer in renal allograft recipients, *Lancet*, 20, 1132, 1989.

34. Zukervar, P., Euvrard, S., Chardonnet, Y., and Thivolet, J., Incidence des papillomes viraux et des cancers malpighiens chez les transplantes renaux, *Nouv. Dermatol.*, 8, 4, 422, 1989.

35. Dyall-Smith, D., Trowell, H., and Dyall-Smith, M. L., Benign human papillomavirus infection in renal transplant recipients, *Int. J. Dermatol.*, 30, 785, 1991.

36. Soler, C., Chardonnet, Y., Euvrard, S., Chignol, M. C., and Thivolet, J., Evaluation of human papillomavirus type 5 on frozen sections of multiple lesions from transplant recipients with in situ hybridization and non isotopic probes, *Dermatology*, 184, 248, 1992.

37. Muller, M., Kelley, G., Fiedler, M., and Gissmann, L., Human papillomavirus type 48, *J. Virol.*, 63, 4907, 1989.

38. Scheurlen, W., Gissman, L., Gross, G., and Zur Hausen, H., Molecular cloning of the two new HPV-types (HPV 37 and HPV 38) from a keratoacanthoma and malignant melanoma, *Int. J. Cancer*, 37, 505, 1986.

39. Kawashima, M., Favre, M., Obalek, S., Jablonska, S., and Orth, G., Premalignant lesions and cancers of the skin in the general population: evaluation of the role of human papillomavirus, *J. Invest. Dermatol.*, 95, 537, 1990.

40. Kawashima, M., Favre, M., Jablonska, S., Obalek, S., and Orth, G., Characterization of a new type of human papillomavirus (HPV) related to HPV5 from a case of actinic keratosis, *Virology*, 154, 389, 1986.

41. Kawashima, M., Jablonska, S., Favre, M., Obalek, S., Croissant, O., and Orth, G., Characterization of a new type of human papillomavirus found in a lesion of Bowen's disease of the skin, *J. Virol.*, 5, 688, 1986.

42. Pfister, H., Gassenmaier, A., and Fuchs, P. G., Demonstration on human papillomavirus DNA in two keratoacanthomas, *Arch. Dermatol. Res.*, 218, 243, 1986.

43. Moy, R., Eliezri, Y. D., Nuovo, G. J., Zitelli, J. A., Bennett, R. G., and Silverstein, S., Human papillomavirus type 16 DNA in periungual squamous cell carcinomas, *J. Am. Med. Assoc.*, 261, 2669, 1989.

44. Eliezri, Y. D., Silverstein, S. J., and Nuovo, G. J., Occurence of human papillomavirus type 16 DNA in cutaneous squamous and basal cell neoplasms, *J. Am. Med. Dermatol.*, 23, 836, 1990.

45. Lutzner, M. A., Epidermodysplasia verruciformis an autosomal recessive disease characterized by viral warts and skin cancer, *Bull. Cancer*, (Paris), 65, 169, 1978.

46. Androphy, E. J., Dvoretzky, I., and Lowy, D. R., X-linked inheritance of epidermodysplasia verruciformis: genetic and virologic studies of a kindred, *Arch. Dermatol.*, 121, 864, 1985.

47. Rajagoplan, K., Bahru, J., Loo, D. S., Tay, C. H., Chin, K. N., and Tan, K. K., Familial epidermodysplasia verruciformis of Lewandowsky and Lutz, *Arch. Dermatol.*, 102, 247, 1972.

48. Wojtulewicz-Kurkus, J., Glinski, W., Jablonska, S., Podobinska, I., and Obalek, S., Identification of HLA antigenes in familial and nonfamilial epidermodysplasia verruciformis, *Dermatologica*, 170, 53, 1985.

49. Jablonska, S., Orth, G., Jarzabek-Chorzelska, M., Rzesa, G., Obalek, S., Glinski, W., Favre, M., and Croissant, O., Epidermodysplasia verruciformis versus disseminated verrucae planae: Is epidermodysplasia verruciformis a generalized infection with wart virus?, *J. Invest. Dermatol.*, 72, 114, 1979.

50. Jablonska, S., Obalek, S., Orth, G., Haftek, M., and Jarzabek-Chorzelska, M., Regression of the lesions of epidermodysplasia verruciformis, *Br. J. Dermatol.*, 107, 109, 1982.

51. Jacyk, W. K., Dreyer, L., and Villiers, E. M., Seborrheic keratoses of black patients with epidermodysplasia verruciformis contain human papillomavirus DNA, *Am. J. Dermatopath.*, 15, 1, 1993.

52. Yabe, Y., Tanimura, Y., Sakai, A., Hitsumoto, T., and Nohara, N., Molecular characteristics and physical state of human papillomavirus DNA change with progressing malignancy: studies in a patient with epidermodysplasia verruciformis, *Int. J. Cancer*, 43, 1022, 1989.

53. Yutsudo, M. and Hakura, A., Human papillomavirus type 17 transcripts expressed in skin carcinoma tissue of a patient with epidermodysplasia verruciformis, *Int. J. Cancer*, 39, 586, 1987.

54. Kiyono, T., Hiraiwa, A., and Ishibashi, M., Differences in transforming activity and coded amino acid sequence among E6 genes of several papillomaviruses associated with epidermodysplasia verruciformis, *Virology*, 186, 628, 1992.

55. Iftner, T., Bierfelder, S., Csapo, Z., and Pfister, H., Involvement of human papillomavirus type 8 genes E6 and E7 in transformation and replication, *J. Virol.*, 62, 3655, 1988.

56. Kiyono, T., Nagashima, K., and Ishibashi, M., The primary structure of major RNA in a rat cell line transfected with type 47 human papillomavirus DNA and the transforming activity of its cDNA and E6 gene, *Virology*, 173, 551, 1989.

57. Pizarro, A., Gamallo, C., Castresana, J. S., Gomez, L., Palacios, J., Benito, N., Espada, J., Fonseca, E., and Contreras, F., p53 protein expression in viral warts from patients with epidermodysplasia verruciformis, *Br. J. Dermatol.*, 132, 513, 1995.

58. Steger, G. and Pfister, H., In vitro expressed HPV 8 E6 protein does not bind, p 53, *Arch. Virol.*, 125, 355, 11992.

59. May, M., Grassmann, K., Pfister, H., and Fuchs, P. G., Transcriptional silencer of the HPV type 8 late promoter interacts alternatively with the viral transactivator E2 or with cellular factors, *J. Virol.*, 68, 3612, 11994.

60. Iftner, T., Fuchs, P. G., and Pfister, H., Two independently transforming functions of human papillomavirus, *Curr. Top. Microbiol. Immunol.*, 144, 167, 1989.

61. Stubenrauch, F., Malejczyk, J., Fuchs, P. G., and Pfister, H., Late promoter of human papillomavirus 8 and its regulation, *J. Virol.*, 66, 3485, 1992.

62. Reh, H. and Pfister, H., Human papillomavirus type 8 contains cis-active positive and negative transcriptional control sequences, *J. Gen. Virol.*, 71, 2457, 1990.

63. Ensser, A. and Pfister, H., Epidermodysplasia verruciformis associated with human papillomaviruses present s subgenus-specific organization of the regulatory genome region, *Nucleic Acids Res.*, 18, 3919, 1990.

64. Fuchs, P. G. and Pfister, H., Papillomaviruses in epidermodysplasia verruciformis, *Papillomavirus Report*, 1, 1, 1990.

65. Horn, S., Pfister, H., and Fuchs, P., Constitutive transcription activator of epidermodysplasia verruciformis-associated human papillomavirus 8, *Virology*, 196, 1, 1993.

66. Zur Hausen, H., Papillomaviruses in human cancers, *Mol. Carcinogenesis*, 1, 147, 1988.

67. Zur Hausen, H., Papillomaviruses as carcinomaviruses, *Adv. Viral. Oncol.*, 8, 1, 1989.

68. Majewski, S., Malejczyk, J., Jablonska, S., Mislewicz, J., Rudnicka, L., Obalek, S., and Orth, G., Natural cell-mediated cytotoxicity against various target cells in patients with epidermodysplasia verruciformis, *J. Am. Acad. Dermatol.*, 22, 423, 1990.

69. Cooper, K. D., Androphy, E. J., Lowy, D. R., and Katz, S. I., Antigen presentation and T cell activation in epidermodysplasia verruciformis, *J. Invest. Dermatol.*, 94, 769, 1990.

70. Mizoguichi, H., O'Shea, J. J., Longo, D. L., Loeffler, C. M., McVicar, D. W., and Ochoa, A. C., Alterations in signal transduction molecules in T lymphocytes from tumor-bearing mice, *Science*, 258, 1795, 1992.

71. Braciale, T. J. and Braciale, V. L., Antigen presentation: structural themes and functional variations, *Immunol. Today*, 12, 124, 1991.

72. Brodski, F. M. and Guagliardi, L. E., The cell biology of antigen processing and presentation, *Ann. Rev. Immunol.*, 9, 707, 1991.

73. Braciale, T. J., Antigen processing for presentation by MHC class I molecules, *Curr. Opin. Immunol.*, 4, 52, 1992.

74. Unanune, E. R., Cellular studies on antigen presentation by class II MHC molecules, *Curr. Opin. Immunol.*, 4, 63, 1992.

75. Karr, R. W., Yu, W., Watts, R., Evans, K. S., and Celis, E., The role of polymorphic HLA-DRβ chain residues in presentation of viral antigens to T cells, *J. Exp. Med.*, 172, 273, 1990.

76. Monaco, J. J., Genes in the MHC that may affect antigen processing, *Curr. Opin. Immunol.*, 4, 70, 1992.

77. Glynne, R., Powis, S. H., Beck, S., Kelly, A., Kerr, L.-A., and Trowsdale, J., A proteasome-related gene between the two ABC transporter loci in the class II region of the human MHC, *Nature*, 353, 357, 1991.

78. Kelly, A., Powis, S. H., Kerr, L.-A., Mockridge, I., Elliott, T., Bastin, J., Uchanska-Ziegler, B., Ziegler, A., Trowsdale, J., and Townsend., Assembly and function of the two ABC transporter proteins encoded in the human major histocompatibility complex, *Nature*, 365, 641, 1992.

79. Han, R., Breitburd, F., Marche, P. N., and Otrh, G., Linkage of regression and malignant conversion of rabbit viral papillomas to MHC class II genes, *Nature*, 356, 66, 1992.

80. Apple, J. R., Erlich, H. A., Klitz, W., Manos, M. M., Becker, T. M., Wheeler, C. M., HLA DR-DQ associations with cervical carcinoma show papillomavirus-type specificity, *Nature Genet.*, 6, 157, 1994.

81. Bonagura, V. R., O'Reilly, M. E., Abramson, A. L., and Steinberg, B. M., Recurrent respiratory papillomatosis (RRP): enriched HLA DQW3 phenotype and decreased class I MHC expression, In: *Immunology of Papillomaviruses*, Ed., B. M. Steinberg, Plenum Press, London, 1993.

82. Restifo, N. P., Esquivel, F., Kawakami, Y., Yewdell, J. W., Mule, J. J., Resenberg, S. A., and Bennink, J. R., Identification of human cancers defective in antigen processing, *J. Exp. Med.*, 177, 265, 1993.

83. Obalek, S., Glinski, W., Haftek, M., Orth, G., and Jablonska, S., Comparative studies on cell-mediated immunity in patients with different warts, *Dermatologica*, 236, 1, 1979.

84. Glinski, W., Obalek, S., Jablonska, S., and Orth, G., T cell defect in patients with epidermodysplasia verruciformis due to human papillomavirus type 3 and 5, *Dermatologica*, 162, 141, 1981.

85. Haftek, M., Jablonska, S., Szymanczyk, J., and Jarzabek-Chorzelska, M., Langerhans cells in epidermodysplasia verruciformis, *Dermatologica*, 174, 173, 1987.

86. Yoshikawa, T. and Streilein, J. W., Genetic basis of the effects of ultraviolet light B on cutaneous immunity. Evidence that polymorphism at the TNFα and Lps loci governs susceptibility, *Immunogenetics*, 32, 398, 1990.

87. Yoshikawa, T., Rae, V., Bruins-Slot, W., Van den Berg, J.-W., Taylor, J. R., and Streilein, J. W., Susceptibility to effects of UVB radiation on induction of contact hypersensitivity as a risk factor for skin cancer in humans, *J. Invest. Dermatol.*, 85, 530, 1990.

88. Noonan, F. P., DeFabo, E. C., and Morrison, H., Cis-urocanic acid, a product formed by ultraviolet B irradiation of the skin, initiates an antigen presentation defect in splenic dendritic cells in vivo, *J. Invest. Dermatol.*, 90, 92, 1988.

89. Ross, J. A., Howie, S. E. M., Norval, M., Maingay, J., and Simpson, T. J., Ultraviolet-irradiated urocanic acid suppresses delayed-type hypersensitivity to herpes simplex virus in mice, *J. Invest. Dermatol.*, 87, 630, 1986.

90. Harriot-Smith, T. G. and Halliday, W. J., Suppression of contact hypersensitivity by short-term ultraviolet irradiation. II. The role of urocanic acid, *Clin. Exp. Immunol.*, 72, 174, 1988.

91. Streilein, J. W., Sunlight and skin-associated lymphoid tissues (SALT): If UVB is the trigger and TNFα is its mediator, what is the message?, *J. Invest. Dermatol.*, 100, 47S, 1993.

92. Enk, A. H. and Katz, S. I., Early molecular events in the induction phase of contact sensitivity, *Proc. Natl. Acad. Sci. U.S.A.*, 89, 1398, 1992.

93. Majewski, S., Hunzelmann, N., Nischt, R., Eckes, B., Rudnicka, L., Orth, G., Krieg, T., and Jablonska, S., TGFβ-1 and TNFα expression in the epidermis of patients with epidermodysplasia verruciformis, *J. Invest. Dermatol.*, 97, 862, 1991.

94. Jacob, C. O., Fronek, Z., Lewis, G. D., Koo, M., Hansen, J. A., and McDevitt, H. O., Heritable major histocompatibility complex class II-associated differences in production of tumor necrosis factor: relevance to genetic predisposition to systemic lupus erythematosus, *Proc. Natl. Acad. Sci. U.S.A.*, 87, 1233, 1990.

95. Aderka, D., Engelman, H., Hernik, V., Skornick, Y., Levo, Y., Wallach, D., and Kushtal, G., Increased serum levels of soluble receptors for tumor necrosis factor in cancer patients, *Cancer Res.*, 51, 5602, 1991.

96. Roberts, A. B. and Sporn, M. B., The transforming growth factor-beta's, in Sporn, M. B., Roberts, E. B. (Eds): *Handbook of Experimental Pharmacology*, Berlin Springer, 95, 419, 1990.

97. Wahl, Sm., Hunt, D. A., Wakefield, L. M., Francis-McCartney, N., Wahl, L. M., Roberts, A. B., and Sporn, M. S., Tranforming growth factor typeβ induces monocyte chemotaxis and growth factor production, *Proc. Natl. Acad. Sci. U.S.A.*, 84, 5788, 1987.

98. Sieling, P. A., Abrams, J. S., Yamamura, M., Salgame, P., Bloom, B. R., Rea, T. H., and Modlin, R. L., Immunosuppressive roles for IL-10 and IL-4 in human infection, *J. Immunol.*, 150, 5501, 1993.

99. Burnstein, H. J. and Abbas, A. K., In vivo role of interleukin 4 in T cell tolerance induced by aqueous protein antigen, *J. Exp. Med.*, 177, 457, 1993.

100. Hynes, R. O., Integrins: versatility, modulation, and signaling in cell adhesion, *Cell*, 69, 11, 1992.

101. Peltonen, J., Larjava, H., Jaakkola, S., Grainick, H., Akiyama, S., Yamada, S., Yamada, K. M., and Uitto, J., Localization of integrin receptors for fibronectin, collagen and laminin in human skin. Variable expression in basal and squamous cell carcinomas, *J. Clin. Invest.*, 84, 1916, 1989.

102. Cerri, A., Tadini, G., Gitto, R., Crosti, L., and Berti, E., Adhesion molecules and skin tumours: a peculiar pattern of integrin expression is present in carcinoma cells, *Eur. J. Dermatol.*, 4, 279, 1992.

103. Demeter, L. M., Stoler, M. H., Sobel, M. E., Broker, T. R., and Chow, L. T., Expression of high-affinity laminin receptor mRNA correlates with cell proliferation rather than invasion in human papillomavirus-associated cervical neoplasms, *Cancer Res.*, 52, 1561, 1992.

104. Androphy, E. J., Dvoretzky, I., and Malnish, A. E., Response of warts in epidermodysplasia verruciformis to treatment with systemic oral and intralesional alpha interferon, *J. Am. Acad. Dermatol.*, 11, 197, 1984.

105. Kanerva, L. O., Johansson, E., Niemi, K. M., Lauharanta, J., and Salo, O. P., Epidermodysplasia verruciformis. Clinical and light- and electromicroscopic observations during etretinale therapy, *Arch. Dermatol. Res.*, 278, 153, 1985.

106. Kowalzick, L. and Mensing, H., Failure of etretinate in epidermodysplasia verruciforms, *Dermatologica*, 173, 75, 1986.

107. Blanchet-Bardon, C. and Lutzner, M. A., Interferon and retinoid treatment of warts, Warts (Human Papillomaviruses), Jablonska, S., Orth, S., (Eds.), J.B. Lippincott, Philadelphia 1985, *Clin. Dermatol.*, 3(4), 195, 1985.

108. Cornell, R. C., Greenway, H. T., Tucker, S. B., Edwards, L., Ashworth, S., Vance, J. C., Tanner, D. J., Taylor, E. L., Smiles, K. A., and Peets, A., Intralesional interferon therapy for basal cell carcinoma, *J. Am. Acad. Dermatol.*, 23, 694, 1990.

109. Edwards, L., Berman, B., Rapini, R. P., Whiting, D. A., Tyring, S., Greenway, H. T., Eyre, S. P., Tanner, D. J., Taylor, E. L., Peets, E., and Smiles, K. A., Treatment of cutaneous squamous cell carcinomas by intralesional interferon alfa-2 b therapy, *Arch. Dermatol.*, 128, 1486, 1992.

110. Jablonska, S., Obalek, S., and Wolska, H., Follow-up of patients with epidermodysplasia verruciformis treated with etretinate, *Dermatologica*, 173, 196, 1986.

111. Bollag, W., Retionoids and interferon: a new promising combination? *Br. J. Hematology*, 79, Suppl. 1, 87, 1991.

112. Majewski, S., Skopinska, M., Bollag, W., and Jablonska, S., Combination of isotretinoin and calcitriol for precancerous and cancerous skin lesions, *Lancet*, 344, 1510, 1994.

113. Majewski, S., Szmurlo, A., Marczak, M., Jablonska, S., and Bollag, W., Inhibition of tumor cell-induced angiegensis by retinoids, 1,25-dihydroxyvitamin D3 and their combination, *Cancer Lett.*, 75, 35, 1993.

114. Majewski, S., Smurlo, A., Marczak, M., Jablonska, S., Bollag, W., Synergistic effect of retinoids and interferon alpha on tumor-induced angiogenesis: antiangiogenic effect on HPV-harboring tumor cell lines, *Int. J. Cancer*, 57:81, 1994.

9

Condyloma Acuminatum and Other HPV-Related Squamous Cell Tumors of the Genitoanal Area

Kari J. Syrjänen

CONTENTS

I.   INTRODUCTION

Until the late 1970s, condyloma acuminatum (genital wart) was regarded as the only manifestation of human papillomavirus (HPV) in the genital tract, recognized as a disease entity since antiquity.[1] Since 1976, however, it has been well established that HPV induces other types of squamous cell lesions as well.[2] These are currently known as flat and inverted condylomas, being frequently associated with precancer lesions (dysplasia, intraepithelial neoplasia), carcinoma *in situ* (CIS), and frankly invasive squamous cell carcinomas of the uterine cervix.[2-4] The same is true with the Bowenoid papulosis lesions, confined to external genitalia of both sexes.[5,6]

During the past 15 years, significant new data on epidemiology, molecular biology, and biological behavior of HPV infections, as well as their intimate associations with a variety of squamous cell tumors have been published.[3,7-20] These data are reviewed in detail in the separate chapters of this volume. So far, 70 different types of HPV have been recognized,[21] of which more than 20 types can infect the genital tract of both sexes. Based on the integration properties and their preferred detection in either benign condylomas/squamous cell papillomas or invasive carcinomas, HPV types have been classified as low risk types (HPV 6,11,40,42,43,44,54,57) and high risk types (HPV types 16,18,31,33,35,39,45,51,52,55,56,58,66).[6,8,15,16,22-26] An increased risk for the development of an invasive cancer has been ascribed to infections by the latter.[15,16,18-21,27] This is well documented also in our 10-year prospective follow-up study, where a significantly higher progression rate was established for genital HPV 16 lesions.[28-31] The data provided by the rapidly progressing molecular biological research have significantly contributed to our understanding of the molecular mechanisms involved, e.g., in cell transformation, by these viruses.[7,9,10,13,16,23,27,32,33] (See also Fuchs and Pfister in this volume).

Until recently, genital HPV infections were regarded as being exclusively a sexually transmitted disease (STD), and their rapid increase has been attributed to strikingly changed sexual habits during the past two decades, i.e., early onset of sexual activity and large number of sexual partners.[34-42] For prevention of this infection (and thereby reducing the risk for genital cancer in both partners), it would be of crucial importance to identify the reservoirs of HPV.[12,20,43-46] Several recent reports on HPV DNA in biopsies or smears derived from the normal female genital tract suggest that these sites might act as such a reservoir.[18,47-57] Despite the strong evidence implicating the role of the male in transmitting HPV infections,[43,58-60] the male reservoirs of the distinct HPV types detectable in the female genital lesions are far from being fully elucidated yet.[61,62] Studies on the male consorts of women with genital HPV lesions (with or without cervical intraepithelial neoplasia, CIN) have disclosed HPV infections in 50–90% of the cases, most being symptomless, i.e., subclinical or latent.[63,64]

It has been suggested that such subclinical and latent infections in the male may represent an appreciable reservoir for the high-risk HPV types involved in the etiology of cervical cancer.[43,58,65] Indeed, the connections between carcinoma of the penis and carcinoma of the uterine cervix have been subjected to an increasing number of epidemiological surveys recently.[66-72] Geographically, the prevalence of these two diseases shows some interesting parallels; penile carcinoma is a rare disease in all western countries,[14] but more common in Thailand, India, China, Puerto Rico, as well as in certain parts of Africa (e.g., Kenya, Tanzania, and Uganda).[73] Also the age distribution of the patients is different in these low- and high-risk countries.[14] For a long time, penile condylomata acuminata have been implicated in pathogenesis of penile cancer in these high-risk countries.[14,73,74]

On the basis of the accumulated data, it has become necessary to revise the previous concepts on genital HPV infections, and to make a clear distinction between (1) clinical, (2) subclinical, and (3) latent infections.[45,46] Because of marked inconsistencies in the usage of the terms subclinical and latent HPV infection in the current literature,[19,75] the diagnostic criteria for the three categories of genital HPV infections were recently outlined.[20,45,46] (Table 1).

This concept will be followed in the present communication, in which the distinct genital HPV lesions are described with special emphasis on their natural history as well as their associations to

TABLE 1   Criteria of the Different Manifestations of HPV
Infections

Diagnostic method	Results obtained by different diagnostic techniques in:		
	Clinical infection	Subclinical infection	Latent infection
Colposcopy	Decisive	Equivocal	Negative
Pap Smear	Decisive	Equivocal	Negative
Histology	Decisive	Equivocal	Negative
Hybridization	Positive	Positive	Positive
PCR-Amplification	Positive	Positive	Positive

genital squamous cell carcinomas in both sexes. The importance of making a distinction between the clinical infections as potentially precancerous lesions in both sexes is underlined.

II.   CLINICAL MANIFESTATIONS OF GENITAL HPV INFECTIONS

A.   Benign Lesions

HPVs induce benign squamous cell proliferations (papillomas) in the skin and in a wide variety of mucosal sites, including the uterine cervix, vulva, penis, anus, larynx, bronchus, esophagus, tongue, and oral cavity. HPV-induced tumors were traditionally considered benign with only a limited growth potential.[14] Their malignant conversion has been recognized as a potential occurrence, however, albeit usually after a long latency period of years or even decades.[14,76] With the recognition of the flat condylomas in the uterine cervix,[2] it became evident that the cervix is the most frequently HPV-affected genital site, far exceeding in frequency the exophytic lesions of the external genitalia.[4,11,12,20,77] Similarly, since the description of flat condylomas and their associations with CIN lesions, it has been amply documented that there are additional genital and perianal HPV lesions which are different from the classical condyloma acuminatum both on gross appearance and on light microscopy.[78] To date, five morphologically distinct, primarily benign anogenital HPV lesions have been recognized: (1) condyloma acuminatum; (2) giant condyloma; (3) Buschke-Löwenstein tumor; (4) flat condyloma, and (5) papulosis/pigmented papulosis lesion.[5,78] All these varieties are found both on the female and male external genitalia and in the adjacent mucosal sites, i.e., in the urethra and the anus as well.

1.   Condyloma Acuminatum

Condylomata acuminata are papillary genital warts which are usually multiple and grow in clusters. In the vast majority of cases, they are readily detectable with the naked eye, appearing grouped around the mucocutaneous junctions. On the male genitalia, they are found primarily on the shaft of the penis, on the prepuce, and on the glans.[5,78,79]

The light microscopic morphology of the classical condyloma accuminatum has been exhaustively described by a number of authors.[80,81] This lesion is characterized by papillomatosis, acanthosis, elongation and thickening of the rete pegs, parakeratosis, and cytoplasmic vacuolization or koilocytosis.[77,78,80,81] The basal cell layers regularly exhibit some proliferation. Elongated dermal papillae, intercellular edema, dilated vessels, and round cell infiltrates are a constant finding. On light microscopy, this lesion is indistinguishable from the aquamous cell papilloma but the latter name is not used for exophytic genital HPV lesions any longer.[76] Condylomata acuminata on the external genitals are differentiated from those in the uterine cervix or vagina, usually by a layer (varying in thickness) of hyperkeratosis on their surface. Occasionally, condylomata may exhibit enlarged and hyperchromatic nuclei with anisokaryosis, pyknosis, and atypical mitotic figures. These conditions have been called as atypical condylomas by some authors,[82] and they are sometimes difficult to differentiate from true dysplasia. However, the regularity of the basal cell layers and the low nuclear-cytoplasmic ratio indicate a benign condition.[82]

When subjected to immunohistochemical staining for HPV structural proteins, the lesions usually express these antigens in abundance.[11,12,20] Positive staining is localized in the intermediate and superficial layers of the epithelial projections, indicating an ongoing productive (high copy number) HPV infection at these sites. Similarly, when examined by *in situ* DNA hybridization, HPV DNA (usually HPV 6 or HPV 11) is amply present at these same sites. More infrequently, HPV DNA can be disclosed in the parabasal cells, but only exceptionally in the basal cells.[83-85]

2.   Giant Condyloma and Buschke-Löwenstein Tumor

Condylomata acuminata of the male genitalia as well as in the vulva may become very large, particularly in patients with immunosuppression, Hodgkin's disease, or sometimes during pregnancy.[5] These unusual venereal warts are characterized by huge size and cauliflower-like appearance. The largest of these frequently show histological atypia,[5,78] in which case they are better known as Buschke-Löwenstein tumors. While describing the giant condylomas in the penis, Buschke and Löwenstein[86] emphasized their close similarities to squamous cell carcinomas. This relationship has been repeatedly described by other authors as well, and giant condylomas have been called carcinoma-like condylomas to underline the difficulty in making a distinction between these two entities.[5,78] It has also been suggested that giant condyloma is a variant of verrucous carcinoma, characterized by slow growth, fungus-like appearance, and ulceration.[87,88]

Histologically, Buschke-Löwenstein tumor is differentiated from the simple giant condyloma by the downgrowth of the acanthotic epithelium into the underlying connective tissue. Malignant inversion, however, is usually absent. There is sometimes a complex histological pattern with large areas of benign giant condyloma (with koilocytosis) intermixed with areas of atypical epithelial cells or even differentiated squamous cell carcinoma (without koilocytosis).[5,78] In an electron microscopic (EM) study, the ultrastructural features of Buschke-Löwenstein tumors were similar to those of squamous cell carcinoma, but dissimilar to those of condyloma acuminatum.[89] These data suggest that EM could be useful in differentiating the Buschke-Löwenstein tumor from large giant condylomas. This is in alignment with the recent discovery of HPV 6 DNA in a number of giant condylomas.[90]

3.   Flat Condyloma

Until 1976, the exophytic condyloma was regarded as the only manifestation of HPV infection in the genital area.[81] In that year, Meisels et al. in Canada,[2] and Purola et al. in Finland,[91] described in the uterine cervix epithelial changes devoid of the papillary contour of condylomata acuminata, but still exhibiting their characteristic cytological features. These new lesions were named flat and inverted (endophytic) condylomas, and since then their HPV etiology has been unequivocally confirmed by electron microscopic demonstration of HPV particles, by immunohistochemical techniques disclosing HPV antigens both in punch biopsy and in PAP smears, and by DNA hybridization experiments with HPV DNA probes.[76]

Except in the uterine cervix and vagina, flat condylomas are found on the vulva and on the male external genitalia as well. Exhaustive descriptions of the light microscopic appearance of the flat and inverted condylomas have been published in recent years, and are needless to repeat in detail here.[11,12,20,76] In brief, flat condyloma is a flat focus of acanthotic squamous epithelium with accentuated rete pegs and elongated dermal papillae. In many cases, there is a striking contrast between the deep and the superficial layers in the epithelium, the latter crowded by koilocytotic cells. The lesion is usually covered with layers varying in thickness of superficial dyskeratotic cells. In principle, two morphological variants of flat condyloma exist, the one with an entirely flat surface, and another one with tiny epithelial projections called spikes or asperities.[11,12,20,78,91] Not infrequently, however, features of both types are encountered, especially in extensive lesions (Figure 1).

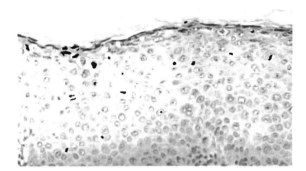

FIGURE 1   A medium power photomicrograph of a typical flat condyloma biopsied from the prepuce. An acanthotic
focus of epithelium is covered by a thin hyperkeratotic layer, under which, a two-to-three cell-thick layer of
epithelium is occupied by koilocytotic cells. No signs of PIN are found in this lesion, which proved to contain
HPV 11 DNA by ISH. (HE, original magnification, ×250).

When changes consistent with dysplasia are encountered and mixed with or adjacent to the flat
condyloma, the lesions have been called atypical condylomas, condylomatous atypias, condyloma
with intraepithelial neoplasia, or condylomatous dysplasias.[2,11,12,20,82,91] Although the nomenclature
is not unified yet, it is generally accepted that HPV lesions are frequently accompanied by cervical,
vaginal, vulvar-, anal-, and penile-intraepithelial neoplasia (CIN, VAIN, VIN, AIN, and PIN), and
occasionally by an invasive squamous cell carcinoma as well[76] (Figure 2 and 3).

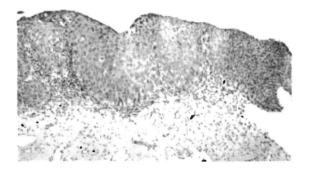

FIGURE 2   A typical flat condyloma associated with high grade CIN III lesion (on the right). Under a thin layer of
flattened parakeratotic cells on the surface, a few koilocytes suggesting HPV are present. There is a large
number of mitotic figures, some close to the uppermost layers of the epithelium. HPV 16 DNA was demonstrated by ISH, and the lesion was successfully eradicated by CO_2-laser. (HE, original magnification, ×100).

Using the immunohistochemical staining for HPV antigens, flat condylomas without intraepithelial neoplasia usually express these antigens in abundance.[11,12,20] In the majority of cases, positive
staining is localized in the intermediate and superficial layers of the epithelium, indicating the
productive HPV infection at these sites. It has been demonstrated that this antigen expression is
inversely related to the grade of the lesions, being usually absent in high grade HPV-CIN lesions.[4,11]
When analyzed by *in situ* DNA hybridization technique, the most intense signals indicating the
localization of HPV DNA are found at the sites of productive infection (Figure 4 and 5). More
infrequently, HPV DNA can be disclosed in the parabasal cells, but only exceptionally in the basal
cells.[83-85] Noteworthy is the fact that HPV DNA seems to be strictly confined to morphologically
altered epithelium, i.e., it is not demonstrable by *in situ* hybridization in the adjacent histologically

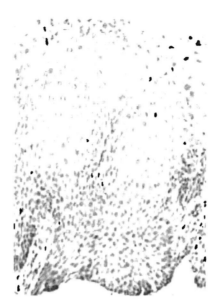

FIGURE 3   A medium power detail of another flat condyloma associated with a CIN II lesion. About one half of the epithelial thickness is occupied by basaloid type of cells, with the upper layers by characteristic koilocytes diagnostic to HPV. In this biopsy, HPV 18 DNA was demonstrated by ISH, and the lesion was shown to progress during the follow-up, necessitating an eradication by conization. (HE, original magnification, ×250).

normal epithelium.[85] This was recently confirmed by using the PCR technique in a series of CIN lesions, where no HPV DNA was disclosed in histologically normal epithelium.[92] Although the HPV type distribution in benign flat condylomas without features of intraepithelial neoplasia is quite similar in both sexes,[93] there seems to be a relative overexpression of HPV 42 in the penile lesions, as pointed out recently.[94] This is consistent with our observations, according to which HPV 42 seems to be frequent finding in male flat condylomas. Beyond doubt, additional HPV types will still be detected in the flat HPV lesions of the anogenital mucosa.[21,92]

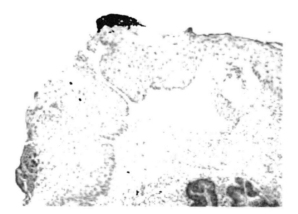

FIGURE 4   A flat condyloma of the uterine cervix devoid of CIN and showing distinct areas of koilocytotic cells in the intermediate and superficial layers. (HE, original magnification, ×100).

4. Endophytic (Inverted) Condyloma

The third type of genital HPV lesion, the inverted or endophytic condyloma is in most respects identical to the flat one, except that it shows as additional features pseudoinvasive penetration into the underlying stroma and/or endocervical gland openings.[2,91] Thus, it shares many of the growth characteristics of the *in situ* carcinoma, with which it actually seems to be associated in a substantial

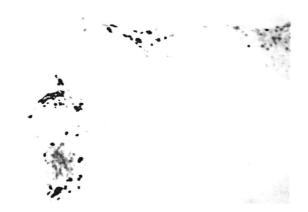

FIGURE 5 The same lesion as in Figure 4, examined by ISH with biotinylated HPV 6 DNA probe. The intense signals indicating the presence of HPV 6 DNA are found localized exactly at the areas of koilocytotic cells, overlying the nuclei in the upper third of the epithelium. (Biohit HPV *in situ* Typing Test® for HPV 6 DNA, no counterstain, original magnification, ×100).

number of cases at least in the uterine cervix. As in making the distinction between *in situ* and microinvasive cancer, special attention should be focused on whether or not any tumor cells are found outside the basement membrane. On the external genitalia, however, inverted condylomas are infrequently (if ever) found. This is most probably due to morphological differences in the epithelium between the uterine cervix and external genitalia. Recently, more and more authors are prone to consider the endophytic condyloma as a variant of the flat condyloma and not as a separate entity.[19,75,76] The author is inclined to share this view.

5. Papulosis and Pigmented Papulosis

Another HPV lesion, encountered exclusively on the external genitalia of both sexes, is called papulosis.[78] By definition, papulosis is an elevated papular focus of acanthotic epithelium, not exhibiting the exophytic papillary structures like condyloma acuminatum. In many cases, a slight papillomatotic contour can be detected.[5,20,78] This epithelial thickening is sometimes quite marked, giving the lesion its clinical outlook of a papule. Frequently, the lesions are covered by superficial parakeratotic or hyperkeratotic cells of varying thickness, sometimes giving the lesion a leukoplakic or acetowhite gross appearance. In cases where intense melanin pigmentation is present in the basal cells, the lesion is brown in color, and can be mixed with seborrhoic keratosis or even nevi.[78] In the later case, the lesions can be called pigmented papulosis. In papulosis lesions, the orderly arrangement of the epithelial layers and preserved cell polarity are the rule.[5,78] Epithelial cells show no or only a slight degree of atypia, and the number of mitotic figures is not increased. In rare instances, clusters of koilocytes are present in the uppermost layers, but otherwise there are no morphological features typical to an HPV infection. According to the experience of the author, many of the papulosis lesions contain HPV types 6 and 11, but also HPV 18, 31, or 33, and frequently with low copy numbers being barely detectable with *in situ* hybridization. Practically nothing is known about the natural history of these lesions as yet.

B. Premalignant Lesions

1. Bowenoid Papulosis

In view of the currently emerging relationship between bowenoid papulosis and Bowen's disease,[5,6,95,96] it is important to draw clinical, histological, and prognostic distinctions between these two entities. Most importantly, bowenoid papulosis lesions show a striking discrepancy between their benign clinical appearance and their histology, which closely resembles that of Bowen's disease.[78] The distinguishing features and the clinical appearances of these two entities are detailed elsewhere in this volume (see Gross).

According to recent data, the glans penis and the vaginal vestibulum were the two most frequently involved sites.[96] The incidence of bowenoid papulosis is certainly much higher than estimated so far. Due to the symptomless course and the inconspicuous clinical appearance, biopsies are rarely done. The clinical diagnoses most often submitted with the biopsy specimens are condyloma acuminatum, psoriasis, lichen ruber, melanotic nevus, and seborrhoeic keratosis.[5,78,96]

Although grossly the lesion appears benign, histologically such lesions show an epithelium with increased cellular atypia and microscopic similarities to Bowen's disease.[5,6,20,78,96,97] By definition, Bowenoid papulosis lesions are intraepithelial neoplasia corresponding to *in situ* squamous cell carcinomas. They are usually characterized by the full-thickness derangement of epithelial cell polarity, hyperchromatic staining pattern of the nuclei, and large number of abnormal mitotic figures.[78,96,97] (Figure 6).

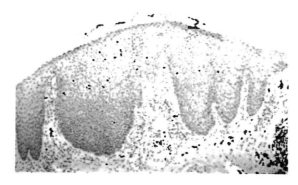

FIGURE 6   A Bowenoid papulosis type of full-thickness (VIN III) lesion from the labia majora, with no morphological evidence for HPV involvement. The epithelium is occupied by basaloid type of cells, with abundant mitotic figures in the intermediate and superficial layers. (HE, original magnification, ×100).

Compared with Bowen's disease, bowenoid papulosis usually shows a lesser degree of epithelial atypia. A further feature of possible value in differentiating between the two entities is the vesicular chromatin pattern and the focal distribution of dysplastic cells in bowenoid papulosis.[5,78] It should be emphasized, however, that bowenoid papulosis represents a clinicopathological entity, in which the diagnosis must be based on clinical examination and light microscopic analysis of the biopsy.

The HPV etiology of this entity has been firmly established by demonstrating characteristic HPV particles, and HPV antigens in these lesions,[96,98] as well as HPV DNA using hybridization techniques.[5,6,95,96] The clinical course of this disease may be unpredictable; some do seem to regress spontaneously, some persist, and probably some may progress to malignancy.[78,96] Bowenoid papulosis is morphologically identical in both sexes, which would be in alignment with the concept on the high-risk male in female genital carcinogenesis. This concept has gained substantial evidence from a recent discovery of the high-risk HPV type 16 DNA in 8/10 biopsies of penile Bowenoid papulosis lesions, two of which also contained sequences of HPV 18.[5,6,78,95] In another recent study, HPV 16 DNA was disclosed in all 12 cases studied with this technique.[96] Other HPV types, including HPV 35, have been recently disclosed in Bowenoid papulosis lesions.[99] It is to be emphasized, however, that no reliable data on the natural history based on prospective follow-up, are available of these lesions in the external genitalia of both sexes as yet. Recently, a number of surveys have been made to detect HPV infections on the penis and in the urethra of the male consorts of the women with genital HPV infections, to elucidate the role of the male as the carrier of HPV infections. The recent literature on this topic was recently subjected to an exhaustive review.[100]

2.   Dysplasia, Intraepithelial Neoplasia, and Squamous Intraepithelial Lesion

The nomenclature for cervical precancer lesions has had a particularly interesting history, beginning in the early 1900s with the classical monograph of Schottländer and Kemauner,[101] and continuing to the present. The traditional World Health Organization (WHO) terminology identifies two types of lesions; dysplasia and carcinoma *in situ*.[102] In the WHO system, dysplasia is regarded as a borderline lesion that may regress to normal, remain unchanged, or progress to carcinoma, whereas carcinoma *in situ* is a lesion that will eventually develop into an invasive carcinoma if left untreated.[102] In the late 1960s, a new terminology was presented, introducing the concept on cervical intraepithelial neoplasia (CIN).[103] Subsequently, this concept has been extended to cover the entire lower female genital tract; VAIN and VIN, for vagina and vulva, respectively. Similarly, anal and penile precancer lesions have been named as AIN and PIN, respectively.

During the 1980s, occasional criticism was presented towards the widely accepted CIN nomenclature.[104] The nomenclature of cervical precancer lesions has been complicated by the current data on HPV and its intimate association with all grades of precancer lesions.[9-12,16,76] In 1987, Richart reported that "current data are consistent with a two-disease system in the genital tract but it is (a human papillomavirus) HPV 6/11 versus HPV 11/18 group system.[11,105] In 1990, he presented a modified terminology for CIN: low-grade CIN with HPV-related changes (old CIN 1) and high-grade CIN (old CIN 2 plus CIN 3).[106] According to his concept, in low-grade CIN with HPV-related changes, the virus resides episomally in the nucleus and the lesion has an uncertain biologic potential, whereas in high-grade CIN, a high-risk HPV has been integrated into the host cell DNA and the lesion is a true cancer precursor.[106]

In 1988, a workshop sponsored by the National Cancer Institute published recommendations and guidelines for reporting the results of cervical/vaginal cytology, known as the Bethesda System.[107] The Bethesda System proposes to replace the terms dysplasia-CIS or CIN with two terms, low-grade squamous intraepithelial lesion (SIL) or high-grade SIL. Low-grade SIL includes lesions that show cellular changes associated with HPV infection or mild (slight) dysplasia (CIN 1). High-grade SIL includes lesions that show moderate dysplasia (CIN II) or severe dysplasia/carcinoma *in situ* (CIN III).[107]

Since its introduction, critical views have been presented against the Bethesda System[108,109] as well as those advocating its adoption for general use.[110] Because we feel that any meaningful terminology should be able to establish a close correlation between the biological behavior and the different grades of lesions, the biological relevance of the Bethesda System was recently tested in our series of over 500 women with genital HPV infections prospectively followed-up since 1981. The cervical biopsies were reclassified as either low-grade or high-grade SIL, and the data obtained by colposcopy, Pap smear, and HPV typing, as well as the biological behavior of the lesions in these two groups, were analyzed.[111]

Altogether, 77.4% (376/486) of the lesions were classified as low-grade SIL lesions, the rest (22.6%) belonged to the high-grade SIL category. The colposcopic appearance was normal significantly more frequently in the low-grade SIL lesions (22.1%) as compared with the high-grade category (8.5%) (p<0.0001). A single Pap smear was clearly an inadequate means to make distinction between the low-grade and high-grade SIL, as evidenced by an almost identical distribution of Pap smear Class III atypias in both categories. Noteworthy was the discovery of normal Pap smears in 8.2% of the high-grade SIL lesions.[111] All six HPV types analyzed[6,11,16,18,31,33] were similarly distributed in both categories, except for HPV 16, which was significantly more frequent in the high-grade SIL (40%) as compared with 12.7% in the low-grade SIL (p<0.0001). Progression was significantly higher (39.1%) in the high-grade SIL category (p<0.0001), and the spontaneous regression rate higher (63.6%) in the low-grade SIL. Again, noteworthy was the fact that 38.2% of the lesions classified as high-grade SIL did regress spontaneously.[111] The results clearly indicate the weakness of the Bethesda classification, when applied to analysis of the natural history of cervical HPV lesions. While abandoning the category of CIN II lesions which seem to possess a progression and regression rate intermediate between those of CIN I and CIN III, the two-grade

Bethesda system leads to a significant loss of prognostically valuable data on the clinical course of the disease, as will be discussed later. Furthermore, it is essential from the patient's point of view that the clinical terminology does not result in overtreatment, which seems to be a definite risk when only two categories of the Bethesda System are used. The author firmly advocates the preservation of the present three-grade terminology (either dysplasia or IN) which has proved effective for many years.

III.   SUBCLINICAL HPV INFECTIONS

During the past few years, reports have been published where HPV DNA has been disclosed in lesions not fulfilling the criteria of the above defined clinical HPV manifestations, or even in the genital tract of healthy women.[56,112-116] However, contradictory reports questioning the existence of HPV DNA in histologically normal epithelium have been published as well.[85,92,113] For proper evaluation of the confusing data, it is essential to define the different manifestations of HPV infections as precisely as possible on the basis of currently available epidemiologic and molecular biological data. The suggested criteria of these three categories are summarized in Table 1.

As in the female genital tract, also in the male genitalia, the term subclinical HPV infection has been ascribed to different issues by different authors.[19,49,50,79,93] Some authors call as subclinical HPV infections those lesions that are not visible on routine inspection, but become visible on peniscopy after acetic acid, and which on histology contain typical HPV-induced changes.[19] There are others who use this term as an equivalent to a flat condyloma.[75] According to our view, however, the term subclinical HPV infection in both sexes should be used for lesions which become visible only by colposcopy (peniscopy) after acetic acid, and which on light microscopy, show minor epithelial changes not consistent with typical flat condylomas.[45,46,79,85] Many times, the diagnosis of subclinical HPV infections is difficult, while abnormalities classifiable only as suspicious to HPV are present in colpo/peniscopy, and not infrequently, in biopsy as well.

As discussed above, subclinical HPV infections should become only visible after acetic acid and, on light microscopy, they are devoid of the characteristic morphological features of the clinical HPV lesions, as outlined above.[20,45,46] In punch biopsy, the slightly acanthotic epithelium might contain superficial dyskeratosis and intermediate cells with slightly vacuolized cystoplasm, but devoid of any nuclear changes characteristic to HPV-induced koilocytosis. (Figure 7). According to experience of the author, the proper assessment of HPV lesions as either clinical or subclinical in the vagina, introitus, vulva, and the entire male genital area is much more difficult than that in the uterine cervix.[20]

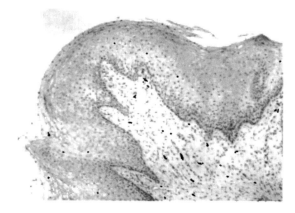

FIGURE 7   A vaginal biopsy with subclinical HPV infection. The epithelium is irregularly acanthotic, with minor spike-like elevations on the surface. The basal cell layer is highly regular, the intermediate layer being composed of small cells with clear cytoplasm. No convincing nuclear abnormalities consistent with koilocytosis is present. The epithelium is covered by a thin layer of parakeratotic cells. When subjected to PCR amplification, however, the biopsy proved to be positive for HPV 6 DNA. (HE, original magnification, ×100).

These difficulties are clearly emphasized by a recent analysis of 58 biopsies derived from different genital lesions classified as subclinical by clinicians.[117] According to our criteria, a total of 20 (35.4%) biopsies had morphological features of HPV infection on light microscopic examination. Flat condyloma was disclosed in 16 cases, endophytic lesions in two, papillary condyloma in one, and a pigmented papulosis in one anal biopsy. CIN or VIN was found in 11 biopsies (19.0%),[117] with all showing morphological features consistent with HPV. HPV DNA was demonstrated, however, in only 3 (5.2%) biopsies by ISH, all being typical flat condylomas. Of significance was the association of HPV 16 with a CIN III lesion. Acanthosis, parakeratosis, dyskeratosis, koilocytosis, and increased mitotic figures were more frequently present in HPV-suggestive lesions than in their nonsuggestive counterparts (p>0.01).[117] In HPV-suggestive lesions, hyperkeratosis was found in 44.4% of the cervical biopsies, as compared with 81.8% in those derived from other genital sites. By definition, true koilocytotic cells did not occur in non-HPV-suggestive lesions.

These revised diagnoses were compared with the original ones settled by different pathologists. In the original assessment, the HPV-related category included 21 cases with diagnosis such as typical condyloma, koilocytotic atypia, papilloma, and mild condylomatous atypia. Of these 21 cases, 10 cases (47.6%) were classified as HPV lesions in our re-examination. On the other hand, 10 of the 37 biopsies (27%) originally classified into the non-HPV-related category, disclosed morphological changes consistent with HPV infection in the new assessment. Undoubtedly, further work is needed to correlate the DNA data with morphology and to establish the histopathological criteria (if any) for the subclinical HPV infections in both sexes.[19,79,93,94,117]

IV. LATENT INFECTIONS

In virology, latent viral infections represent cases where viral genome (DNA or RNA) is present in an otherwise normal target tissue. Accordingly, the term latent HPV infection should be preserved for the cases where HPV DNA is found (by hybridization or PCR) in biopsies which by all histological criteria are classifiable as normal epithelium.[20,45,46] Evidently, the assessment of whether epithelium is normal or not should always be based on careful histopathologic examination of a directed punch biopsy. It is important to realize, however, that some inherent limitations (i.e., false negative findings) are confined to punch biopsies as well. These are mostly due to the fact that the biopsy is not invariably derived from the most representative area of the epithelium. In our practice, however, a repeated examination would affirm the presence or absence of HPV lesion in most cases.[79,118,119]

Latent HPV infections exist in different mucosal sites beyond any doubt. HPV DNA and even viral particles have been shown to persist in histologically normal laryngeal and genital epithelium as well as in the normal skin.[56] In a recent study using PCR and ISH, HPV 6 and 11 DNA could be localized in penile epithelium lacking the characteristic koilocytotic cells.[120] As will be discussed later, however, the detection of HPV DNA in normal epithelium is significantly dependent on the technique used, i.e., the type of hybridization or use of PCR.[19,20,45,46,121] The clinical importance of such an HPV reservoir in the male will be discussed later.

Apart from the males, even more evidence is available to indicate the existence of latent HPV infections in women.[18,47-57] We recently surveyed 100 women who were classified as HPV-negative in the latest mass-screening by Pap smears.[122] All women were invited for re-examination, and 262 biopsies were taken from the cervix (n = 30), vagina (n = 212), and anus (n = 20). The most frequent histological finding was acanthosis (69.1%), followed by vacuolization of the epithelial cells (60.3%). True koilocytosis was seen in only 6.5% (17/262) of the biopsies. Altogether, morphological evidence for HPV infection was found in 18/262 (5.6%) of the biopsies, with flat condyloma in 14 and papillary condyloma in 4 samples. The frequency of morphologically distinct HPV lesions was highest in the anus (15%), followed by the vagina (6.6%) and the cervix (3.3%).[122] CIN was discovered in five biopsies. Seven samples were found to contain HPV DNA by ISH using a cocktail probe for HPV 6, 11, 16, and 18. We randomly selected 93 biopsy samples from 40 women for PCR to detect sequences of HPV 6, 11, 16, and 18. Altogether, 33 out of the 93 biopsies contained amplified HPV DNA (33.5%), the commonest type being HPV 11 (18/33; 54.5%), followed by HPV 18 (11/33; 33.3%). The HPV DNA detection rate was highest (50%) in the cervical biopsy samples and lowest (28.6%) in the anal biopsies.[122] This detection of latent HPV infection by PCR in 35.5% of these Pap-negative women clearly indicates that a single normal Pap smear is far from an adequate means to declare a women HPV-free. This should have important implications while evaluating the studies where HPV DNA has been reported in healthy (= Pap smear-negative) women.[18,47-57,85]

V.   BIOLOGICAL BEHAVIOR OF GENITAL HPV INFECTIONS

A.   Condyloma Acuminatum and Related Lesions

Condyloma acuminatum has been extensively characterized in the external genitalia of both sexes, but the lesion has remained more controversial in the vagina and cervix.[123] It is generally accepted that condylomata acuminata on the external genitalia frequently undergo spontaneous regression, albeit the growth of some may be enhanced by pregnancy and some chronic diseases, including immunosuppression.[14,76] On the other hand, numerous case reports are available on malignant transformation of condylomata acuminata in external genitalia.[14,74] According to such a survey in Uganda (a high risk country for cervical and penile cancer), a high rate of malignant transformation was observed in patients over 40 years of age (6/36 cases), as contrasted to none of the 210 cases in the younger age groups.[74] The authors concluded that condylomata acuminata might represent precancerous lesions showing a low risk and long time interval to malignancy in young, and a high risk and short latency period in later age.[14] More detailed reviews on the substantial literature on the malignant transformation of genital condylomata acuminata are to be found in the recent monographs.[76,124-127]

The clinical course of giant condyloma is distinct from that of the usual condyloma acuminatum, albeit identical at the onset. Nodular areas of induration gradually develop, leading to fistulas with putrid-smelling purulent discharge exuding from the lesion. External genitals may eventually be overgrown with luxuriant condylomatous masses which are extremely hard to eradicate.[128] By 1977, a total of 65 cases of giant condylomas had been reported to have transformed into an invasive squamous cell carcinoma.[128] This literature has been exhaustively cited, the reader being referred to pertinent reviews.[14,76,124-127] These reports usually describe the development of giant condyloma over prolonged periods, their macroscopic carcinoma-like appearance, as well as the histologic demonstration of their invasive growth pattern. The ultrastructure of giant condylomas seems to be practically identical with that of the squamous cell carcinoma, further emphasizing the neoplastic character of this tumor.[89]

As compared with the follow-up studies of HPV lesions in the uterine cervix, surprisingly few studies are available on the natural history of condylomata acuminata in the external genitals.[129] Some data are available, however, as derived from the recent clinical trials where genital warts have been treated with interferon or other chemotherapeutic agents, and where a placebo series has been included.[76,119,124-127,129] These studies are summarized in separate chapters of this volume (see Gross, Barrasso, and von Krogh).

Even in such studies, however, difficulties may arise in interpreting whether the regression of genital warts in the placebo series is indeed spontaneous or induced by iatrogenic manipulation or by local host immune reactions. This is well exemplified by a study of Eron et al.,[130] in which the spontaneous regression of genital condylomata was assessed in 149 male and female patients randomized to the placebo arm of a double-blind clinical trial of alpha$_{2B}$-interferon. Overall, 17% of the 149 subjects who received placebo showed complete regression of their condylomata within 16 weeks of clinical diagnosis.[130] However, since the placebo group received intralesional injections, which may have locally stimulated cell-mediated immune response, it is not clear that regression of the warts in this group was truly spontaneous. Our own experience from two multi-institutional international trials of interferon treatment of external genital warts is quite similar.[131,132] Furthermore, it is important to realize that the disappearance of visible condylomata does not necessarily mean disappearance of HPV, as recently pointed out.[20,45,46] Thus, the term wart regression should be used instead of cure in cases where the complete clearance of HPV DNA has not been affirmed.

B.   Cervical Precancer Lesions

Cervical cancer is an appropriate model disease known to develop through well characterized precancer lesions, known as dysplasia, intraepithelial neoplasia, or squamous intraepithelial lesion, as discussed above. Of central importance in (1) preventing and (2) predicting the development of cervical cancer is the assessment of the biology of these precancer lesions. The time-honored means to prevent the development of cervical cancer is provided by covering mass-screening programs by Pap smears, proven to be effective in dramatically reducing the prevalence of this disease, e.g., in Scandinavian countries since the 1960s.[133,134] A Pap smear also provides a means to assess the prevalence of CIN lesions, which seems to have increased throughout the 1970s and 1980s.[135,136] Based on analysis of almost 800,000 Pap smears in 1981, the prevalence of biopsy-proved CIN lesions (all grades) in the teenage population was 13.3/1,000.[136] This, of course, is a much higher figure than the prevalence of invasive cervical cancer, which is currently 2.7/100,000, e.g., in Finland.[137] Accordingly, the vast majority of cervical precancer lesions never progress to an invasive cancer; they are either eradicated after detection by Pap smear or regress spontaneously.

The accurate prediction of the development of cervical cancer from an individual precancer lesion is a much more complicated issue, however. This key issue is appropriately approached only by prospective follow-up studies, a large number of such studies having been completed even before the connection between HPV and CIN was established (see detailed reviews in 11, 12, 13). The data from these follow-up studies are hard to interpret, however, as recently discussed by Kataja.[138] This is because of a number of reasons, including (1) the different study populations, (2) different methods of follow-up (i.e., Pap smear or biopsy), (3) the length of the follow-up period, and (4) the reproducibility problems of grading the precancer lesions.[138] These problems are well illustrated by the highly divergent figures for progression rates from CIN 1 to carcinoma *in situ*, ranging from 0 to 64% in these classical follow-up studies.[139-148]

C.   Follow-Up of Genital HPV Lesions

The recognition of the association between HPV and CIN has further complicated the assessment of the natural history of this disease. The connection of a viral infection with a spectrum of distinct morphological manifestations (CIN) in itself is hard to approach, and the scene is rendered more complex by the recognition of subclinical and latent HPV infections.[20,45,46,129]

The several methodological and conceptual problems encountered in the natural history studies conducted so far were discussed in a recent review by Koutsky et al.[129] These issues are fully appreciated by the author, and thus they are shortly listed here before proceeding with the discussion of the follow-up data available from these studies. First, in the studies where biopsy was used to classify the lesions to be followed-up, the biopsy (1) may not have sampled the highest grade of lesions, and (2) it may have modified the natural history of the infection. The first argument is easy to agree, and this kind of bias inevitably leads to a certain degree of misclassification, being hard to completely avoid even with multiple biopsies. The second point is more controversial, and data are available to indicate that even repeated biopsies during the follow-up do not interfere (or do so insignificantly) with the natural history of CIN lesions.[28,144,145,147]

Secondly, in studies that did not use biopsy, cytologic findings may not necessarily reflect the underlying histologic abnormality. Thus, it is difficult (if not impossible) to interpret the meaning of cytologic progression from mild to moderate or severe dysplasia presented in such studies. It is well established that a single Pap smear is (1) not a reliable indicator of HPV,[20,45,46,149] nor (2) is a single normal smear a complete reassurance of an HPV-free epithelium.[149] Furthermore, third, in cytologic specimens showing koilocytosis, it is sometimes impossible to distinguish between those with and those without CIN, as correctly pointed out.[129] Thus, the definition of progression on the basis of cytology alone using the change from HPV without CIN to those showing evidence of HPV with CIN as the only criteria, is problematic. Ideally, each follow-up examination should include colposcopy, Pap smear, and punch biopsy with hybridization (or PCR) as a confirmation if necessary.[28-30]

Fourth, since the invasive cervical cancer cannot ethically be an endpoint of prospective follow-up studies, the most critical step in the progression of HPV infection cannot be subjected to cohort studies.[28-30,129,138] Accordingly, the follow-up must be terminated whenever CIN III lesion is encountered, leaving the progression rate of CIN III (or carcinoma *in situ*) to invasive carcinoma a controversial issue.[139-148]

1.   Early Prospective Studies

Until the mid 1980s, the natural history of cytologically defined cervical HPV infections in relation to the development of CIN has been studied among three cohorts of women (see reviews in 76, 124, 125, 126, 127). Results from these three studies are remarkably consistent. Progression from HPV-NCIN (i.e., koilocytosis without CIN) to CIN I or greater was reported for 18 (8%) of 232 women followed by Syrjänen et al. for an average of 25 months,[28,150] for 26 (8%) of 314 women followed by de Brux et al.[151] for 15 to 18 months, and for 113 (13%) of 846 women followed for up to six years by Mitchell et al.[152] In the latter study, 30 cases of carcinoma *in situ* were observed, (as compared with only 1.9 cases expected in the general population), giving a relative risk of 15.6[152] Campion et al.[153] found that 22 (56%) of 39 women with HPV 16-associated CIN I progressed to CIN III, whereas only one (4%) of 26 women with HPV 6 progressed to CIN III. The most extensive of these follow-up studies (albeit retrospective) was reported by deBrux et al.,[154] based on observations of 2,466 women out of 7,257 cases diagnosed among 1,036,020 Pap smears between 1979–1982. During a 42-month follow-up period, 10% progression rate was found in 1,269 women with HPV-CIN I, and in 17% of 762 women with HPV-CIN II.[154] On the other hand, the spontaneous regression rates were 53% and 39% in these cohorts, respectively. As evident from these figures, the progression rates in these different studies are remarkably constant, varying from 8 to 17%, depending on the length of the follow-up time. This is fully consonant with our experience from an over 10-year follow-up of 530 women in Kuopio.

2.   Kuopio Follow-Up Study

To elucidate the natural history (i.e., the clinical behavior without treatment) of genital HPV infections, a prospective follow-up study of the women infected with this virus was started by our clinic in 1981. During 1981–1985, more than 500 women were invited to participate in the study, and their genital HPV lesions have been followed-up for a mean of 9 years (M ± SD, 104 + 41 months) by now, using colposcopy, Pap smears, and punch biopsies, but without any kind of therapy.[28,29,31,45,46,138,150,155,156] Undoubtedly, the nationwide mass-screening program for detection of cervical precancer lesions has contributed to the willingness of the women to participate in such a long-term follow-up program, and made it possible to collect and keep going such a unique series of patients for over 15 years by now.

The results of this extensive study have been reported in a series of previous publications.[28-31,45,46,138,150,155,156] The prospective follow-up data accumulated until now are summarized in Figure 8. There are two major trends emerging, when individual patients are followed-up for a prolonged period. The rate of spontaneous regression increases in parallel with the extent of the follow-up time, from 28% at 25 months of mean follow-up, to 56% at 57 months, up to 63.8% after 83 months of observation.[138] In practice, this means that a marked difference exists in the regression rates obtained when the follow-up is continued for 2 years, 4 years, and up to 6 years. After that, however, the regression rate does not seem to increase any longer, as evident in Figure 8.

From the clinical point of view, even more important is the progression of HPV lesions towards carcinoma *in situ*. As repeatedly emphasized, the main attention should be focused on predicting

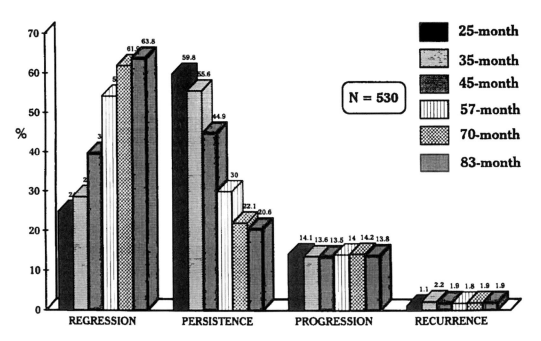

FIGURE 8   Natural history of Cervical HPV Infections during a long-term prospective follow-up.

the lesions eventually progressing among the clinical lesions.[20,45,46] In contrast to the increasing trend in regression as a function of time, no such trend can be observed in progression rate. As evident from Figure 8, the progression rate remains unchanged (around 14%) after 25 months of mean follow-up time. In practice, this means that the lesions destined to clinical progression do so quite rapidly, almost invariably during the first two years from the diagnosis. This should have important clinical implications while planning the strategies for diagnosis, treatment, and follow-up of gynecological HPV infections.[157]

3.   Recent Follow-Up Studies

The number of prospective follow-up studies carried out for genital HPV infections (mainly focused on cervical lesions) has increased during the late 1980s.[158-174] Because of the difficulties discussed above, the results of these studies are hard to interpret and subject to mutual comparison. A summary of the recent follow-up studies is made in Table 2.

The major clinical impact of these studies would be to give the definite answers to two key questions: (1) what is the spontaneous regression rate of HPV lesions of different grades, and (2) what is the inherent potential of different grades of HPV lesions to progress towards an invasive cancer. As evident from the figures in Table 2, no such unanimous answers can be obtained from these extensive studies, unfortunately. Let's consider the clinical regression first. Fairly unanimous agreement seems to exist in that the regression rate for HPV lesions without CIN is substantial, i.e., ranging from 21%[165] up to 78%.[172] In many of the follow-up studies with the longest duration, however, these figures have not been determined.[159,160,164,166-169,171,173,174] According to our experience from the Kuopio study, we would be prone to agree that the vast majority (two thirds) of these lesions will eventually regress when controlled long enough.[111] Even more controversial are the data on regression rates of HPV-CIN I lesions, the figures extending from 3.6%[165] to 85.3%.[167] Here again, these data were not recorded in the majority of these studies, and notable differences in categorizing criteria exist between the studies. The regression data for HPV-CIN II lesions are even more meager, being available in only four of these reports.[111,166,167,173] It seems evident, however, that even the CIN II lesions possess a substantial regression tendency, ranging from 25%[173] to

TABLE 2   Natural History of Genital HPV Infections as Established by Follow-Up Studies

Reference number	Number of patients	Follow-up time (month)	Rate of regression (%)				Rate of progression (%)			
			HPV	CIN I	CIN II	CIN III	NORMAL	HPV	CIN I	CIN II
158	51	12	47.0	n.d.	n.d.	n.d.	n.d.	11.8	n.d.	n.d.
159	30	24	n.d.	83.0	n.d.	n.d.	16.7	n.d.	n.d.	n.d.
160	20	28	n.d.	n.d.	n.d.	n.d.	5.0	15.0	n.d.	n.d.
161	45	11	40.0	n.d.	n.d.	n.d.	n.d.	33.3	n.d.	n.d.
162	12	4	50.0	n.d.	n.d.	n.d.	n.d.	n.d.	n.d.	n.d.
163	50	6	22.4	n.d.	n.d.	n.d.	13.6	3.5	n.d.	n.d.
164	415	36	n.d.	3.6	n.d.	n.d.	n.d.	n.d.	22.2	n.d.
165	82	18	21.4	26.6	42.8	n.d.	21.7	9.7	n.d.	n.d.
166	38	36	n.d.	85.3[b]	n.d.	n.d.	n.d.	n.d.	73.3[a]	57.1[a]
167	146	18	n.d.	n.d.	60.8	33.3	n.d.	n.d.	14.7[a]	39.2[a]
168	2.709[c]	60	n.d.	n.d.	n.d.	n.d.	0.65[d]	n.d.	n.d.	n.d.
169	101	73	n.d.	13.3	n.d.	n.d.	n.d.	n.d.	13.0[e]	n.d.
170	100	120	47.0	77.3[f]	n.d.	n.d.	n.d.	49.0	n.d.	n.d.
171	525	54	n.d.	n.d.	n.d.	n.d.	n.d.	n.d.	7.8[f]	n.d.
172	91	9	78.3[g]	n.d.	n.d.	n.d.	n.d.	3.4[g]	n.d.	0.0
173	24	2–65	n.d.	37.5	25.0	n.d.	n.d.	n.d.	4.2	16.7
174	241	25	n.d.	n.d.	n.d.	n.d.	3.0	28.0[h]	n.d.	n.d.
111	487	70	66.7	55.7	52.9	14.3	n.d.	6.3	14.2	20.6

HPV, HPV without CIN; n.d., not defined; [a]Includes both persistence and progression; [b]Includes CIN 0 and CIN I lesions; [c]Pap smears only; [d]Progression to CIN III or invasive carcinoma; [e]Progression defined by PAP smear only; [f]Includes both CIN I and CIN II cases; [g]Low Grade SIL lesions; [h]Women with positive test for HPV.

60.8%.[167] Suprisingly few reports are able to give the data on regression rate of HPV-CIN III lesions.[111,166] This is explained by the fact that for safety reasons, most authors are apt to institute an immediate treatment for CIN III lesions, a policy that cannot be protested against with any reasonable arguments. The general impression is obtained, however, that the regression tendency for CIN III lesions is significantly lower than that of the lower grade lesions.

Of even greater clinical significance are the lesions with potential to progress, as discussed before.[20,45,46,76] From the above studies, progression data are available even for women assesses as normal at the onset of the follow-up.[159,160,163,165,168,174] As could be expected, the progression rates for such cases (i.e., the development of HPV lesion of any grade) is relatively low, ranging from 0.65%[168] to 21.7%,[165] even after a lengthy observation period. As with the regression, the deviation is marked in the figures of progression for HPV lesions without CIN; from 3.4%[172] to 49%.[170] Some of these discrepancies are due to different criteria of categorization, as indicated by the superscripts in Table 2. The studies are surprisingly consistent, however, in reporting the progression rates of HPV-CIN I. If the extreme of 73.3% (due to different ranking) is ignored, the range is quite narrow, from 4.2%[173] to 22.2%,[165] the majority setting around 10%.[111,167,169,171] Too little data are available to draw definite conclusions from the progression tendency of HPV-CIN II. Because of the ranking differences, the two highest figures, 39.2% and 57.1%[166,167] cannot be compared with those of our study (20.6%).[111] As pointed out before, the progression rate of CIN III is ethically unjustified to establish by prospective follow-up.

VI. HPV INFECTIONS AND GENITAL CANCER

A. Risk Factors for Clinical HPV Infections

Because of the fact that cervical (and other genital) squamous cell carcinomas only develop through the successive grades of precancer lesions (intraepithelial neoplasia), the development of a clinically manifest HPV lesion (usually flat condyloma) is a prerequisite for such a sequence of events.[11,12,20,45,46] Accordingly, searching for the risk factors predisposing the women and men for the development of clinical HPV infections may have implications in evaluating the subsequent risk for genital cancer. During the past few years, a number of epidemiological studies focusing on these issues have been conducted, as discussed in detail elsewhere in this volume (see Galloway and Koutsky).

Our experience from the Kuopio follow-up study was summarized in the recent monograph of Kataja.[138] Accordingly, the most important independent risk factor for clinical HPV infection was the number of sexual partners during the past two years. The adjusted prevalence odds ratio for women having had 5 or more sexual partners was 12.1 as compared to those with no or only one partner. Independent effect on the risk was also exerted by age, current smoking, genital warts in sexual partner(s), increasing frequency of sexual intercourse per week, previous normal Pap smear (protective), regular use of IUD (protective), and good personal hygiene practices (protective). Strong univariate effects were also associated with previous CIN, previous STD, and previous warts, as well as with age at first intercourse. These associations could mainly be explained by adjusting for other sexual variables.[138]

B. Risk Factors for Progression

Apart from regression and progression as the two opposite behavioral patterns of HPV infections, a number of other disease patterns can be distinguished. Indeed, genital HPV infections seem to run an extremely fluctuating course, a passage from a manifest to a subclinical or latent infection being frequently encountered in individual patients when examined at 6-month intervals for prolonged periods.[45,46] Such a fluctuation is clearly established by HPV typing as well, while showing a frequent change from one HPV type to another in individual patients during a longitudinal study.[175,176]

Indeed, at least six behavioral patterns are recognized in our prospective follow-up series.[45] These include the following: (1) Early regressors are women, in whom the lesion disappears quite quickly, i.e., sometimes during the period elapsed from the invitation (the Pap smear diagnostic to HPV) to the first attendance at the clinic, which usually takes from a few weeks to 2 months. (2) Persistors are the patients whose HPV lesion remains morphologically unchanged for a prolonged time without regression or progression at repeated examinations at 6-month intervals. Such a persistence of a single HPV type for years has been clearly demonstrated by hybridization techniques and PCR.[177,178] (3) Quite a substantial percentage of the patients are fluctuators, with their lesions alternatively disappearing and reappearing during the long follow-up. (4) Progression, when destined to develop, usually is evident during the first two years of the follow-up, as evidenced by the settling of the progression rate at a constant level of about 14% after the mean follow-up of about two years (Figure 8). (5) Late regressors are women in whom the lesion abruptly disappears after a prolonged follow-up period. This is reflected in the constantly increased rate of regression (over 65% in 9 years), as a direct function of the extent of the follow-up time (Figure 8). (6) Most unfortunate are the recurrators, i.e., women whose lesion after having been eradicated by conization because of rapid progression into CIS, will recur after a variable period of post-treatment follow-up.

Bearing in mind the recent epidemiological data (discussed in detail by Galloway and Koutsky in this volume), only a small minority (approximately 2–3%) of women bear a clinical HPV infection,[133,134] while the vast majority have the infection as latent or subclinical.[20,45,46] This is suggested by the data on routine mass-screening on one hand,[133] and the estimated lifetime risk of 80% for genital HPV infections by the age of 80 years.[134] Of major clinical importance would be to elaborate accurate means to predict, among the clinical infections, those high-risk lesions possessing the potential for progression to carcinoma *in situ* and eventually to invasive carcinomas.[45,46]

During the past couple of years, data on such risk factors are gradually emerging from a number of studies.[179-181] The detection of HPV DNA by either dot blot hybridization or PCR was a significant predictor of subsequent development of CIN in women with an abnormal Pap smear but not shown CIN on initial colposcopic examination.[179] There are others, however, who could not find any difference in the detection rate of HPV DNA in women who developed an invasive cancer and in those who did not.[180] In one study, the persistence of HPV 16 DNA and expression of mRNA could be shown in a patient throughout the precancer lesions and in the subsequent invasive cervical cancer.[181] It seems that, as a risk factor for progression, more important than the mere detection of HPV DNA is the assessment of the distinct HPV types. Here, we are facing the question about the practical value of HPV typing in disease prognostication.[182] Although there is ample evidence to indicate that HPV 16 is associated with significantly higher risk (>5-fold) for progression as compared with HPV 6/11 or HPV DNA-negative lesions,[136] there still seems to be too many exceptions of this rule (e.g., HPV 6/11 found in invasive carcinomas, HPV 16 in regressing lesions etc.) to justify the systematic use of HPV typing (with any technique) as a routine screening method.[182] Furthermore, recent evidence suggests that infection by HPV 16 as well as the progression of such infections to CIN III might be genetically determined, while shown to be intimately linked with HLA class II antigens, i.e., HLA-RD5.[183] It should be emphasized that data on the natural history and risk factors for the male HPV lesions and their progression are scanty or missing.[100]

As part of our prospective cohort study, the prognostic factors of female genital HPV infections were recently summarized by Kataja.[138] Accordingly, as established by the life-table analysis used to assess the clinical course, progression and regression were significantly related to grade of the lesion at the time of diagnosis ($p<0.00001$, and $p = 0.0005$, respectively), and clinical progression to the cellular atypia in the first Pap smear ($p = 0.006$).[31,155] On the other hand, the Pap smear or HPV type were not of predictive value for spontaneous regression, and a colposcopic pattern did predict the clinical course (either regression or progression) quite poorly.[31,138,155] Data in alignment with our experience recently came out from an extensive cohort study in Toronto.[184] Based on analysis of 176,808 Pap smears from 70,236 women, the relative risks for the development of cervical cancer in a subsequent smear were 1.48, 3.42, 20.9, and 71.5 for women with minimal, mild, moderate, and severe dysplasia, respectively.[184] The results strongly suggest that the grade of precancer lesion is significantly related to the development of cervical cancer. This is in complete agreement with our data, indicating that the progression rate is directly related to the grade of CIN[31,138] (see also Table 2). Taken together, if prognostication is to be practiced, the two single most important prognostic factors predicting clinical progression with a high grade of accuracy are (1) the histological grade of precancer lesion at the time of diagnosis, and (2) the presence of HPV type 16 in any lesion. Self-evidently, the highest risk is associated with high grade CIN lesions containing HPV 16 DNA.[138,182]

C. Epidemiologic Associations

1. Cancer of the Uterine Cervix

It can be argued that in countries like Finland, where the age-adjusted incidence rates of cervical cancer have dramatically declined since 1950s (from $16/10^5$ to $5/10^5$ in 1980, attributable to the nationwide mass-screening program effective since the early 1960s), carcinoma of the uterine cervix does not any longer represent such a major clinical problem as it did in the early 1960s. The same applies to other Nordic countries, except Norway. However, WHO estimates that the annual worldwide incidence of cervical carcinoma is about 450,000 cases, and other squamous cell carcinomas of the genital tract account for some 150,000 additional cases.[185-187] Even with adequate medical intervention, 45 to 50% of these patients eventually die of their disease. Worldwide, there are certain high-risk areas for this malignancy, including Latin America, Tropical Africa, and some parts of China.[37-42,188] Not incidentally, the prevalence and incidence of genital HPV infections in those countries seem to be particularly high.

Epidemiological evidence strongly suggests that cervical carcinomas derive from a sexually transmitted disease.[14,185-187,189] Thus, many of the risk factors for cervical cancer are similar to those found to predispose the women to HPV infections.[11,12,37,39-41] These include the onset of sexual relations at an early age, sexual promiscuity, lower socioeconomic status, poor sexual hygiene, and multiple episodes of other venereal infections.[138,190] Although many of the molecular mechanisms remain to be solved, the association of different genital carcinomas (in both sexes) with HPV is quite convincing at the moment.[76,124-127]

2. Cancer of the Penis

Practically all penile cancers are squamous cell carcinomas, and grossly they may be nodular, exophytic, or fungating. The geographic distribution of penile cancer is peculiar. Although rare in the U.S. and in Europe, penile cancer is fairly common in many developing countries of Africa, Central and South America, where circumcision is not practiced and poor hygiene abounds.[191] Cancer of the penis accounts for 2% of all malignant tumors of the male genitourinary tract, but represents less than 0.1% of all male cancers in North America. In Finland, penile cancer is an extreme rarity, the annual number of only 12 to 16 new cases having been diagnosed in this country between 1956 and 1988.[192] This gives an age-adjusted incidence of 0.4 to 0.9 per 100,000. In 1988, the age-adjusted incidence was 0.4, the highest age-specific incidence (2.4) falling into the age-group of 65–69 year-old males.[192]

Although the epidemiology of penile cancer is incompletely understood as yet, one of the recognized risk factors seems to be the absence of circumcision. Also a definite geographic clustering of penile and cervical cancer has been reported, e.g., in China.[193] In most studies, smegma, phimosis (75–90% of all cases), inflammation, and a history of STDs (27%) have been regarded as contributing factors.[194] The epidemiological data unequivocally show that some of the world's high-risk areas for penile cancer are in Brazil. Here, generally younger patients (33–35 years) are affected when compared with the cases in the U.S. and Europe (mean age 65 years).[195] Extremely high prevalence rates have been found in rural regions of the northern part of Brazil (6.8 per

100,000) as contrasted to industrialized urban regions in the south (2.9 per 100,000)[195] Carcinoma of the penis is the second most frequent malignancy of the males in Bali, another high-risk country, occurring in young men.[196] These authors found evidence on HPV involvement in 75% of penile carcinomas in that country.

Recently, a case-control study was initiated in the Henan Province in the People's Republic of China, an area with a high mortality rates for this malignancy.[197] Strongly associated with the risk were all conditions restricting the mobility of the foreskin, including phimosis and paraphimosis. Similarly, poor hygiene practices also appeared to increase the risk, especially when smegma was detectable on physical examination. A sexual relationship outside marriage was associated with relative risk (RR) of 1.7, exceeding the number of lifetime sexual partners. Risk was also increased among subjects reporting a previous genital disease, condyloma in particular.[197] These data support the role of sexually transmitted agent (HPV) in the etiology of penile cancer in this high-risk area. Interestingly, similar observations were reported in a low-incidence country, Finland as well, where all 269 penile cancer patients reported to the Finnish Cancer Registry between 1955 and 1977 were analyzed for epidemiological risk factors.[192] Cancer of the penis seems to be a disease of elderly males which does not show any systematic geographic variation within Finland in terms of risk. The most frequent predisposing factors were phimosis, present in 44% of cases, and penile condylomas, detected in 20% of cases.[192]

3.   Precancer Lesions and Genital Cancer in Sexual Partners

The number of sexual partners is an established risk factor for both cervical cancer[198] and the acquisition of STDs, HPV infections included.[138] This was recently well documented among female college students, in whom the relative risk for having an STD was 8.1 in those with more than 5 sexual partners.[199] According to this line of thinking, HPV as an STD and its close associations with genital precancer lesions, a large number of epidemiological studies have been completed, searching for a common etiologic agent for both the penile cancer and carcinoma of the uterine cervix.[76]

Among the female sexual partners of the males with penile cancer, a significant excess of deaths due to carcinoma of the uterine cervix has been recorded.[66-69] There are also reports where these two malignancies have been detected in married couples.[67,200] Interestingly, a recent epidemiologic survey on penile carcinomas in Finland (a low-risk country for both penile and cervical cancer), could not establish an increased risk for cervical cancer among wives of these males.[201] This might indicate that different factors are involved in the development of genital carcinomas in the high-risk and low-risk countries, as suggested also in large epidemiological studies.[196,197]

High-risk HPV types are equally involved in the precancer lesions of the uterine cervix, vagina, and vulva, as well as on the penis, and these same types are also present in invasive carcinomas of these mucosal sites. This is paralleled by the concurrent presence of HPV 16 DNA in genital lesions of the sexual partners.[5,6,95] From the epidemiological standpoint, this concordance of HPV types between the sexual couples has become of prime importance. To evaluate the concordance of (1) genital HPV lesions and (2) viral types in HPV-infected women and their male sexual partners, a series of 282 prospectively followed-up women and their male partners were examined by peniscopy and punch biopsy.[93] Of the males, 199 (70.6%) showed histological evidence for HPV infection, 89.4% of which were flat lesions. HPV DNA was found in 181 (38.0%) of the 476 biopsies examined by ISH, exophytic warts (26 cases) and PIN lesions (20 cases) were the most frequently HPV DNA-positive (92.3 and 80%, respectively). HPV DNA was also detected in 76 (31.3%) flat lesions histologically not equivocal HPV, i.e., in subclinical infections. Of the 271 sexual couples subjected to HPV typing, both partners were ISH positive in 66 (24.4%) cases, but only 15 (5.5%) couples had an identical HPV type in their genital tract. Of the 20 couples with a PIN lesion, both partners were positive in 8 (40%) cases, 3 (15%) having the same type.[93]

The number of studies analyzing penile HPV infections in the sexual partners of women who have genital HPV infections has increased rapidly. These studies were recently discussed in detail.[100]

As pointed out before, the detection rate of penile HPV lesions is completely dependent on the detection technique used, whether peniscopy, biopsy, hybridization, or PCR. Studies are few, however, in which the concordance of specific HPV types in sexual couples have been analyzed. The tentative findings of low concordance[93,94] cast some doubt on the concept that HPV is invariably a sexually transmitted infection. It should be realized, however, that the concordance figures are dependent on the study design, i.e., whether the sexual partners are monogamous or not.[93,94,202] From the clinical point of view, prospective follow-up studies on male HPV infections are mandatory to fully elucidate their natural history.[100]

VII. CONCLUSIONS

A large number of mucosal HPV types affects the genital tract mucosa, inducing either clinical, subclinical, or latent infections at these sites. The former can be diagnosed by clinical detection techniques, whereas the latter can only be established by demonstrating HPV DNA in a normal epithelium. In both sexes, low-risk (HPV 6 and 11) and high-risk (HPV 16 and 18) HPV types can be differentiated, with markedly divergent malignant potential. Squamous cell carcinoma of the uterine cervix is the most frequent malignant tumour in women worldwide. Penile carcinomas are distinct rarities in most Western countries, but highly prevalent in some other geographical areas. These two malignancies are frequently associated with the high-risk HPV types, strongly suggesting that HPV is a major risk factor (acting synergistically with other carcinogenic agents) for both the cervical and penile squamous cell cancer. The epidemiology of female HPV infections is extensively studied, but still incompletely understood. The data on the males are more scanty. The possibility clearly exists, however, that normal genital mucosa (cervix, vagina, vulva, penis, urethra, prostate) contains a major reservoir of HPV, with potential for transmission by sexual intercourse.

The feasibility of active preventive measures to interrupt the transmission remains an open issue. There is evidence that eradication of the female HPV lesions by laser, cryotherapy, or conization gives excellent (>90%) cure rates, which can hardly be improved by treating the male sexual partners. Agreement exists that clinical HPV lesions should be eradicated. The same applies to the established precancer lesions (CIN, VAIN, VIN, PIN, bowenoid papulosis) even if subclinical, to interfere with the process of malignant transformation. More problematic are the entirely benign lesions (flat condylomas without IN), and those acetowhite (subclinical) lesions which on light microscopy only present minor epithelial changes and contain the low-risk HPV types (HPV 6, 11, 42, etc.). It is evident that no practical means exist to eradicate the latent HPV infections with no epithelial abnormalities. This does not seem feasible either, because (1) probably all people show it in some stage of their life, and (2) because genital squamous cell cancer only develops through the well-established precancer lesions, which can be eradicated whenever detected.

According to current understanding, early diagnosis and treatment of all suspicious lesions (whether clinical or subclinical) remains mandatory to prevent genital cancer, and possibly to reduce the risk for a similar lesion in the sexual partner. Whether special attention should be focused on the detection of "high-risk partners" bearing (1) high-risk lesions (IN, bowenoid papulosis), or (2) subclinical infections with the high-risk HPV types 16 and 18, remains under debate. The former can be accomplished by carefully conducting colpo/peniscopic examination with acetic acid and directed punch biopsy. Viral typing of the directed biopsy or cellular scraping by DNA hybridization or PCR is mandatory to confirm or exclude the high-risk HPV types. Discovery of the high-risk lesions containing HPV 16 DNA will probably enable us to identify the patients (and their partners) at increased risk for malignant transformation, and thus would contribute to early detection and prevention of genital cancer in both sexes.

ACKNOWLEDGMENTS

The original studies of the author included in this review have been supported during the past several years by research grants from the Finnish Cancer Society, by PHS grant number 5 RO1

CA 42010-03 awarded by the National Cancer Institute, DHHS, a research grant from the Social Insurance Institution of Finland, a joint research grant from Fabriques de Tabac Reunies S.A., and British-American Tobacco Company Ltd., and a Research Contract (# 1041051) from the Medical Research Council of the Academy of Finland.

REFERENCES

1. Oriel, J. D., Genital warts, *Sex. Trans. Dis.*, 8, 326, 1981.
2. Meisels, A., Fortin, R., Roy, M., Condylomatous lesions of cervix and vagina. I. Cytologic patterns, *Acta Cytol.*, 20, 505, 1976.
3. Syrjänen, K. J., Heinonen, U. M., Kauraniemi, T., Cytological evidence of the association of condylomatous lesions with the dysplastic and neoplastic changes in uterine cervix, *Acta Cytol.*, 25, 17, 1981.
4. Syrjänen, K. J., Human papillomavirus (HPV) lesions in association with cervical dysplasias and neoplasias, *Obstet. Gynecol.*, 62, 617, 1983.
5. Gross, G., Lesions of the male and female external genitalia associated with human papillomaviruses, in *Papillomaviruses and Human Disease*, Syrjänen, K. J., Gissmann, L., Koss, L., Eds., Springer Verlag, Heidelberg, 1987, 197.
6. Ikenberg, H., Gissmann, L., Gross, G., Grussendorf-Conen, E-I., zur Hausen, H., Human papillomavirus type 16-related DNA in genital Bowen's disease and bowenoid papulosis, *Int. J. Cancer*, 32, 563, 1983.
7. Broker, T. R., Botchan, M., Papillomaviruses: Retrospectives and prospectives, *Cancer Cells*, 4, 17, 1986.
8. Gissmann, L., Boshart, M., Dürst, M., Ikenberg, H., Wagner, D., zur Hausen, H., Presence of Human papillomavirus in genital tumors, *J. Inv. Dermatol.*, 83, 26s, 1984.
9. Pfister, H., Biology and biochemistry of papillomaviruses, *Rev. Physiol. Biochem. Pharmacol.*, 99, 112, 1984.
10. Smith, K. T., Campo, M. S., Papillomaviruses and their involvement in oncogenesis, *Biomed. Pharmacother.*, 39, 405, 1985.
11. Syrjänen, K. J., Current concepts on Human papillomavirus (HPV) infections in the genital tract and their relationship to intraepithelial neoplasia and squamous cell carcinoma, *Obstet. Gynecol. Surv.*, 39, 252, 1984.
12. Syrjänen, K. J., Human papillomavirus (HPV) infections of the female genital tract and their associations with intraepithelial neoplasia and squamous cell carcinoma, *Pathol. Annu.*, 21, 53, 1986.
13. Syrjänen, K. J., Papillomaviruses and Cancer, in *Papillomaviruses and Human Disease*, Syrjänen, K. J., Gissmann, L., Koss, L., Eds., Springer Verlag, Heidelberg, 1987, 468.
14. zur Hausen, H., Human papillomaviruses and their possible role in squamous cell carcinomas, *Curr. Topics Microbiol. Immunol.*, 78, 1, 1977.
15. zur Hausen, H., Human genital cancer: Synergism between two virus infections or synergism between a virus infection and initiating events?, *Lancet*, II, 1370, 1982.
16. zur Hausen, H., Papillomaviruses in human cancers, *Mol. Carcin.*, 1, 147, 1988.
17. McCance, D. J., Human papillomavirus (HPV) infections in the aetiology of cervical cancer, *Cancer Surv.*, 7, 499, 1988.
18. Meanwell, C. A., The epidemiology of human papillomavirus infection in relation to cervical cancer, *Cancer Surv.*, 7, 481, 1988.
19. Roman, A., Fife, K. H., Human papillomaviruses: Are we ready to type, *Clin. Microbiol. Rev.*, 2, 166, 1989.
20. Syrjänen, K. J., Genital Human papillomavirus (HPV) infections and their associations with squamous cell cancer: Reappraisal of the morphologic, epidemiologic and DNA data, in *Progress in Surgical Pathology*, Fenoglio-Preiser, C. M., Wolff, M., Rilke, F. Eds., Field and Wood, New York, 1992, Vol. XII, 217.
21. de Villiers, E.-M., Laboratory techniques in the investigation of human papillomavirus infection, *Genitour. Med.*, 68, 50, 1992.
22. DiPaolo, J. A., Woodworth, C. D., Popescu, N. C., Notario, V., Doniger, J., Induction of human cervical squamous cell carcinoma by sequential transfection with human papillomavirus 16 DNA and viral Harvey ras, *Oncogene*, 4, 395, 1989.

23. zur Hausen, H., Papillomaviruses in anogenital cancer as a model to understand the role of viruses in human cancers, *Cancer Res.*, 49, 4677, 1989.
24. Cannizzaro, L. A., Dürst, M., Mendez, M. J., Hecht, B. K., Hecht, F., Regional chromosome localization of human papillomavirus integration sites near fragile sites, oncogenes, and cancer chromosome breakpoints, *Cancer Gen. Cytogen.*, 33, 93, 1988.
25. Dürst, M., Croce, C. M., Gissmann, L., Schwarz, E., Huebner, K., Papillomavirus sequences integrate near cellular oncogenes in some cervical carcinomas, *Genetics*, 84, 1070, 1987.
26. Mincheva, A., Gissmann, L., zur Hausen, H., Chromosomal integrated sites of human papillomavirus DNA in three cervical cancer cell lines mapped by *in situ* hybridization, *Med. Microbiol. Immunol.*, 176, 245, 1987.
27. Pfister, H., Fuchs, P. G., Papillomaviruses: Particles, genome organisation and proteins, in *Papillomaviruses and Human Disease*, Syrjänen, K. J., Gissmann, L., Koss, L., Eds., Springer Verlag, Heidelberg, 1987, 1.
28. Syrjänen, K., Väyrynen, M., Saarikoski, S., Mäntyjärvi, R., Parkkinen, S., Hippeläinen, M., Castrén, O., Natural history of cervical Human papillomavirus (HPV) infections based on prospective follow-up, *Br. J. Obstet. Gynaecol.*, 92, 1086, 1985.
29. Syrjänen, K., de Villiers E-M., Väyrynen, M., Mäntyjärvi, R., Parkkinen, S., Saarikoski, S., Castrén, O., Cervical papillomavirus infection progressing to invasive cancer in less than three years. *Lancet*, I, 510, 1985.
30. Syrjänen, K., Mäntyjärvi, R., Parkkinen, S., Väyrynen, M., Saarikoski, S., Syrjänen, S., Castrén, O., Prospective follow-up in assessment of the biological behaviour of cervical HPV-associated dysplastic lesions, *Banbury Report*, 21, 167, 1986.
31. Kataja, V., Syrjänen, K., Mäntyjärvi, R., Väyrynen, M., Syrjänen, S., Saarikoski, S., Parkkinen, S., Yliskoski, M., Salonen, J.T., Castrén, O., Prospective follow-up of cervical HPV infections. Life-Table analysis of histopathological, cytological and colposcopic data, *Eur. J. Epidemiol.*, 5, 1, 1989.
32. Schwarz, E., Transcription of Papillomavirus genomes, in *Papillomaviruses and Human Disease*, Syrjänen, K. J., Gissmann, L., Koss, L., Eds., Springer Verlag, Heidelberg, 1987, 444, 1987.
33. Spalholz, B. A., Howley, P. M., Papillomavirus-host cell interactions, *Adv. Virol. Oncol.*, 8, 27, 1989.
34. Chuang, T.-Y., Perry, H. O., Kurland, L. T., Ilstrup, D. M., Condyloma acuminatum in Rochester, Minn, 1950-1978. I. Epidemiology and clinical features, *Arch. Dermatol.*, 120, 469, 1984.
35. Oriel, J. D., Genital and anal papillomavirus infections in human males, in *Papillomaviruses and Human Disease*, Syrjänen, K. J., Gissmann, L., Koss, L., Eds., Springer Verlag, Heidelberg, 1987, 182.
36. Syrjänen, K., Väyrynen, M., Castren, O., Yliskoski, M., Mäntyjärvi, R., Pyrhönen, S., Saarikoski, S., Sexual behaviour of the females with human papillomavirus (HPV) lesions in the uterine cervix, *Br. J. Venereal Dis.*, 60, 243, 1984.
37. Donnan, S. P. B., Wong, F. W. S., Ho, S. C., Lau, E. M. C., Takashi, K., Esteve, J., Reproductive and sexual risk factors and human papillomavirus infection in cervical cancer among Hong Kong Chinese, *Int. J. Epidemiol.*, 18, 32, 1989.
38. Schmauz, R., Okong, P., de Villiers, E.-M., Dennin, R., Brade, L., Lwanga, S. K., Owor, R., Multiple infections in cases of cervical cancer from a high-incidence area in tropical Africa, *Int. J. Cancer*, 43, 805, 1989.
39. Villa, L. L., Franco, E. L. F., Epidemiologic correlates of cervical neoplasia and risk of human papillomavirus infection in asymptomatic women in Brazil, *J. Nat. Cancer Instit.*, 81, 332, 1989.
40. Reeves, W. C., Rawls, W. E., Brinton, L. A., Epidemiology of genital papillomaviruses and cervical cancer, *Rev. Infect. Dis.*, 11, 426, 1989.
41. Zhang, Z. F., Parkin, D. M., Yu, S. Z., Esteve, J., Yang, X. Z., Risk factors for cancer of the cervix in a rural Chinese population, *Int. J. Cancer*, 43, 762, 1989.
42. Ji, H., Syrjänen, S., Syrjänen, K., Wu, A., Chang, F., In situ hybridization analysis of HPV DNA in cervical precancer and cervical cancers from China, *Arch. Gynecol. Obstet.*, 247, 21, 1990.
43. Barrasso, R., de Brux, J., Croissant, O., Orth, G., High prevalence of papillomavirus-associated penile intraepithelial neoplasia in sexual partners of women with cervical intraepithelial neoplasia, *N. Eng. J. Med.*, 317, 916, 1987.
44. Campion, M. J., Singer, A., Clarkson, P. K., Increased risk of cervical neoplasia in consorts of men with penile condylomata acuminata, *Lancet*, I, 943, 1985.
45. Syrjänen, K. J., Epidemiology of Human papillomavirus (HPV) infections and their associations with genital squamous cell cancer, *Acta Pathol. Microbiol. Immunol. Scand.*, 97, 957, 1989.

46. Syrjänen, K.J., Natural history of genital HPV infections. *Papillomavirus Report*, 1(4), 1, 1990.
47. de Villiers, E.-M., Schneider, A., Miklaw, H., Papendick, U., Wagner, D., Wesch, H., Wahrendorf, J., zur Hausen, H., Human papillomavirus infections in women with and without abnormal cervical cytology, *Lancet*, II, 703, 1987.
48. Grussendorf, E.-I., de Villiers, E.-M., Gissmann, L., Human papillomavirus genomes in penile smears of healthy men, *Lancet*, II, 1092, 1986.
49. Macnab, J. C. M., Walkinshaw, S. A., Cordiner, J. W., Clements, J. B., Human papillomavirus in clinically and histologically normal tissue of patients with genital cancer, *N. Eng. J. Med.*, 315, 1052, 1986.
50. Wickenden, C., Malcolm, A. D. B., Steele, A., Coleman, D. V., Screening for wart virus infection in normal and abnormal cervices by DNA hybridization of cervical scrapes, *Lancet*, I, 65, 1985.
51. Toon, P. G., Arrand, J. R., Wilson, L. P., Sharp, D. S., Human papillomavirus infection of the uterine cervix of women without cytological signs of neoplasia, *Br. Med. J.*, 293, 1261, 1986.
52. Lörincz, A. T., Temple, G. F., Patterson, J. A., Jenson, A. B., Kurman, R. J., Lancaster, W. D., Correlation of cellular atypia and human papillomavirus deoxyribonucleic acid sequences in exfoliated cells of the uterine cervix, *Obstet. Gynecol.*, 68, 508, 1986.
53. Schneider, A., Hotz, M., Gissmann, L., Increased prevalence of human papillomaviruses in the lower genital tract of pregnant women, *Int. J. Cancer*, 40, 198, 1987.
54. Wickenden, C., Malcolm, A. D. B., Byrne, M., Smith, C., Anderson, M. C., Coleman, D. V., Prevalence of HPV DNA and viral copy numbers in cervical scrapes from women with normal and abnormal cervices, *J. Pathol.*, 153, 127, 1987.
55. Gergely, L., Czegledy, J., Hernady, Z., Human papillomavirus frequency in normal cervical tissue, *Lancet*, II, 513, 1987.
56. Ferenczy, A., Mitao, M., Nagai, N., Silverstein, S. J., Crum, C. P., Latent papillomavirus and recurring genital warts, *N. Eng. J. Med.*, 313, 784, 1985.
57. Cox, M. F., Meanwell, C. A., Maitland, N. J., Blackledge, G., Scully, C., Jordan, J. A., Human papillomavirus type-16 homologous DNA in normal human ectocervix, *Lancet*, II, 157, 1986.
58. Levine, R. V., Crum, C. P., Herman, E., Cervical papillomavirus infection and intraepithelial neoplasia: a study of male sexual partners, *Obstet. Gynecol.*, 64, 16, 1984.
59. Krebs, H.-B., Schneider, V., Human papillomavirus-associated lesions of the penis: Colposcopy, cytology, and histology, *Clin. Obstet. Gynecol.*, 70, 299, 1987.
60. Rosenberg, S. K., Greenberg, M. G., Reid, R., Sexually transmitted papillomavirus infection in men, *Obstet. Gynecol. Clin. N. Am.*, 14, 495, 1987.
61. Krebs, H. B., Genital HPV infections in men, *Clin. Obstetr. Gynecol.*, 32, 180, 1989.
62. Rotola, A., Di Luca, D., Savioli, A., Simone, R., Secchiero, P., Reggiani, A., Cassai, E., Presence and physical state of HPV DNA in prostate and urinary-tract tissues, *Int. J. Cancer*, 52, 359, 1992.
63. Sand, P. K., Bowen, L. W., Blischke, S. O., Ostergard, D. R., Evaluation of male consorts of women with genital human papilloma virus infection, *Obstet. Gynecol.*, 68, 679, 1986.
64. Kennedy, L., Buntine, D. W., O'Connor, D., Frazer, I. H., Human papillomavirus — a study of male sexual partners, *Med. J. Aust.*, 149, 309, 1988.
65. Sedlacek, T. V., Cunnane, M., Carpiniello, V., Colposcopy in the diagnosis of penile condyloma, *Am. J. Obstet. Gynecol.*, 154, 494, 1986.
66. Martinez, I., Relationship of squamous cell carcinoma of the cervix uteri to squamous cell carcinoma of the penis among Puerto Rican women married to men with penile carcinoma, *Cancer*, 24, 777, 1969.
67. Goldberg, H. M., Pell-Ilderton, R., Daw, E., Saleh, N., Concurrent squamous cell carcinoma of the cervix and penis in a married couple, *Br. J. Obstet. Gynaecol.*, 86, 585, 1979.
68. Graham, S., Priore, R., Graham, M., Browne, R., Burnett, W., West, D., Genital cancer in wives of penile cancer patients, *Cancer*, 44, 1970, 1979.
69. Cocks, P. S., Peel, K. R., Cartwright, R. A., Adib, R., Carcinoma of penis and cervix, *Lancet*, II, 855, 1980.
70. Smith, P. G., Kinlen, L. J., White, G. C., Adelstein, A. M., Fox, A. J., Mortality of wives of men dying with cancer of the penis, *Br. J. Cancer*, 41, 422, 1980.
71. Fine, R. M., The penile condyloma cancer connection, *Int. J. Dermatol.*, 26, 289, 1987.
72. Hellberg, D., Nilsson, S., Genital cancer among wives of men with penile cancer. A study between 1958 and 1982, *Br. J. Obstet. Gynecol.*, 96, 321, 1989.

73. Schmauz, R., Findlay, M., Lalwak, A., Katsumbira, N., Buxton, E., Variation in the appearance of giant condyloma in an Ugandan series of cases of carcinoma of the penis, *Cancer*, 40, 1686, 1977.

74. Schmauz, R., Owor, R., Epidemiology of malignant degeneration of condylomata acumimata in Uganda, *Pathol. Res. Prac.*, 170, 91, 1980.

75. Schneider, A., Latent and subclinical genital HPV infections, *Papillomavirus Report*, 1(3), 2, 1990.

76. Syrjänen, K., Gissmann, L., Koss, L. G., *Papillomaviruses and Human Disease*, Eds., Springer Verlag, Heidelberg, 1987, 1-518.

77. Syrjänen, K. J., Morphologic survey of the condylomatous lesions in dysplastic and neoplastic epithelium of the uterine cervix, *Arch. Gynaecol.*, 227, 153, 1979.

78. Gross, G., Ikenberg, H., Gissmann, L., Hagedorn, M., Papillomavirus infection of the anogenital region: correlation between histology, clinical picture and virus type. Proposal of a new nomenclature, *J. Inv. Dermatol.*, 85, 147, 1985.

79. Hippeläinen, M., Yliskoski, M., Saarikoski, S., Syrjänen, S., Syrjänen, K., Genital human papillomavirus lesions of the male sexual partners: the diagnostic accuracy of peniscopy, *Genitour. Med.*, 67, 291, 1991.

80. Pitkin, R. M., Kent, T. H., Papillary squamous lesions of the uterine cervix. A difficult problem in diagnosis, *Am. J. Obstet. Gynecol.*, 85, 440, 1963.

81. Woodruff, J. D., Peterson, W. F., Condyloma acuminata of the cervix, *Am. J. Obstet. Gynecol.*, 75, 1354, 1958.

82. Meisels, A., Roy, M., Fortier, M., Morin, C., Casas-Cordero, M., Shah, K. V., Turgeon, H., Human papillomavirus infection of the cervix. The atypical condyloma, *Acta Cytol.*, 25, 1677, 1981.

83. Syrjänen, S., Syrjänen, K., Mäntyjärvi, R., Parkkinen, S., Väyrynen, M., Saarikoski, S., Castrén, O., Human papillomavirus (HPV) DNA sequences demonstrated by *in situ* DNA hybridization in serial paraffin-embedded cervical biopsies, *Arch. Gynaecol.*, 239:39, 1986.

84. Syrjänen, S., Syrjänen, K., An improved *in situ* DNA hybridization protocol for detection of Human papillomavirus (HPV) DNA sequences in paraffin-embedded sections, *J. Virol. Meth.*, 14, 293, 1986.

85. Syrjänen, K., Syrjänen, S., Concept on the existence of Human papillomavirus (HPV) DNA in histologically normal squamous epithelium of the genital tract should be re-evaluated, *Acta Obstet. Gynecol. Scand.*, 68, 613, 1989.

86. Buschke, A., Löwenstein, L., Beziehungen der spizen Kondylome zu den Carcinomen des Penis, *Arch. Dermatol.*, 163, 30, 1932.

87. Weed, J. C., Lozier, C., Daniel, S. J., Human papillomavirus in multifocal invasive female genital tract malignancy, *Obstet. Gynecol.*, 62, 583, 1983.

88. Väyrynen, M., Romppanen, T., Koskela, E., Castrén, O., Syrjänen, K., Verrucous squamous cell carcinoma of the female genital tract. Report of three cases and survey of the literature, *Int. J. Gynaecol. Obstet.*, 19, 351, 1981.

89. Hull, M. T., Eble, J. N., Priest, J. B., Mulcahy, J. J., Ultrastructure of Buschke-Löwenstein tumor, *J. Urol.*, 126, 485, 1981.

90. De Villiers, E. M., Schneider, A., Gross, G., zur Hausen, H., Analysis of benign and malignant urogenital tumors for human papillomavirus infection by labelling cellular DNA, *Med. Microbiol. Immunol.*, 174, 281, 1986.

91. Purola, E., Savia, E., Cytology of gynecologic condyloma accuminatum, *Acta Cytol.*, 21, 26, 1977.

92. Cornelissen, M. T. E., Tweel, J. G. V. D., Struyk, A. H. B., Jebbink, M. F., Briot, M., Noordaa, J. V. D., Schegget, J. T., Localization of human papillomavirus type 16 DNA using the polymerase chain reaction in the cervix uteri of women with cervical intraepithelial neoplasia, *J. Gen. Virol.*, 70, 2555, 1989.

93. Hippeläinen, M., Yliskoski, M., Syrjänen, S., Saastamoinen, J., Saarikoski, S., Hippeläinen, M., Syrjänen, K., Concordance of genital Human papillomavirus (HPV) lesions and viral types in HPV-infected women and their male sexual partner, *Br. Med. J.*, 1993; Submitted.

94. Barrasso, R., HPV-related genital lesions in men, in *The Epidemiology of Cervival Cancer and Human Papillomavirus*, Munoz, N., Bosch, F. X., Shah, K. V., Meheus, A., Eds., International Agency for Research on Cancer, Lyon, 1992, 85.

95. Gross, G., Ikenberg, H., de Villiers, E. M., Schneider, A., Wagner, D., Gissmann, L., Bowenoid papulosis: a venereally transmissible disease as reservoir for HPV 16, in *Origins of Female Genital Cancer: Virological and Epidemiological Aspects. Banbury Report*, zur Hausen, H., Peto, R., Eds., Cold Spring Harbor Laboratory, New York, 1986, 149.

96. Gross, G., Hagedorn, M., Ikenberg, H., Rufli, T., Dahlet, C., Grosshans, E., Gissmann, L., Bowenoid papulosis. Presence of human papillomavirus (HPV) structural antigens and of HPV 16-related DNA sequences, *Arch. Dermatol.*, 121, 858, 1985.

97. Wade, T. R., Kopf, A.W., Ackerman, A. B., Bowenoid papulosis in the genitalia, *Arch. Dermatol.*, 115, 306, 1979.

98. Guillet, G. Y., Braun, L., Masse, R., Aftimos, J., Geniaux, M., Texier, L., Bowenoid papulosis. Demonstration of Human papillomavirus (HPV) with anti-HPV immune serum, *Arch. Dermatol.*, 120, 514, 1984.

99. Rüdlinger, R., Grob, R., Yu, Y. X., Schnyder, U. W., Human papillomavirus-35-positive bowenoid papulosis of the anogenital area and concurrent human papillomavirus-35-positive verruca with bowenoid dysplasia of the periungual area, *Arch. Dermatol.*, 125, 655, 1989.

100. Syrjänen, K. J., Association of HPV with penile cancer, in *Genital Warts — Human papillomavirus Infection*, Mindel, A., Ed., Edward Arnold, Kent, 1995, 163–197.

101. Schottländer, J., Kemauner, F., Zur Kenntnis des Uteruskarzinoms: Monographische Studie über Morphologie, Entwicklung, Wachstum. *Beiträgen zur Klinik der Erkrankung*, S. Karger, Berlin, 1912.

102. Riotton, G., Christopherson, W. M., *Cytology of the Female Genital Tract*, World Health Organization, Geneva, 1973.

103. Richart, R. M., Cervical intraepithelial neoplasia, *Pathol. Ann.*, 8, 301, 1973.

104. Giacomini, G., Simi, U., CIN or not CIN, *Acta Cytol.*, 27, 543, 1983.

105. Richart, R. M., Causes and management of cervical intraepithelial neoplasia, *Cancer*, 60, 1951, 1987.

106. Richart, R. M., A modified terminology for cervical intraepithelial neoplasia, *Obstet. Gynecol.*, 75, 131, 1990.

107. National Cancer Institute Workshop: The 1988 Bethesda System for reporting cervical/vaginal cytologic diagnoses, *Acta Cytol.*, 33, 567, 1989.

108. Giacomini, G., Simi, U., Nomenclature for the cytodiagnosis of cervical intraepithelial lesions, *Acta Cytol.*, 35, 483, 1991.

109. Herbst, A. L., The Bethesda system for cervical/vaginal cytologic diagnosis: a note of caution, *Obstet. Gynecol.*, 76, 449, 1990.

110. Kurman, R. J., Malkasian, G. D., Sedlis, A., Solomon, D., From Papanicoau to Bethesda: The rational for a new cervical cytologic classification, *Obstet. Gynecol.*, 77, 779, 1991.

111. Syrjänen, K., Kataja, V., Yliskoski, M., Chang, F., Syrjänen, S., Saarikoski, S., Natural history of cervical HPV lesions with special emphasis on the biologic relevance of the Bethesda System, *Obstet. Gynecol.*, 79, 675, 1992.

112. Czegledy, J., Gergely, L., Endrödi, I., Detection of human papillomavirus deoxyribonucleic acid by filter in situ hybridization during pregnancy, *J. Med. Virol.*, 28, 250, 1989.

113. Kulski, J. K., Pakoczy, D P., Sterrett, G. F., Pixley, E. C., Human papillomavirus coinfections of the vulva and uterine cervix, *J. Med. Virol.*, 27, 244, 1989.

114. Nuovo, G. J., Cottral, S., Richart, R., Occult human papillomavirus infection of the uterine cervix in postmenopausal women, *Am. J. Obstet. Gynecol.*, 160, 340, 1989.

115. Colgan, T. J., Percy, M. E., Suri, M., Shier, R. M., Andrews, D. F., Lickrish, G. M., Human papillomavirus infection of morphologically normal cervical epithelium adjacent to squamous dysplasia and invasive carcinoma, *Human Pathol.*, 20, 316, 1989.

116. Choo, K. B., Shen, H. D., Leung, W. Y., Lee, Y. N., A distinct difference in the prevalence of papillomavirus infection in cytologically normal and neoplastic cells of the uterine cervix, *Clin. Med. J.*, 42, 1, 1988.

117. Ji, H., Syrjänen, S., Matinlompolo, T., Huovinen, K., Fuju, C., Syrjänen, K., Subclinical HPV infections in the lower female genital tract: Histological evaluation and detection of HPV DNA by in situ hybridization with biotinylated probes, *Cervix lower female gen. tract*, 7, 255, 1989.

118. Yliskoski, M., Saarikoski, S., Syrjänen, K., Conization for CIN associated with Human papillomavirus infection, *Arch. Gynecol. Obstet.*, 249, 59, 1991.

119. Yliskoski, M., Syrjänen, K., Syrjänen, S., Saarikoski, S., Nethersell, A., Systemic α-interferon (Wellferon®) treatment of genital Human papillomavirus (HPV) type 6, 11, 16 and 18 infections. Double-blind, placebo-controlled trial, *Gynecol. Oncol.*, 43, 55, 1991.

120. Nuovo, G. J., Becker, J., Margiotta, M., MacConnell, P., Comite, S., Hochman H., Histological distribution of polymerase chain reaction-amplified human papillomavirus 6 and 11 DNA in penile lesions, *Am. J. Surg. Pathol.*, 16, 269, 1992.

121. Syrjänen, S., Syrjänen, K., Human papillomavirus (HPV) infections of the genital tract. Clinical Significance and diagnosis by PCR, in, *Frontiers in Virology: Diagnosis of Human Viruses by Polymerase Chain Reaction Technology*, Becker, Y., Darai, G, Eds., Springer-Verlag, Heidelberg, 1992, 185.

122. Syrjänen, S., Saastamoinen, J., Chang, F., Ji, H., Syrjänen, K., Colposcopy, punch biopsy, in situ DNA hybridization and polymerase chain reaction in searching for genital Human papillomavirus (HPV) infections in women with normal PAP smears, *J. Med. Virol.*, 31, 259, 1990.

123. Qizilbash, A. H., Papillary squamous tumors of the uterine cervix. A clinical and pathologic study of 21 cases, *Am. J. Clin. Pathol.*, 61, 508, 1974.

124. von Krogh, G., Rylander, E., Eds., *Genital Papilloma Virus Infection: A Survey for the Clinician,* Conpharm, A. B., Karlstad, 1989.

125. de Palo, G., Rilke, F., zur Hausen, H., Eds., *Herpes and Papilloma Viruses*, (vol II), Serono Symposia Publications, Raven Press, Vol 46, 1988.

126. Gross, G., Jablonska, S., Pfister, H., Stegner, H. E., Eds., *Genital Papillomavirus Infections: Modern Diagnosis and Treatment*, Springer Verlag, Heidelberg, 1990.

127. Monsonego, J., Ed., *Papillomaviruses in Human Pathology. Recent Progress in Epidermoid Precancers*, Serono Symposia Publications, Raven Press, Vol 78, 1990.

128. Boxer, R. J., Skinner, D. G., Condylomata acuminata and squamous cell carcinoma, *Urology*, 9, 72, 1977.

129. Koutsky, L., Galloway, D., Holmes, K. K., Epidemiology of genital human papillomavirus infection, *Epidemiol. Rev.*, 10, 122, 1988.

130. Eron, L. J., Franklin, J., Tucker, S., Interferon therapy for condylomata acuminata, *N. Eng. J. Med.*, 315, 1059, 1986.

131. Belli, L., Frazer, I., Hogan, P., Kennedy, L., O'Connor, D., Hersey, P., Law, C., Arseneau, J., Dascal, A., Eiley, S., Ferenczy, A., Mendelson, J., Bouchard, C., Fortier, M., Champoux, F., Roy, M., van de Berg, G. M., Stolz, E., Freeman, K., Syrjänen, K., Barclay, C., Boland, K., Fauchere, S., Kroon, M., Walker, M., Ryff, J. Ch., Smith, P., Wahl, M., Scott, K., Recurrent condylomata acuminata treated with recombinant interferon alfa-2a: A multicenter double-blind placebo-controlled clinical trial, *J. Am. Med. Assoc.*, 265, 2684, 1991.

132. Maw, R. D., Disnmore, W., Horner, T., Lawther, H., Rinne, E., Lassus, A., Paavonen, J., Aho, M., Nieminen, P., Vesterinen, E., Tuimala, R. J., Juuakka, T., Saastamoinen, J., Syrjänen, S. M., Syrjänen, K. J., Walker, M., Ryff, J. C., Smith, C., Budde, M., Blackburn, N., Ellmen, J., Wahl, M., Comparison of interferon alpha-2a and podophyllin in the treatment of primary condylomata acuminata, *Genitour, Med.*, 67, 394, 1991.

133. Syrjänen, K., Yliskoski, M., Kataja, V., Hippeläinen, M., Syrjänen, S., Saarikoski, S., Ryhänen, A., Prevalence of genital human papillomavirus (HPV) infections in a mass-screened Finnish female population aged 20-65 years, *Int. J. STD AIDS*, 1, 410, 1990.

134. Syrjänen, K., Hakama, M., Saarikoski, S., Väyrynen, M., Yliskoski, M., Syrjänen, S., Kataja, V., Castren, O., Prevalence, incidence and estimated life-time risk of cervical human papillomavirus (HPV) infections in nonselected Finnish female population, *Sex. Trans. Dis.*, 17, 15, 1990.

135. Fredricsson, B., Nasiell, M., Sennerstam, R., Wadås, A-M., Is there a changing epidemiology of premalignant lesions of the cervix, *Acta Obstetr. Gynecol. Scand.*, 56, 435, 1977.

136. Sadeghi, S. B., Hsieh, E. W., Gunn, S. W., Prevalence of cervical intraepithelial neoplasia in sexually active teenagers and young adults. Results of data analysis of mass papanicolaou screening of 796,337 women in the United States, *Am. J. Obstet. Gynecol.*, 148, 726, 1984.

137. Finnish Cancer Registry, *Cancer incidence in Finland 1988*, Cancer Statistics of the National Agency for Welfare and Health, Helsinki, 1991, pp. 8-16.

138. Kataja, V., Genital Human papillomavirus (HPV) infections. Prevalence, incidence, risk factors and prognosis, *Kuopio University Publications Department of Medical Sciences*, 13, 1992.

139. Varga, A., The relationship of cervical dysplasia to in situ and invasive carcinoma of the cervix, *Am. J. Obstet. Gynecol.*, 95, 759, 1966.

140. Hall, J. E., Walton, L., Dysplasia of the cervix. A prospective study of 206 cases, *Am. J. Obstet. Gynecol.*, 100, 662, 1968.

141. Spriggs, A. I., natural history of cervical dysplasia, *Clin. Obstet. Gynaecol.*, 8, 65, 1981.

142. Villa Santa, U., Diagnosis and prognosis of cervical dysplasia, *Obstet. Gynecol.*, 38, 811, 1971.

143. Sedlis, A., Cohen, A., Sall, S., The fate of cervical dysplasia, *Am. J. Obstet. Gynecol.*, 107, 1065, 1970.

144. Nasiell, K., Nasiell, M., Vaclavinkova, V., Behavior of moderate cervical dysplasia during long-term follow-up, *Obstet. Gynecol.*, 61, 609, 1983.

145. Nasiell, K., Roger, V., Nasiell, M., Behavior of mild cervical dysplasia during long-term follow-up, *Obstet. Gynecol.*, 67, 665, 1986.

146. Richart, R. M., Barron, B. A., A follow-up study of patients with cervical dysplasia, *Am. J. Obstet. Gynecol.*, 105, 386, 1969.

147. Stern E., Neely, P. M., Dysplasia of the uterine cervix. Incidence of regression, recurrence, and cancer, *Cancer*, 17, 508, 1964.

148. Fox, C. H., Biologic behavior of dysplasia and carcinoma in situ, *Am. J. Obstet. Gynecol.*, 99, 960, 1967.

149. Starreveld, A. A., Romanowski, B., Hill, G. B., Koch, M., Pearce, K. I., The latency period of carcinoma in situ of the cervix, *Obstet. Gynecol.*, 62, 348, 1983.

150. Syrjänen, K., Mäntyjärvi, R., Väyrynen, M., Syrjänen, S., Parkkinen, S., Yliskoski, M., Saarikoski, S., Castren, O., Human papillomavirus (HPV) infections involved in the neoplastic process of the uterine cervix as established by prospective follow-up of 513 women for two years, *Eur. J. Gynaecol. Oncol.*, 8, 5, 1987.

151. deBrux, J., Ionesco, M., Cochard, B., Masson, M. F., Kaeding, H., Epidemiologie, morphologie, evolution des condylomes cervicaux, *Gynecologie*, 32, 413, 1981.

152. Mitchell, H., Drake, M., Medley, G., Prospective evaluation of risk of cervical cancer after cytological evidence of human papillomavirus infection, *Lancet* I, 573, 1986.

153. Campion, M. J., McCance, D. J., Cuzick, J., Singer, A., Progressive potential of mild cervical atypia: Prospective cytological, colposcopic, and virological study, *Lancet* II, 237, 1986.

154. deBrux, J., Orth, G., Croissant, O., Cochard, B., Ionesco, M., Lesions condylomateuses du col uterin: evolution chez 2466 patients, *Bull. Cancer*, 70, 410, 1983.

155. Kataja, V., Syrjänen, K., Syrjänen, S., Mäntyjärvi, R., Yliskoski, M., Saarikoski, S., Mäntyjärvi, R., Salonen, J. T., Prospective follow-up of genital HPV infections: Survival analysis of the HPV typing data, *Eur. J. Epidemiol.*, 6, 9, 1990.

156. Syrjänen, K., Mäntyjärvi, R., Saarikoski, S., Väyrynen, M., Syrjänen, S., Parkkinen, S., Yliskoski, M., Saastamoinen, J., Castrén, O., Factors associated with progression of cervical Human papillomavirus (HPV) infections into carcinoma in situ during a long-term prospective follow-up, *Br. J. Obstet. Gynaecol.*, 95, 1096, 1988.

157. Raymond, C. A., For women infected with papillomavirus, close watch counseled, *J. Am. Med. Assoc.*, 257, 2398, 1987.

158. Evans, A. S., Monaghan, J. M., Spontaneous resolution of cervical warty atypia: the relevance of clinical and nuclear DNA features: a prospective study, *Br. J. Obstet. Gynaecol.*, 92, 165, 1985.

159. Cheetham, D., Smith, J., Wilson, C., Munday, P. E., Coleman, D. V., Clinical significance of human papillomavirus infection of the uterine cervix in the development of cervical intraepithelial neoplasia, *Br. J. Ven. Dis.*, 60, 182, 1984.

160. Lorincz, A. T., Schiffman, M. H., Jaffurs, W. J., Marlow, J., Quinn, A. P., Temple, G. F., Temporal associations of human papillomavirus infection with cervical cytologic abnormalities, *Am. J. Obstet. Gynecol.*, 162, 645, 1990.

161. Nash, J. D., Burke, T. W., Hoskins, W. J., Biologic course of cervical human papillomavirus infection, *Obstet. Gynecol.*, 69, 160, 1987.

162. Alberico, S., Facca, M. C., Mandruzzato, G. P., Di Bonito, L., Colautti, I., Patriarca, S., Recurrence incidence in follow-up of patients affected by condylomatosis of the uterine cervix with VCE (viral cytopathic effect), *Eur. J. Gynaecol. Obstet.*, 3, 222, 1985.

163. Walker, P. G., Singer, A., Dyson, J. L., Oriel, J. D., Natural history of cervical epithelial abnormalities in patients with vulvar warts, *Br. J. Ven. Dis.*, 59, 327, 1983.

164. Franceschi, S., Doll, R., Gallwey, J., La Vecchia, C., Peto, R., Spriggs, A. I., Genital warts and cervical neoplasia: An epidemiological study, *Br. J. Cancer*, 48, 621, 1983.

165. Kitchener, H. C., Neilson, L., Burnett, R. A., Young, L., Macnab, J. C. M., Prospective serial study of viral change in the cervix and correlation with human papillomavirus genome status, *Br. J. Obstet. Gynecol.*, 98, 1042, 1991.

166. Hörding, U., Daugaard, S., Bock, J. E., Sebbelov, A. M., Norrild, B., HPV 11, 16 and 18 DNA sequences in cervical swabs from women with cervical dysplasia; prevalence and associated risk of progression, *Eur. J. Obstet. Gynecol. Rep. Biol.*, 40, 43, 1991.

167. Courtial, I., Bremond, A., Aknin, D., Regression spontanee des condylomes plan du col uterin, *J. Gynecol. Obstet. Biol. Rep.*, 20, 527, 1991.

168. de Villiers, E.-M., Wagner, R., Schneider, A., Wesch, H., Munz, F., zur Hausen H., Human papillomavirus DNA in women without and with cytological abnormalities: results of a 5-year follow-up study, *Gynecol. Oncol.*, 44, 33, 1992.

169. Hirschowitz, L., Raffle, A .E., Mackenzie, E. F. D., Hughes, A. O., Long term follow up of women with borderline cervical smear test results: effects of age and viral infection on progression to high grade dyskaryosis, *Br. Med. J.*, 304, 1209, 1992.

170. Handley, J., Lawther, H., Horner, T., Maw, R., Dinsmore, W., Ten year follow-up study of women presenting to a genitourinary medicine clinic with anogenital warts, *Int. J. STD AIDS*, 3, 28, 1992.

171. Carmichael, J. A., The management of minor degrees of cervical dysplasia associated with the human papilloma virus, *Yale J. Biol. Med.*, 64, 591, 1991.

172. Montz, F. J., Monk, B. J., Fowler, J. M., Nguyen, L., Natural history of the minimally abnormal Papanicolaou smear, *Obstet. Gynecol.*, 80, 385, 1992.

173. Pich, A., Margaria, E., Ghiringhello, B., Navone, R., In situ hybridization for human papillomavirus as a method of predicting the evolution of cervical intraepithelial neoplasia, *Arch. Gynecol. Obstet.*, 252, 11, 1992.

174. Koutsky, L. A., Holmes, K. K., Critchlow, C. W., Stevens, C. E., Paavonen, J., Beckmann, A. M., DeRouen, T. A., Galloway, D. A., Vernon, D., Kiviat, N., A cohort study of the risk of cervical intraepithelial neoplasia grade 2 or 3 in relation to papillomavirus infection, *N. Eng. J. Med.*, 327, 1272, 1992.

175. Schneider, A., Kirchhoff, T., Meinhardt, G., Gissmann, L., Repeated evaluation of human papillomavirus 16 status in cervical swabs of young women with a history of normal Papanicolaou smears, *Obstet. Gynecol.*, 79, 683, 1992.

176. Rosenfeld, W. D., Rose, E., Vermund, S. H., Schreiber, K., Burk, R. D., Follow-up evaluation of cervicovaginal human papillomavirus infection in adolescents, *J. Pediat.*, 121, 307, 1992.

177. Wilson, R. W., Chenggis, M. L., Unger, E. R., Longitudinal study of human papillomavirus infection of the female urogenital tract by in situ hybridization, *Arch. Lab. Med.*, 114, 155, 1990.

178. Konno, R., Sato, S., Yajima, A., Progression of squamous cell carcinoma of the uterine cervix from cervical intraepithelial neoplasia infected with human papillomavirus: A retrospective follow-up study by *in situ* hybridization and polymerase chain reaction, *Int. J. Gynecol. Pathol.*, 11, 105, 1992.

179. Nuovo, G. J., Moritz, J., Walsh, L. L., MacConnell, P., Koulos, J., Predictive value of human papillomavirus DNA detection by filter hybridization and polymerase chain reaction in women with negative results of colposcopic examination, *Am. J. Clin. Pathol.*, 98, 489, 1992.

180. Caussy, D., Marrett, L. D., Worth, A. J., McBride, M., Rawls, W. E., Human papillomavirus and cervical intraepithelial neoplasia in women who subsequently had invasive cancer, *Can. Med. Assoc. J.*, 142, 311, 1990.

181. Wilbur, D. C., Bonfiglio, T. A., Stoler, M. H., Continuity of human papillomavirus (HPV) type between neoplastic precursors and invasive cervical carcinoma, *Am. J. Surg. Pathol.*, 12, 182, 1988.

182. Syrjänen, K., The long-term consequences of genital HPV infections in Women, Editorial, *Ann. Med.*, 24, 233, 1992.

183. Syrjänen, K., Nurmi, T., Mäntyjärvi, R., Ilonen, J., Syrjänen, S., Surcel, H.-M., Yliskoski, M., Väyrynen, M., Saarikoski, S., HLA types in women with human papillomavirus (HPV)-associated cervical precancer lesions with established natural history, *Cytopathology*, 7, 99, 1996.

184. Narod, S. A., Thompson, D. W., Jain, M., Wall, C., Green, L. M., Miller, A. B., Dysplasia and the natural history of cervical cancer: Early results of the Toronto cohort study, *Eur. J. Cancer*, 27, 1411, 1991.

185. Brinton, L. A., Current epidemiological studies-Emerging hypotheses, *Banbury Report*, 21, 17, 1986.

186. Doll, R., Implications of epidemiological evidence for future progress, *Banbury Report*, 21, 321, 1986.

187. Vessey, M. P., Epidemiology of cervical cancer: Role of hormonal factors, cigarette smoking and occupation, *Banbury Report*, 21, 29, 1986.

188. Fuju, C., Syrjänen, S., Shen, Q., Ji, H., Syrjänen, K., Detection of Human papillomavirus (HPV) in genital warts and carcinomas by DNA in situ hybridization in Chinese patients, *Cytopathology*, 1, 97, 1990.

189. Singer, A., Reid, B. L., Coppleson, M., A hypothesis. The role of a high-risk male in the etiology of cervical carcinoma, *Am. J. Obstet. Gynecol.*, 126, 110, 1976.

190. Syrjänen, K., Väyrynen, M., Castren, O., Yliskoski, M., Mäntyjärvi, R., Pyrhönen, S., Saarikoski, S., Sexual behaviour of the females with Human papillomavirus (HPV) lesions in the uterine cervix, *Br. J. Ven. Dis.*, 60, 243, 1984.

191. Waterhouse, J., Muir, C., Correa, P., Powell, J., *Cancer in Five Continents, Volume 4*, International Agency for Research on Cancer, Lyon, 1982, 123–34.

192. Maiche, A. G., Epidemiological aspects of cancer of the penis in Finland, *Eur. J. Cancer Prev.*, 1, 153, 1992.

193. Li, J. Y., Li, F. P., Blot, W. J., Miller, R. W., Fraumeni, J. F., Jr., Correlation between cancers of the uterine cervix and penis in Caina, *J. Nat. Cancer Instit.*, 69, 1063, 1982.

194. Narayana, A. S., Olney, L. E., Loening, S. A., Weimar, G. W., Culp, D. A., Carcioma of the penis, *Cancer*, 49, 2185, 1982.

195. Berg, J. W., Lampe, J. G., High-risk factors in gynecologic cancer, *Cancer*, 48, 429, 1981.

196. Boon, M., Susanti, I., Tasche, M. J. A., Kok, L. P., Human papillomavirus (HPV)-associated male and female genital carcinomas in a Hindu population. The male as vector and victim, *Cancer*, 64, 559, 1989.

197. Brinton, L. A., Jun-Yao, L., Shou-De, R., Huang, S., Sheng, X. B., Bal-Gao, S., Zhe-Jun, Z., Schiffman, M. H., Dawsey, S., Risk factors for penile cancer: Results from a case-control study in China, *Int. J. Cancer*, 47, 504, 1991.

198. Brinton, L. A., Reeves, W. C., Brenes, M. M., Herrero, R., Gaitan, E., Tenorio, F., The male factor in the etiology of cervical cancer among sexually monogamous women, *Int. J. Cancer*, 44, 199, 1989.

199. Joffe, G. P., Foxman, B., Schmidt, A. J., Farris, K. B., Carter, R. J., Neumann, S., Tolo, K.-A., Walters, A. M., Multiple partners and partner choice as risk factors for sexually transmitted disease among female college students, *Sex. Trans. Dis.*, 19, 272, 1992.

200. Cocks, P. S., Adib, R. S., Hunt, K. M., Concurrent carcinoma of penis and carcinoma-in situ of the cervix in a married couple. Case report, *Br. J. Obstet. Gynecol.*, 89, 408, 1982.

201. Maiche, A. G., Pyrhönen, S., Risk of cervical cancer among wives of men with carcinoma of the penis, *Acta Oncol.*, 29, 569, 1990.

202. Schneider, A., Sawada, E., Gissmann, L., Shah, K., Human papillomaviruses in women with a history of abnormal papanicolaou smears and in their male partners, *Obstetr. Gynecol.*, 69, 554, 1987.

10

HPV-Related Squamous Cell Tumors of the Airways and Esophagus: Epidemiology and Malignant Potential

Stina Syrjänen

CONTENTS

I. INTRODUCTION

Tumors of the squamous cell origin are the most common neoplasms of the oral cavity and upper respiratory tract. Controversy exists as to whether all of them are true neoplasms or if some of them rather represent hyperplasias reactive to tissue injury. The broad and loosely defined category of squamous cell papillomas refers to the low power and/or gross architecture and does not necessarily imply a neoplastic origin. These lesions are important not only for the diagnostic problems they represent, but also because papillomas of the sino-nasal tract and larynx

0-8493-7356-5/97/$0.00+$.50
© 1997 by CRC Press, Inc.

are therapeutically quite refractory. Furthermore, clinical data implicate that squamous cell papillomas in those areas may progress to malignancy.

Squamous cell carcinoma originating from the mucous membranes of the upper aerodigestive tract is by far the most frequent tumor occurring primarily in the head and neck. In the Western world, the incidence of head and neck squamous cell carcinoma is generally low, accounting for approximately 5% of the new cancer cases. The larynx, oral cavity, and pharynx are most commonly involved. It is likely that the pathogenesis of head and neck cancer is multifactoral. Both tobacco and alcohol are important risk factors, although they cannot solely explain carcinomas of this region. The association of squamous cell carcinoma of the cervix and HPV is well established. HPV has been detected in aerodigestive tract carcinomas as well as in the normal mucosa. The tumors seem to have revealed an HPV predilection for specific sites. In the future, the main important task is to find out what proportion of the tumors have an HPV etiology.

This chapter discusses both the benign and malignant lesions of the aerodigestive tract, and which evidence is available for a human papillomavirus (HPV) etiology or involvement.

II.   SINO-NASAL PAPILLOMAS AND CARCINOMAS

Papillomas of the sino-nasal cavity occur in two predominant patterns with distinct clinical and histological features.[1] Fungiform or exophytic papillomas arise from the nasal septum, are rarely recurrent, and have little propensity for malignant transformation. Inverted papillomas, on the other hand, usually develop on the lateral nasal wall either as isolated or multifocal lesions and spread from the nose to the paranasal sinuses. They have a tendency for both clinical recurrence and progression to malignancy. Several synonyms have been used for inverted sino-nasal papillomas, including Schneiderian, transitional cell, cylindrical and Ewing's papillomas.[1] In a proportion of cases, nasal squamous cell carcinoma and inverted papilloma occur in the same patient, either simultaneously at initial presentation or as a subsequent development.

Although the pathobiology of sinonasal papillomas still remains unclear, recent evidence suggests an HPV involvement. HPV etiology was first suggested by Syrjänen et al. (1983), while describing morphological similarities to exophytic genital condylomas and showing expression of HPV structural antigens in such lesions.[2] To date, HPV 6, 11, 16, 18 and 57b have been identified in inverted papillomas and HPV 6, 11, and 57b in squamous cell papillomas. Reported prevalence rates of HPV types 6 and 11 in inverted papillomas vary from 0 to 86%. HPV 6, 16, and 18 have been detected in sporadic cases of squamous cell carcinomas arising from inverted papillomas. Table 1 summarizes the evidence on HPV involvement (i.e., detection of HPV DNA) in sino-nasal papillomas and carcinomas collected from the available literature.[3-19] Future studies are needed on the natural history of HPV-associated nasal lesions as well as the mode of HPV transmission and prevention of the infections.

III.   BRONCHIAL PAPILLOMAS AND CARCINOMAS

Papillary lesions of the bronchus comprise a group of tumors with different degrees of malignancy ranging from benign squamous cell papillomas to exophytic squamous cell carcinomas. Solitary squamous cell papillomas are extremely rare and largely found in adults, in contrast to squamous papillomatosis encountered in children. It was estimated that approximately 50% of the solitary adult papillomas eventually become malignant.[20]

Following the recognition that koilocytotic (or condylomatous) change in the squamous epithelium of the genital tract was induced by HPV infection, Syrjänen first started screening the possible HPV-induced changes in the bronchial mucosa.[21] He described changes consistent with a papillary, inverted, and flat condyloma in the adjacent bronchial mucosa of 25% of squamous cell carcinomas.[22] Stremlau et al. first reported HPV 16 DNA in an anaplastic lung carcinoma from a patient who had a cervical carcinoma 9 years previously.[23]

TABLE 1 Detection of HPV DNA in Sino-Nasal Papillomas and Carcinomas

Author	Year	Type of lesion	Number of cases	HPV 6	HPV 6/11	HPV 11	HPV 16	HPV 16/18	HPV 18	HPV positivity total (%)	Technique
Syrjänen	1987	IP	14			7	1			50	IS
	1987	SSC	3				3			100	IS
Respler	1987	IP	2			2				100	SB
Bradsma	1988	IP	2				1			50	SB
Weber	1988	IP	21			11				52	IS
Brandwein	1989	IP	7		3			1		57	IS
Ishibashi	1990	IP	7	1						14	SB
Furuta	1991	IP	26			3				12	DB, IS
		SSC	2				1			50	PCR
Judd	1991	SSC	8	1						12	PCR
		IP	12							0	PCR
		P	7			3				43	PCR
Fu	1992	IP	9		8					89	IS
McLachlin	1992	IP	15		6					40	IS
		P	5		3					60	PCR
Kashima	1992	IP	29	2		5				24	PCR
		P	26	3		1				15	PCR
		SSC	24						1	4	PCR
Furuta	1992	SSC	49				6		1	14	PCR
Ogura	1992	IP	3							0	DB, SB
		SP	2		1					50	DB, SB
Sarkar	1992	SCC, P	35				1			3	IS, PCR
Wu	1993	P, SCC	22 x						57b	86	IS, PCR
Tang	1994	WP, SCC	30		6					20	IS

Note: IP, inverted papilloma; SSC, squamous cell papilloma; P, squamous cell carcinoma; DB, dot blot hybridization; IS, *in situ* hybridization; PCR, polymerase chain reaction; SB, southern blot hybridization; x) 19 cases were HPV 57b positive.

In the subsequent studies, Syrjänen et al.[24] showed HPV DNA in 5 of 99 bronchial squamous cell carcinomas by *in situ* hybridization technique using a mixed probe of HPV types 6, 11, 16, 18, and 30. When subjected to type-specific *in situ* hybridization, HPV types 6, 11, and 16 DNA was disclosed in 9 of 113 lesions.[25] Studies of Bejui-Thivolet et al.[26,27] as well as of Yousem et al.[28] expanded these observations. Two cases of squamous cell carcinomas developing after a long history of laryngotracheal papillomatosis have also been reported. In one case, PV antigen was detected[29] and in the other, the presence of HPV 11 DNA.[30]

Recently, DiLorenzo et al. detected transcriptionally active HPV 6a DNA in a lung carcinoma of a patient with recurrent laryngeal papillomatosis.[31] Carcinoma cells contained episomal HPV 6a genome with a duplication of the upstream regulatory region (URR), the late region, and a portion of the early region. Interestingly, HPV 6a genome found in the benign laryngeal papilloma of the same patient did not contain this duplication.[31] Popper and co-workers analyzed 31 solitary bronchial squamous cell papillomas with variable degrees of dysplasia, one combined with larynx papilloma and small cell carcinoma in the contralateral lung, and 12 papillomas combined with invasive squamous cell carcinoma. Benign papillomas showed an association with HPV type 11 and rarely with type 6, whereas type 16 or 18, sometimes in combination with type 31/33/35, was found in papillomas associated with carcinoma.[32] Recently, HPV DNA was detected using consensus primer PCR in 2 squamous cell carcinomas and importantly, only in tumor but not normal lung tissue.[33] The detection rates of HPV DNA in bronchial papillomas and carcinomas are summarized in Table 2.[23-36]

In essence, all these studies based on either Southern blot hybridization, *in situ* hybridization or PCR methods indicate that HPV is unlikely to play a role in most lung cancers. Nevertheless, the data suggest that HPV may be important in a small subset of SCC.

IV. LARYNGEAL PAPILLOMAS/CARCINOMAS

The search for the cause of laryngeal papilloma started with Ullman who in 1923 reported on a successful transfer of an agent from human laryngeal papillomas to the vagina of a dog and to his own arm.[37] Some 50 years later, Boyle et al. identified Papova viral particles on electron microscopy.[38] Since 1981, the involvement of HPV infection, mostly types 6 and/or 11 (from 67 up to 97%), in both juvenile and adult papillomas is well established as summarized in Table 3.[39-72] Quite recently, Rihkanen et al. analyzed laryngeal papillomas and the surrounding normal appearing mucosa of the larynx for the presence of HPV by *in situ* hybridization and PCR.[73] All except one papilloma contained HPV DNA; 9 were HPV 6/11 positive and 1 positive for HPV 16. The normal appearing mucosa harbored HPV DNA in 8 of 11 cases. The authors suggest that the persistence of HPV DNA in the adjacent normal epithelium is consistent with the frequent recurrence of these lesions.[73]

The epidemiology of the laryngeal papillomas is still not completely understood. A relationship between juvenile-onset papillomas and maternal genital HPV infections has been proposed. It is unknown whether adult-onset laryngeal papilloma is acquired at birth or later in life by autoinoculation or orogenital sexual contact.[74,75]

Although the majority of laryngeal papillomas are entirely benign, several reports are available on invasive laryngeal papillomas and occurrence of dysplastic changes up to 20–40% of the cases as well as malignant transformation of the previously benign laryngeal papillomas. Laryngeal papillomas can also prove fatal by extending into the lower respiratory tract.[50,53,74] Malignant changes are likely to occur in severe papillomatosis of long duration with signs of spread throughout the respiratory tract. Despite this clear association of previous laryngeal papillomas to subsequent carcinomas, HPV sequences are relatively rarely found in laryngeal carcinomas and the results from different series are controversial. Table 3 summarizes the studies available on the detection of HPV DNA in laryngeal lesions.

Syrjänen et al., in 1982, demonstrated HPV capsid antigen in 36% of laryngeal carcinomas.[76] This antigen was also detected in 14 out of 20 patients with carcinoma *in situ*.[77] Using *in situ*

TABLE 2 Detection of HPV DNA In Broncial Papillomas and Carcinomas

Author	Year	Type of lesion	Number of cases	HPV DNA 6	HPV 6/11	HPV 11	HPV 16	HPV 16/18	HPV 18	HPV positivity total (%)	Technique
Stremlau	1985	SSC	9							0	SB
		LSSC	7							0	SB
		ASCC	2							0	SB
		AnSCC	5							20	SB
Bryne	1987	SCC	1			1				100	SB
Syrjänen	1987	SCC	99							5	IS
Syrjänen	1989	SCC	131	2				5		7	IS
Kerley	1989	P	1			1				100	IS
Carey	1990	P	15				1			7	IS
Bejui-Thivolet	1990	M	10	1						10	IS
		SCC	33	1		1	1		3	18	IS
	1990	SCC	1			1				100	IS
Popper	1992	P	6		6					100	IS
		SSC	5						5[a,b]	100	IS
DiLorenzo	1992	SSC	1	1						100	IS
Yousem	1992	M	17		1			1		12	IS
		SCC	20		1			2		15	IS
		AdSSC	12							0	IS
		ASSC	16							0	IS
		SSSC	4							0	IS
		LSSC	6		1					17	IS
		P	2		2					100	IS
Popper	1994	P	20	3		6			2	55	PCR
		SSC	11						1	9	PCR

Note: AdSSC; adenocarcinoma; ASSC, alveolar carcinoma; AnSCC, anaplastic carcinoma; SSCC, small cell carcinoma; LSSC, large cell carcinoma; SSC, squamous cell carcinoma; P, squamous cell papilloma; M, squamous cell metaplasia; DB, Dot Blot hybridization; IS, in situ hybridization; PCR, polymerase chain reaction; SB, southern blot hybridization; [a] Three additional cases with HPV 31/33/35; [b] Two additional cases with HPV 31/33/35.

TABLE 3 Detection of HPV DNA in Laryngal Papillomas and Carcinomas

Author	Year	Type of lesion	Number of cases	HPV 6	HPV 6/11	HPV 11	HPV 16	HPV 16/18	HPV 18	HPV positivity total (%)	Technique
Lancaster	1981	JP	5	x)						100	SB
Abramson	1985	VCA	5				5			100	SB
Scheurlen	1986	SCC	36				1			3	SB
Brandsma	1986	VCA	6				3			50	SB, DB
Syrjänen	1987	SCC	116	5[a]		9	6			13	IS
Terry	1987	JP	10	10[b]		9				100	IS
Zarod	1988	SCC	1	1						100	SB
Corbitt	1988	JP	8	4		3				87	SB
	1988	AP	6	6						100	SB
Brandsma	1989	SCC	60			3	3			10	SB
		CO	53			2				4	SB
Levi	1989	JP	19	13		3				84	PCR
Ward	1989	JP, SCC	4	4						100	SB
Lindberg	1989	JP, SCC	2			2				100	IS
		AP, SCC	2							0	IS
Tsutsumi	1989	AP	20			8				40	IS
Quiney	1989	AP	31	19[b]		17				61	IS
		JP	14	7[b]		8				57	IS
Ishibashi	1990	SCC	3							0	SB
Bryan	1990	JP	6	2		3				83	PCR
Lindeberg	1990	AP	20		19					95	IS
Hsiao	1990	AP	2							0	SB
		JP	5	5						100	SB
Hoshikawa	1990	SSC	34	1			7			21	PCR
Perez-Ayala	1990	SSC	48				26			54	PCR
Dickens	1990	JP	6			5				83	DB
		AP	21	3		10	3			72	DB

Author	Year	Type	n					%	Method
Ocura	1991	SCC	28				3	11	PCR
Morgan	1991	SCC	10	1			4	50	PCR
McGullough	1991	SCC	1				1	100	SB
Rimell	1992	AP	11	11				100	IS
		JP	9	9				100	IS
Arndt	1992	SCC	27		12			14	IS
Answar	1993	SSC	43				3	40	PCR, DB
Arndt	1993	SSC	100	1	5		15	32	PCR, SB
Doyle	1994	IP, SSA	1	1			1	100	PCR, SB
Clayman	1994	SSC	65					46	PCR
Gale	1994	IP		25					
		AP		36				77	
Hartley	1994	AP	28	11			6	61	
Grogoulu	1994	SSC	40			2	9	28	PCR, DB
Fouret	1995	DSP	57					10	PCR, DB

Note: SSC, squamous cell carcinoma; AP, adult squamous cell papilloma; CO, normal tissue; JP, juvenile squamous cell papilloma; DB, dot blot hybridization; IS, *in situ* hybridization; PCR, polymerase chain reaction; SB, southern blot hybridization; VCA, verrucous carcinoma; *5 cases with double infections; ᵇdouble infections. x) 5 positive samples, typing not possible.

hybridization, Syrjänen et al.[43] found HPV DNA in 15 out of 116 laryngeal carcinomas (13%). HPV 11 was the single most frequent type followed by HPV 16 (5.2%). Abramson et al.[46] described HPV 16 DNA in five patients with verrucous carcinoma but in none of the four cases of squamous cell carcinomas. The role of HPV in laryngeal malignancy has also been doubted by Scheurlen et al.[41] and Ostrow et al.[78] Although HPV 30 was isolated from a laryngeal carcinoma, subsequent studies failed to demonstrate this HPV type in any of the laryngeal carcinomas.[79]

The recent utilization of PCR techniques has resulted in an increased detection of HPV infection in laryngeal carcinomas. With this method, the rate of detection of HPV infection in laryngeal cancer has varied from 11 to 75%.[57,60,61,80] Recently, Snijders and co-workers analyzed the presence of HPV in 185 biopsy samples of squamous cell carcinoma of digestive and respiratory tracts. HPV DNA was found in 18% of laryngeal carcinomas. However, the copy number of HPV was very low suggesting a nonclonal HPV association with these carcinomas.[81]

Of significance are the recent studies where HPV DNA was detected in entirely normal tissues of the larynx. Bryan et al. analyzed 14 biopsies from normal nasopharyngeal mucosa and 9 cases proved to be either HPV 6- or HPV 11-positive.[54] Similarly, Brandsma and Abramson detected HPV DNA in 2 biopsies out of 51 normal laryngeal tissues analyzed.[47] Rihkanen and co-workers found HPV DNA in 8 biopsy samples among the analyzed 41 normal tissues.[82] Nunes and co-workers have determined the prevalence of HPV in normal larynges obtained by autopsy. HPV type 11 was detected in three specimens out of 12 samples analyzed with PCR.[83]

These contradictory results clearly indicate that the mere presence of HPV DNA in malignant or other tissue is insufficient to infer a causative involvement of HPV. It might be that HPV may merely increase the target cell population that runs the risk of undergoing malignant transformation.

V.   HPV INFECTIONS IN ORAL MUCOSA

Different types of HPV have been demonstrated in a variety of benign oral lesions, including squamous cell papilloma/condyloma, verruca vulgaris, focal epithelial hyperplasia, papillary hyperplasia, fibrous hyperplasia, lichen planus, and leukoplakia.[84-87] Among the known HPV types, HPV 1, 2, 4, 6, 7, 11, 13, 16, 18, 32, and 57 have been found in different types of oral lesions. Of these, HPV 13 and HPV 32 seem to be exclusively confined to a specific oral lesion known as focal epithelial hyperplasia. Recently, the possible etiological role of HPV infection in the pathogenesis of oral precancer lesions and cancer has been suggested by the discovery of HPV-suggestive lesions in oral cancer specimens as well as by DNA-hybridization studies disclosing HPV 11, 16, and 18 DNA in oral precancer lesions and squamous cell cancer.[88-90] However, since it is now clear that HPV DNA is harbored by normal oral mucosa as well as in premalignant and malignant lesions, such an association may not necessarily implicate a causal relationship.

A.   Normal Mucosa

The examination of apparently healthy oral mucosa from normal adults by DNA hybridization confirmed the existence of latent HPV infections in the oral cavity, too. Using Southern blot hybridization, HPV 16-related virus could be detected in more than 40% of biopsies from normal oral mucosa.[91,92] Recently, Kellokoski et al. found HPV DNA in 2.6% of cytological scrapings taken from 334 women with past or present genital HPV infection using a dot blot hybridization. By clinical inspection, only three tiny exophytic growths similar to condyloma were diagnosed in these patients.[93,94] By Southern blot hybridization, 15% of the biopsies taken from clinically normal buccal mucosa contained HPV DNA. The PCR technique increased the positivity of HPV DNA in these biopsies to 21.8%. Only one subject had the same HPV type both in genitalia and oral mucosa.[95] Recently, Buchwald and co-workers analyzed the presence of HPV DNA in 61 oral smears and 48 nasal smears. HPV was not found in the oral mucosa, while a single individual harbored HPV in nasal mucosa.[96] The presence of HPV DNA in the oral mucosal smears of postmenopausal women have also been analyzed. None of the 100 samples were HPV DNA positive with consensus primer PCR.[97]

B.   Papilloma and Condyloma Acuminatum

Oral squamous cell papilloma is a benign tumor, which can occur at any age.[85,87] In the early 1980s, HPV etiology of oral papillomas was suggested by demonstration of HPV particles and HPV antigens.[98,99] Only in the past few years, DNA hybridization studies have revealed HPV DNA sequences in 35 to 100% of oral papillomas with mainly of HPV 6 and HPV 11.[100-103]

Occasional case reports on oral condyloma acuminatum have been published as well.[101,104,105] Originally, oral condyloma was regarded as a lesion transmitted via oral sex.[106] However, its differentiation from the squamous cell papilloma is difficult or impossible and largely academic.

C.   Common Wart

Common wart or verruca vulgaris is one of the most common skin lesions, especially in children. Occasional case reports have been published on common warts in the oral cavity. Oral verruca vulgaris is clearly HPV-related mainly with HPV 2 and HPV 4.[98,99,107] In HIV infected subjects, oral warts have been shown to contain HPV 7 which is usually found in butchers' warts.[108,109] Recently, a novel type HPV 57 was identified in an oral wart.[110] Because of the discrepancy in the nomenclature and histological criteria of papilloma, condyloma, and verruca vulgaris, the interpretation of the different studies is difficult.

D.   Focal Epithelial Hyperplasia

Focal epithelial hyperplasia (FEH) or Heck's disease is a benign lesion of the oral mucosa characterized by multiple (or solitary) painless, soft papules. Following the isolation and characterization of two new HPV types, designated as HPV 13[111] and HPV 32,[112] from FEH lesions, it soon became apparent that FEH is a manifestation of HPV infection in the oral cavity in individuals with a genetic predisposition, like epidermodysplasia verruciformis lesions of the skin. More than 90% of the biopsies derived from FEH have been demonstrated to contain either HPV 13 or 32 DNA.[89,113,114] Notably, these two HPV types have only been occasionally detected in other oral lesions, but never outside the oral cavity, strongly indicating that these two types of HPV are pathognomonic to FEH. The positive signals obtained by hybridization with HPV 6, 11, and 16 are most probably due to the close relatedness of these HPV types to HPV 13. Recently, HPV 13 DNA was detected in a clinically and histologically typical oral condyloma (Syrjänen unpublished data).

E.   Lichen Planus

Lichen planus is one of the most common epithelial diseases affecting oral mucosa. The possible viral etiology is proposed by the recent demonstration of HPV in a high percentage of oral lichen planus. Using immunoperoxidase technique, HPV structural proteins have been shown in these lesions.[115] With the DNA hybridization methods, HPV 11, 16, and 16-related types have been found.[74,85] By the PCR technique, 65% of erosive oral lichen planus samples contained 6, 11, or 16 DNA.[116] However, Kashima et al. could not demonstrate HPV 6, 11, 16, 18, or 31 DNA in their HPV antigen-positive oral lesions suggesting that another HPV type was involved in these lesions.[115] In spite of the preliminary evidence on HPV involvement in lichen planus, the etiological role of this virus remains to be established.

F.   Oral Leukoplakia

Oral leukoplakia is a whitish lesion histologically showing a variety of epithelial changes ranging from harmless epithelial hyperplasia to various degrees of dysplasia. HPV antigens and DNA have been demonstrated in oral leukoplakia lesions.[115,117,118] According to these reports HPV 6, 11, and 16 sequences could be detected in some cases of the leukoplakias studied. On the basis of the present knowledge, however, the role of HPV in the etiology of oral leukoplakia is not clear as yet.

G.   Precancer Lesions and Cancer

The possibility of HPV in the etiology of oral cancer was first appreciated in 1983 by Syrjänen et al.[88] Of the 40 oral carcinoma specimens, 16 (40%) cases showed HPV-suggestive lesions. When these samples were subjected to immunohistochemical staining, 8/16 showed positive reactivity for HPV structural proteins, the positive staining being confined to the epithelium adjacent to the invasive carcinomas. The same series of biopsies was later analyzed for the presence of HPV DNA by ISH-and PCR techniques; 12/40 (30%) disclosed HPV 11, 16, or 18 DNA sequences.[119] In another series, Syrjänen and co-workers found HPV 6, 11, 16, and 18 DNA in 6 of 51 oral carcinomas and 6 of 21 epithelial dysplasias.[120] Similarly, Löning and co-authors reported HPV 11 and 16 DNA in 3 of 6 oral carcinomas.[100] de Villiers et al. detected HPV 2 in one and HPV 16 in two of their seven tongue carcinomas. Interestingly, the HPV 2 differed from the established HPV 2 prototype.[121] Furthermore, the HPV 16 in one carcinoma differed somewhat from the HPV 16 prototype and it is likely that this is the same type as the HPV 16-related virus identified in 46% of carcinomas of the tongue/floor of mouth in a recent report.[86] Accordingly, HPV 16 seems to be the most frequent type associated with oral carcinomas. This was also confirmed by the recent studies of Chang et al.[119] who found HPV 16 DNA in 76.4% of their 17 oral squamous cell carcinomas. HPV 16 has also been reported in the lymph node metastasis from a lingual carcinoma.[78] In a recent case of an immunosuppressed adult male, HPV-associated bowenoid papulosis developed on his genitals, accompanied by skin warts, oral papules, and lingual carcinoma.[122] The genital lesion was HPV 16 associated; HPV 11 was found in the skin lesions, while both HPV 11 and HPV 16 were found in the oral carcinoma. An additional case of bowenoid papulosis of the oral cavity has recently been described.[123] The most important evidence against HPV as the sole etiological agent in oral carcinoma is, however, the demonstration of HPV DNA in a range of benign oral lesions, and in normal mucosa.[90,91] Recent studies on head and neck tumors have revealed an HPV predilection for specific sites.[81] Recently Snijders and co-workers analyzed 221 squamous cell carcinoma of the aerodigestive tract. After applying HPV GP5+/6+ general primer mediated PCR assay, 32% of the samples scored positive. The HPV prevalence rate ranged from about 70% in tonsillar SSC down to 10% in hypopharyngeal SCC. Approximately 60% of the oral cancer proved to be HPV positive. HPV 16 was by far the most predominant type for all sites. In addition, HPV 6, 7, 33, 35, and 59 were detected infrequently. It has been shown that the HPV prevalence rate is higher in oral cancer patients younger than 60 years.[124,125] Oral carcinomas as others in aerodigestive tract appear to have low copy numbers of HPV. In addition, *in situ* hybridization studies have shown that HPV DNA positivity is focal indicating a nonclonal association of the tumor with HPV.

H.   Verrucous Carcinoma

Verrucous carcinoma of the oral cavity is a distinct variant of well-differentiated squamous cell carcinoma. The development of this entity has been linked with heavy use of tobacco products and betel chewing. The viral etiology of verrucous carcinomas at other body sites (e.g., larynx and anogenital area) has been suspected for a long time. Morphological features showing papillomatosis, dyskeratosis, and koilocytosis suggest an HPV etiology. This hypothesis was further supported by the demonstration of HPV DNA in these lesions.[126] Adler-Storthz et al. examined 9 oral verrucous carcinomas and found 3 positive for HPV 2. More cases must be analyzed, however, before final conclusions can be made.

VI. ESOPHAGUS

Squamous cell papilloma of the esophagus is a rare lesion that is being appreciated with increasing frequency, however. Since the first report by Adler in 1959,[127] more than 60 cases have been reported worldwide. In 1968, Weitzner and Hentel estimated the incidence of true papillomas of the esophagus as being between 0.01 and 0.04% in their review of autopsy studies.[128] The etiology of esophageal papillomas was regarded as unknown until the early 1980s, when the first evidence on the possible HPV involvement in the development of this tumor was reported.[129] First, HPV antigens were disclosed in such a lesion by immunohistochemistry. This was subsequently confirmed by other groups.[130] Furthermore, HPV DNA has been convincingly demonstrated in several squamous cell papillomas.[131] Cutsem et al.[132] described a squamous cell papilloma of the esophagus with malignant degeneration in which the presence of HPV was demonstrated by immunohistochemistry and transmission electron microscopy.[114] They were unable, however, to detect HPV DNA with *in situ* hybridization. More recently, Chang et al. analyzed 12 esophageal papillomas for the presence of HPV by *in situ* hybridization and PCR, but no viral DNA was detected.[133] These contradictory results suggest that esophageal papillomas might harbor still unidentified HPV types.

The development of malignancy from a pre-existing squamous cell papilloma is well known in bronchial and laryngeal mucosa. There are also reports in which esophageal carcinomas were antedated by esophageal papillomas.[134,135] HPV genome has been detected in three cases of esophageal carcinoma in Australian patients by Kulski et al. using filter *in situ* hybridization with a probe mixture containing HPV types 11, 13, 16, and 18.[136] By contrast, Kiyabu et al. were unable to detect HPV 16 or 18 invasive carcinoma of the esophagus in North American patients using PCR.[137] Similarly, Loke et al. could not detect any HPV DNA in 37 esophageal carcinoma in Hong Kong by *in situ* or dot blot hybridization.[138] Recently, Williamson et al., 1991, detected HPV DNA in 10/14 (71%) of esophageal carcinomas by PCR.[139] Benamouzig et al. described HPV infection in 5 out of 12 esophageal carcinoma.[140]

Quite recently, the systematic study on esophageal precancer and cancer lesions collected from the high-incidence area for esophageal carcinoma in China showed that HPV DNA was detectable in 43% of these lesions by *in situ* hybridization and in 72% by filter *in situ* hybridization,[141] Furthermore, PV-like particles located in the nuclei of koilocytotic cells were demonstrated in 2 of the 5 specimens previously shown to be HPV-positive by *in situ* hybridization.[141] Using PCR, 49.0% (25/51) of the esophageal cancer specimens were demonstrated to contain HPV DNA sequences.[142] In another series, Chang et al. detected HPV DNA in 9 out of 20 esophageal carcinomas by Southern blot hybridization under low stringency conditions. Of these, 8 samples presented positive hybridization with the probe cocktail of HPV types 11, 16, and 18 under high stringency conditions as well. HPV DNA sequences in these carcinomas appear to be present mainly as an integrated form.[142] These results support the concept of HPV as a possible etiologic agent in esophageal carcinogenesis. However, the controversial results in the detection rate of HPV in esophageal carcinomas suggest geographic variations in HPV infections. So far, esophageal HPV infections in control population remains incompletely studied.

VII. NONSEXUAL TRANSMISSION OF HPV

Classically, HPV infections have been regarded as a sexually transmitted disease. Current evidence implies, however, that other modes of transmission have to be considered. These include autoinoculation, perinatal infection, infection in utero, casual social contact, and sexual abuse. Several studies have indicated that nonsexual transmission of high risk HPVs is possible. HPV DNA has been detected in nine vulval samples out of 61 women who had no history of sexual intercourse.[143] Similarly HPV DNA was detected in five and three vulval scrapings taken from 24 and 15 asymptomatic virgins, respectively.[144,145] Some recent studies have also shown a low concordance of genital HPV infections between heterosexual partners. Hippeläinen et al. reported that HPV DNA was more frequently detected in the male partners of woman with HPV 6 or 11 (62% and

50%) than with other types (range 18–33%). Of the 270 couples typed by *in situ* hybridization, both partners were HPV positive in 66 (24%) cases but only 15 of these had identical HPV types in their genital tract.[146] These results were confirmed by a DNA sequencing study of Ho et al. who investigated the occurrence of HPV 16 genomic variants in 8 HPV 16 positive husband and wife couples. While four of these couples had identical HPV genomic variants, four had mismatched variants.[148]

In children, condylomata acuminata has been suggested as an indicator of sexual abuse.[148-150] However, recent studies indicate that there are at least two different modes of HPV infection in infants, namely sexual abuse and vertical transmission. In a study of four cases with childhood condylomas, only one had evidence of a sexual abuse.[151] In another study of 500 children, it was shown that sexual abuse does not explain the occurrence of all lesions. Children with genital warts not associated with sexual abuse were one year younger (the age ranges of one to six years) than those sexually abused.[152]

Several studies suggest that neonates can acquire HPV infection as they pass through an infected birth canal. Pakarian et al. showed that 50% of children born to HPV-infected mothers were positive at 24 h and 25% remained positive at six weeks.[153] Similarly Fredericks and co-workers showed that 54% of infants born to HPV 18 infected mothers were also HPV 18 positive.[154] Similar transmission rate was reported also by Sedlacek and co-workers.[155] Puranen et al. have studied the presence of HPV DNA in oral mucosa of 98 children born to mothers with genital HPV infection.[156] The mean age of the children was $4.0 + 2.8$ years. HPV DNA was found in 31 of the oral scrapings. At the time of the delivery, 5 mothers had genital HPV infection with the same virus type as found in her child. In the additional 11 mothers, genital HPV infection with the same virus type as in the child was diagnosed a few months before or after delivery. Mothers of 25 children shown to be negative for oral HPV were also HPV DNA negative at the time of delivery.[156]

Recently, perinatal vertical HPV transmission has been suspected, when it was found that caesarean section delivery was not effective in protecting children from the mother-fetus HPV transmission. Armbruster-Moraes and co-workers have analyzed amniotic fluid from 37 pregnant women with cervical HPV infection. HPV DNA was found in 24 of 37 samples by using consensus primer PCR.[157] Puranen and co-workers have studied vertical transmission of HPV in newborn babies. Nasopharyngeal aspirates were taken just after the birth and analyzed by PCR. HPV DNA was detected in 11 samples taken from 19 babies born by vaginal delivery to mothers with genital infection. Interestingly, 10 out of 28 samples taken from the children born by caesarean section were also positive. Identical sequences have been identified both in the mothers and their babies. These preliminary results indicate that transplacental infection is possible.[158] For review of non-sexual acquistion of human genital papillomaviruses see reference 159.

HPV infections of the aerodigestive tract have to be considered when analyzing the significance of serological response to HPV infection and its associations with cervical cancer. The possibility of acquiring high risk HPV infections at birth is of crucial importance when planning the vaccination programs.

VIII. CONCLUSIONS

As with anogenital HPV infections, current data suggest that HPV 6 and HPV 11 are the two most frequent HPV types associated with benign papillomatous lesions of the airways and HPV 16 and 18 are found in squamous cell carcinomas. In the aerodigestive tract, the presence of HPV DNA has been shown to be focal by *in situ* hybridization. Also the copy numbers in these cancers are low. This indicates a nonclonal association of the tumor with HPV. If this is shown to be true, HPV is not needed for the maintenance of the malignant state. A hit and run theory has been proposed several times. If this mechanism exists *in vivo*, HPV negative carcinomas might have developed from HPV containing precursors. Both the respiratory, oral, and esophageal mucosa is continuously exposed to high levels of a large number of environmental agents such as cigarette smoke, alcohol, occupational exposures, numerous pollutants, and various microorganisms. Whether these environmental agents act synergistically with HPV remains to be proved. Epidemiological follow-up studies are necessary to understand the role of HPV in pathogenesis of aerodigestive tract carcinomas. Furthermore, the prevalence, incidence, and natural history of HPV infections in aerodigestive tract should be known to recognize the HPV associated high risk lesions in this area.

REFERENCES

1. Batsakis JC. The pathology of head and neck tumors. Nasal cavity and paranasal sinuses. V. *Head Neck Surg.* 2:410, 1980.
2. Syrjänen KJ, Pyrhönen S, Syrjänen SM. Evidence suggesting human papillomavirus (HPV) etiology for the squamous cell papilloma of the paranasal sinus. *Arch. Geschwulstforsh.* 53:77, 1983.
3. Syrjänen S, Happonen R-P, Virolainen E, Siivonen L, Syrjänen K. Detection of human papillomavirus (HPV) structural antigens and DNA types in inverted papillomas and squamous cell carcinomas of the nasal cavities and paranasal sinuses. *Acta Otolaryngol. (Stockholm)* 104:334, 1987.
4. Respler DS, Jahn A, Pater A, Pater M. Isolation and charaterization of papillomavirus DNA from nasal inverting (Schneiderian) papillomas. *Ann. Otol. Rhinol. Laryngol.* 96:170, 1987.
5. Brandsma JL, Steinberg BM, Abramson AL, Winkler B. Presence of human papillomavirus type 16 related sequences in verrucous carcinoma of the larynx. *Cancer Res.* 46:2185–2188, 1986.
6. Weber SR, Shillitoe E, Robbins T, Luna M, Batsakis J, Donovan D, Adler-Storthz K. Prevalence of human papillomavirus in inverted nasal papillomas. *Arch. Otolaryngol. Head Neck Surg.* 114:23, 1988.
7. Brandwein M, Steinberg B, Thung S, Biller H, Dilorenzo T, Galli R. Human papillomavirus 6/11 and 16/18 in Schneiderian inverted papillomas. *Cancer* 63:1708, 1989.
8. Ishibashi T, Matsushima S, Tsunokawa Y, Nomura Y, Sugimura T, Terada M. Human papillomavirus DNA in squamous cell carcinoma of the upper aerodigestive tract. *Arch. Otolaryngol. Head Neck Surg.* 116:294, 1990.
9. Furuta Y, Shinohara T, Sano K, Nagashima K, Inoue K, Tananka K, Inuyama Y. Molecular pathologic study of human papillomavirus infection in inverted papilloma and squamous cell carcinoma of the nasal cavities and paranasal sinuses. *Laryngoscope* 101:79, 1991.
10. Judd R, Zaki SR, Coffield LM, Evatt BL. Human papillomavirus type 6 detected by the polymerase chain reaction in invasive sinonasal papillary squamous cell carcinoma. *Arch. Pathol. Lab. Med.* 115:1150, 1991.
11. Judd R, Zaki SR, Coffield LM, Evatt BL. Sinonasal papillomas and human papillomavirus. *Human Pathol.* 22:550, 1991.
12. Fu YS, Hoover L, Franklin M, Cheng L, Stoler M. Human papillomavirus identified by nucleic acid hybridization in concomitant nasal and genital papillomas. *Laryngoscope* 102:1014, 1992.
13. McLachlin CM, Kandell RA, Colgan TJ, Swanson DB; Witterick IJ, Ngan BY. Prevalence of human papillomavirus in sinonasal papillomas: A study using polymerase chain reaction and in situ hybridization. *Mod. Patol.* 5:406, 1992.
14. Kashima H, Kesssis T, Hruban RH, Wu TC, Zinreich J, Shah KV. Human papillomavirus in sinonasal papillomas and squamous cell carcinoma. *Laryngoscope* 102:973, 1992.
15. Furuta Y, Takasu T, Asai T, Shinohara T, Sawa H, Nagashima K, Inuyama Y. Detection of human papillomavirus DNA in carcinomas of the nasal cavities and paranasal sinuses by polymerase chain reaction. *Cancer* 69:353, 1992.
16. Oqura H, Kawakami T, Fujiwara T, Sakai A, Saito R, Watnabe S, Masuda Y, Yabe Y. Detection of human papillomavirus type 6f genome in nasal papillomatosis. *Acta Otolaryngol. (Stockholm)* 112:115, 1992.
17. Sarkar FH, Vischer DW, Kintanar EB, Zarbo RJ, Crissman JD. Sinonasal Schneiderian Papillomas: Human papillomavirus typing by polymerase chain reaction. *Mod. Patol.* 5:329–332, 1992.
18. Wu TC, Trujullo JM, Kashima HK, Mounths P. Association of human papillomavirus with nasal neoplasia. *Lancet* 341:522–524, 1993.
19. Tang AC, Grignon DJ, MacRae DL. The association of human papillomavirus with Schneiderian: A DNA in situ hybridization study. *J. Otolaryngol.* 23:292–297, 1994.
20. WHO. Histological typing of lung tumors 2nd edn. Geneva. *WHO* 21 1981.
21. Syrjänen KJ. Condylomatous changes in neoplastic broncial epithelium. Report of a case. *Respiration* 98:299, 1979.

22. Syrjänen KJ. Epithelial lesions suggestive of a condylomatous origin found closely associated with invasive broncial squamous cell carcinomas. *Respiration* 40:150, 1980.

23. Stremlau A, Gissman L, Ikenberg H, Stark M, Bannasch P, zur Hausen H. Human papillomavirus type 16 related DNA in an anaplastic carcinoma of the lung. *Cancer* 55:1737, 1985.

24. Syrjänen KJ, Syrjänen SM. Human papillomavirus DNA in broncial squamous cell carcinoma (letter). *Lancet* I:168, 1987.

25. Syrjänen KJ, Syrjänen SM, Kellokoski J, Kärjä J, Mäntyjärvi R. Human papillomavirus (HPV) type 6 and 16 DNA sequences in broncial squamous cell carcinomas demonstrated by in situ DNA hybridization. *Lung* 167:33, 1989.

26. Bejui-Thivolet F, Liagre N, Chignol MC, Chardonnet Y, Patricot LM. Detection of human papillomavirus DNA in squamous bronchial metaplasia and squamous cell carcinomas of the lung by in situ hybridization using biotinylated probes in paraffin-embedded specimens. *Hum. Pathol.* 21:111, 1990.

27. Bejui-Thivolet F, Chardonnet Y, Patricot LM. Human papillomavirus type 11 DNA in papillary squamous cell lung carcinoma. *Virchows Arch. Pathol. Anat. Histopathol.* 417:457, 1990.

28. Yousem SA, Ohori P, Sonmez-Alpan E. Occurence of human papillomavirus DNA in primary lung neoplasms. *Cancer* 69:693, 1992.

29. Helmut R, Strate RW. Squamous cell carcinoma of the lung in a nonirradiated, nonsmoking patient with juvenile laryngotracheal papillomatosis. *Am. J. Surg. Pathol.* 11:643, 1987.

30. Bryne JC, Tsao MS, Fraser RS, Howley PM. Human papillomavirus 11DNA in a patient with chronic laryngotracheobroncial papillomatosis and metastatic squamous cell carcinoma of the lung. *N. England J. Med.* 317:873, 1987.

31. DiLorenzo TP, Tamsen A, Abramson AL, Steinberg BM. Human papillomavirus type 6a DNA in the lung carcinoma of a patient with recurrent laryngeal papillomatosis is characterized by a partial dublication. *J. Gen. Virol.* 73:423, 1992.

32. Popper HH, El-Shabrawi Y, Wöckel W, Höfler G, Kenner L, Jüttner-Smolle FM, Pongratz MG. Prognostic importance of human papillomavirus typing in squamous cell papilloma of the bronchus: Comparison in situ hybridization and the polymerase chain reaction. *Human Pathol.* 25:1191-1197, 1994.

33. Fong KW, Schonrock J, Frazer IM, Zimmerman PV, Smith PJ. Human papillomavirus not found in squamous and large cell lung carcinomas by polymerase chain reaction. *Cancer* 73:2740, 1994.

34. Kerley SW, Buchon-Zalles C, Moran J, Fishback JL. Chronic cavitary respiratory papillomatosis. *Arch. Pathol. Lab. Med.* 113:1166, 1989.

35. Carey FA, Salter DM, Kerr KM, Lamb D. An investigation into the role of human papillomavirus in endobroncial papillary squamous tumors. *Resp. Med.* 84:445, 1990.

36. Popper HH, Wirnsberger G, Juttner-Smolle FM, Pongratz MG, Sommergutter M. The predictive value of human papilloma virus (HPV) typing in the prognosis of broncial squamous cell papillomas. *Histopathology* 21:323-330, 1992.

37. Ullman EV. On the etiology of the laryngeal papilloma. *Acta Otolaryngol. (Stockholm)* 5:317, 1923.

38. Boyle WF, Riggs JL, Oshiro LS, Lennette EH. Electron microscopic identification of papova virus in laryngeal papilloma. *Laryngoscope* 83:1102, 1973.

39. Lancaster WD, Jenson AB. Evidence for papillomavirus genus-specific antigens and DNA in laryngeal papilloma. *Intervirology* 15:204, 1981.

40. Abramson A, Brandsma J, Steinberg B, Winkler B. Verrucous carcinoma of the larynx. *Arch. Otolaryngol.* 111:709, 1985.

41. Scheurlen W, Stremlau A, Gissman L, Höhn D, Zenner H-P, zur Hausen. Rearranged HPV 16 molecules in an anal and in a laryngeal carcinoma. *Int. J. Cancer* 38:671, 1986.

42. Brandsma JL, Steinberg BM, Abramson AL, Winkler B. Presence of human papillomavirus type 16 related sequences in verrucous carcinoma of the larynx. *Cancer Res.* 46:2185, 1986.

43. Syrjänen S, Syrjänen K, Mäntyjärvi R, Collan Y, Kärjä J. Human papillomavirus DNA in squamous cell carcinomas of the larynx demonstrated by in situ DNA hybridization. *ORL Otolaryngol. Rel. Spec.* 49:175, 1987.

44. Terry RM, Lewis FA, Griffiths S, Wells M, Bird CC. Demonstration of human papillomavirus types 6 and 11 in juvenile laryngeal papillomatosis by in situ DNA hybridization. *J. Pathol.* 153:245, 1987.

45. Zarod AP, Rutherford JD, Corbitt G. Malignant progression of laryngeal papilloma associated with human papillomavirus virus type 6 (HPV-6) DNA. *J. Clin. Pathol.* 41:280, 1988.

46. Corbitt G, Zarod AP, Arrand JR, Longson M, Farrington WT. Human papillomavirus (HPV) genotypes associated with laryngeal papilloma. *J. Clin. Pathol.* 41:284, 1988.

47. Brandsma JL, Abramson AL. Association of papillomavirus with cancers of the head and neck. *Arch. Otolaryngol. Head Neck Surg.* 115:621, 1989.

48. Levi JE, Delcelo R, Alberti VN, Torloni H, Villa LV. Human papillomavirus DNA in respiratory papillomatosis detected by in situ hybridization and the polymerase chain reaction. *Am. J. Pathol.* 135:1179, 1989.

49. Ward P, Mounts P. Heterogeneity in mRNA of human papillomavirus type-6 subtypes in respiratory tract lesions. *Virology* 168:1, 1989.

50. Lindeberg H, Syrjänen S, Kärjä J, Syrjänen K. Human papillomavirus type 11 DNA in squamous cell carcinomas and pre-existing multiple laryngeal papillomas. *Acta Otolaryngol. (Stockholm)* 107:141, 1989.

51. Tsutsumi K, Nakajima T, Gotoh M, Shimosato Y, Tsunokawa Y, Terada M, Ebihara S, Ono I. In situ hybridization and immunohistochemical study of human papillomavirus infection in adult laryngeal papillomas. *Laryngoscope* 99:80, 1989.

52. Quiney RE, Wells M, Lewis FA, Terry RM, Michaels L, Croft CB. Laryngeal papillomatosis: correlation between severity of disease and presence of HPV 6 and 11 detected by in situ DNA hybridization. *J. Clin. Pathol.* 42:694, 1989.

53. Ishibashi T, Matsushima S, Tsunokawa Y, Asai M, Nomura Y, Sugimura T, Terada M. Human papillomavirus DNA in squamous cell carcinoma of the upper aerodigestive tract. *Arch. Otolaryngol. Head Neck Surg.* 116:294, 1990.

54. Bryan RL, Bevan IS, Crocker J, Young LS. Detection of HPV 6 and 11 in tumors of the upper respiratory tract using the polymerase chain reaction. *Clin. Otolaryngol.* 15:177, 1990.

55. Lindeberg H, Johansen L. The presence of human papillomavirus (HPV) in solitary adult laryngeal papillomas demonstrated by in situ DNA hybridization with sulphonated probes. *Clin. Otolaryngol.* 15:367, 1990.

56. Hsiao TY, Chen JY, Lee SY, Hsu MM. Detection of human papillomavirus (HPV) DNA in laryngeal papilloma. *J. Formosan Med. Assoc.* 89:293, 1990.

57. Hoshikwa T, Nakjajima T, Uhara H, Gotoh M, Shimosato Y, Tsutsumi K, Ono I, Ebihara S. Detection of human papillomavirus DNA in laryngeal squamous carcinomas by polymerase chain reaction. *Laryngoscope* 100:647–650, 1990.

58. Perez-Ayala M, Ruiz-Cabello F, Esteban F, Concha A, Redondo M, Oliva MR, Cabrera T, Carrido F. Presence of HPV 16 sequences in laryngeal carcinomas. *Int. J. Cancer* 46:8–11, 1990.

59. Dickens P, Srivastava G, Loke SL, Larkin S. Human papillomavirus 6, 11 and 16 in laryngeal papillomas. *J. Pathol.* 165:243, 1991.

60. Ogura H, Watanabe S, Fukushima K, Masuda Y, Fujiwara T, Yabe Y. Presence of human papillomavirus type 18 DNA in a pharyngeal and laryngeal carcinoma. *Jap. J. Cancer Res.* 82:1184, 1991.

61. Morgan DW, Abdullan V, Quiney R, Myint S. Human papilloma virus and carcinoma of the laryngopharyngx. *J. Laryngol. Otol.* 105:288, 1991.

62. McCullough DW, McNicol PJ. Laryngeal carcinoma associated with human papillomavirus type 16. *J. Otolaryngol.* 20:97–99, 1991.

63. Rimell F, Maisel R, Dayton V. In situ hybridization and laryngeal papillomas. *Ann. Otol. Rhinol. Laryngol.* 101:119, 1992.

64. Arndt O, Zeise K, Bauer I, Brock J. Humane Papillomviren (HPV) vom Typ 6/11 und 16/18 in Plattenepithelkarzinomen des oberen Atmungs- und Verauungstraktes. Eine In-situ-Hynbridisierungsstudie. *Laryngol. Rinol. Otol.* 71:500, 1992.

65. Anwar K, Nakahuki K, Imai H, Naiki H, Inuzuka M. Over-expression of p53 protein in human laryngeal carcinoma. *Int. J. Cancer* 53:952–956, 1993.

66. Arndt O, Brock J, Kundt G, Müllender A. Der Nachweis humaner Papillomavirus DNA in formalifixierten invasiven Plattenepithelkarzinomen des Larynx mit der Polymerase Chain Reaction (PCR). *Laryngol. Rhinol. Otol.* 73:527–532, 1994.

67. Doyle DJ, Henderson LA, LeJeune FE, Miller RH. Changes in human papillomavirus typing of recurrent respiratory papillomatosis progressing to malignant neoplasm. *Arch. Otolaryngol. Head Neck Surg.* 120:1273–1276, 1994.

68. Clayman GL, Stewart MG, Weber RS, El-Naggar AK, Grimm EA. Human papillomavirus in laryngeal and hypopharyngeal carcinomas. *Arch. Orolaryngol. Head Neck Surg.* 120:743–748.

69. Gale N, Poljak M, Kambic V, Ferluga D, Fischinger J. Laryngeal papillomatosis: molecular, histopathological, and clinical evaluation. *Virchows Archiv.* 425:291–295, 1994.

70. Hartley C, Hamilton J, Birzgalis AR, Farrington WT. Recurrent respiratory papillomatosis - the Manchester experience, 1974-1992. *J. Laryngol. Otol.* 108:226–229, 1994.

71. Gourgoulis V, Rassidakis G, Karameris A, Giatromanolaki A, Barbatis C, Kittas C. Expression of p53 protein in laryngeal squamous cell carcinoma and dysplasia: possible correlation with human papillomavirus infection and clinicopathological findings. *Virchows Archiv.* 425:481–489, 1994.

72. Fouret P, Dabit D, Sibony M, Alili D, Commo F, Saint-Guily JL, Callard P. Short communication. Expression of p53 protein related to the presence of human papillomavirus infection in precancer lesions of the larynx. *Am. J. Pathol.* 146:599–604, 1995.

73. Rihkanen H, Aaltonen LM, Syrjänen SM. Human papillomavirus in laryngeal papillomas and in adjacent normal epithelium. *Clin. Otolaryngol.* 18:470, 1993.

74. Mounths B, Shah K. Respiratory papillomatosis: etiological relation to genital tract papillomaviruses. *Prog. Med. Virol.* 20:90, 1984.

75. Smith EM, Johnson SR, Cripe TP, Pignatari S, Turek L. Perinatal vertical transmission of human papillomavirus and subsequent development of respiratory tract papillomatosis. *Ann. Rhinol. Laryngol.* 100:479, 1991.

76. Syrjänen K, Syrjänen S, Pyrhönen S. Human papillomavirus (HPV9) antigens in lesions of laryngeal squamous cell carcinomas. *ORL Otolaryngol. Rel. Spec.* 44:323, 1982.

77. Kashima H, Mounts P, Kuhajda F, Loury M. Demonstration of human papillomavirus capsid antigens in carcinoma in situ of the larynx. *Ann. Otol. Rhinol. Laryngol.* 95:603, 1986.

78. Ostrow RS, Manias DA, Fong WJ, Zachow KR, Faras AJ. A survey of human cancers for human papillomavirus DNA by filter hybridization. *Cancer* 59:429, 1987.

79. Kahn T, Schwarz E, zur Hausen H. Molecular cloning and characterization of the DNA of a new human papillomavirus (HPV 30) from a laryngeal carcinoma. *Inter. J. Cancer* 37:61, 1986.

80. Kiyabu MT, Shibata D, Arnheim N, Martin WJ, Fitzgibbons PL. Detection of human papillomavirus in formalin-fixed, invasive squamous carcinomas using the polymerase chain reaction. *Am. J. Surg. Pathol.* 13:221, 1989.

81. Snijedrs PJF, Cromme FV, van den Brule AJC, Schrijnemakers HFJ, Snow GB, Meijer CJLM, Walboomers JMM. Prevalence and expression of human papillomavirus in tonsillar carcinomas, indicating a possible viral etiology. *Int. J. Cancer* 51:845, 1992.

82. Rihkanen H, Peltomaa J, Syrjänen S. Prevalence of human papillomavirus (HPV) in vocal cords without laryngeal papillomas. *Acta Otolaryngol.* 114:348–351, 1994.

83. Nunez DA, Astley SM, Lewist FA, Wells M. Human papilloma viruses: a study of their prevalence in the normal larynx. *J. Laryngol. Otol.* 108:319–320, 1993.

84. Scully C, Prime SS, Maitland N. Papillomaviruses: Their possible role in oral disease. *Oral Sur. Oral Med. Oral Pathol.* 60:166, 1985.

85. Syrjänen SM. Human papillomavirus infection in the oral cavity. In: Syrjänen KJ, Gissman L, Koss LG. Eds. *Papillomavirus and Human Disease* Heidelberg: Springer-Verlag, 104, 1987.

86. Scully C, Cox MF, Prime SS, Maitland NJ. Papillomaviruses: The current status in relation to oral disease. *Oral Sur. Oral Med. Oral Pathol.* 65:526, 1988.

87. Chang F, Syrjänen S, Kellokoski J, Syrjänen K. Human papillomavirus (HPV) infections and their associations with oral disease. *J. Oral Pathol. Med.* 20:305, 1991.

88. Syrjänen K, Syrjänen S, Lamberg M, Pyrhönen S, Nuutinen J. Morphological and immunohistochemical evidence suggesting human papillomavirus (HPV) involvement in oral squamous cell carcinogenesis. *Int. J. Oral Surg.* 12:418, 1983

89. Syrjänen S, Syrjänen K, Ikenberg H, Gissman L, Lamberg M. A human papillomavirus closely related to HPV 13 found in a focal epithelial hyperplasia lesion (Heck disease). *Archiv. Dermatol. Res.* 276:199, 1984.

90. Lindberg H, Fey SJ, Ottosen PD, Larsen PM. Human papilloma virus (HPV) and carcinomas of the head and neck. *Clin. Otolaryngol.* 13:447, 1988.

91. Maitland NJ, Cox MF, Lynas C, Prime SS, Meanwell CA, Scully C. Detection of human papillomavirus DNA in biopsies of human oral tissue. *Br. J. Cancer* 56:245, 1987.

92. Jalal H, Sanders CM, Prime SS, Scully C, Maitland NJ. Detection of human papillomavirus type 16 DNA in oral squames from normal young adults. *J. Oral Pathol. Med.* 21:465, 1992.

93. Kellokoski J, Syrjänen S, Syrjänen KJ, Oral mucosal changes in women with genital HPV infection. *J. Oral Pathol. Med.* 19:142, 1990.

94. Kellokoski J, Syrjänen S, Yliskoski M, Syrjänen K. Dot blot hybridization in detection of human papillomavirus (HPV) infections in oral cavity in women with genital infections. *J. Oral Microbiol. Immunol.* 7:19, 1992.

95. Kellokoski J, Syrjänen S, Chang F, Yliskoski M, Syrjänen KJ. Southern blot hybridization and PCR in detection of oral human papillomavirus (HPV) infections in women with genital HPV infections. *J. Oral Pathol. Med.* 21:459, 1992.

96. Eike A, Buchwald C, Rolighed J, Lindberg H. Human papillomavirus (HPV) is rarely present in normal oral and nasal mucosa. *Clin. Oncol.* 20:171, 1995.

97. Leimola-Virtanen R; Syrjänen S. Failure to detect human papillomvirus (HPV) DNA in oral mucosa of postmenopausal women. *Clin. Infect. Dis.* 22:593, 1996.

98. Adler-Storthz K, Newland JR, Tessin BA, Yeudall WA, Shillitoe EJ. Identification of human papillomavirus types in oral verruca vulgaris. *J. Oral Pathol. Med.* 15:230, 1986.

99. Eversole LR, Laipis PJ, Green TL. Human papillomavirus type 2 DNA in oral and labial verruca vulcaris. *J. Cutaneous Pathol.* 14:319, 1987.

100. Löning T, Ikenberg H, Becker J, Gissman L, Hoepper I, zur Hausen H. Analysis of oral papillomas, leukoplakias, and invasive carcinomas for human papillomavirus type related DNA. *J. Inv. Dermatol.* 83:417, 1985.

101. Syrjänen SM, Syrjänen KJ, Happonen R-P, Lamberg MA. In situ DNA hybridization analysis of human papillomavirus (HPV) sequences in benign oral mucosal lesions. *Arch. Dermatol. Res.* 279:543, 1987.

102. Eversole LR, Stone CE, Beckman AM. Oral squamous cell papillomas: Detection of HPV DNA by in situ hybridization. *Oral Sur. Oral Med. Oral Pathol.* 65:545, 1988.

103. Young SK, Min KW. In situ hybridization analysis of oral papillomas, leukoplakias and carcinomas for human papillomavirus. *Oral Sur. Oral Med. Oral Pathol.* 71:726, 1991.

104. Syrjänen SM, Syrjänen K, Lamberg MA. Detection of human papillomavirus DNA in oral mucosal lesions using in situ DNA-hybridization applied on paraffin sections. *Oral Sur. Oral Med. Oral Pathol.* 62:660, 1986.

105. Eversole LR, Laipis PJ, Merrell P, Choi E. Demonstration of human papillomavirus DNA in oral condyloma acuminatum. *J. Oral Pathol. Med.* 16:266, 1987.

106. Knapp MJ, Uohara GI. Oral condyloma acuminatum. *Oral Sur. Oral Med. Oral Pathol.* 23:538, 1967.

107. Lutzner M, Kuffer R, Blanchet-Bardon C, Croissant O. Different papillomaviruses as the causes of oral warts. *Arch. Dermatol.* 118:393, 1982.

108. Greenspan D, de Villiers EM, Greenspan JS, De Souza YG, zur Hausen H. Unusual HPV types in oral warts in association with HPV infection. *J. Oral Pathol.* 17:482, 1988.

109. Syrjänen S, Von Krogh G, Kellokoski J, Syrjänen K. Two different human papillomavirus (HPV) types associated with oral mucosal lesions in an HIV-seropositive man. *J. Oral Pathol. Med.* 18:366, 1989.

110. De Villiers EM, Hirsch-Behnam A, von Knebel-Doeberitz C, Neumann CH, zur Hausen H. Two newly identified human papillomavirus types (HPV 40 and 57) isolated from mucosal lesions. *Virology* 171:248, 1989.

111. Pfister H, Hettich I, Runne U, Gissman L, Chilf G. Characterization of human papillomavirus type 13 from focal epithelial hyperplasia Heck lesions. *J. Virol.* 47:363, 1983.

112. Beaudenon S, Praetorius F, Kremsdorf D. A new type of human papillomavirus associated with oral focal epithelial hyperplasia. *J. Inv. Dermatol.* 88:130, 1987.

113. Henke R-P, Guerin-Reverchon I, Milde-Langosch K, Stromme-Koppang H, Löning T. *In situ* detection of human papillomavirus types 13 and 32 in focal epithelial hyperplasia of the oral mucosa. *J. Oral Pathol. Med.* 18:419, 1989.

114. Garlick JA, Calderon S, Buchner A, Mitrani-Rosenbaum S. Detection of human papillomavirus in focal epithelial hyperplasia. *J. Oral Pathol. Med.* 18:172, 1989.

115. Kashima HK, Kutcher M, Kesis T, Levin LS, De Villiers E-M, Shah K. Human papillomavirus in squamous cell carcinoma, leukoplakia, lichen planus, and clinically normal epithelium of the oral cavity. *Ann. Otol. Rhinol. Laryngol.* 99:55, 1990.

116. Jontell M, Watts S, Wallström M, Levin L, Sloberg K. Human papillomavirus in erosive lichen planus. *J. Oral Path. Med.* 19:273, 1990.

117. Löning T, Reichart P, Staquet MJ, Becker J, Thivolet J. Occurrence of papillomavirus structural antigens in oral papillomas and leukoplakias. *J. Oral Pathol. Med.* 13:155, 1984.

118. Gassenmeier A, Hornstein OP: Presence of human papillomavirus DNA in benign and precancerous oral leukoplakias and squamous cell carcinomas. *Dermatologica* 176:224, 1988.

119. Chang F, Syrjänen S, Nuutinen J, Kärjä J, Syrjänen K. Detection of human papillomavirus (HPV) DNA in oral squamous cell carcinomas by in situ hybridization and polymerase chain reaction. *Arch. Dermatol. Res.* 4:550, 1990.

120. Syrjänen SM, Syrjänen KJ, Happonen RP. Human papillomavirus (HPV) DNA sequences in oral precancerous lesions and squamous cell carcinoma demonstrated by in situ hybridization. *J. Oral Pathol. Med.* 17:273, 1988.

121. De Villiers E-M, Weidauer H, Otto H, Zur Hausen H. Papillomavirus DNA in human tongue carcinomas. *Int. J. Cancer* 36:575, 1985.

122. Lookingbill DP, Kreider JW, Howett MK, Olmstead PM, Conner GH. Human papillomavirus type 16 in bowenoid papulosis, intraoral papillomas, and squamous cell carcinoma of the tongue. *Arch. Dermatol.* 123:363, 1987.

123. Kratochvill FJ, Cioffi GA, Auclair PL, Rathbun WA. Virus-associated dysplasia (bowenoid papulosis?) of the oral cavity. *Oral Sur. Oral Med. Oral Pathol.* 68:312, 1989.

124. Cruz IBF, Snijders PJF, Seenbergen RDM, Meijer CJLM, Snow GB, Walboomers JMM, van der Waal I. Age-dependence of human papillomavirus DNA presence in oral squamous cell carcinomas. *Eur. J. Cancer Oral Oncol. Part B*. 32B:55, 1996.

125. Balaram P, Nalinakumari KR, Abraham E, Balan A, Hareendran NK, Bernhard H-U, Chan S-Y. Human papillomaviruses in 91 oral cancers from Indian betel quid chewers - high prevalence and multiplicity of infections. *Int. J. Cancer* 61:450, 1995.

126. Adler-Storthz K, Newland JR, Tessin BA, Yeudall WA, Shillitoe EJ. Human papillomavirus type 2 DNA in oral verrucous carcinoma. *J. Oral Pathol. Med.* 15:472, 1986.

127. Adler RH, Carberry DM, Ross CA. Papilloma of the esophagus. Association with hiatal hernia. *J. Thorac. Cardiovasc. Sur.* 37:625, 1959.

128. Weitzner S, Hentel W. Squamous papilloma of the esophagus: Case report and review of the literature. *Am. J. Gastroenterol.* 50:391, 1968.

129. Syrjänen K, Pyrhönen S, Aukee S, Koskela E. Squamous cell papilloma of the esophagus: a tumor probably caused by human papillomavirus (HPV). *Diagn. Histopathol.* 5:291, 1982.

130. Winkler B, Capo V, Reumann W. Human papillomavirus infection of the esophagus: a clinicopathologic study with demonstration of papillomavirus antigen by the immunoperoxidase technique. *Cancer* 55:149, 1985.

131. Politoske EJ. Squamous cell papilloma of the esophagus associated with human papillomavirus. *Gastroenterology* 102:668, 1992.

132. Van Cutsem E, Geboes K, Visser L, Devos R, Janssens J, Lerut T, Vantrappen G. *Eur. J. Gastroenterol. Hepatol.* 3:561, 1991.

133. Chang F, Janatuinen E, Pikkarainen P, Syrjänen S, Syrjänen K. Esophageal squamous cell papillomas. Failure to detect human papillomavirus DNA by in situ hybridization and polymerase chain reaction. *Scand. J. Gastroenterol.* 26:535, 1991.

134. de Borges RF, Acevedo F, Miralles E, Mijares P. Squamous papilloma of the esophagus diagnosed by cytology. Report of a case with concurrent occult epidermoid carcinoma. *Acta Cytol.* 30:487, 1986.

135. Hille JJ, Margolius KA, Markowitz S, Isaacson C. Human papillomavirus infection related to esophageal carcinoma in black South Africans. *S. Afr. Med. J.* 69:441, 1986.

136. Kulski J, Demeter T, Sterret GF, Shilkin KB. Human papillomavirus DNA in esophageal carcinoma. *Lancet* 2:683, 1986.

137. Kiyabu MT, Shibata D, Arnheim N, Martin WJ, Fitzgibbons Pl, Detection of human papillomavirus in formalin-fixed, invasive squamous carcinoma using the polymerase chain reaction. *Am. J. Surg. Pathol.* 13:221, 1989.

138. Loke SL, Ma L, Wong M, Srivastava G, Lo I, Bird CC. Human papillomavirus in esophageal squamous cell carcinoma. *J. Clin. Pathol.* 43:909, 1990.

139. Williamson AI, Jaskiesicz K, Gunning A. The detection of human papillomavirus in esophageal lesions. *Anticancer Res.* 11:263, 1991.

140. Benamouzig R, Pigot F, Quiroga G, Validire P, Chaussade S, Catalan F, Couturier D. Human papillomavirus infection in esophageal squamous cell carcinoma in Western countries. *Int. J. Cancer* 50:549, 1992.

141. Chang F, Syrjänen S, Shen Q, Ji H, Syrjänen K. Human papillomavirus (HPV) DNA in esophageal precancer lesions and squamous cell carcinomas from China. *Int. J. Cancer* 45:21, 1990.

142. Chang F, Shen Q, Zhou J, Wang C, Wang D, Syrjänen S, Syrjänen K. Detection of human papillomavirus DNA in cytologic specimens derived from esophageal precancer lesions and cancer. *Scand. J. Gastroenterol.* 25:383, 1990.

143. Gutman LT, Claire K, Herman-Giddens ME, Johnston WW, Phelps WC. Evaluation of sexually abused and nonabused young girls for intravaginal human papillomavirus infection. *Am. J. Dis. Child* 146:694, 1992.

144. Kudiclka J, Sneider A, Braun R. Antibodies against the human papillomavirus type 16 early proteins in human sera: correlation of anti-E7 reactivity with cervical cancer. *J. Natl. Cancer Inst.* 81:1698, 1989.

145. Ley C, Bauer HM, Reingold A, Schiffman MH, Chambers JC, Tashiro CJ, Manos MM. Determinants of genital human papillomavirus infection in young women. *J. Natl. Cancer Inst.* 83:997, 1991.

146. Hippeläinen MI, Yliskoski M, Syrjänen S, Saastamoinen J, Hippeläinen M, Saarikoski S, Syrjänen K. Low concordance of genital human papillomavirus lesions and viral types in HPV infected women and their sexual partners. *Sex. Trans. Dis.* 21:76, 1994.

147. Ho L, Tay S-K, Chan S-Y, Bernard HU. Sequence variants of human papillomavirus type 16 from couples suggest sexual transmission with low infectivity and polyclonality in genital neoplasia. *J. Inf. Dis.* 168:803, 1993.

148. Lacey CIN. Genital warts in children. *Papillomavirus Report* 2:31, 1991.

149. Gutman LT. Sexual abuse and human papillomavirus infection. *J. Ped.* 116:495, 1990.

150. Herman-Giddens ME, Gutman LT, Berson NL. The Duke Child Protection Team. Association of coexisting vaginal infection and multiple abusers in female children with genital warts. *Sex. Trans. Dis.* 54:63, 1988.

151. Sait MA, Garg BR. Condylomata acuminata in children:report of 4 cases. *Genitour. Med.* 61:338, 1985.

152. Ingram DL, Everett VD, Lyna PR, White ST, Rockwell LA. Epidemiology of adult sexually transmitted disease agents in children being evaluated for sexual abuse. *Ped. Inf. Dis. J.* 11:945, 1992.

153. Pakarian F, Kaye J, Cason J, Kell B, Jewers R, Derias NW, Raju, KS, Best JM. Cancer associated human papillomaviruses: perinatal transmission and persistence. *Br. J. Obstet. Gynaecol.* 101:514, 1994.

154. Fredericks BD, Balkin A, Daniel HW, Schonrock J, Ward B, Frazer IH. Transmission of human papillomavirus from mother to child. *Aust. N. Z. J. Obstet. Gynecol.* 33:30, 1993.

155. Sedlacek TV, Lindheim S, Eder C, Hasty L, Woodland M, Ludomirsky A. Rando RF. Mechanism for human papillomavirus transmission at birth. *Am. J. Obstet. Gynecol.* 161:55, 1989.

156. Puranen M, Yliskoski M, Saarikoski S, Syrjänen K, Syrjänen S. Vertical transmission of human papillomavirus from infected mothers to their newborn babies and persistence of the virus in childhood. *Am. J. Obstet. Gynecol.* 174:694, 1996.

157. Armbruster-Moraes E, Ioshimoto LM, Leao E, Zugaib M. Presence of human papillomavirus DNA in amniotic fluids of pregnant women with cervical lesions. *Gynecol. Oncol.* 54:152-158, 1994.

158. Puranen M, Yliskoski M, Saarikoski S, Syrjänen K, Syrjänen S. Vertical transmission of human papillomavirus from infected mothers to their newborn babies and persistence of the virus in childhood. *14th International Papillomavirus Conference Quebec, Canada* 1995.

159. Cason J, Kaye JN, Best JM. Non-sexual acquisition of human genital papillomaviruses. *Papillomavirus Report* 1:1 1995.

V. Immunological Modulation

11

The Regulatory Influence of Immunological Host Responses

Jacek Malejczyk, Slawomir Majewski, and Stefania Jablonska

CONTENTS

I.   INTRODUCTION

Mucosal or cutaneous lesions induced by human papillomaviruses (HPV) usually display a benign course with spontaneous regression; however, some of them may persist even for a long time. By infection with high risk HPV types, such lesions may undergo malignant conversion.[1,2] Little is known as to what factors are decisive for such a variable natural course of HPV-associated lesions.

Immortalization and malignant transformation of HPV-harboring cells appears to be under control of an intracellular genetic surveillance mechanism.[3,4] However, there is a growing evidence that development and persistence of the lesions may also depend on host immune defense reactions (immune surveillance).

The concept of specific antiviral/antitumor immune surveillance is based on assumption that viral proteins display antigenic properties, and virus-infected or transformed cells present novel "alien" antigens (virus- or tumor-associated antigens) which are not detectable in normal cells. These antigens are recognized by immunocompetent cells and are able to elicit specific antiviral and antitumor immunological responses.

There are several lines of evidence for existence of immune surveillance that may control papillomavirus infection and development of papillomavirus-associated lesions:

1. Induction of specific humoral and cellular immunity in papillomavirus-infected subjects[5-8] or transgenic animals expressing papillomavirus proteins.[9]
2. Regression of the papillomavirus-associated lesions mediated by infiltrating mononuclear immune cells.[10-12]
3. An increased incidence of the papillomavirus-associated lesions in immunosuppressed or immunodeficient humans[13,14] and animals.[15]

The concept of the role of immune surveillance in control of HPV infection and HPV-associated neoplasia is summarized in Figure 1. According to this concept, the host immune system normally controls HPV infection and rejects HPV-harboring neoplastic cells. Inability to eradicate the virus and HPV-associated lesions due to immunosuppression, immunodeficiency, or immunotolerance may result in widespread HPV infection and persistence of the disease. Genomic instability of the cells infected with high risk HPV types leading to their malignant transformation may in addition result in loss of antigenicity and/or in resistance to immune effector mechanisms thus facilitating an unopposed tumor growth.

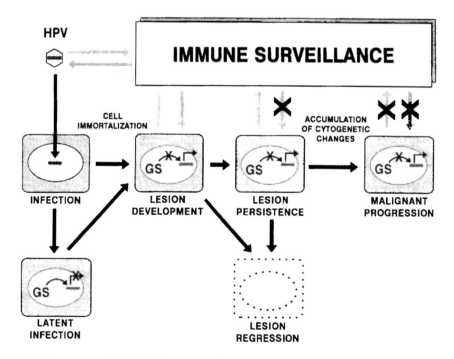

FIGURE 1   The concept of anti-HPV immune surveillance. Explanations are in text; GS = genetic surveillance.

Specific immunological responses against viruses and tumor cells require antigen processing and presentation by specialized antigen presenting cells (APC). Antigen presentation is necessary for activation of specific T helper (Th) lymphocyte clones that, in turn, stimulate specific cytotoxic T lymphocyte (CTL) clones and specific antibody production by B lymphocytes. Furthermore, immunological surveillance against viral infections and neoplasia also involves participation of natural cytotoxic cells and immunoregulatory/antitumor cytokines. Elucidation of these immune surveillance mechanisms that are actively involved in resistance against HPV infections and neoplasia may be helpful for better understanding the mechanisms of disease progression and may constitute a basis for new strategies of immunotherapy and vaccination for HPV-associated tumors.

II. ANTIGEN PRESENTATION AND INDUCTION OF SPECIFIC IMMUNE RESPONSES AGAINST HPV

Putative antigens that may be responsible for induction of specific immune response against HPV and HPV-harboring cells include both capsid and regulatory proteins encoded by late and early HPV open reading frames, respectively.[11,16] Although HPV-related proteins appear to be the main antigens involved in anti-HPV immune response, participation of some HPV-unrelated cellular neoantigens cannot be excluded.

A. Presentation of HPV-Specific Antigens

Antigen recognition and specific activation of T lymphocytes requires antigens processed into small oligopeptide fragments (antigenic epitopes) and presented in assembly with class I or class II major histocompatibility complex (MHC) molecules.[17,18] MHC class I molecules (e.g., HLA-A, -B, and -C) present intracellularly expressed antigens and are essential for triggering CD8+ CTL responses and target cell killing whereas class II molecules (e.g., HLA-DR, -DQ, and -DP) participate in presentation of exogenous extracellular antigens and are necessary for stimulation of CD4+ (Th) lymphocyte responses.

MHC class I molecules are expressed on almost all nucleated cell types.[17,18] Endogenously expressed antigens (intracellular pathogens and normal cell proteins) are cleaved by the cytosol proteasome system into 8–9 aminoacid oligopeptides which are translocated into the endoplasmic reticulum by TAP-1/2 transporter proteins which are encoded within MHC class II region and belong to a superfamily of ATP-binding transporters.[19] In endoplasmic reticulum, the antigenic peptides are captured by MHC class I molecules and consecutively transferred onto the cell surface (Figure 2A).

On the other hand, antigen processing and presentation to CD4+ Th lymphocytes is accomplished by specialized "professional" APC that constitutively express class II molecules.[17,18] As "professional" APC may serve dendritic/Langerhans cells, macrophages/monocytes, and B lymphocytes.[20,21] APC uptakes exogenous antigens (viral particles or viral proteins released by the infected cells), internalizes them by endocytosis, and proteolytically processes by lysosomal enzymes into 12–20 amino acid oligopeptides. The antigenic oligopeptides are then bound by class II MHC molecules and are transferred to the APC surface (Figure 2B).

Intraepithelial Langerhans cells (LC) appear to be the main APC involved in presentation of antigens in the skin.[22] Thus, the proper function of these cells may be crucial for induction of specific anti-HPV immune response and lesion rejection. Indeed, the number of LC was found to be normal in regressing genital warts[12] and an increased density of LC has been associated with a more favorable prognosis in some HPV-associated laryngeal lesions.[23] On the other hand, analysis of LC in a variety of persistent HPV-associated lesions has shown that their number is usually significantly decreased as compared to uninvolved skin.[24-27] This suggests that loss of LC may be an important phenomenon facilitating development and persistence of HPV-associated lesions. However, it is not known whether a decrease of LC numbers is a prerequisite for lesion development. The mechanism of this decrease is also unclear. It may be associated with virus replication,[26]

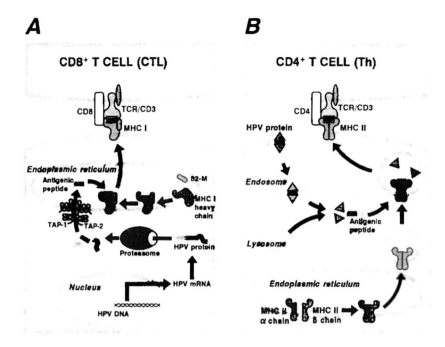

FIGURE 2   Simplified scheme of antigen processing and presentation in context of MHC class I (A) and II (B) molecules. Explanations are in text; β2-M = β2-microglobulin.

nevertheless, it cannot be excluded that a reduced number of LC in the skin could also be attributed to their enhanced physiological migration to regional lymph nodes.[28]

1.   A Significance of MHC Polymorphism

Both class I and II MHC genes display a high degree of polymorphism of the sequences responsible for antigenic peptide binding.[29,30] This polymorphism results in selectivity of peptide capture and implies that certain MHC class I or II allele products are able to present a limited number (1,000–2,000) of different peptides displaying particular "acceptable" amino acid sequences.[31,32] Therefore, it is plausible that in individuals displaying a particular combination of MHC alleles, presentation of a given antigenic peptide may not be equally efficient. Accordingly, some individuals may be more susceptible to certain pathogens including HPV infection and, in consequence, to HPV-associated neoplasia.

The evidence for existence of tumor "susceptible" and "resistant" MHC phenotype has recently come from the studies in rabbits experimentally infected with Shope cottontail rabbit papillomavirus (CRPV).[33,34] Restriction fragment length polymorphism (RFLP) studies of rabbit MHC have revealed a strong linkage between malignant CRPV-induced papilloma progression and class II MHC DRα PuII fragment. On the other hand, regression of papillomas was associated with DQα EcoRI fragment phenotype.

Studies in humans have revealed that similar links may also exist in patients with HPV-associated cancers. Wank and Thomssen[35] have reported that cervical cancer in South German population is strongly connected to MHC class II HLA-DQw3 and DR5 antigens, the latter possibly being a result of a linkage disequilibrium between DQw3 and DR5. On the other hand, HLA-DR6 phenotype was associated with a relative resistance to the disease. Furthermore, analysis of DQB1 genes coding for HLA-DQw3 has shown a preferential increase in the frequencies of DQB1*0301 and *0303 alleles and the absence of DQB1*0302 allele in cervical cancer patients.[36] An increased prevalence of HLA-DQw3 in patients with cervical cancer has been confirmed in Norwegian[37] and African-American[38] populations. In the latter group, a statistically significant increase in a relative risk was seen for DQB1*0303 and *0604 alleles, while a decreased risk was associated with DQB1*0201 and DQB1*0301/*0501 heterozygote. A relationship to HLA-DQw3 has also been reported in patients with recurrent respiratory papillomatosis.[39] On the other hand, cervical cancer in the Hispanic population was significantly associated with DRB1*1501/DQB1*0602 haplotypes.[40] HLA-DR13 haplotypes were negatively associated and these associations were HPV 16-type specific. Another interesting association has also been reported in renal transplant recipients suffering from HPV-related skin cancers. In these patients, development of cancer was strongly associated with HLA-DR7 and was accompanied by the absence of switch from IgM to IgG antibodies directed against HPV8 L1 protein.[41]

These results strongly suggest that some specific MHC class II haplotypes may affect the risk of development of some HPV-associated malignant and benign lesions by influencing specific anti-HPV immune responses. A similar risk may also be associated with MHC class I molecules. Such possible associations have been reported for HLA-A11 and HLA-B14[39] as well as HLA-B7[42,43] genotypes. In patients with cervical carcinomas, HLA-B7 was also associated with poorer clinical outcome.[43] The possible explanation for this phenomenon is that some oncogenic HPV may display a genetic variability resulting in modifications of antigenic epitope which is specific for the HLA-B7 molecule.[42] This modification alters the structure of the peptide making its presentation in the context of HLA-B7 molecule impossible. This, in turn, may affect the neoplastic cells recognition by specific CD8+ CTL and may result in an unopposed tumor growth.

The results of the studies on MHC class I and II associations with HPV-induced neoplasia strongly suggest that HLA typing as well as sequence analysis of possible HPV-associated antigenic epitopes may serve to identify persons at risk of malignant conversion and may be useful in prognostication of the disease course. Furthermore, analysis of HLA polymorphism and HPV variability appears to be necessary for optimization of anti-HPV vaccination procedures.

2.   Mapping of Specific HPV-Associated Antigenic Epitopes

During recent years, several methods of studying the antigenic peptides have been developed[44] leading to identification of certain sequence motifs containing specific MHC class I and II anchor residues.[31,32,45] Mapping and identification of such antigenic epitopes that may be presented in context of MHC molecules and that may trigger the specific T cell responses appear to be the crucial step for development of both preventive and therapeutic HPV-specific vaccines.

The presence of HPV sequences containing antigenic peptide motifs has been first demonstrated using the murine system. In these studies, the respective HPV peptides binding murine MHC class I molecules have been recognized and their effectiveness for triggering the T cell responses has been confirmed using the specific CTL assays.[46-48] Furthermore, it has been found that vaccination with a putative HPV16 E7 epitope resulted in rejection of syngeneic tumor cells expressing HPV 16 sequences.[47]

Several HPV16 E6 and E7 as well as HPV6 and 11 E7 peptide sequences presented in context of different human HLA-A molecules have also been identified.[49-52] Some of these peptides have also been demonstrated as targets for the specific CTL clones,[49,52] thus providing evidence for their possible application for immunotherapy. Interestingly, not all peptides predicted on a basis of the presence of specific anchor residues were able to bind to the relevant HLA-A molecules.[50] On the other hand, studies in mice have revealed that HPV peptides that do not contain specific MHC binding motifs may also be presented and may trigger CTL responses.[48]

Attempts are undertaken for identification of HPV-derived MHC class II-specific peptides capable of specific induction of CD4+ Th cells. Using an overlapping peptide system in a mouse model, some MHC class II-restricted antigenic determinants have been demonstrated for HPV16 E7 and L1 proteins on a basis of induction of T cell proliferative responses and T cell-dependent antibody production by B cells.[53-56] Mapping of antigenic epitopes for BPV E7 protein using responding T cells from vaccinated cattle has also been reported.[57] Likewise, certain Th cell stimulatory epitopes have been identified in the human system for HPV16 L1, L6, E7,[58,59] as well as HPV1 E4 protein.[60]

These studies have revealed MHC class II and HPV type restriction of anti-HPV peptide response. However, although some HLA-DR4, -DR7, and -DQ7-restricted antigenic epitopes have already been identified,[58,60] other HPV peptide motifs specific for certain human MHC class II alleles that might be useful for vaccine preparation are still unidentified.

3.   Changes in MHC Molecule Expression as an Important Event in Progression of HPV-Associated Tumors

MHC molecules are crucial for antigen presentation and activation of T cells. It is therefore plausible that any abrogation of MHC expression may result in a disturbed antigen presentation and lack of induction of specific anti-HPV immune responses leading to an unopposed tumor growth. Indeed, in a very high proportion of cervical carcinomas as well as HPV-associated cutaneous lesions MHC class I expression has been found to be reduced or absent.[26,61-64] Furthermore, loss of MHC class I expression in cervical lesions was found to be accompanied by a reduced numbers of infiltrating CD8+ T cells[65] and was associated with an increased malignancy and poorer prognosis.[43,66,67] On the other hand, no apparent reduction in MHC class I expression was noted in benign HPV-induced anogenital lesions.[64,68] These observations strongly suggest that loss of MHC class I expression may be an important factor favoring growth of HPV-associated neoplasia.

The mechanisms of abrogation of MHC class I expression in HPV-associated tumors are poorly understood. Down regulation of MHC class I molecules may be associated with an abrogated β2-microglobulin or heavy chain mRNA expression[69,70] that might be due to viral infection and/or oncogene overexpression.[71] However, there is no clear evidence so far that MHC class I downregulation may be due to HPV gene expression. Furthermore, studies by Cromme and collaborators[63] have revealed that absence of MHC class I molecules in HPV-associated cervical cancers was due to abrogation of post-transcriptional mechanisms and was not related to HPV E7 transcription or *c-myc* overexpression. However, the same group revealed that downregulation of MHC class I protein in cervical carcinoma cells strongly correlated with loss of the TAP-1 transporter protein.[66,72] Inasmuch as TAP transporters participate in antigenic peptide transportation into the endoplasmic reticulum (see Figure 2A), their loss may indeed result in destabilization and degradation of MHC class I molecules. These results strongly imply the role of TAP proteins in the presentation of HPV-related antigenic peptides and evaluation of their expression might be of prognostic importance.

Little is known about a possible abrogation of MHC class II molecules. Normal keratinocytes do not constitutively express these molecules; however, they may be induced by several immuno-regulatory cytokines released by, e.g., inflammatory leukocytes.[73] Studies on MHC class II molecules on HPV-harboring epithelial cells have revealed that their expression may be upregulated in some lesions including cervical carcinomas[62,64,74] and that this upregulation was associated with the presence of leukocytic infiltrates.[26,65,68]

Expression of MHC class II molecules by lesional epithelia appears to not have a significant prognostic value. However, it might be speculated that MHC class II molecule expression on keratinocytes or other epithelial cells may facilitate their killing by a subset of CD4+ CTL.[75] Furthermore, the presence of functional MHC class II molecules may enable keratinocytes to present antigens to infiltrating Th cells. However, the keratinocytes are not professional APC and therefore they may present antigens in a tolerogenic way that might result in induction of T cell anergy.[76,77]

4.   Other APC Molecules and Factors Participating in Antigen Presentation and T Cell Activation

Although MHC molecules play a primary role in antigen presentation and T cell activation, participation of other cell-associated molecules and some soluble factors also appear to be necessary. The molecules that are expressed by APC and are also involved in antigen presentation are intercellular adhesion molecule 1 (ICAM-1), leukocyte function antigen 3 (LFA-3), and B7.1/B7.2, which are recognized and bound by respective LFA-1, LFA-2, and CD28/CTLA-4 molecules present on lymphocytes.[78,79] Furthermore, activation of T cells also requires costimulation by a variety of immunoregulatory cytokines produced by APC.[80] Both adhesion molecules and cytokines provide a costimulatory signal to T cells and are necessary for effective activation of specific immune responses.

ICAM-1 is not constitutively expressed by normal keratinocytes and cervical epithelium; however, its expression may be induced by some cytokines such as interferon γ (IFN-γ), tumor necrosis factor α (TNF-α), and IL-1.[73,81] Indeed, ICAM-1 has been reported to be expressed in HPV-associated lesions and was usually related to the presence of immune infiltrates.[12,26,28,82] Interestingly, ICAM-1 expression has also been demonstrated in HPV16-harboring cervical and vulval cell lines such as CaSki, SiHa, and SKv.[82,83] The nature of this "spontaneous" ICAM-1 expression in these cell lines is unclear. It is plausible, however, that it may be due to some autocrine stimulation as found for SKv cells in which ICAM-1 expression has been found to be due to autocrine activation by TNF-α.[83]

The presence of ICAM-1 on keratinocytes appears to facilitate T cell binding[84,85] and has been reported to be necessary for activation of CD8[+] CTL and target cell killing.[86] Thus, ICAM-1 expression by HPV-harboring neoplastic cells may be an advantageous event enhancing induction of specific T cell responses and lesion regression.

There is little known about expression and a possible role of B7 molecules in induction of anti-HPV immune responses. However, the evidence for such a role has come recently from the studies of Chen and collaborators.[87,88] Using an experimental system, they found that HPV E7-harboring murine cells cotransfected with B7 were able to elicit specific host immune responses and regression of the transplanted tumors. This finding may be of special interest in view of immunotherapy with "attenuated" tumor cells as stimulators of specific anti-tumor immunity.

B. Activation and Regulatory Role of Specific T Helper Cells

Activation of CD4[+] Th cells is mediated by specific T cell receptors (TCR) associated with CD3 complex molecules that recognize antigenic determinants presented by APC in context of MHC class II molecules as well as by accessory molecules and cytokines.[79,89,90] Proper activation of Th cells leads to their proliferation, recruitment to the site of reaction, and production of immunoregulatory cytokines that are necessary for further induction of the effector cell-mediated and humoral immunity. Accordingly, CD4[+] Th cells were found to be a predominant cell type in the infiltrates of regressing HPV-associated genital lesions[12,91] or in delayed-type hypersensitivity reaction to HPV16 E7 protein in preimmunized mice.[92,93] These CD4[+] Th cells are a source of immuno-regulatory cytokines and their presence appears to be necessary for local stimulation of effector CTL, NK cells, and macrophages which, in turn, are responsible for direct killing of HPV-harboring keratinocytes.

Studies on Th cell function have revealed the existence of at least two different populations of CD4[+] cells differing in immunoregulatory cytokine production and an ability to support either cellular or humoral effector mechanisms (Figure 3).[89,90] Depending on the nature of APC and costimulatory cytokines, they may differentiate into type 1 (Th1) or type 2 (Th2) cells. Th1 cells produce IL-2, IL-15, IFN-γ, and TNF-β and stimulate the effector cells responsible for cell-mediated or delayed-type hypersensitivity (DTH), i.e., CTL, macrophages, and NK cells. On the other hand, Th2 cells release IL-4, IL-5, IL-6, IL-10, and IL-13 and provide a help for immunoglobulin synthesis by B cells. Furthermore, Th2 cytokines (IL-4, IL-10, and IL-13) exert an inhibitory effect on production of cytokines by Th1 cells, thus inhibiting cell-mediated immunity reactions.[89,90] On the contrary, the function of Th2 cells may be downregulated by IFN-γ. Accordingly, a normal immune response appears to be dependent on a proper balance between Th1 and Th2 activities. Inasmuch as cellular immunity, namely cell-mediated cytotoxicity mechanisms, that play a crucial role in eradication of virus-infected and neoplastic cells, are dependent on the cytokines released by Th1 cells, enhanced activity of Th2 cells may lead to suppression of specific anti-viral and anti-tumor responses.

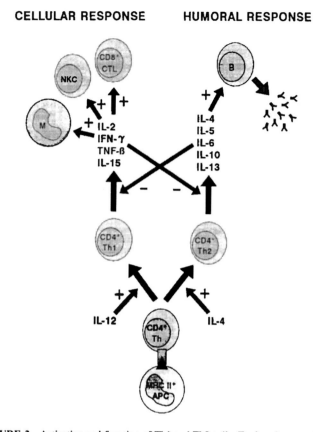

FIGURE 3 Activation and function of Th1 and Th2 cells. Explanations are in text.

The role of Th1 and Th2 cells in maintaining the anti-HPV immunity is as yet poorly recognized. HPV16 E7 has been found to elicit both Th1 and Th2 responses in the immunized mice.[94] Furthermore, a preliminary analysis of cytokine profile of T cells present in infiltrates mediating regression of HPV-associated lesions has revealed a high prevalence of Th1 phenotype.[95] Since Th1 cells are likely to play a crucial role in regression of HPV-associated lesions, it is intriguing to speculate that lesion persistence and progression might be related to abrogation of Th1 cell function and/or suppressive activity of Th2 cells.

An excellent model for the study on a possible suppressive mechanisms responsive for lesion persistence and malignant progression appears to be *epidermodysplasia verruciformis* (EV) characterized by specific immunotolerance against the disease-specific HPV (EV HPV) types.[96] This immunotolerance is manifested by T cell unresponsiveness to EV HPV-harboring keratinocytes.[97] Although the mechanism of this unresponsiveness is unknown, participation of some immunosuppressive factors cannot be excluded. The keratinocytes from EV lesions have been found to express and release transforming growth factor β (TGF-β),[98] and this cytokine has been reported to exert a strong inhibitory effect on proliferation of T cells and to abrogate Th1 cell functions.[99-101] Thus, TGF-β that has been demonstrated to be produced by some HPV-harboring tumor cell lines[102,103] may, at least partially, account for abrogation of local activation of T cells and for HPV-associated lesion progression.

A way by which HPV antigen(s) is delivered to the organism may also influence induction of the regulatory T cell responses. It has been found that priming of immunocompetent mice with low amounts of HPV16 E7 protein resulted in sustained immune unresponsiveness and loss of Th1-stimulated cell-mediated immunity against transplanted syngeneic HPV16 E7-harboring keratinocytes.[104]

In conclusion, analysis of activation status and functional phenotype of intralesional and circulating specific Th cells may be of some clinical and prognostic value. This may be supported by the most recent observation by Kadish and collaborators[105] that Th proliferatory responses to HPV16 E6 and E7 antigenic peptides are prerequisite of cervical lesion regression. Th1/Th2 cell function may be also a possible target for immunomodulatory treatment and should be considered as an important factor in course of anti-HPV vaccination.

III. EFFECTOR MECHANISMS OF ANTI-HPV IMMUNE SURVEILLANCE

The effector mechanisms involved in immune surveillance against HPV include humoral (antibody) response, cell-mediated cytotoxicity reactions, and participation of some immunoregulatory/antitumor cytokines. Antibody response appears to be significant for neutralization of virus particles and prevention of the spread of infection. On the other hand, cell-mediated cytotoxicity reactions and antitumor cytokines are the main factors involved in eradication of neoplastic cells and lesion regression.

A. The Role and Significance of Humoral Response

The specific humoral responses against HPV late and early gene products have been detected in patients with various HPV infections as well as in the experimental systems.[5-8,10] In a majority of studies, antibodies were detected by Western blotting or enzyme-linked immunosorbent assays (ELISA) using bacterially expressed fusion proteins or synthetic peptides as an antigen. However, such antigens, especially L1 and L2 fusion proteins and peptides, usually do not express native conformational epitopes that might serve as a real target for anti-HPV humoral response *in vivo*. Therefore, detection of antibodies against native capsid antigens that neutralize virus particles and may prevent HPV appears to be of higher diagnostic and prognostic value. Recently, production of empty virus-like particles (VLP) displaying native conformational epitopes has been developed using a recombinant baculovirus/insect cell expression system.[106,107] A similar system has also been used in attempts to obtain native HPV early proteins.[108,109]

Intact HPV capsid proteins and VLP have been found to elicit a specific humoral response in a variety of experimental systems.[106,110-114] A high prevalence of anti-capsid or anti-VLP antibodies has also been found in sera of patients with various HPV-associated benign and malignant lesions.[113,115-117] These antibodies appear to be of limited significance for immune control of tumor cell growth and progression. However, both polyclonal and monoclonal anti-capsid antibodies were demonstrated to specifically neutralize virus particles[112,113,118-121] and to prevent their infectivity *in vivo*.[119,120] This constitutes a basis for preparation of effective prophylactic vaccines for protection against HPV infections. Accordingly, preimmunization of rabbits with CRPV native L1 protein or VLP resulted in their significant resistance to CRVP infection.[122,123]

The biological significance of humoral response against HPV early proteins also appears to be limited. However, detection of these antibodies might be of some diagnostic and prognostic value. It has been reported that the prevalence of antibodies against certain HPV early proteins is significantly higher in patients with malignant cervical carcinomas than in asymptomatic control persons and patients with low grade CIN.[124-129] The studies on possible prognostic significance of serum antibodies against different HPV early proteins require, however, further standardization of the specific antibody detection methods.

B. The Role of Cell-Mediated Cytotoxicity

Cytotoxic effector cells are present among the leukocytes infiltrating HPV-associated lesions and appear to be the main effectors responsible for destruction of HPV-harboring cells. The important cells involved in elimination of HPV-infected neoplastic cells are CTL, natural cytotoxic cells, and macrophages.

1.   The Role of Cytotoxic T Lymphocytes (CTL)

CD8[+] CTL are considered to be the most important cells responsible for antigen-specific MHC-restricted eradication of tumor and virus-infected cells. CD8[+] CTL specifically recognize the target cells on a basis of antigenic peptides presented by MHC class I molecules.[79,81] Some of such HPV E6 and E7 protein-derived peptides have already been demonstrated to trigger the specific CTL cytotoxic response,[130,131] suggesting that these proteins may be tumor rejection antigens. Cytotoxic properties may also be attributed to some subsets of CD4[+] T cells.[75]

The role of CTL has been documented for the first time on the Shope papilloma-carcinoma model.[132] These studies have revealed that lymphocytes isolated from lymph nodes of rabbits in which CRPV-induced lesions had regressed are able to invade and destroy lesional tissues in an *in vitro* system. Furthermore, it has been found that preimmunization of mice with cells transfected with HPV16 E6 or E7 resulted in regression of syngeneic HPV16 E6 or E7-expressing tumors.[130,131] Rejection of these E6 or E7 expressing tumor cells depended on CD8[+] CTL, and their specific lysis could be demonstrated *in vitro* using lymphocytes isolated from regressor animals. Similar results were also obtained in rats preimmunized with vaccinia virus recombinants expressing HPV16 E6 or E7[133] and in mice preimmunized with HPV16 E7 peptide constituting CTL epitope.[47]

Generation of specific cytotoxicity of human CTL against target cells presenting HPV-associated antigenic epitopes has also been reported.[49,52] However, lack of a suitable MHC class I-compatible HPV-expressing cell system hampers the studies on evaluation of the specific CTL responses in the patients. There exists a possibility of using as targets autologous Epstein-Barr virus-immortalized lymphoblastoid B cell lines infected with recombinant HPV open reading frame containing vaccinia virus.[52] A possible significance of this system for evaluation of patients' anti-HPV CTL-mediated cytotoxicity needs, however, to be confirmed.

While the most CTL display specific T cell antigen receptors (TCR) composed of α and β chains, the cytotoxic activity is also a property of T cells expressing TCR composed of γ and δ chains (γδT cells).[134,135] These cells may be present in the epidermis[79,134] and therefore may play an important role in eradication of HPV-infected cells. Most recently, cytotoxic γδT cell lines specific against Shope carcinoma cells have been established from rabbits bearing Shope papillomas and carcinomas.[136] However, a possible role of human γδT cells in cytotoxicity against HPV-associated tumors is still unknown.

2.   The Role of Natural Cytotoxic Cells

Natural cytotoxic lymphoid cells are defined by spontaneous, MHC-unrestricted ability to recognize and lyse a variety of tumor and virus-infected cells, and are therefore considered to constitute the first line of host defense against neoplasia and viral infections.[137,138] They are heterogenous in respect of the phenotype; however, the most common are natural killer (NK) cells having large granular lymphocyte morphology, displaying neither T nor B cell markers, and sharing CD16 and CD56 molecules.[139] Natural cytotoxic ability may be also displayed by some CD3[+] CD56[+] T lymphocytes mostly γδT cells,[134,140] as well as by activated macrophages/monocytes.[141] A lytic activity of natural cytotoxic cells may be upregulated by several factors, such as IL-2,[142] interferons (IFN),[143] IL-6,[144] and IL-12.[145] A prolonged stimulation of lymphocytes with IL-2 leads to generation of the so called lymphokine-activated killer (LAK) cells with a very high cytotoxic potential and a very broad spectrum of target cell recognition.[146] These LAK cells are mostly derived from precursors with NK cell characteristics; however, a proportion of them may also share T cell markers.

Normal human keratinocytes (NHK) are resistant to NK cell-mediated cytotoxicity.[83,147] However, in the *in vitro* systems, nonadherent CD16[+] NK cells have been found to recognize and kill HPV16-harboring SKv cells established from bowenoid papulosis[83,148] and EV-derived HPV5-harboring keratinocytes.[147] On the contrary, the majority of HPV16 DNA-immortalized cervical epithelial cells as well as some HPV16- and HPV18-positive cervical carcinoma cell lines were found to be resistant.[83,149] However, these cells were found to be susceptible to LAK cells.[149-151]

These data together with the observations that the cells with natural cytotoxic phenotype are present in leukocyte infiltrates mediating regression of HPV-associated lesions[65,152-154] may strongly imply that these cells are actively involved in eradication of HPV-induced neoplasia.

The specific target structures recognized by natural cytotoxic cells and triggering the cytotoxic reaction are still unrecognized. It is known that NK cell-target interactions may involve participation of some adhesion molecules.[139] Indeed, expression of ICAM-1 by SKv cells has been found to be crucial for their recognition and killing by unstimulated NK cells.[83] Inasmsuch as NHK are resistant to lysis by NK cells, it is also plausible that susceptibility of HPV-harboring cells to natural cell-mediated cytotoxicity is linked to virus infection. It has been demonstrated that transfection of murine 3T3 cells with DNA coding for a HPV16 E7 oncoprotein having a functional pRB binding domain results in their susceptibility to lysis by activated macrophages.[155] The mechanism of E7-induced susceptibility as well as a possible role of other HPV proteins remain, however, to be elucidated.

Determination of NK cell cytotoxicity against disease-specific HPV-harboring target cells may be of clinical relevance. While NK cell activity against standard K562 erythroleukemic target cells has been found to be preserved, a significant decrease of NK cell cytotoxicity against HPV16- and HPV5-harboring targets has been reported in patients with persistent HPV16-associated anogenital lesions[148,156] and EV,[147] respectively. This decrease was found to be associated with inability of effector cells to recognize and bind HPV16-harboring SKv cells.[156] Moreover, while patients' NK cell cytotoxicity against K562 erythroleukemic cells could be upregulated by IL-2 or IFNs, lysis of SKv cells was not increased. This HPV-harboring target-restricted defect of NK cell activity was found to be reversible after successful surgical treatment or spontaneous regression of the lesions.[156] It is therefore plausible that abrogation of NK cell activity depends on persisting lesions and may be related to some circulating blocking factor(s) originating from HPV-transformed cells. Indeed, the presence of such yet uncharacterized factor(s) inhibiting lysis of SKv cells has been demonstrated in patients' sera[147] and culture supernatants from SKv cells.[157] Detection of such blocking factor(s) might be of prognostic value and might also serve as targets for a potential therapeutical intervention.

NK cell activity has also been evaluated in CIN2 patients treated with IFNα.[158] It has been found that patients in whom IFNα treatment resulted in lesion regression had a significantly higher baseline NK cell activity which was further increased during treatment. On the contrary, nonresponding patients had low NK cell activity and no increase could be seen. This further suggests that NK cell cytotoxicity evaluation might be of some prognostic value.

3. Modulation of Sensitivity to Cell-Mediated Cytotoxicity as a Possible Tool for Facilitating Lesion Regression

Immunohistochemical and histopathological analysis have demonstrated that potentially cytotoxic CD8+ CTL, CD16+ CD56+ NK cells, and macrophages are present in immune infiltrates in HPV-associated lesions.[65,152-154,159-161] Although CTL present in cervical cancer infiltrates were found to be inactive on a basis of their low expression of granule cytolysins,[162] these cells appear to retain lytic capabilities, inasmuch as in vitro expanded IL-2 stimulated tumor-infiltrating lymphocytes from cervical carcinomas were found to be able to efficiently kill heterologous tumor cells.[163,164] This strongly suggests that persistence and progression of HPV-associated lesions may be due to abrogated CTL stimulation and/or loss of susceptibility of HPV-harboring malignant cells to cell-mediated cytotoxicity.

Lack of CTL stimulation and loss of sensitivity to CTL could be primarily associated with loss of functional class I MHC molecules.[165] A decreased susceptibility might be also due to lowered expression of some accessory adhesion molecules such as ICAM-1.[166] It is therefore possible that the susceptibility of target cells to recognition and lysis by effector cytotoxic cells might be increased by upregulating MHC and/or adhesion molecule expression. Expression of MHC class I and II molecules as well as ICAM-1 in HPV-16-harboring keratinocytes was found to be strongly upregulated by treatment with IFN-γ and TNF-α,[82,83,166] and target cell pretreatment with IFN-γ has been demonstrated to enhance CTL-mediated lysis of allogeneic keratinocytes,[86] as well as result in an increased susceptibility of HPV-harboring cells to lysis by LAK cells.[151] This implies that local application of these cytokines and other similarly acting agents might be helpful in treatment of some persistent and progressively growing HPV-associated lesions. Furthermore, such local or systemic application of immunomodulatory cytokines might also be used as adjuvant treatment to therapeutic vaccination.

Loss of sensitivity to lysis may also result from an increased tumor cell resistance to soluble cytotoxic factors (cytolysins) released by infiltrating cytotoxic cells. Therefore, another therapeutic possibility could be application of factors that would interfere with the resistance mechanisms. Leukoregulin, a 50 kDa lymphokine which increases tumor cell membrane permeability,[167] appears to be a possible candidate. This cytokine has been reported to significantly enhance the susceptibility of HPV16 DNA-immortalized epithelial cells and cervical carcinoma cells to lysis by both NK and LAK cells.[149,150]

C.   The Role of Immunoregulatory/Antitumor Cytokines

Normal keratinocytes are a significant source of a variety of immunoregulatory cytokines.[168,169] Some of these keratinocyte-derived cytokines may also exert direct and indirect antiviral and antitumor effects, thus being an important factor in surveillance against HPV-associated neoplasia. Some cytokines locally released by infiltrating leukocytes may play a crucial role in anti-HPV responses.

1.   Direct Effects of Cytokines on HPV-Infected Cell Growth

The main immunoregulatory/antitumor cytokines shown to have a direct effect on HPV-associated neoplasia are TNFα, TGFβ, IL-1, IL-6, interferons, and leukoregulin (Table 1). Some of these cytokines were found to inhibit growth of premalignant HPV-harboring cell lines.[102,103,170,171] and this effect may be, at least partially, due to downregulation of HPV E6 and E7 oncoprotein expression.[83,102,103,172-175] Antiproliferative effects of these cytokines may also be associated with inhibition of some cellular protooncogene, e.g., *c-myc*,[176,177] and/or stimulation of antioncogene, e.g., pRB,[178] expression. TNFα may also exert direct cytotoxic effect on HPV-harboring cells inasmuch as expression of this cytokine by infiltrating immune cells has been found to be associated with apoptotic cell death in regressing Shope papillomas.[179] On the contrary, in some instances, TNFα, IL-1, and IL-6 may be also responsible for indirect stimulation of HPV-harboring important and malignant cell growth.[175,180] These cytokines were found to induce expression of TGFα and amphiregulin, two epidermal growth factor receptor ligands that, in turn, stimulated cell proliferation in an autocrine manner. It should be stressed, however, that data on stimulatory effects of TNFα, IL-1, and IL-6 were obtained in other cell culture conditions. Thus, the way by which HPV-infected cells respond to some antitumor cytokines may depend on some other, yet unidentified, factors. Their identification is necessary regarding a possible therapeutic application of antitumor cytokines.

Immunoregulatory/antitumor cytokines, i.e., TNF-α, TGF-β, and IL-6, that may exert some direct or indirect antitumor activity, were also found to be spontaneously expressed and released by HPV-harboring cells.[98,170,181] The nature of this spontaneous expression is unknown. Nevertheless, it provides evidence for existence of autocrine regulatory mechanisms that may inhibit expression of HPV genes and prevent accelerated proliferation of the infected/immortalized cells. This mechanism might explain a slow, self-limited growth of some premalignant as well as potentially malignant HPV-associated lesions.

A progressive growth of some HPV-associated tumors may be, at least partially, related to cell escape from autocrine or paracrine cytokine-mediated surveillance. Unlike nontumorigenic HPV DNA-immortalized keratinocytes and cervical epithelial cell lines, highly tumorigenic cervical carcinoma cell lines were found to be resistant to antiproliferative and anti-HPV effects of

TABLE 1   Direct Effects of Cytokines with Potent Antitumor Properties in HPV-Harboring Cells

Cytokine	Effect on HPV E6/E7 expression	Effect on cell growth	Other direct effects
TNF-α and β	–	– or +	Upregulation of MHC and adhesion molecule expression; induction of chemokine, IL-1, IL-6, and other cytokine expression
INF-α, β, and γ	–	–	Upregulation of MHC and adhesion molecule expression
TGF-β	–	–	?
IL-1	–	0 or +	Induction of chemokine and IL-6 expression
Leukoregulin	–	–	Increase of susceptibility to NK/LAK cell-mediated cytotoxicity

Note: – = Inhibitory effect; + = stimulatory effect; 0 = no apparent effect.

TGF-β.[102,103] An example of the escape from autocrine cytokine control is also an acquirement of resistance to autocrine antiproliferative activity of TNF-α by HPV16-harboring SKv cell lines that is associated with an accelerated *in vitro* growth and an increased tumorigenicity in *nu/nu* mice.[182] This resistance to TNF-α and an increased cell tumorigenicity were found to be associated with a decreased expression of a TNF receptor (TNF-R)[182] as well as with an increased shedding rate of extracellular ligand-binding TNF-R domain.[183,184] This soluble TNF-R (sTNF-R) binds to and neutralizes TNF-α activity, and was found to stimulate *in vitro* proliferation of TNF-sensitive and weakly tumorigenic SKv cells.[184] This effect appears to be probably due to protection against autocrine TNF-α-mediated growth inhibition.

Release of sTNF-R by some HPV-harboring cells strongly implies that detection of this factor may be of some clinical and prognostic value. Indeed, we found significantly increased levels of circulating sTNF-R in some patients with various HPV-associated long-lasting and progressive lesion.[183,185] High levels of circulating sTNF-R correlated with a high grade of cervical carcinoma and, interestingly, were also present in some patients with benign HPV6/11-associated anogenital condylomas.[185] The clinical relevance of these findings remains to be elucidated; nevertheless, it is conceivable that high levels of circulating sTNF-R might facilitate growth of HPV-associated lesions.

2.   The Role of Cytokines Released by HPV-Infected Cells in Induction of Tumor Regression

Besides their apparent direct antitumor and antiviral effects, immunoregulatory cytokines released by HPV-infected keratinocytes may be also involved in inducing the immune cell-mediated mechanisms leading to regression of the lesions (Figure 4). It is plausible that HPV-harboring cell-derived TNFα plays a crucial role in initiation of the inflammatory response. This cytokine has been found to induce expression of monocyte chemoattractant protein (MCP-1), a member of the chemokine family, in nontumorigenic HPV18-harboring HeLa-fibroblast hybrids.[173] MCP-1 is a strong activator and chemoattractant for monocytes/macrophages[186] as well as T cells[187] and may play an important role in induction of regression of HPV-associated lesions. Accordingly, expression of MCP-1 in highly tumorigenic HeLa cells transfected with full length MCP-1 cDNA resulted in induction of strong macrophage infiltrations and tumor growth retardation after transplantation of the cells into *nu/nu* mice.[188] Leukocytes attracted by chemokines into the tumor tissue may be additionally stimulated by other keratinocyte-derived cytokines such as IL-1 and IL-6. Accordingly, HPV16-harboring SKv cells were found to spontaneously produce IL-6 which, in turn, stimulated their lysis by NK cells[181] via IL-2-dependent mechanism.[144] Furthermore, cytokines released by HPV-transformed keratinocytes may stimulate expression of adhesion molecules on endothelial cells thus facilitating leukocyte migration into the epidermis.[189] Such upregulation of functional ICAM-1 and vascular cell-adhesion molecule-1 (VCAM) on endothelia has been reported by Coleman and Stanley[190] in CIN2/3 lesions.

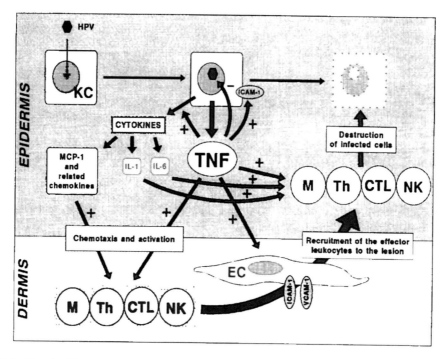

FIGURE 4 The role of immunoregulatory cytokines released by HPV-infected cells in induction of regression of HPV-associated lesions. KC = keratinocyte, NK = natural killer cell, CTL = cytotoxic T lymphocyte, M = macrophage, Th = T helper lymphocyte, EC = endothelial cell.

Any impairment of local cytokine production by HPV-harboring keratinocytes might result in a decreased leukocyte infiltration and less efficient elimination of the infected cells. Indeed, inability to express MCP-1,[173] IL-1,[191] or IL-6[192] has been found to be associated with more malignant phenotypes of several HPV-transformed cell lines. A decreased cytokine production has also been reported in cervical cells immortalized with potentially oncogenic HPV types.[193] The mechanism of this abrogated cytokine release is unknown and may be related to yet unidentified host genome alterations accompanying transformation of HPV-harboring cells.

It is tempting to speculate that local immunotherapy with some, especially chemotactic/activatory cytokines could be of some therapeutic significance and may be helpful in induction of regression of some persisting lesions. Local or systemic treatment of HPV-associated lesions with different types of IFN has been found to be associated with a higher rate of regression[194] and is already introduced into a clinical practice.

IV. SUMMARY AND CONCLUSIONS

Immune surveillance mechanisms play an important role in controlling the natural course of HPV infections. Humoral immune responses, mainly neutralizing anticapsid antibodies, are involved in prevention of infection and control of virus dissemination. On the other hand, cell-mediated cytotoxicity reactions are responsible for eradication of HPV-infected cells and are involved in lesion regression. The immunological host regulatory mechanisms are also related to the action of cytokines derived both from infected keratinocytes and infiltrating leukocytes. These cytokines may affect HPV gene expression and influence infected cell growth and differentiation. Accordingly, tumorigenic progression of HPV-associated lesions appears to be associated with an escape from immune surveillance and the most important mechanisms of this escape include loss of susceptibility to cell-mediated cytotoxicity and disregulation of immunoregulatory and antitumor cytokine network.

The studies on immunological responses against HPV and HPV-harboring neoplastic cells provide a theoretical and practical basis for the development of both prophylactic and therapeutic vaccination using, e.g., VLP and HPV early protein-derived antigenic peptides, respectively. They also provide a basis for possible application of other therapeutic modalities, e.g., local or systemic cytokine immunotherapies.

At present, practical application might include the following tests:

1. Detection of anticapsid antibodies is of some clinical value for diagnosis of HPV infection and of great importance for epidemiological studies.
2. Detection of antibodies to E6 and 7 oncoproteins, reflecting progression of HPV-associated tumors, could be of prognostic value. The seroepidemiological studies of these antibodies, especially if performed simultaneously by different methods, could also be useful in screening for anogenital malignancy.
3. Evaluation of nonspecific parameters of cellular immunity, e.g., CD4/CD8 ratio, lymphocyte transformation with mitogens, IL-2 receptor level, etc., may provide some information on general immunological status of the patient, which could be important for prognostication. Evaluation of circulating immune suppressor factors such as sTNF-R which was found to correlate with progression of the lesions, could also be of some practical significance.
4. Assessment of anti-HPV cell-mediated cytotoxicity appears to be important for prognostication. It may be evaluated with the use of NK cell-susceptible HPV-harboring target cells. In the future, it could also be possible to detect and evaluate the activity of specific CTL using HLA-matched HPV E6/7 antigen-expressing cells.
5. Immunohistopathological detection of HLA and adhesion molecule (ICAM-1) expression in HPV-infected cells might provide information on their potential susceptibility to cell-mediated cytotoxicity.
6. Determination of HLA class I and II polymorphism might be helpful assessing oncogenic risk factors, especially for cervical cancer, and for preparation of proper antigenic peptides suitable for vaccination.

ACKNOWLEDGMENTS

We would like to express our gratitude to Prof. Dr. Marek Jakobisiak for his generous help during preparation of the manuscript. We would also like to thank all colleagues who provided us with their results prior to publication. The original work presented in this chapter was supported by the State Committee for Scientific Research (KBN) grant No. 6 P207 039 06.

REFERENCES

1. Kiviat, N. B. and Koutsky, L. A., Specific human papillomavirus types as the casual agents of most cervical intraepithelial neoplasia: implications for current views and treatment, *J. Natl. Cancer Inst.*, 85, 934, 1993.
2. Obalek, S., Jablonska, S., Beaudenon, S., Walczak, L., and Orth, G., Bowenoid papulosis of the male and female genitalia: risk of cervical neoplasia, *J. Am. Acad. Dermatol.*, 14, 433, 1986.
3. zur Hausen, H., Papillomaviruses in anogenital cancer as a model to understand the role of viruses in human cancers, *Cancer Res.*, 49, 4677, 1989.
4. Howley, P. M., Role of human papillomaviruses in human cancer, *Cancer Res.*, 51, 5019s, 1991.
5. Pfister, H., Immunobiology of papillomaviruses and prospects for vaccination, in *Papillomaviruses and Human Cancer*, Pfister, H., Ed., CRC Press, Boca Raton, FL, 1990, 239.
6. Galloway, D. A. and Jenison, S. A., Characterization of the humoral immune response to genital papillomaviruses, *Mol. Biol. Med.*, 7, 59, 1990.

7. Tindle, R. W. and Frazer, I. H., Immune response to genital tract infections with human papillomaviruses, *Aust. N. Z. J. Obstet. Gynaecol.*, 30, 370, 1990.
8. Wu. T.-C., Immunology of the human papilloma virus in relation to cancer, *Curr. Opin. Immunol.*, 6, 746, 1994.
9. Frazer, I. H., Leippe, D. M., Dunn, L. A., Liem, A., Tindle, R. W., Fernando, G. J. P., Phelps, W. C., and Lambert, P. F., Immunological responses in human papillomavirus 16 E6/E7-transgenic mice to E7 protein correlate with the presence of skin disease, *Cancer Res.*, 55, 2635, 1995.
10. Jablonska, S., Majewski, S., and Malejczyk, J., HPV infection and immunological responses, in *Genitoanal Papilloma Virus Infection,* von Krogh, G., Rylander, E., Eds., Conpharm AG, Karlstad, 1989, 289.
11. Frazer, I. and Tindle, R., Cell-mediated immunity to papillomaviruses, *Papillomavirus Rep.*, 3, 53, 1992.
12. Coleman, N., Birley, H. D., Renton, A. M., Hanna, N. F., Ryait, B. K., Byrne, M., Taylor-Robinson, D., and Stanley, M. A., Immunological events in regressing genital warts, *Am. J. Clin. Pathol.*, 102, 768, 1994.
13. Benton, C., Shahidullah, H., and Hunter, J., Human papillomavirus in the immunosuppressed, *Papillomavirus Rep.*, 3, 23, 1992.
14. Petry, K. U., Scheffel, D., Bode, U., Gabrysiak, T., Kochel, H., Kupsch, E., Glaubitz, M., Nieseret, S., Kuhnle, H., and Schedel, I., Cellular immunodeficiency enhances the progression of human papillomavirus-associated lesions, *Int. J. Cancer*, 57, 836, 1994.
15. Jarrett, W. S. H., Murphy, J., O'Neil, B. W., and Laird, H. M., Virus-induced papillomas of the alimentary tract of cattle, *Int. J. Cancer*, 22, 323, 1978.
16. Dillner, J., Antibody responses to defined HPV epitopes in cervical neoplasia, *Papillomavirus Rep.*, 5, 35, 1994.
17. Germain, R. N., The biochemistry and cell biology of antigen processing and presentation, *Ann. Rev. Immunol.*, 11, 403, 1993.
18. Germain, R. N., MHC-dependent antigen processing and peptide presentation: providing ligands for T lymphocyte activation, *Cell*, 76, 287, 1994.
19. Momburg, F., Neefjes, J. J., and Hämmerling, G. J., Peptide selection by MHC-encoded TAP transporters, *Curr. Opin. Immunol.*, 6, 32, 1994.
20. van Rooijen, N., Antigen processing and presentation *in vivo*: the microenvironment as a crucial factor, *Immunol. Today*, 11, 436, 1990.
21. Knight, S. C. and Stagg, A. J., Antigen-presenting cell types, *Curr. Opin. Immunol.*, 5, 374, 1993.
22. Hamilos, D. L., Immunocompetent dendritic cells, in *The Year in Immunology, Vol. 3*, Cruse, J. M. and Lewis, R. E., Eds., S. Karger, Basel, 1988, 89.
23. van Rensburg, E. J., van Heerden, W. F., and Raubenheimer, E. J., Langerhans cells and human papillomaviruses in oesophageal and laryngeal carcinomas, *In Vivo*, 7, 229, 1993.
24. Bhawan, J., Dayal, Y., and Bhan, A. K., Langerhans cells in molluscum contagiosum, verruca vulgaris, plantar wart, and condyloma acuminatum, *J. Am. Acad. Dermatol.*, 15, 645, 1986.
25. Viac, J., Soler, C., Chardonnet, Y., Euvrard, S., and Schmitt, D., Expression of immune associated surface antigens of keratinocytes in human papillomavirus-derived lesions, *Immunobiol.*, 188, 392, 1993.
26. Lehtinen, M., Rantala, I., Toivonen, A., Luoto, H., Aine, R., Lauslahti, K., Yla-Outinen, A., Romppanen, U., and Paavonen, J., Depletion of Langerhans cells in cervical HPV infection is associated with replication of the virus, *AMPIS*, 101, 833, 1993.
27. Morelli, A. E., Belardi, G., DiPaola, G., Paredes, A., and Fainboim, L., Cellular subsets and epithelial ICAM-1 and HLA-DR expression in human papillomavirus infection of the vulva, *Acta Derm. Venereol.*, 74, 45, 1994.
28. Austyn, J. M. and Larsen, C. P., Migration patterns of dendritic leukocytes: implications for transplantation, *Transplantation*, 149, 1, 1990.
29. Zemmour, J. and Parham, P., HLA class I nucleotide sequences, *Immunobiology*, 187, 70, 1993.
30. Marsh, S. G. and Bodmer, J. G., HLA class II nucleotide sequences, *Tissue Antigens*, 40, 229, 1992.
31. Engelhard, V. H., Structure of peptides associated with MHC class I molecules, *Curr. Opin. Immunol.*, 6, 13, 1994.
32. Sinigaglia, F. and Hammer, J., Defining rules for the peptide-MHC class II interaction, *Curr. Opin. Immunol.*, 6, 52, 1994.

33. Han, R., Breiburd, F., Marche, P. N., and Orth, G., Linkage of regression and malignant conversion of rabbit viral papillomas to MHC class II genes, *Nature,* 156, 66, 1992.

34. Han, R., Breiburd, F., Marche, P. N., and Orth, G., Analysis of the nucleotide sequence variation of the antigen-binding domain of DR α and DQ α molecules as related to the evolution of papillomavirus-induced warts in rabbits, *J. Invest. Dermatol.,* 103, 376, 1994.

35. Wank, R. and Thommsen, C., High risk of squamous cell carcinoma of the cervix for women with HLA-DQw3, *Nature,* 352, 723, 1991.

36. Wank, R., Schendel, D. J., and Thommsen, C., HLA antigens and cervical carcinoma, *Nature,* 356, 22, 1992.

37. Helland, Å., Børresen, A. L., Kærn, J., Rønningen, K. S., and Thorsby, E., HLA antigens and cervical carcinoma, *Nature,* 356, 23, 1992.

38. Gregoire, L., Lawrence, W. D., Kukuruga, D., Eisenbrey, A. B., and Lancaster, W. D., Association between HLA-DQB1 alleles and risk for cervical cancer in African-American women, *Int. J. Cancer,* 57, 504, 1994.

39. Bonagura, V. R., O'Reilly, M. E., Abramson, A. L., and Steinberg, B. M., Recurrent respsiratory papillomatosis (RRP): enriched HLA DQw3 phenotype and decreased class I MHC expression, in *Immunology of Human Papillomaviruses,* Stanley, M. A., Ed., Plenum Press, New York, 1994, 195.

40. Apple, R. J., Erlich, H. A., Klitz, W., Manos, M. M., Becker, T. M., and Wheeler, C. M., HLA DR-DQ associations with cervical carcinoma show papillomavirus-type specificity, *Nature Genet.,* 6, 157, 1994.

41. Bavinck, J. N. B., Gissman, L., Claas, F. J. H., van der Woude, F. J., Persijn, G. G., ter Schegget, J., Vermeer, B. J., Johmus, I., Müller, M., Steger, G., Gebert, S., and Pfister, H., Relation between skin cancer, humoral response to human papillomavsiruses, and HLA class II molecules and renal transplant recipients, *J. Immunol.,* 151, 1579, 1993.

42. Ellis, J. R. M., Keating, P. J., Baird, J., Hounsell, E. F., Renouf, D. V., Rowe, M., Hopkins, D., Duggan-Keen, M. F., Bartholomew, J. S., Young, L. S., and Stern, P. L., The association of an HPV16 oncogene variant with HLA-B7 has implications for vaccine design in cervical cancer, *Nature Med.,* 1, 464, 1995.

43. Keating, P. J., Cromme, F. V., Duggan-Keen, M. F., Snijders, P. J., Walboomeers, J. M., Hunter, R. D., Dyer, P. A., and Stern, P. L., Frequency of downregulation of individual HLA-A and -B alleles in cervical carcinomas in relation to TAP-1 expression, *Br. J. Cancer,* 72, 405, 1995.

44. Joyce, S. and Nathenson, S. G., Methods to study peptides associated with MHC class I molecules, *Curr. Opin. Immunol.,* 6, 24, 1994.

45. Rötzschke, O. and Falk, K., Origin, structure and motifs of naturally processed MHC class II ligands, *Curr. Opin, Immunol.,* 6, 45, 1994.

46. Stauss, H. J., Davies, H., Sadovnikova, E., Chain, B., Horowitz, N., and Sinclair, C., Induction of cytotoxic T lymphocytes with peptides *in vitro:* identification of candidate T-cell epitopes in human papilloma virus, *Proc. Natl. Acad. Sci. U.S.A.,* 89, 7871, 1992.

47. Feltkamp, M. C. W., Smits, H. L., Vierboom, M. P. M., Minnaar, R. P., de Jongh, B. M., Drijfhout, J. W., ter Schegget, J., Melief, C. J. M., and Kast, W. M., Vaccination with cytotoxic T lymphocyte epitope-containing peptide protects against a tumor induced by human papillomavirus type 16-trans-formed clls, *Eur. J. Immunol.,* 23, 2242, 1993.

48. Sadovnikova, E., Zhu, X., Collins, S. M., Zhou, J., Voudsen, K., Crawford, L., Beverley, P., and Stauss, H. J., Limitations of predictive motifs revealed by cytotoxic T lymphocyte epitope mapping of the human papilloma virus E7 protein, *Int. Immunol.,* 6, 289, 1994.

49. Kast, M. W., Brandt, R. P. M., Drijfhout, J. W., and Melief, C. J. M., Human leukocyte antigen-A2.1 restricted candidate cytotoxic T lymphocyte epitopes of human papillomavisrus type 16 E6 and E7 proteins identified by using the processing-defective human cell line T2, *J. Immunother.,* 14, 115, 1993.

50. Kast, M. W., Brandt, R. P. M., Sidney, J., Drijfhout, J. W., Kubo, R. T., Grey, H. M., Melief, C. J. M., and Sette, A., Role of HLA-A motifs in identification of potential CTL epitopes in human papillomavirus type 16 E6 and E7 proteins, *J. Immunol.,* 152, 3904, 1994.

51. Bartholomew, J. S., Stacey, S. N., Coles, B., Burt, D. J., Arrand, J. R., and Stern, P. L., Identification of a naturally processed HLA A0201-restricted viral peptide from cells expressing human papillomavirus type 16 E6 oncoprotein, *Eur. J. Immunol.,* 24, 3175, 1994.

52. Tarpey, I., Stacey, S., Hickling, J., Birley, H. D. L., Renton, A., McIndoe, A., and Davies, D. H., Human cytotoxic T lymphocytes stimulated by endogenously processed human papillomavirus type II E7 recognize a peptide containing a HLA-A2 (A*0201) motif, *Immunology,* 81, 222, 1994.

53. Davies, D. H., Hill, C. M., Rothbard, J. B., and Chain, B. M., Definition of murine T helper cell determinants in the major capsid protein of human papillomavirus type 16, *J. Gen. Virol.*, 71, 2691, 1990.

54. Comeford, S. A., McCance, D. J., Dougan, G., and Tite, J. P., Identification of T- and B-cell epitopes of the E7 protein of human papillomavirus type 16, *J. Virol.*, 65, 4681, 1991.

55. Tindle, R. W., Fernando, G. J., Sterling, J. C., and Frazer, I. H., A "public" T-helper epitope of the E7 transforming protein of human papillomavirus 16 provides cognate help for several E7 B-cell epitopes from cervical cancer-associatged human papillomavirus genotypes, *Proc. Natl. Acad. Sci. U.S.A.*, 88, 5887, 1991.

56. Shepperd, P. S., Tran, T. T., Rowe, A. J., Cridland, J. C., Comeford, S. A., Chapman, M. G., and Rayfield, L. S., T cell responses to the human papillomavirus type 16 to E7 protein in mice of different haplotypes, *J. Gen. Virol.*, 73, 1269, 1992.

57. McGarvie, G. M., Grindlay, G. J., Chandrachud, L. M., O'Neill, B. W., Jarrett, W. F., and Campo, M. S., T cell responses to BPV-4 E7 during infection and mapping of T cell epitopes, *Virology*, 206, 504, 1995.

58. Strang, G., Hickling, J. K., McIndoe, G. A. J., Howland, K., Wilkinson, D., Ikeda, H., and Rothbard, J. B., Human T cell responses to human papillomavirus type 16 L1 and E6 synthetic peptides: identification of T cell determinants, HLA-DR restriction and virus type specificity, *J. Gen. Virol.*, 71, 423, 1990.

59. Kadish, A. S., Romney, S. L., Ledwidge, R., Tindle, R., Fernando, G. J. P., Zee, S., Y., van Ranst, M. A., and Birk, R. D., Cell-mediated immune responses to E7 peptides of human papillomavirus (HPV) type 16 are dependent on the HPV type infecting the cervix whereas serological reactivity in not type-specific, *J. Gen. Virol.*, 75, 2277, 1994.

60. Steele, J. C., Stankovic, T., and Gallimore, P. H., Production and characterization of human proliferative T-cell clones specific for human papillomavirus type I E4 protein, *J. Virol.*, 67, 2799, 1993.

61. Connor, M. E. and Stern, P. L., Loss of MHC class-I expression in cervical carcinomas, *Int. J. Cancer*, 46, 1029, 1990.

62. Cromme, F. V., Meijer, C. J. L. M., Snijders, P. J. F., Uyterlinde, A., Kenemans, P., Helmerhost, T., Stern, P. L., van den Brule, A. J. C., and Walboomers, J. M., Analysis of MHC class I and II expression in relation to presence of HPV genotypes in premalignant and malignant cervical lesions, *Br. J. Cancer*, 68, 1372, 1993.

63. Cromme, F. V., Snijders, P. J. F., van den Brule, A. J. C., Kenemans, P., Meijer, C. J. L. M., and Walboomers, J. M. M., MHC class I expression in HPV 16 positive cervical carcinomas is post-transcriptionally controlled and independent from *c-myc* overexpression, *Oncogene*, 8, 2969, 1993.

64. Glew, S. S., Conner, M. E., Snijders, P. J., Stanbridge, C. M., Buckley, C. H., Walboomers, J. M., Meijer, C. J., and Stern, P. L., HLA expression in pre-invasive cervical neoplasia in relation to human papilloma virus infection, *Eur. J. Cancer*, 29A, 1963, 1993.

65. Hilders, C. G., Houbiers, J. G., van Ravenswaay-Claasen, H. H., Veldhuizen, R. W., and Fleuren, G. J., Associations between HLA-expression and infiltration of immune cells in cervical carcinoma, *Lab. Invest.*, 69, 651, 1993.

66. Torres, L. M., Cabrera, T., Concha, A., Oliva, M. R., Ruiz-Cabello, F., and Garrido, F., HLA class I expression and HPV-16 sequences in premalignant and malignant lesions of the cervix, *Tissue Antigens*, 41, 65, 1993.

67. Cromme, F. V., van Bommel, P. F. J., Walboomers, J. M. M., Gallee, M. P. W., Stern, P. L., Kenemans, P., Helmerhost, T., Stukart, M. J., and Meijer, C. J. L. M., Differences in MHC and TAP-1 expression in cervical cancer lymph node metastases as compared to the primary tumours, *Br. J. Cancer*, 69, 1176, 1994.

68. Johmus, I., Dürst, M., Reid, R., Altmann, A., Bijward, K. E., Gissman, L., and Jenson, A. B., Major histocompatibility complex and human papillomavirus type 16 E7 expression in high-grade vulvar lesions, *Hum. Pathol.*, 24, 519, 1993.

69. D'Urso, C. M., Wang, Z., Cao, Y., Takake, R., Zeff, R., and Ferrone, S., Lack of HLA class I antigen expression by cultured melanoma cells FO-1 due to a defect in β2-microglobulin expression, *J. Clin. Invest.*, 87, 284, 1991.

70. Lassam, N. and Jay, G., Suppression of MHC class I RNA in highly oncogenic cells occurs at the level of transcription initiation, *J. Immunol.*, 143, 3792, 1989.

71. Maudsley, D. J. and Pound, J. D., Modulation of MHC antigen expression by viruses and oncogenes, *Immunol. Today*, 12, 429, 1991.

72. Cromme, F. V., Airey, J., Heemels, M.-T., Ploegh, H. L., Keating, P. J., Stern, P. L., Meijer, C. J. L. M., and Walboomers, J. M. M., Loss of transporter protein, encoded by the TAP-1 gene, is highly correlated with loss of HLA expression in cervical carcinomas, *J. Exp. Med.*, 179, 335, 1994.

73. Nickoloff, B. J. and Turka, L. A., Keratinocytes: immunocytes of the integument, *Am. J. Pathol.*, 143, 325, 1993.

74. Glew, S. S., Duggan-Keen, M., Cabrera, T., and Stern, P. L., HLA class II antigen expression in human papillomavirus-associated cervical cancer, *Cancer Res.*, 52, 4009, 1992.

75. Hahn, S., Gehri, R., and Erb, P., Mechanism and biological significance of CD4-mediated cytotoxicity, *Immunol. Rev.*, 146, 57, 1995.

76. Gaspari, A. A., Jenkins, M. K., and Katz, S. I., Class II MHC-bearing keratinocytes induce antigen-specific unresponsiveness for hapten specific TH-1 cells, *J. Immunol.*, 141, 2216, 1988.

77. Bal, V., McIndoe, A., Denton, G., Hudson, D., Lombardi, G., Lamb, J., Lechler, R., Antigen presentation by keratinocytes induces tolerance in human T cells, *Eur. J. Immunol.*, 20, 1893, 1990.

78. Guinan, E. C., Gribben, J. G., Boussiotis, V. A., Freeman, G. J., and Nadler, L. M., Pivotal role of the B7:CD28 pathway in transplantation tolerance and tumor immunity, *Blood*, 84, 3261, 1994.

79. Siu, G., Springer, E. A., and Hedrick, S. M., The biology of the T-cell antigen receptor and its role in the skin immune system, *J. Invest. Dermatol.*, 94, 91S, 1990.

80. Zhou, L.-J. and Tedder, T. F., A distinct pattern of cytokine gene expression by human CD83⁺ blood dendritic cells, *Blood*, 86, 3295, 1995.

81. Norris, D. A. Cytokine modulation of adhesion molecules in the regulation of immunologic cytotoxicity of epidermal targets, *J. Invest. Dermatol.*, 95, 111S, 1990.

82. Coleman, N., Greenfield, I. M., Hare, J., Kruger-Gray, H., Chain, B. M., and Stanley, M. A., Characterization and functional analysis of the expression of intercellular adhesion molecule-1 in human papillomavirus-related disease of cervical keratinocytes, *Am. J. Pathol.*, 143, 355, 1993.

83. Malejczyk, J., Majewski, S., Malejczyk, M., Skopinska, M., Hyc, A., Breitburd, F., Orth, G., and Jablonska, S., Autocrine expression of intercellular adhesion molecule-1 confers susceptibility of human papillomavirus-harboring keratinocytes to NK cell-mediated cytotoxicity: a regulatory role of tumor necrosis factor-α, submitted for publication.

84. Dustin, M. L., Singer, K. H., Tuck, D. T., and Springer, T. A., Adhesion of T lymphoblasts to epidermal keratinocytes is regulated by interferon γ and is mediated by intercellular adhesion molecule 1 (ICAM-1), *J. Exp. Med.*, 167, 1323, 1988.

85. Caughman, S. W., Lian-Jie, L., and Degitz, K., Characterization and functional analysis of interferon-γ-induced intercellular adhesion molecule-1 expression in human keratinocytes and A-431 cells, *J. Invest. Dermatol.*, 94, 22S, 1990.

86. Symington, F. W. and Santos, E. B., Lysis of human keratinocytes by allogeneic HLA class I-specific cytotoxic T cells: keratinocyste ICAM-1 (CD54) and T cell LFA-1 (CD11a/CD18) mediate enhanced lysis of IFN-γ-treated keratinocytes, *J. Immunol.*, 146, 2169, 1991.

87. Chen, L., Ashe, S., Brady, W. A., Hellström, I., Hellström, K. E., Ledbetter, J. A., McGowan, P., and Linsley, P. S., Costimulation of antitumor immunity by the B7 counterreceptor for the T lymphocyte molecules CD28 and CTLA-4, *Cell*, 71, 1093, 1992.

88. Chen, L., McGowan, P., Ashe, S., Johnston, J., Li, Y. W., Hellström, I., and Hellström, K. E., Tumor immunogenicity determines the effect of B7 costimulation on T cell-mediated tumor immunity, *J. Exp. Med.*, 179, 523, 1994.

89. Seder, R. A. and Paul, W. E., Acquisition of lymhokine-producing phenotype by CD4⁺ T cells, *Annu. Rev. Immunol.*, 12, 635, 1994.

90. Reiner, S. L. and Seder, R. A., T helper cell differentiation in immune response, *Curr. Opin. Immunol.*, 7, 360, 1995.

91. Viac, J., Chardonnet, Y., Chignol, M. C., and Schmidtt, D., Papilloma viruses, warts, carcinoma and Langerhans cells, *In Vivo*, 7, 207, 1993.

92. McLean, C. S., Sterling, J. S., Mowat, J., Nash, A. A., and Stanley, M. A., Delayed-type hypersensitivity response to the human papillomavirus type 16 E7 protein in a mouse model, *J. Gen. Virol.*, 74, 239, 1993.

93. Chambers, M. A., Stacey, S. N., Arrand, J. R., and Stanley, M. A., Delayed-type hypersensistivity response to human papillomavirus type 16 E6 protein in a mouse model, *J. Gen. Virol.*, 75, 165, 1994.

94. Tindle, R. W., Herd, K., Londono, P., Fernando, G. J., Chatfield, S. N., Malcolm, K., and Dougan, G., Chimeric hepatitis B core antigen particles containing B- and Th-epitopes of human papillomavirus type 16 E7 protein induce specific antibody and T-helper responses in immunised mice, *Virology*, 200, 547, 1994.

95. Stanley, M. A., personal communication, 1995.

96. Jablonska, S. and Majewski, S., Epidermodysplasia verruciformis: immunological and clinical aspects, *Curr. Top. Microbiol. Immunol.*, 186, 157, 1994.

97. Cooper, K. D., Androphy, E. J., Lowy, D. R., and Katz, S. I., Antigen presentation and T cell activation in epidermodysplasia verruciformis, *J. Invest. Dermatol.*, 94, 769, 1990.

98. Majewski, S., Hunzelmann, N., Nischt, R., Eckes, B., Rudnicka, L., Orth, G., Krieg, T., and Jablonska, S., TGFβ-1 and TNFα expression in the epidermis of patients with epidermodysplasia verruciformis, *J. Invest. Dermatol.*, 97, 862, 1991.

99. Rodland, K. D., Muldoon, L. L., and Magun, B. E., Cellular mechanisms of TGF-β action, *J. Invest. Dermatol.*, 94, 33S, 1990.

100. Barral, N. M., Barral, A., Brownell, C. E., Skeiky, Y. A., Ellingsworth, L. R., Twardzik, D. R., and Reed, S. G., Transforming growth factor-beta in leishmanial infection: a parasite escape mechanism, *Science*, 257, 545, 1992.

101. Yamamoto, H., Hirayama, M., Genyea, C., and Kaplan, J., TGF-β mediates natural suppressor activity of IL-2 activated lymphocytes, *J. Immunol.*, 152, 3842, 1994.

102. Woodworth, C. D., Notario, V., and DiPaolo, J. A., Transforming growth factors beta 1 and 2 transcriptionally regulate human papillomavirus (HPV) type 16 early gene expression in HPV-immortalized human genital epithelial cells, *J. Virol.*, 64, 4767, 1990.

103. Braun, L., Dürst, M., Mikumo, R., and Gruppuso, P., Differential response of nontumorigenic and tumorigenic human papillomavirus type 16-positive epithelial cells to transforming growth factor β₁, *Cancer Res.*, 50, 7324, 1990.

104. Chambers, M. A., Wei, Z., Coleman, N., Nash, A. A., and Stanley, M. A., "Natural" presentation of human papillomavirus type-16 E7 protein to immunocompetent mice results in antigen-specific sensitization or sustained unresponsiveness, *Eur. J. Immunol.*, 24, 738, 1994.

105. Kadish, A., personal communication, 1995.

106. Kirnbauer, R., Booy, F., Cheng, N., Lowy, D. R., Schiller, J. T., Papillomavirus L1 major capsid protein self-assembles into virus like particles that are highly immunogenic, *Proc. Natl. Acad. Sci. U.S.A.*, 89, 12180, 1992.

107. Rose, R. C., Bonnez, W., Reichman, R. C., and Garcea, R. L., Expression of human papillomavirus type 11 L1 protein in insect cells: *in vivo* and *in vitro* assembly of viruslike particles, *J. Virol.*, 67, 1936, 1993.

108. Park, D. S., Selvey, L. A., Kelsall, S. R., and Frazer, I. H., Human papillomavirus type 16 E6, E7 and L1 and type 18 E7 proteins produced by recombinant baculoviruses, *J. Virol. Methods*, 45, 303, 1993.

109. Bream, G. L., Ohmstede, C. A., and Phelps, W. C., Characterization of human papillomavirus type 11 E1 and E2 proteins expressed in insect cells, *J. Virol.*, 67, 2655, 1993.

110. Ghim, S. J. and Jenson, A. B., Identification of conformational epitopes of the BPV-1 capsid recognized by competitive inhibition of sera from infected or immunized animals, *Pathology*, 61, 138, 1993.

111. Rose, R. C., Bonnez, W., Da-Rin, C., McCance, D. J., and Reichman, R. C., Serological differentiation of human papillomavirus types 11, 16 and 18 using recombinant virus-like particles, *J. Gen. Virol.*, 75, 2445, 1994.

112. Christensen, N. D., Hopfl, R., DiAngelo, S. L., Cladel, N. M., Patrick, S. D., Welsh, P. A., Budgeon, L. R., Reed, C. A., and Kreider, J. W., Assembled baculovirus-expressed human papillomavirus type 11 L1 capsid protein virus-like particles are recognized by neutralizing monoclonal antibodies and induce high titres of neutralizing antibodies, *J. Gen. Virol.*, 75, 2271, 1994.

113. Rose, R. C., Reichman, R. C., and Bonnez, W., Human papillomavirus (HPV) type 11 recombinant virus-like particles indice the formation of neutralizing antibodies and detect HPV-specific antibodies in human sera, *J. Gen. Virol.*, 75, 2075, 1994.

114. Hines, J. F., Ghim, S. J., Christensen, N. D., Krieder, J. W., Barnes, W. A., Schiegel, R., and Jenson, A. B., Role of conformational epitopes expressed by human papillomavirus major capsid proteins in the serological detection of infection and prophylactic vaccination, *Gynecol. Oncol.*, 55, 13, 1994.

115. Kirnbauer, R., Hubbert, N. L., Wheeler, C. M., Becker, T. M., Lowy, D. R., and Schiller, J. T., A virus-like particle enzyme-linked immunosorbent assay detects serum antibodies in a majority of women infected with human papillomavirus type 16, *J. Natl. Cancer Inst.*, 86, 494, 1994.

116. Bonnez, W., Da-Rin, C., Rose, R. C., Tyring, S. K., and Reichman, R. C., Evolution of antibody response to human papillomavirus type 11 (HPV-11) in proteins with condyloma acuminatum according to treatment response, *J. Med. Virol.*, 39, 340, 1993.

117. Heino, P., Eklund, C., Fredriksson-Shanazarian, V., Goldman, S., Schiller, J. T., and Dillner, J., Association of serum immunoglobulin G antibodies against human papillomavirus type 16 capsids with anal epidermoid carcinoma, *J. Natl. Cancer Inst.*, 87, 437, 1995.

118. Christensen, N. D., Kreider, J. W., Shah, K. V., and Rando, R. F., Detection of human serum antibodies that neutralize infectious human papillomavirus type 11 virions, *J. Gen. Virol.*, 73, 1261, 1992.

119. Christensen, N. D., Kirnbauer, R., Schiller, J. T., Ghim,. S. J., Schlegel, R., Jenson, A. B., and Kreider, J. W., Human papillomavisrus types 6 and 11 have antigenically distinct strongly immunogenic conformationally dependent neutralizing epitopes, *Virology*, 205, 329, 1994.

120. Christensen, N. D., Cladel, N. M., and Reed, C. A., Postattachment neutralization of papillomaviruses by monoclonal and polyclonal antibodies, *Virology*, 207, 136, 1995.

121. Roden, R. B., Weissinger, E. M., Henderson, D. W., Booy, F., Kirnbauer, R., Mushinski, J. F., Lowy, D. R., and Schiller, J. T., Neutralization of bovine papillomavirus by antibodies to L1 and L2 capsid proteins, *J. Virol.*, 68, 7570, 1994.

122. Lin, Y. L., Borenstein, L. A., Ahmed, R., and Wettstein, F. O., Cottontail rabbit papillomavirus L1 protein-based vaccines: protection is achieved only with a full-length, nondenatured product, *J. Virol.*, 67, 4154, 1993.

123. Breitburd, F., Kirnbauer, R. Hubbert, N. L., Nonnenmacher, B., Trin-Dinh-Desmarquet, C., Orth, G., Schiller, J. T., and Lowy, D. R., Immunization with virus-like particles from cottontail rabbit papillomavirus (CRPV) can protect against experimental CRPV infection, *J. Virol.*, 69, 3959, 1995.

124. Jochmus-Kudielka, I., Schneider, A., Braun, R., Kimmig, R., Koldovsky, U., Schneweis, K. E., Seedorf, K., and Gissmann, L., Antibodies against the human papillomavirus type 16 early proteins in human sera: correlation of anti-E7 reactivity with cervical cancer, *J. Natl. Cancer Inst.*, 81, 1698, 1989.

125. Viscidi, R. P., Sun, Y., Tsuzaki, B., Bosch, F. X., Munoz, N., Shah, K. V., Serologic response in human papillomavirus-associated invasive cervical cancer, *Int. J. Cancer*, 55, 780, 1993.

126. Onda, T., Kanda, T., Zamma, S., Yasugi, T., Watanabe, S., Kawana, T., Ueda, K., Yoshikawa, H., Taketani, Y., and Yoshike, K., Association of antibodies against human papillomavirus 16 E4 and E7 proteins with cervical cancer positive for human papillomavirus DNA, *Int. J. Cancer*, 54, 624, 1993.

127. Ghosh, A. K., Smith, N. K., Stacey, S. N., Glew, S. S., Connor, M. E., Arrand, J. R., and Stern, P. L., Serological response to HPV 16 in cervical dysplasia and neoplasia: correlation of antibodies to E6 with cervical cancer, *Int. J. Cancer*, 53, 591, 1993.

128. Dillner, J., Lenner, P., Lehtinen, M., Eklund, C., Heino, P., Wiklund, F., Hallmans, G., and Stendahl, U., A population-based seroepidemiological study of cervical cancer, *Cancer Res.*, 54, 134, 1994.

129. Dillner, J., Wiklund, F., Lenner, P., Eklund, C., Frederiksson-Shanazarian, V., Schiller, J. T., Hibma, M., Hallmans, G., and Stendahl, U., Antibodies against linear and conformational epitopes of human papillomavirus type 16 that independently associate with incident cervical cancer, *Int. J. Cancer*, 60, 377, 1995.

130. Chen, L., Thomas, E. K., Hu, S.-L., Hellström, I., and Hellström, K. E., Human papillomavirus type 16 nucleoprotein E7 is a tumor rejection antigen, *Proc. Natl. Acad. Sci. U.S.A.*, 88, 110, 1991.

131. Chen, L., Mizuno, M. T., Singhal, M. C., Hu, S.-L., Galloway, D. A., Hellström, I., and Hellström, K. E., Induction of cytotoxic T lymphocytes specific for a syngeneic tumor expressing the E6 oncoprotein of human papillomavirus type 16, *J. Immunol.*, 148, 2617, 1992.

132. Hellström, I., Evans, C. A., and Hellström, K. E., Cellular immunity, and its serum-mediated inhibition in Shope-virus-induced rabbit papillomatosis, *Int. J. Cancer*, 4, 601, 1969.

133. Meneguzzi, G., Cerni, C., Kieny, M. P., and Lathe, P., Immunization against human papillomavirus type 16 tumor cells with recombinant vaccinia viruses expressing E6 and E7, *Virology*, 181, 62, 1991.

134. Haas, W., Pereira, P., and Tonegawa, S., Gamma/delta cells, *Annu. Rev. Immunol.*, 11, 637, 1993.

135. Kronenberg, M., Antigens recognized by γδ T cells, *Curr. Opin. Immunol.*, 6, 64, 1994.

136. Kim, C. J., Isono, T., Tomoyoshi, T., and Seto, A., Variable region sequences for T-cell receptor-gamma and -delta chains of rabbit killer cell lines against Shope carcinoma cells, *Cancer Lett.*, 89, 37, 1995.

137. Reynolds, C. W. and Wiltrout, R. H., Eds., *Functions of the Natural Immune System,* Plenum Publishing Corp., New York, 1989.

138. Welsh, R. M., Regulation of virus infections by natural killer cells, *Nat. Immun. Cell Growth Regul.,* 5, 169, 1986.

139. Storkus, W. J. and Dawson, J. R., Target structures involved in natural killing (NK) characteristics, distribution, and candidate molecules, *Crit. Rev. Immunol.,* 10, 393, 1991.

140. Hersey, P. and Bolhuis, R., "Nonspecific" MHC-unrestricted killer cells and their receptors, *Immunol. Today,* 8, 233, 1987.

141. Philip, R. and Epstein, L. B., Tumor necrosis factor as immunomodulator and mediator of monocyte cytotoxicity induced by itself, γ-interferon and interleukin-1, *Nature,* 323, 86, 1986.

142. Henney, C. S., Kuribayashi, K., Kern, D. E., and Gillis, D., Interleukin-2 augments natural killer cell activity, *Nature,* 291, 335, 1981.

143. Herbermann, R. B., Ortaldo, J. R., and Bonnard, G. D., Augmentation by interferon of human natural and antibody-dependent cell-mediated cytotoxicity, *Nature,* 227, 221, 1979.

144. Luger, T. A., Kruttmann, J., Kirnbauer, R., Urbanski, A., Schwarz, T., Klappacher, G., Köck, A., Micksche, M., Malejczyk, J., Schauer, E., May, L. T., and Sehgal, P. B., IFN-β_2 IL-6 augments the activity of human natural killer cells, *J. Immunol.,* 143, 1206, 1989.

145. Banks, R. E., Patel, P. M., and Selby, P. J., Interleukin 12: a new clinical player in cytokine therapy, *Br. J. Cancer,* 71, 655, 1995.

146. Yagita, M. and Grimm, E. A., Current understanding of the lymphokine-activated killer cell phenomenon, *Prog. Exp. Tumor Res.,* 32, 213, 1988.

147. Majewski, S., Malejczyk, J., Jablonska, S., Misiewicz, J., Rudnicka, L., Obalek, S., and Orth, G., Natural cell-mediated cytotoxicity against various target cells in patients with epidermodysplasia verruciforms, *J. Am. Acad. Dermatol.,* 22, 243, 1990.

148. Malejczyk, J., Majewski, S., Jablonska, S., Rogozinski, T. T., and Orth, G., Abrogated NK-cell lysis of human papillomavirus (HPV)-16-bearing keratinocytes in patients with pre-cancerous and cancerous HPV-induced anogenital lesions, *Int. J. Cancer,* 43, 209, 2989.

149. Furbert-Harris, P. M., Evan, C. H., Woodworth, C. D., and DiPaolo, J. A., Loss of leukoregulin upregulation of natural killer but not lymphokine-activated killer lymphocytotoxicity in human papillomavirus 16 DNA-immortalized cervical epithelial cells, *J. Natl. Cancer Inst.,* 81, 1080, 1989.

150. Evans, C. H., Flugelman, A. A., and DiPaolo, J. A., Cytokine modulation of immune defenses in cervical cancer, *Oncology,* 50, 245, 1993.

151. Wu, R., Coleman, N., Higgins, G., Choolun, E., and Stanley, M. A., Lymphocyte-mediated cytotoxicity to HPV16 infected cervical keratinocytes, in *Immunology of Human Papillomaviruses,* Stanley, M. A., Ed., Plenum Press, New York, 1994, 255.

152. Syrjänen, K., Väyrynen, M., Mäntyjärvi, R., Castren, O., and Saarikoski, S., Natural killer (NK) cells with HNK-1 phenotype in the cervical biopsies of women follow-up for human papillomavirus (HPV) lesions, *Acta Obstet. Gynecol. Scand.,* 65, 139, 1986.

153. Tay, S. K., Jenkins, D., and Singer, A., Natural killer cells in cervical intraepithelial neoplasia and human papillomavirus infection, *Br. J. Obstet. Gynaecol.,* 94, 901, 1987.

154. Bishop, P. E., McMillan, A., and Fletcher, S., An immunohistological study of spontaneous regression of condylomata acuminata, *Genitourin. Med.,* 66, 901, 1987.

155. Banks, L., Moreau, F., Voudsen, K., Pim, D., and Matlashewski, G., Expression of the human papillomavirus E7 oncogene during cell transformation is sufficient to induce susceptibility to lysis by activated macrophages, *J. Immunol.,* 146, 2037, 1991.

156. Malejczyk, J., Malejczyk, M., Majewski, S., Orth, G., and Jablonska, S., NK-cell activity in patients with HPV16-associated anogenital tumors: defective recognition of HPV16-harboring keratinocytes and restricted unresponsiveness to immunostimulatory cytokines, *Int. J. Cancer,* 54, 917, 1993.

157. Jablonska, S., Majewski, S., and Malejczyk, J., Die Immunologie von HPV-Infektionen und der Mechanismus einer latenten Infektion, *Hautarzt,* 43, 305, 1992.

158. Garzetti, G. G., Ciavattini, A., Romanini, C., Goreti, G., Tranquilli, A. L., Muzzioli, M., and Fabris, N., Interferon alpha 2b treatment of cervical intraepithelial neoplasia grade 2: modulation of natural killer cell, *Gynecol. Obstet. Invest.,* 37, 304, 1994.

159. Iwatsuki, K., Tagami, H., Takigawa, M., and Yamada, M., Plane warts under spontaneous regression. Immunopathologic study on cellular constituents leading to the inflammatory reaction, *Arch. Dermatol.,* 122, 655, 1986.

160. Tay, S. K., Jenkins, D., Maddox, P., and Singer, A., Lymphocyte phenotypes in cervical intraepithelial neoplasia and human papillomavirus infection, *Br. J. Obstet. Gynaecol.*, 94, 16, 1987.

161. Tay, S. K., Jenkins, D., Maddox, P., Hogg, N., and Singer, A., Tissue macrophage response in human papillomavirus infection and cervical intrepithelial neoplasia, *Br. J. Obstet. Gynaecol.*, 94, 1094, 1987.

162. Cromme, F. V., Walboomers, J. M. M., Stukart, M. J., Kummer, J. A., Leonhart, A. M., Helmerhorst, T. J. M., and Meijer, C. J. L. M., Lack of granzyme expression in T-lymphocytes indicates poor CTL activation in HPV-associated cervical carcinomas, submitted for publication.

163. Ghosh, A. K. and Moore, M., Tumour-infiltrating lymphocytes in cervical carcinoma, *Eur. J. Cancer*, 28A, 1910, 1992.

164. Ghosh, A. K. Glenville, S., Bartholomew, J., and Stern, P. L., Analysis of tumour-infiltrating lymphocytes in cervical carcinoma, in *Immunology of Human Papillomaviruses*, Stanley, M. A., Ed., Plenum Press, New York, 1994, 249.

165. Duggan-Keen, M., Keating, P., Cromme, F. V., Walboomers, J. M. M., and Stern, P. L., Alterations in major histocompatibility complex expression in cervical cancer: possible consequences for immunotherapy, *Papillomavirus Rep.*, 5, 3, 1994.

166. Majewski, S., Bretburd, F., Orth, G., and Jablonska, S., Regulation of MHC class I, class II and ICAM-1 expression by cytokines and retinoids in HPV-harboring keratinocyte lines, in *Immunology of Human Papillomaviruses*, Stanley, M. A., Ed., Plenum Press, New York, 1994, 207.

167. Barnett, S. C. and Evans, C. H., Leukoregulin-increased plasma membrane permeability and associated ionic fluxes, *Cancer Res.*, 46, 2686, 1986.

168. Luger, T. A., Epidermal cytokines, *Acta Derm. Venereol.*, 69 (Suppl. 151), 61, 1989.

169. Luger, T. A. and Schwarz, T., Epidermal cell-derived cytokines, in *Skin Immune System (SIS)*, Bos, J. D., Ed., CRC Press, Boca Raton, FL., 1990, 257.

170. Malejczyk, J., Malejczyk, M., Köck, A., Urbanski, A., Majewski, S., Hunzelmann, N., Jablonska, S., Orth, G., and Luger, T. A., Autocrine growth limitation of human papillomavirus type 16-harboring keratinocytes by constitutively released tumor necrosis factor-α, *J. Immunol.*, 149, 2702, 1992.

171. Villa, L. L., Vieira, K. B. L., Pei, X.-F., and Schlegel, R., Differential effect of tumor necrosis factor on proliferation of primary human keratinocytes and cell lines containing human papillomavirus types 16 and 18, *Mol. Carcinogenesis*, 6, 5, 1992.

172. Woodworth, C. D., Lichti, U., Simpson, S., Evans, C. H., and DiPaolo, J. A., Leukoregulin and gamma-interferon inhibit human papillomavirus type 16 gene transcription in human papillomavirus-immortalized human cervical cell, *Cancer Res.*, 52, 456, 1992.

173. Rösl, F., Lengert, M., Albrecht, J., Kleine, K., Zawatzky, R., Achraven, B., and zur Hausen, H., Differential regulation of the JE gene encoding the monocyte chemoattractant protein (MCP-1) in cervical carcinoma cells and derived hybrids, *J. Virol.*, 68, 2142, 1994.

174. Kyo, S., Inoue, M., Hayasaka, N., Inoue, T., Yutsudo, M., Tanizawa, O., and Hakura, A., Regulation of early gene expression of human papillomavirus type 16 by inflammatory cytokines, *Virology*, 200, 130, 1994.

175. Woodworth, C. D., McMullin, E., Iglesias, M., and Plowman, G. D., Interleukin 1α and tumor necrosis factor α stimulate autocrine amphiregulin expression and proliferation of human papillomavirus-immortalized and carcinoma-derived cervical epithelial cells, *Proc. Natl. Acad. Sci. U.S.A.*, 92, 2840, 1995.

176. Yarden, A. and Kimchi, A., Tumor necrosis factor reduces *c-myc* expression and cooperates with interferon-gamma in HeLa cells, *Science*, 234, 1419, 1986.

177. Malejczyk, J., unpublished observation.

178. Arany, I., Rady, P., and Tyring, S. K., Interferon treatment enhances the expression of underphosphorylated (biologically-active) retinoblastoma protein in human papillomavirus-infected cells through the inhibitory TGFβ1/IFNβ cytokine pathway, *Antiviral. Res.*, 23, 131, 1994.

179. Hagari, Y., Budgeon, L. R., Pickel, M. D., and Kreider, J. W., Association of tumor necrosis factor-α gene expression and apoptotic cell death with regression of Shope papillomas, *J. Invest. Dermatol.*, 104, 526, 1995.

180. Iglesias, M., Plowman, G. D., and Woodworth, C. D., Interleukin-6 and interleukin-6 soluble receptor regulate proliferation of normal, human papillomavirus-immortalized, and carcinoma-derived cervical cells *in vitro*, *Am. J. Pathol.*, 146, 944, 1995.

181. Malejczyk, J., Malejczyk, M., Urbanski, A., Köck, A., Jablonska, S., Orth, G., and Luger, T. A., Constitutive release of IL-6 by human papillomavirus type 16 (HPV16)-harboring keratinocytes: a mechanism augmenting the NK-cell-mediated lysis of HPV-bearing neoplastic cells, *Cell. Immunol.,* 136, 155, 1991.

182. Malejczyk, J., Malejczyk, M., Majewski, S., Breitburd, F., Luger, T. A., Jablonska, S., and Orth, G., Increased tumorigenicity of human papillomavirus type 16-harboring keratinocytes is associated with resistance to endogenous tumor necrosis factor-α-mediated growth limitation, *Int. J. Cancer,* 56, 593, 1994.

183. Malejczyk, J., Malejczyk, M., Majewski, S., Hyc, A., Breitburd, F., Orth, G., and Jablonska, S., Release of soluble tumor necrosis factor-α (TNF-α) receptor by HPV-associated neoplastic cells, in *Immunology of Human Papillomaviruses,* Stanley, M. A., Ed., Plenum Press, New York, 1994, 315.

184. Malejczyk, J., Malejczyk, M., Breitburd, F., Majewski, S., Schwarz, A., Expert-Besançon, N., Jablonska, S., Orth, G., and Luger, T. A., Progressive growth of human papillomavirus type 16-transformed keratinocytes is associated with an increased release of soluble tumour necrosis factor (TNF) receptor, *Br. J. Cancer,* in press.

185. Malejczyk, M. and Malejczyk, J., unpublished observations.

186. Miller, M. D. and Krangel, M. S., Biology and biochemistry of the chemokines: a family of chemotactic and inflammatory cytokines, *CRC Crit. Rev. Immunol.,* 12, 17, 1992.

187. Taub, D. D., Proost, P., Murphy, W. J., Anver, M., Longo, D. L., van Damme, J., and Oppenheim, J. J., Monocyste chemotactic protein-1 (MCP-1), -2, and -3 are chemotactic for human T lymphocytes, *J. Clin. Invest.,* 95, 1370, 1995.

188. Kleine, K., König, G., Kreutzer, J., Komitowski, D., zur Hausen, H., and Rösl, F., The effect of the JE (MCP-1) gene, which encodes monocyte chemoattractant protein-1 on the growth and derived somatic cell hybrids of HeLa-cells in nude mice, *Mol. Carcinogensis.,* 14, 179, 1995.

189. Springer, T. A., Traffic signals for lymphocyte recirculation and leukocyte emigration: the multistep paradigm, *Cell,* 76, 301, 1994.

190. Coleman, N. and Stanley, M. A., Characterization and functional analysis of the expression of vascular adhesion molecules in human papillomavirus-related disease of the cervix, *Cancer,* 74, 884, 1994.

191. Merrick, D. T. and McDougall, J. K., personal communication, 1993.

192. Fuze, A., Simizu, B., van Ranst, M., Obdenakker, G., and van Damme, J., The induction of IL-5 and gelatinase-B by II-1 in mouse cell lines transformed with bovine papillomavirus: decreased production in tumorigenic cells, *Lymphokine Cytokine Res.,* 11, 215, 1992.

193. Woodworth, C. D. and Simpson, S., Comparative lymphokine secretion by cultured normal human cervical keratinocytes, papillomavirus-immortalized, and carcinoma cell lines, *Am. J. Pathol.,* 142, 1544, 1993.

194. Cirelli, R. and Tyring, S. K., Interferons in human papillomavirus infections, *Antiviral. Res.,* 24, 191, 1994.

12

HPV-Related Disease in Immunosuppressed Individuals

Joel Palefsky

CONTENTS

I. INTRODUCTION

The association between human papillomaviruses (HPV) and epithelial cancer is now well established. Recent advances in technologies for the detection of HPV have revealed that anogenital HPV infection in sexually active young women is common,[1] and that the number of women who harbor HPV DNA at any one time far exceeds the number with HPV-associated disease. Accordingly, HPV infection is likely to be necessary but insufficient for most cases of anogenital cancer. Cofactors in the development of HPV-associated disease likely play an important role in anogenital disease pathogenesis, and may include smoking,[2-4] oral contraceptives,[5] chronic irritation,[3] and other sexually transmitted agents.[6] In recent years, it has also become clear that the outcome of HPV infection results from a complex interaction between host and viral factors at the cellular and tissue levels. At the cellular level, the HPV E6 and E7 proteins bind and inactivate important negative regulators of cell growth, the p53[7-10] and retinoblastoma gene products,[11,12] respectively, and in turn, cellular transcription factors play an important role in regulating HPV protein expression. At the tissue level, the host immune response likely plays an important role.

The role of host immunity in preventing development of HPV-associated disease was first noted in the context of epidermodysplasia verruciformis, a hereditary skin disorder associated with immune dysfunction that in conjunction with ultraviolet irradiation and HPV infection, is associated with a high incidence of epithelial cancer. With the growing practice of organ transplantation and new immunosuppressive regimens, skin cancers associated with HPV and iatrogenic immunosuppression are also being reported. Fortunately, the number of such HPV-associated cancers remains relatively small. With the advent of the HIV epidemic, however, the importance of immunosuppression as a cofactor for HPV-associated disease has increased dramatically, as a large number of individuals with HPV infection and HIV-associated immunosuppression may be at risk for development of HPV-associated epithelial neoplasia.

II.   IMMUNE RESPONSE TO HPV INFECTION

Several lines of evidence suggest that the immune response plays an important role in the control of HPV. Most convincing is the observation of an altered clinical course of HPV infection among those with immune deficiencies. The nature of the immune response to HPV remains poorly elucidated. To date, most studies of the immune response to HPV, whether cellular or humoral, have been difficult to interpret and inconsistent from group to group for a variety of reasons: (1) variability of the target antigens and assays from laboratory to laboratory, (2) inadequate assessment of HPV type-specificity, and (3) incomplete characterization of the study population. For example, there are over 65 HPV types, some of which share extensive homology at the amino acid level. Some of these are ubiquitous, such as HPV 1 and 2, which are associated with hand and foot warts. Use of an antigen to study genital HPV infection that has cross-reactivity with other HPV types may therefore result in false-positive results. With the advent of molecular biologic techniques, efforts have been made to address the issue of type-specificity using cloned putative HPV antigens and mapping the precise epitopes with deletion techniques and synthetic peptides. Both type-common and type-specific epitopes of a variety of different HPV proteins have been identified,[13-15] and reactivity was most commonly detected to the L1 fusion protein.

In general, use of these assays in large populations has produced surprising results that have been difficult to reconcile with our current notion that HPV is primarily a sexually transmitted pathogen.[16] Antibodies to the HPV 16 E4 protein were found to be widespread, having been detected in 30% of the children who were tested.[17] In other studies, antibodies to HPV 16 proteins were detected in over one half of all patients attending an STD clinic and in almost as many children with no history of sexual activity.[18] The reason for the widespread positivity remains unclear. While it could indicate that acquisition of genital HPV types is not sexual in nature, it seems likelier that the detected antibody response reflects reactivity to either nongenital HPV types, or to non-HPV antigens. Perhaps most important is the detection of antibodies in large numbers of women who appear to have HPV-associated disease, including cancer,[19] suggesting that HPV antibodies may be exerting little protective effect. As such, cell-mediated immunity (CMI) may play a more important role in defense against HPV than humoral immunity.

Studies of CMI to HPV have suffered many of the same limitations as humoral studies, and as a result, we still know very little about CMI to HPV. CMI has been measured in a variety of ways, including descriptive studies of mononuclear infiltrates in HPV-associated lesions, leukocyte migration inhibition assays, T cell proliferation assays, cell-mediated cytotoxicity, and natural killer (NK) cell activity. Previous studies have shown lymphocyte proliferative responses,[20] lymphokine release[21] and cytotoxic responses to papillomavirus virions.[22] Temporary HPV-specific stimulation has been demonstrated during regression of plane warts in immunologically intact subjects using leukocyte migration inhibition assays,[23] and Morison showed that the leukocyte migration inhibition tests of many people were positive after resolution of a wart.[24] Conversely, weak or negative responses were obtained among those with longstanding warts,[25] suggesting that the persistence of disease represents a failure of CMI.

Evidence is now accumulating for both a T cell proliferative response to HPV antigens, as well as a cell-mediated cytotoxic response. In one study, a lymphoproliferative assay was performed to elicit T cell responses in control subjects and those with dysplastic cervical smears.[26] A few patients and controls responded weakly to the fusion protein whereas a larger number responded to HPV 1 or HPV 2 virions. Studies with synthetic peptides containing putative T cell epitopes of the HPV 16 L1 and E6 proteins[27] demonstrated both type-specific and cross-reactive responses with other

HPV strains. Tindle et al.[28] point to the importance of T cell responses to a particular epitope of the E7 protein. Mice immunized with the E7 peptide "DRAHYNI" demonstrated a T cell proliferative response to the peptide and parent E7 protein. This peptide defines a T cell helper epitope for B cell proliferation. This and other immunodominant regions of E7 were also described by others in proliferative studies performed in BALB/c mice.[29] In this study, the authors note that the response to these epitopes varied from mouse strain to mouse strain. Altmann et al. recently reported generation of T cell clones from peripheral mononuclear blood cells using E7 synthetic peptides that exhibited a proliferative response to 3 different E7 epitopes. These cells were shown to express the CD4 surface glycoprotein, and were presumably recognized in the context of MHC class II molecules.[30] To date, however, little remains known about the T cell proliferative response in humans.

In addition to T cell proliferative response, several compelling reasons suggest that cell-mediated cytotoxicity could be a critical effector mechanism in immunity to HPV. First, cytotoxic T lymphocytes (CTL) are the key effector cells against many intracellular organisms. Second, other viral infections stimulate production of a large repertoire of CTL[31,32] and in selected instances, it has been demonstrated by adoptive transfer that CTL play an important role in anti-viral defense. CTL recognize viral proteins that are synthesized endogenously in infected cells, processed into peptides, and transported to the cell surface in association with MHC molecules. These viral epitopes are recognized primarily by CD8 CTL in the context of MHC class I molecules and target-effector cell binding occurs through the aid of adhesion proteins, such as LFA 1 and ICAM-1. CTL then release preformed cytolytic constituents from intracellular granules destroying cells that harbor viruses. As yet there is no direct evidence for MHC-restricted CTL in modulating HPV infection or HPV-associated disease. However, fragmentary evidence is now emerging linking several HPV proteins to possible induction of anti-viral CTL. Altmann et al.[30] have reported that T cell clones generated from human PBMC using E7 synthetic peptides exhibit specific CTL activity toward EBV-transformed autologous lymphocytes in the presence of the E7 peptides. Evidence is also emerging in animal models that links several HPV proteins to possible induction of anti-viral CTL. Protection from an HPV 16 E7-bearing syngeneic tumor could be induced in mice immunized with fibroblasts transfected with the E7 protein. If the animals were depleted of CD8 cells, no anti-tumor protective effect, and presumably no CTL, was noted.[33] Mice immunized with vaccinia virus expressing a full-length L1 transcript also produced splenic CTL which killed P815 cells expressing L1 after being restimulated with these cells.[34] Lastly, studies by Chen et al. have shown that tumor cells in mice may also be inhibited by CTL directed against the E6 protein,[35] demonstrating that multiple HPV proteins may be capable of eliciting a CTL response.

Although a cytotoxic T cell (CTL) response could therefore be one of the mechanisms of immunity to HPV, as yet there is little direct evidence for MHC-restricted CTL in modulating HPV infection or HPV-associated disease in humans. Certainly, it seems reasonable to assume that MHC-restricted CTL emerge during the course of HPV infection and that their failure to develop, failure to persist, or other inherent mechanisms that suppress their action, could play a critical role in the development of HPV disease, including cervical intraepithelial neoplasia (CIN) and possibly squamous cell cancer (SCC). Because different HPV proteins are expressed at different stages of HPV-associated disease, it is also reasonable to surmise that the specificity of CTL response may change in the course of disease progression or regression.

III. HPV-ASSOCIATED DISEASE IN IMMUNOSUPPRESSED INDIVIDUALS

A. Epidermodysplasia Verruciformis

Epidermodysplasia verruciformis (EV) was the first human disease in which HPV-associated malignancy was linked to immunosuppression. This rare X-linked recessive familial condition is characterized by numerous red-brown macules and flat warts that are typically infected with HPV 5 or

8,[36-38] although a wide variety of HPV types may be detected.[39,40] These lesions demonstrate a high rate of progression to squamous cell carcinoma, frequently in areas exposed to the sun.[36,41,42]

Patients with EV appear to have a wide range of immunologic defects. These include decreased cell-mediated cytotoxicity,[43] reduced dinitrochlorobenzene sensitivity, reduced erythrocyte rosette formation,[36,44] and a decreased number of T-helper cells.[45] NK activity was increased in about one half of the patients. Langerhans cells and their ability to present antigen were found to be intact in EV patients.[46] However, circulating T cells in that study were unresponsive to virally-infected epidermal cells, suggesting that the abnormality was in the circulating T-cell arm of the immune system.

EV has also been diagnosed in the setting of other conditions associated with immunosuppression, suggesting that the skin lesions of this disease are specifically associated with immunosuppression per se, and not necessarily with the genetic defects associated with the heritable disorder described above. These include iatrogenic immunosuppression associated with renal transplantation,[47,48] Hodgkin's disease,[49] systemic lupus erythematosis,[50] and human immunodeficiency virus infection.[51]

B.   HPV-Associated Cancers in Iatrogenically Immunosuppressed Individuals

Up to 6% of all transplant recipients have been shown to develop neoplasms during lifetime follow-up, with 1% dying of these tumors.[52] The earliest recognition of an association between iatrogenic immunosuppression and increased incidence of HPV-associated disease was made in the setting of women undergoing renal transplantation; women who underwent renal transplants with iatrogenic immunosuppression had an incidence of cervical cancer 5 times higher and vulvar cancer 100 times higher than that of age-matched controls.[53] Other studies have demonstrated increased rates of vulvar and cervical carcinoma as well.[54] In addition to increased rates of anogenital disease associated with HPV infection, a high proportion, ranging from 75–92% of renal transplant patients with graft survival over 5 years, have been shown to have cutaneous HPV infection.[48,55] Similar to EV patients, these lesions have been shown to harbor a wide variety of HPV types[48,56] and as described above, EV itself may be found among renal transplant recipients. Lastly, other HPV-associated tumors have been described as well in transplant recipients, including tumors of the head and neck[57] and bladder.[58]

Few studies have been performed to date in which the magnitude of risk attributable to immunosuppression has been quantified using age-matched controls. Clearly, the risk of anogenital and cutaneous HPV-associated disease is increased in immunosuppressed individuals, as is the variety of HPV types found in these lesions when compared to individuals with normal immunity. However, the role of immunosuppression in the pathogenesis of other diseases such as head and neck and bladder cancer is difficult to ascertain, because of the relatively small numbers of patients. It also remains unclear whether HPV-associated disease progresses more rapidly and whether HPV types that are normally nononcogenic may behave more aggressively in this setting.

C.   HPV-Related Anogenital Cancers in HIV-Associated Immunosuppression

Individuals with HIV infection appear to be at increased risk of HPV-associated anogenital disease for three reasons: (1) they are at increased risk of acquiring the etiologic agent, i.e., HPV, since acquisition of both HIV and HPV is associated with many of the same risk factors, including sexual transmission; (2) they have attenuated defense against viral infection as indicated by frequency and severity of herpes simplex virus and recurrences and cytomegalovirus disease; and (3) they have attenuated tumor surveillance as indicated by increased incidence of tumors such as Kaposi's sarcoma and non-Hodgkin's lymphoma. As described below, issues of concern in HIV-positive individuals include high prevalence of anogenital HPV infection, infection with multiple HPV types, multifocal HPV-associated anogenital disease, rapid progression of HPV-associated disease, and high likelihood of disease recurrence.

1. HPV-Associated Anogenital Cancers in HIV-Positive Men

An association between anal cancer and condyloma has been observed[3,59-62] suggesting that HPV may be an important factor in the pathogenesis of anal cancer, similar to its role in cervical cancer. This has been confirmed by several studies that demonstrated HPV directly in anal cancer tissues, and similar to cervical cancer, the predominant HPV type was HPV 16.[63-67]

Prior to the HIV epidemic, anal cancer was predominantly a disease of older women, with a female to male ratio of 2:1 to 3:1.[68,69] Receptive anal intercourse was shown to be an important risk for anal cancer in men, consistent with both its association with anal condyloma and with HPV infection.[70] However, even though the incidence of anal cancer was elevated in men with a history of receptive anal intercourse, it was still a relatively uncommon disease. Since the onset of the HIV epidemic, however, the number of new cases of anal cancer has increased more than seven-fold among single, never married men aged 20–49 in the San Francisco Bay area compared to the period spanning 1973–1978.[71] In this group, the incidence of anal cancer is approximately 8/100,000 (A. Hauser, personal communication, Surveillance, Epidemiology and End Results Program, Northern California Cancer Center), close to that of cervical cancer among American women.[72] However, assuming that a disproportionate number of cases in single, never-married men is occurring in HIV-positive homosexual men, it is likely that the incidence of anal cancer among the latter is several-fold higher than that of cervical cancer in women.

Consistent with the change in anal cancer incidence since the onset of the HIV epidemic, striking differences have been found between HIV-positive and HIV-negative men with respect to prevalence of anal HPV infection and potentially precancerous anal cytologic abnormalities. Employing techniques similar to those used for the assessment of cervical disease, anal swabs have been used to collect material for cytology and HPV DNA hybridization.[73-75] Both high level HPV infection indicative of active HPV replication as determined by ViraPap/Viratype™ positivity, or low level infection as indicated by the detection of HPV DNA by polymerase chain reaction only, were sought. Not surpisingly, a higher proportion of anal samples were found to have low level infection than high level infection.[73] However, most studies to date have concentrated on the detection of high level HPV infection. HIV-associated immunosuppression was shown to be an important risk factor for high level HPV infection, since the prevalence of HPV infection has been shown to increase with increasing immunosuppression as measured by absolute CD4 counts,[73,75] and the highest prevalence of anal HPV infection has been found among men with symptomatic (Centers for Disease Control group IV) HIV disease.[74] In general, the HPV types found in the anal canal mirrored those found in the cervix, but the proportion of men with multiple HPV types also increased with increasing degrees of immunosuppression.[73,74] Together, these data suggest that HIV-positive men are likelier to have high level anal HPV infection than HIV-negative men. While this may reflect higher exposure risk, the increased prevalence of high level HPV infection found in more immunosuppressed individuals suggests that attenuated immunity may be playing an important role in permitting active replication of HPV DNA.

Likewise, the prevalence of abnormal anal cytology, and AIN in particular, has been shown to increase with increasing degrees of immunosuppression.[73,74] Studies in Australia have also shown that detection of clinical anal lesions was likelier among men with symptomatic HIV infection.[76] Among HIV-positive men, the proportion of those with anal HPV infection who develop anal cytologic abnormalities is higher than among HIV-negative men, and this proportion increases as absolute CD4 levels decrease (J. Palefsky, unpublished data) (Figure 1). Combined with the observation that relatively few HIV-negative men with HPV infection develop anal disease, these data indicate that while HPV infection is common in HIV-negative and HIV-positive men with a history of receptive anal intercourse, development of potentially precancerous anal cytologic abnormalities in conjunction with anal HPV infection is largely an HIV-associated phenomenon. These data also may help to explain the increase in anal cancer in men with a history of receptive anal intercourse that has been observed since the onset of the HIV epidemic despite the high prevalence of anal HPV infection in that population prior to the epidemic.

The natural history of anal HPV infection and potentially precancerous disease remains poorly characterized, but available data suggest that precancerous changes may progress rapidly in the setting of advanced immunosuppression. Among men with symptomatic (Centers for Disease Control group IV) HIV disease, the proportion of the study population with anal HPV infection increased from 60 to 89% over a 17 month period, and those with anal cytologic abnormalities increased from 27 to 65%.[71] The proportion of subjects with anal intraepithelial neoplasia (AIN) rose from 8 to 32%, with high grade AIN increasing from 0 to 16%.

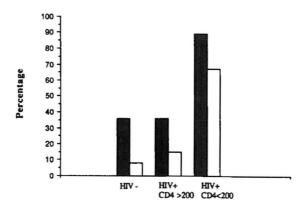

FIGURE 1 Percentage of men positive for anal HPV infection and anal cytologic abnormalities. Black bars indicate anal HPV infection and white bars indicate abnormal anal cytology.

Since a large proportion of high grade AIN occurs in individuals with advanced immunosuppression, many of whom have limited survival time, the clinical significance of these findings remains uncertain. However, despite the long time periods that may be required for invasive cancer to develop, as described previously, the incidence of anal cancer in this population has clearly increased. Moreover, since progression to invasive cancer may take a period of years, recent improvements in survival time for those with advanced HIV disease may result in a further increase in morbidity and mortality from this disease in the future. Similar to cervical cancer, anal cancer may be preventable using anal cytology and anoscopy as screening techniques. Because these tests are relatively inexpensive and non invasive, and treatment of anal disease is relatively non invasive, a strong case could be made for screening individuals at risk who retain a good Karnofsky performance status and are expected to survive for several more years. At a minimum, this should include all such HIV-positive individuals who have absolute CD4 counts of less than 200/mm³, and it may also be of value to screen individuals with higher CD4 counts as well.

To obtain material for anal cytology, a Dacron™ swab is moistened in tap water or saline and inserted to the anorectal junction. The swab is rotated and pressed against the wall of the anal canal as it is withdrawn, and the collected material smeared onto a glass slide and immediately preserved in alcohol to avoid air-drying. The slide is stained with Papanicolaou stain, and the criteria used to grade anal cytology are the same as those for cervical cytology.[74] Similar to cervical cytology, anal cytology has limited sensitivity, i.e., approximately 75%, when compared to the gold standard, which remains histopathology obtained by anoscopically-directed biopsy.[74]

A strategy for screening would therefore consist of performing anal cytology for individuals meeting the criteria described above. An individual with normal cytology should probably be re-screened on a regular basis, e.g., every six months, particularly as his immune status deteriorates. Abnormal results, including atypia, should prompt anoscopy followed by anoscopically directed biopsy, since unlike cervical atypia, atypia, on anal cytology is likely to be HPV-associated and may reflect the presence of a bona fide HPV-associated lesion. Application of 3 to 5% acetic acid may improve diagnostic sensitivity of anoscopy, as does magnification. Anoscopic criteria for determining which areas should be biopsied include those showing vascular punctation, leukoplakia, papillations, or other topographic irregularity (Figures 2 and 3). Unlike the cervix, distinguishing between condyloma and intraepithelial neoplasia may be very difficult in the anal canal, and suspicious areas should be biopsied regardless of their clinical appearance. Lesions may occur anywhere within the anal canal, and are often found at the anorectal junction. Disease may also be found on the exterior surface of the anus, and lesions at this location should also be biopsied.

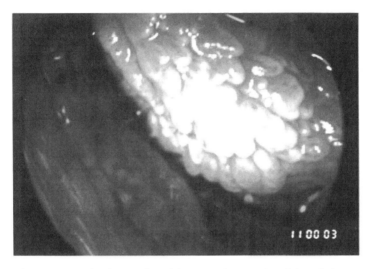

FIGURE 2   Anoscopic appearance of an intra-anal condyloma acuminatum, viewed through the anoscope at 16× magnification after application of 5% acetic acid. The lesion appears acetowhite and demonstrates extensive papillation.

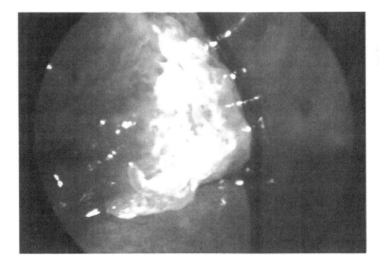

FIGURE 3   Anoscopic appearance of an anal intraepithelial neoplasia grade 2, viewed through the anoscope at 16× magnification after application of 5% acetic acid. In contrast to the lesion shown in Figure 2, this lesion is flatter, well-demarcated and demonstrates vasular punctation. Of note, the clinical appearances of anal condyloma acuminatum and anal intraepithelial neoplasia frequently overlap, and biopsy is necessary to establish a definitive diagnosis.

Experience with treatment of anal disease in the setting of HIV infection is also very limited. To date, most clinicians treat AIN and anal condyloma in HIV-positive individuals in the same manner as anal condyloma in HIV-negative individuals, i.e., with ablation of the diseased tissue. This may be accomplished in a variety of ways, including liquid nitrogen, electrocautery, and surgical excision. Although a high recurrence rate would be predicted, there have been no treatment follow-up studies published yet. There are also few guidelines as to which lesions require therapy; although it would seem prudent to treat all cases of AIN, it is not yet clear that all cases of condyloma require therapy given their low likelihood of progression to invasive cancer and high likelihood of recurrence. If a decision not to treat condyloma is made, affected individuals should be followed carefully to ensure that AIN does not develop at a later date.

2.   HPV-Associated Anogenital Cancers in HIV-Positive Women

Most of the considerations described for anal disease in HIV-positive men apply to cervical disease in HIV-positive women as well. Several early case reports documented a high incidence of genital HPV infection and HPV-associated disease in HIV-positive women.[77,78] Several subsequent studies of larger cohorts then demonstrated that the prevalence of both cervical HPV infection and HPV-associated cervical disease is increased among HIV-positive women compared to HIV-negative women.[79-83] In one study of 67 women, of whom 35 were HIV-positive, nearly one half of the latter were shown to have cervical HPV infection by Southern blot hybridization, compared to one quarter of HIV-negative women.[80] In a study of Nairobi prostitutes, however, no significant differences were found in HIV-positive and negative women with respect to the prevalence of either HPV infection or CIN. However, 93% of the HIV-positive women had asymptomatic (Centers for Disease Control group II) HIV disease. These data and data from other studies[80,84] suggest that as with anal disease in men, much of the increased risk associated with HIV may occur with more advanced immunosuppression. In one of these studies,[80] 73% of HIV-positive symptomatic women had HPV infection compared to 18% of asymptomatic HIV-positive women, and 11 of 22 (50%) of symptomatic HIV-positive women had cervical lesions compared to 3 of 13 (25%) of asymptomatic HIV-positive women. Of note, the prevalence of HPV-associated disease in HIV-infected populations may vary considerably; in one study, 18 of 19 (95%) of asymptomatic HIV-positive women were reported to have abnormalities of the lower genital tract.[85] In general, however, most investigators report a prevalence that is closer to that described above. Together, these studies indicate that HPV-associated cervical disease is very common among HIV-infected women, and in a meta-analysis of five controlled studies, an odds ratio of 4.9 (95% confidence interval, 3.0–8.2) for having cervical neoplasia[86] was reported among HIV-positive women.

As of January 1, 1993, the Centers for Disease Control in the U.S. expanded the AIDS case definition to include invasive cervical cancer among HIV-positive women. If the prevalence of HPV infection and HPV-associated disease are elevated in HIV-positive women, then it might be expected that the incidence of cervical cancer would be elevated as well. To date, however, there has not been a significant increase in the number of reported cases of cervical cancer among HIV-positive women, and there are several explanations for this: (1) in the U.S., most women will have their cervical lesion detected by Pap smear and will be treated before cancer develops, and (2) as with anal disease in men, the natural history of cervical disease may exceed the survival time of many HIV-positive women. This is true as well in Africa, where two studies of HIV-positive women have failed to show an increased risk of cervical cancer although the prevalence of HIV antibody positivity was higher among women with cervical cancer than noncancer controls.[87,88]

Once cervical cancer does develop in a HIV-positive woman, its behavior may be more aggressive than usual. In one case report, a HIV-positive patient with stage IIB cervical cancer was described who initially responded well to standard radiation therapy but relapsed at a periclitoral site within 2 months.[89] Within 3 months, the patient died of disseminated carcinomatosis despite chemotherapy with cisplatin, bleomycin, and mitomycin C.

Based on the above information, it would seem reasonable to screen HIV-positive women with Pap smears at least as often as is currently recommended by the American Cancer Society for sexually active women, i.e., on an annual basis. Women considered to be at particularly high risk, e.g., those with multiple sexual partners, women with symptomatic HIV disease, and women with CD4 counts less than 500/mm^3 could be screened more often, e.g., every 6 months. In addition to ruling out cervical disease, the clinician must be very careful to rule out disease in other anogenital areas, including the vulva, vagina, and anus, because of the possibility of multifocal HPV -associated disease. Detection of a lesion on colposcopy should be confirmed histopathologically, and treated according to standard guidelines. At this time, it is unclear if HIV-positive women require routine colposcopy in addition to routine Pap smear screening; one study suggested that the diagnostic sensitivity of cervical cytology was especially low among HIV-positive women,[90] but this has not been confirmed in other published reports. Once a lesion is demonstrated by colposcopically-directed biopsy, it should be treated aggressively, provided that an aggressive approach is warranted by the clinical status of the patient. As with anal disease in HIV-positive men, treatment is similar to disease in HIV-negative patients, and follow-up must be performed frequently because of the high risk of lesion recurrence.

IV. CONCLUSION

Several mechanisms may explain why immunosuppressed individuals are at increased risk of HPV-associated disease. Clearly, one of the features shared by each of the diseases described above is attenuated T cell immunity that has widespread effects on the immune response to a wide variety of antigens, including HPV antigens. For example, a soluble factor produced by CD8 cells in HIV-positive individuals may be responsible for down-regulating T helper cell responses to a variety of antigens.[91] Attenuated T cell immunity to HPV in these diseases is therefore but one manifestation of a broadly abnormal immune system. Other mechanisms may also be operative in individuals with immunosuppression secondary to HIV infection. First, transactivation of HIV promoters by the HPV 16 E6 protein has been reported[92] raising the possibility of direct interaction between HIV and HPV. Mitigating against this possibility, however, is the paucity of evidence demonstrating co-infection of HIV and HPV in the epithelial cells of the anogenital tract. Second, alterations in cytokine levels, including Il-2 and Il-4 have been reported in HIV infection.[93] Cytokines secreted by epithelial cells may play an important role in modulating immune response to viral infection[94-95] and also play a role in regulating epithelial cell growth.[96] Accordingly, soluble autocrine and paracrine factors may affect HPV gene expression and perturbations in levels of these factors associated with HIV infection may also play a role in determining the outcome of HPV-associated disease.

Therapy of HPV-associated disease in HIV-positive individuals is likely to be highly problematic due to the multifocal nature of HPV-associated diseases and high probability of disease recurrence after treatment. At this time, the mainstay of therapy remains the removal of HPV-infected tissue as is currently the norm in HIV-negative individuals, using methods such as surgical excision, laser, electrocautery, cryotherapy, podophyllin or podophyllotoxin, or trichloroacetic acid. Based on the considerations described above, approaches that modulate HIV infection may also be of value in the therapy of HPV-associated disease. Although there is little supporting evidence to date, medications such as zidovudine may retard the development of HPV-associated disease in HIV-positive individuals through generalized improvement in immune function. Other approaches that may be of value in the future may include administration of cytokines and/or interferon, and further studies to define their effects on the course of HPV-associated disease are needed.

REFERENCES

1. Ley, C.; Bauer, H. M.; Reingold, A.; Schiffman, M. H.; Chambers, J. C.; Tashiro, C. J.; Manos, M. M., Determinants of genital human papillomavirus infection in young women, *J Natl Cancer Inst*, 83, 997, 1991.
2. Daling, J. R.; Sherman, K. J.; Hislop, T. G.; Maden, C.; Mandelson, M. T.; Beckmann, A. M.; Weiss, N. S., Cigarette smoking and the risk of anogenital cancer, *Am J Epidemiol*, 135, 180, 1992.

3. Holly, E. A.; Whittemore, A. S.; Aston, D. A.; Ahn, D. K.; Nickoloff, B. J.; Kristiansen, J. J., Anal cancer incidence: genital warts, anal fissure or fistula, hemorrhoids, and smoking, *J Natl Cancer Inst*, 81, 1726, 1989.

4. Rabkin, C. S.; Biggar, R. J.; Melbye, M.; Curtis, R. E., Second primary cancers following anal and cervical carcinoma: evidence of shared etiologic factors, *Am J Epidemiol*, 136, 54, 1992.

5. Negrini, B. P.; Schiffman, M. H.; Kurman, R. J.; Barnes, W.; Lannom, L.; Malley, K.; Brinton, L. A.; Delgado, G.; Jones, S.; Tchabo, J. G., Oral contraceptive use, human papillomavirus infection, and risk of early cytological abnormalities of the cervix, *Cancer Res*, 50, 4670, 1990.

6. Koutsky, L. A.; Holmes, K. K.; Critchlow, C. W.; Stevens, C. E.; Paavonen, J.; Beckmann, A. M.; DeRouen, T. A.; Galloway, D. A.; Vernon, D.; Kiviat, N. B., A cohort study of the risk of cervical intraepithelial neoplasia grade 2 or 3 in relation to papillomavirus infection, *N Engl J Med*, 327, 1272, 1992.

7. Hubbert, N. L.; Sedman, S. A.; Schiller, J. T., Human papillomavirus type 16 E6 increases the degradation rate of p53 in human keratinocytes, *J Virol*, 66, 6237, 1992.

8. Crook, T.; Tidy, J. A.; Vousden, K. H., Degradation of p53 can be targeted by HPV E6 sequences distinct from those required for p53 binding and trans-activation, *Cell*, 67, 547, 1991.

9. Lechner, M. S.; Mack, D. H.; Finicle, A. B.; Crook, T.; Vousden, K. H.; Laimins, L. A., Human papillomavirus E6 proteins bind p53 in vivo and abrogate p53-mediated repression of transcription, *Embo J*, 11, 3045, 1992.

10. Werness, B. A.; Levine, A. J.; Howley, P. M., Association of human papillomavirus types 16 and 18 E6 proteins with p53, *Science*, 248, 76, 1990.

11. Dyson, N.; Howley, P. M.; Munger, K.; Harlow, E., The human papilloma virus-16 E7 oncoprotein is able to bind to the retinoblastoma gene product, *Science*, 243, 934, 1989.

12. Munger, K.; Werness, B. A.; Dyson, N.; Phelps, W. C.; Harlow, E.; Howley, P. M., Complex formation of human papillomavirus E7 proteins with the retinoblastoma tumor suppressor gene product, *Embo J*, 8, 4099, 1989.

13. Jenison, S. A.; Yu, X. P.; Valentine, J. M.; Galloway, D. A., Human antibodies react with an epitope of the human papillomavirus type 6b L1 open reading frame which is distinct from the type-common epitope, *J Virol*, 63, 809, 1989.

14. Cason, J.; Patel, D.; Naylor, J.; Lunney, D.; Shepherd, P. S.; Best, J. M.; McCance, D. J., Identification of immunogenic regions of the major coat protein of human papillomavirus type 16 that contain type-restricted epitopes, *J. Gen. Virol.*, 70, 2973, 1989.

15. Tindle, R. W.; Smith, J. A.; Geysen, H. M.; Selvey, L. A.; Frazer, I. H., Identification of B epitopes in human papillomavirus type 16 E7 open reading frame protein, *J Gen Virol*, 71, 1347, 1990.

16. Schiffman, M. H., Recent progress in defining the epidemiology of human papillomavirus infection and cervical neoplasia, *J Natl Cancer Inst*, 84, 394, 1992.

17. Jenison, S. A.; Firzlaff, J. M.; Langenberg, A.; Galloway, D. A., Identification of immunoreactive antigens of human papillomavirus type 6b by using Escherichia coli-expressed fusion proteins, *J Virol*, 62, 2115, 1988.

18. Jenison, S. A.; Yu, X. P.; Valentine, J. M.; Koutsky, L. A.; Christiansen, A. E.; Beckmann, A. M.; Galloway, D. A., Evidence of prevalent genital-type human papillomavirus infections in adults and children, *J Infect Dis*, 162, 60, 1990.

19. Jochmus, K. I.; Schneider, A.; Braun, R.; Kimmig, R.; Koldovsky, U.; Schneweis, K. E.; Seedorf, K.; Gissmann, L., Antibodies against the human papillomavirus type 16 early proteins in human sera: correlation of anti-E7 reactivity with cervical cancer, *J Natl Cancer Inst*, 81, 1698, 1989.

20. Walter, M.; Gissman, L.; Zentgraf, H.; Kirchner, H., Measurement of cell-mediated immunity against bovine papilloma virus by lymphoproliferative reactions, *Immunobiology*, 174, 244, 1987.

21. Haftek, M.; Jablonska, S.; Orth, G., Specific cell-mediated immunity in patients with epidermodysplasia verruciformis and plane warts, *Dermatologica*, 170, 2, 1985.

22. Iwatsuki, K.; Tagami, H.; Takagawa, M.; Yameda, M., Plane warts under spontaneous regression, *Arch. Derm.*, 122, 655, 1986.

23. Rogozinski, T. T.; Jablonska, S.; Jarzabek-Chorzelska, M., Role of cell-mediated immunity in spontaneous regression of plane warts, *Int J Dermatol*, 27, 322, 1988.

24. Morison, W. L., Viral warts, herpes simplex and herpes zoster in patients with secondary immune deficiencies and neoplasms, *Br J Dermatol*, 92, 625, 1975.

25. Ivanyi, L.; Morison, W. L., In vitro lymphocyte stimulation by wart antigens in man, *Br J Dermatol*, 94, 523, 1976.

26. Cubie, H. A.; Norval, M.; Crawford, L.; Banks, L.; Crook, T., Lymphoproliferative response to fusion proteins of human papillomaviruses in patients with cervical intraepithelial neoplasia, *Epidemiol Infect*, 103, 625, 1989.

27. Strang, G.; Hickling, J. K.; McIndoe, A. J.; Howland, K.; Wilkinson, D.; Ikeda, H.; Rothbard, J. B., Identification of T cell determinants, HLA-DR restriction and virus type specificity, *J Gen Virol*, 71, 423, 1990.

28. Tindle, R. W.; Fernando, G. J.; Sterling, J. C.; Frazer, I. H., A "public" T-helper epitope of the E7 transforming protein of human papillomavirus 16 provides cognate help for several E7 B-cell epitopes from cervical cancer-associated human papillomavirus genotypes, *Proc Natl Acad Sci U.S.A.*, 88, 5887, 1991.

29. Shepherd, P.; Lunny, D.; Brookes, R.; Palmer, T.; McCance, D., The detection of human papillomaviruses in cervical biopsies by immunohistochemistry and in situ hybridization, *Scand J Immunol*, 11, 69, 1992.

30. Altmann, A.; Jochmus-Kudielka, I.; Frank, R.; et al., Definition of immunogenic determinants of the human papillomavirus type 16 nucleoprotein E7, *Eur J Can*, 28:, 326, 1992.

31. Rouse, B. T.; Norley, S.; Martin, S., Antiviral cytotoxic T lymphocyte induction and vaccination, *Rev Infect Dis*, 10, 16, 1988.

32. Pasternack, M. S., Cytotoxic T-lymphocytes, *Adv Intern Med*, 33, 17, 1988.

33. Chen, L. P.; Thomas, E. K.; Hu, S. L.; Hellstrom, I.; Hellstrom, K. E., Human papillomavirus type 16 nucleoprotein E7 is a tumor rejection antigen, *Proc Natl Acad Sci U.S.A.*, 88, 110, 1991.

34. Zhou, J. A.; McIndoe, A.; Davies, H.; Sun, X. Y.; Crawford, L., The induction of cytotoxic T-lymphocyte precursor cells by recombinant vaccinia virus expressing human papillomavirus type 16 L1, *Virology*, 181, 203, 1991.

35. Chen, L.; Mizuno, M. T.; Singhal, M. C.; Hu, S. L.; Galloway, D. A.; Hellstrom, I.; Hellstrom, K. E., Induction of cytotoxic T lymphocytes specific for a syngeneic tumor expressing the E6 oncoprotein of human papillomavirus type 16, *J Immunol*, 148, 2617, 1992.

36. Lutzner, M. A.; Blancet-Bardon, C.; Orth, G., Clinical observations, virologic studies, and treatment trials in patients with epidermodysplasia verruciformis, a disease induced by specific papillomaviruses, *J Inv Dermatol*, 83, 18, 1984.

37. Androphy, E. J.; Dvortzky, I.; Lowy, D. R., X-linked inheritance of epidermodysplasia verruciformis: genetic and virologic studies of a kindred, *Arch Dermatol*, 121, 864, 1985.

38. Jablonska, S., Wart viruses: Human papillomaviruses, *Sem Dermatol*, 3, 120, 1984.

39. Kanda, R.; Tanigaki, T.; Kitano, Y.; Yoshikawa, K.; Yutsudo, M.; Hakura, A., Types of human papillomavirus isolated from Japanese patients with epidermodysplasia verruciformis, *Br J Dermatol*, 121, 463, 1989.

40. Obalek, S.; Favre, M.; Szymanczyk, J.; Misiewicz, J.; Jablonska, S.; Orth, G., Human papillomavirus (HPV) types specific of epidermodysplasia verruciformis detected in warts induced by HPV3 or HPV3-related types in immunosuppressed patients, *J Invest Dermatol*, 98, 936, 1992.

41. Jablonska, S.; Dabrowski, J.; Jakowicz, K., Epidermodysplasia verruciformis as a model in studies on the role of papillomaviruses in oncogenesis, *Cancer Res.*, 32, 583, 1987.

42. Salmon, R.; Thompson, C.; Rose, B.; Kelly, G.; Cossart, Y., Epidermodysplasia verruciformis associated with multiple squamous cell carcinomas, *Aust J Dermatol*, 29, 9, 1988.

43. Majewski, S.; Malejczyk, J.; Jablonska, S.; Misiewicz, J.; Rudnicka, L.; Obalek, S.; Orth, G., Natural cell-mediated cytotoxicity against various target cells in patients with epidermodysplasia verruciformis, *J Am Acad Dermatol*, 22, 423, 1990.

44. Glinski, W.; Obalek, S.; Jablonska, S.; Orth, G., T cell defect in patients with epidermodysplasia verruciformis due to human papillomavirus type 3 and 5, *Dermatologica*, 162, 141, 1981.

45. Majewski, S.; Skopinska-Rosewska, E.; Jablonska, S.; Wasik, M.; Misiewicz, J.; Orth, G., Partial defects of cell-mediated immunity in patients with epidermodysplasia verruciformis, *J Am Acad Dermatol*, 15, 966, 1986.

46. Cooper, K. D.; Androphy, E. J.; Lowy, D.; Katz, S. I., Antigen presentation and T-cell activation in epidermodysplasia verruciformis, *J Invest Dermatol*, 94, 769, 1990.

47. Rudlinger, R.; Bunney, M. H.; Smith, I. W.; Hunter, J. A., Detection of a human papilloma virus type 5 DNA in a renal allograft patient from Scotland, *Dermatologica*, 177, 280, 1988.

48. Barr, B. B. B.; Benton, E. C.; McLaren, K.; Bunney, M. H.; Smith, I. W.; Blessing, K.; Hunter, J. A., Papillomavirus infection and skin cancer in renal allograft recipients, *Lancet*, 2, 224, 1989.

49. Gross, G.; Ellinger, K.; Roussaki, A.; Fuchs, P. G.; Peter, H. H.; Pfister, H., Epidermodysplasia verruciformis in a patient with Hodgkin's disease: characterization of a new papillomavirus type and interferon treatment, *J Invest Dermatol*, 91, 43, 1988.

50. Tanagaki, T.; Kanda, R.; Sato, K., Epidermodsyplasia verruciformis in a patient with systemic lupus erythematosis, *Arch Dermatol Res*, 278, 247, 1986.

51. Berger, T. G.; Sawchuk, W. S.; Leonardi, C.; Langenberg, A.; Tappero, J.; Leboit, P. E., Epidermodysplasia verruciformis-associated papillomavirus infection complicating human immunodeficiency virus disease, *Br J Dermatol*, 124, 79, 1991.

52. Penn, I., Occurrence of cancers in immunosuppressed organ transplant recipients, *Clin Transpl*, 1990, 53, 1990.

53. Penn, I., Cancers of the anogenital regions in renal transplant recipients, *Cancer*, 58, 611, 1986.

54. Penn, I., Secondary neoplasms as a consequence of transplantation and cancer therapy, *Cancer Detect Prev*, 12, 39, 1988.

55. Dyall, S. D.; Trowell, H.; Dyall, S. M., Benign human papillomavirus infection in renal transplant recipients, *Int J Dermatol*, 30, 785, 1991.

56. van der Leest, R.; Zachow, K.; Bender, M.; Pass, F.; Faras, A., Human papillomavirus heterogeneity in 36 renal transplant recipients, *Arch Dermatol*, 123, 354, 1987.

57. Bradford, C. R.; Hoffman, H. T.; Wolf, G. T.; Carey, T. E.; Baker, S. R.; McClatchey, K. D., Squamous carcinoma of the head and neck in organ transplant recipients: possible role of oncogenic viruses, *Laryngoscope*, 100, 190, 1990.

58. Querci; della; Rovere; G; Oliver, R. T.; McCance, D. J.; Castro, J. E., Development of bladder tumour containing HPV type 11 DNA after renal transplantation, *Br J Urol*, 62, 36, 1988.

59. Gillatt, D. A.; Teasdale, C., Squamous cell carcinoma of the anus arising within condyloma acuminatum, *Eur J Surg Oncol*, 11, 369, 1985.

60. Ejeckam, G. C.; Idikio, H. A.; Nayak, V.; Gardiner, J. P., Malignant transformation in an anal condyloma acuminatum, *Can J Surg*, 26, 170, 1983.

61. Sturm, J. T.; Christenson, C. E.; Uecker, J. H.; Perry, J. F. J., Squamous cell carcinoma of the anus arising in a giant condyloma acuminatum. Report of a case, *Dis Colon Rectum*, 18, 147, 1975.

62. Daling, J. R.; Weiss, N. S.; Hislop, T. G.; Maden, C.; Coates, R. J.; Sherman, K. J.; Ashley, R. L.; Beagrie, M.; Ryan, J. A.; Corey, L., Sexual practices, sexually transmitted diseases and the incidence of anal cancer, *New Engl J Med*, 317, 973, 1987.

63. Koulos, J.; Symmans, F.; Chumas, J.; Nuovo, G., Human papillomavirus detection in adenocarcinoma of the anus, *Modern Pathology*, 4, 58, 1991.

64. Palefsky, J. M.; Holly, E. A.; Gonzales, J.; Berline, J.; Ahn, D. K.; Greenspan, J. S., Detection of human papillomavirus DNA in anal intraepithelial neoplasia and anal cancer, *Cancer Res*, 51, 1014, 1991.

65. Zaki, S. R.; Judd, R.; Coffield, L. M.; Greer, P.; Rolston, F.; Evatt, B. L., Human papillomavirus infection and anal carcinoma. Retrospective analysis by in situ hybridization and the polymerase chain reaction, *Am J Pathol*, 140, 1345, 1992.

66. Beckmann, A. M.; Daling, J. R.; Sherman, K. J.; Maden, C.; Miller, B. A.; Coates, R. J.; Kiviat, N. B.; Myerson, D.; Weiss, N. S.; Hislop, T. G., Human papillomavirus infection and anal cancer, *Int J Cancer*, 43, 1042, 1989.

67. Gal, A. A.; Saul, S. H.; Stoler, M. H., In situ hybridization analysis of human papillomavirus in anal squamous cell carcinoma, *Modern Pathology*, 2, 439, 1989.

68. Walz, B. in *Colon, Rectal and Anal Surgery*; Kodner, I. J., Fry, R. D., and Roe, J. P., Eds., CV Mosby, St. Louis, 1985, p 198.

69. Hughes, E.; Cuthbertson, A. M.; Killingback, M. K., Eds.; in *Colorectal Surgery*; Churchill-Livingstone, New York, 1983, p 413.

70. Daling, J. R.; Weiss, N. S.; Klopfenstein, L. L.; Cochran, L. E.; Chow, W. H.; Daifuku, R., Correlates of homosexual behavior and the incidence of anal cancer, *J Am Med Assoc*, 247, 1988, 1982.

71. Palefsky, J. M.; Holly, E. A.; Gonzales, J.; Lamborn, K.; Hollander, H., Natural history of anal cytologic abnormalities and papillomavirus infection among homosexual men with Group IV HIV disease, *J AIDS*, 5, 1258, 1992.

72. Qualters, J. R.; Lee, N. C.; Smith, R. A.; Aubert, R. E., Breast and cervical cancer surveillance, United States, 1973-1987, *MMWR*, 41, 1, 1992.

73. Caussy, D.; Goedert, J. J.; Palefsky, J.; Gonzales, J.; Rabkin, C. S.; DiGioia, R. A.; Sanchez, W. C.; Grossman, R. J.; Colclough, G.; Wiktor, S. Z., Interaction of human immunodeficiency and papilloma viruses: association with anal epithelial abnormality in homosexual men, *Int J Cancer*, 46, 214, 1990.

74. Palefsky, J. M.; Gonzales, J.; Greenblatt, R. M.; Ahn, D. K.; Hollander, H., Anal intraepithelial neoplasia and anal papillomavirus infection among homosexual males with group IV HIV disease, *J Am Med Assoc*, 263, 2911, 1990.

75. Critchlow, C. W.; Holmes, K. K.; Wood, R.; Krueger, L.; Dunphy, C.; Vernon, D. A.; Daling, J. R.; Kiviat, N. B., Association of human immunodeficiency virus and anal human papillomavirus infection among homosexual men, *Arch Intern Med*, 152, 1673, 1992.

76. Law, C. L.; Qassim, M.; Thompson, C. H.; Rose, B. R.; Grace, J.; Morris, B. J.; Cossart, Y. E., Factors associated with clinical and sub-clinical anal human papillomavirus infection in homosexual men, *Genitourin Med*, 67, 92, 1991.

77. Sillman, F. H.; Stanek, A.; Sedlis, A.; Rosenthal, J.; Lanks, K. W.; Bushhagen, D.; Nicastri, A.; Boyce, J., The relationship between human papillomavirus and lower genital intraepithelial neoplasia in immunosuppressed women, *J Obstet Gynecol*, 150, 300, 1984.

78. Sillman, F. H.; Sedlis, A., Anogenital papillomavirus infection and neoplasia in immunodeficient women, *Obstet Gynecol Clin North Am*, 14, 537, 1987.

79. Maiman, M.; Fruchter, R. G.; Serur, E.; Remy, J. C.; Feuer, G.; Boyce, J., Human immunodeficiency virus infection and cervical neoplasia, *Gynecol Oncol*, 38, 377, 1990.

80. Feingold, A. R.; Vermund, S. H.; Burk, R. D.; Kelley, K. F.; Schrager, L. K.; Schreiber, K.; Munk, G.; Friedland, G. H.; Klein, R. S., Cervical cytologic abnormalities and papillomavirus in women infected with human immunodeficiency virus, *J Acquir Immune Defic Syndr*, 3, 896, 1990.

81. Schrager, L. K.; Friedland, G. H.; Maude, D.; Schreiber, K.; Adachi, A.; Pizzuti, D. J.; Koss, L. G.; Klein, R. S., Cervical and vaginal squamous cell abnormalities in women infected with human immunodeficiency virus, *J Acquir Immune Defic Syndr*, 2, 570, 1989.

82. Schafer, A.; Friedmann, W.; Mielke, M.; Schwartlander, B.; Koch, M. A., The increased frequency of cervical dysplasia-neoplasia in women infected with the human immunodeficiency virus is related to the degree of immunosuppression, *Am J Obstet Gynecol*, 164, 593, 1991.

83. Laga, M.; Icenogle, J. P.; Marsella, R.; Manoka, A. T.; Nzila, N.; Ryder, R. W.; Vermund, S. H.; Heyward, W. L.; Nelson, A.; Reeves, W. C., Genital papillomavirus infection and cervical dysplasia--opportunistic complications of HIV infection, *Int J Cancer*, 50, 45, 1992.

84. Johnson, J. C.; Burnett, A. F.; Willet, G. D.; Young, M. A.; Doniger, J., High frequency of latent and clinical human papillomavirus cervical infections in immunocompromised human immunodeficiency virus-infected women, *Obstetr Gynecol*, 79, 321, 1992.

85. Byrne, M. A.; Taylor, R. D.; Munday, P. E.; Harris, J. R., The common occurrence of human papillomavirus infection and intraepithelial neoplasia in women infected by HIV, *Aids*, 3, 379, 1989.

86. Mandelblatt, J. S.; Fahs, M.; Garibaldi, K.; Senie, R. T.; Peterson, H. B., Association between HIV infection and cervical neoplasia: implications for clinical care of women at risk for both conditions, *Aids*, 6, 173, 1992.

87. ter Meulen, J.; Eberhardt, H. C.; Luande, J.; Mgaya, H. N.; Chang, C. J.; Mtiro, H.; Mhina, M.; Kashaija, P.; Ockert, S.; Yu, X.; et al., Human papillomavirus (HPV) infection, HIV infection and cervical cancer in Tanzania, east Africa, *Int J Cancer*, 51, 515, 1992.

88. Rogo, K. O.; Kavoo, L., Human immunodeficiency virus seroprevalence among cervical cancer patients, *Gynecol Oncol*, 37, 87, 1990.

89. Rellihan, M. A.; Dooley, D. P.; Burke, T. W.; Berkland, M. E.; Longfield, R. N., Rapidly progressing cervical cancer in a patient with human immunodeficiency virus infection, *Gynecol Oncol*, 36, 435, 1990.

90. Maiman, M.; Tarricone, N.; Vieira, J.; Suarez, J.; Serur, E.; Boyce, J. G., Colposcopic evaluation of human immunodeficiency virus-seropositive women, *Obstetr Gynecol*, 78, 84, 1991.

91. Clerici, M.; Roilides, E.; Via, C. S.; Pizzo, P. A.; Shearer, G. M., A factor from CD8 cells of human immunodeficiency virus-infected patients suppresses HLA self-restricted T helper cell responses, *Proc Natl Acad Sci U.S.A.*, 89, 8424, 1992.

92. Desaintes, C.; Hallez, S.; Van, A. P.; Burny, A., Transcriptional activation of several heterologous promoters by the E6 protein of human papillomavirus type 16, *J Virol*, 66, 325, 1992.

93. Shearer, G.; Clerici, M., TH1 and TH2 cytokine production in HIV infection., *Eighth Interational Conference on AIDS, Amsterdam, the Netherlands*, Abstract # WeA1047, We53, 1992.

94. Malejczyk, J.; Malejczyk, M.; Urbanski, A.; Kock, A.; Jablonska, S.; Orth, G.; Luger, T. A., Constitutive release of IL6 by human papillomavirus type 16 (HPV16)-harboring keratinocytes: a mechanism augmenting the NK-cell-mediated lysis of HPV-bearing neoplastic cells, *Cell Immunol*, 136, 155, 1991.

95. Majewski, S.; Hunzelmann, N.; Nischt, R.; Eckes, B.; Rudnicka, L.; Orth, G.; Krieg, T.; Jablonska, S., TGF beta-1 and TNF alpha expression in the epidermis of patients with epidermodysplasia verruciformis, *J Invest Dermatol*, 97, 862, 1991.

96. Krueger, J.; Ray, A.; Tamm, I.; Sehgal, P. B., Expression and function of interleukin-6 in epithelial cells, *J Cell Biochem*, 45, 327, 1991.

VI. Clinical Presentation
and Evaluation

13

Skin Warts: Gross Morphology and Histology

Gerd Gross and Stefania Jablonska

CONTENTS

GROSS MORPHOLOGY

HISTOLOGY

Gross Morphology

I. INTRODUCTION

The traditional classification of skin warts is based on clinical appearance and location. It includes the following three clinical types: deep plantar warts (myrmecia), common warts (verrucae vulgares), and flat warts (verrucae planae). Disclosure of the plurality of HPV types associated with skin warts raised the problem of the relationship of clinical morphology to distinct types of HPV. This was first suggested by the characterization of distinct HPVs from different types of lesions: HPV 1 from deep plantar warts,[1] HPV 2 from common hand warts,[1] and HPV 3 from flat warts[2] and flat wartlike lesions of patients with epidermodysplasia verruciformis (EV).[3] At present, more than 70 types of HPV are recognized, with several subtypes of them. Some HPV types are specifically associated with skin warts: HPV 1–4, 7, 10, 26–28, and 41. A great number of other HPV types are associated with EV (see Chapter 8 by Majewski et al. in this volume).

Due to the multiplicity of types, the problem of specific or preferential association of distinct HPVs with warts differing in morphology and location is still controversial. For instance, myrmeciae are often not distinguished from common or mosaic warts in spite of their very precise histologic and clinical description by Lyell and Miles.[4] Therefore, this chapter tries to present the available data on the association of different types of skin warts with distinct HPVs on the basis of morphological features (Table 1). Such recognition might be important because of the differences in clinical course, contagiousness, and response to treatment.

Most often warts are few in number and small in size. In some instances they may grow exuberantly and become very large or warts may spread, leading to innumerable lesions which are often confluent (Figure 1).

TABLE 1   Correlation Between HPV Types, Preferential Location, and Morphological Characteristics

Type of skin lesion	HPV type	Preferential location	Morphological characteristics
Myrmecia	1	Soles, palms	Rough horny surface, horny collar
Common Warts	2,4,7,26,27, 29,57	Extremities	
typical	2 or 4	Usually hands	Rough surface, irregular, hyperkeratotic (1-10 mm) hyperkeratotic
mosaic	2	Soles	Multiple, confluent with polygnal outlines
endophytic	4	Soles, palms	Punctate lesions, horny wall surrounding a central depression
butcher's wart	7[a]	Hands	Large, cauliflower-like, proliferative, friable
Flat Warts	3,10,27-29,41	Face, brow, backs of hands, knees	Superficial, multiple, flat smooth surface, irregular outlines
Intermediate Warts	10,28	Backs of hands	Flatter surface than common warts, linear arrangement

[a] In warty lesions of the oral mucosa and facial skin of HIV positive patients

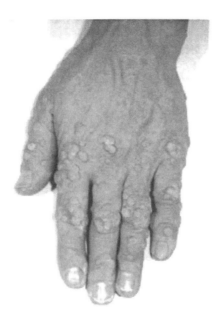

FIGURE 1   Multiple, partially confluent common warts (HPV 2) on the dorsum of the hand of a patient suffering from chronic lymphatic leukemia.

II.   CLINICAL TYPES OF SKIN WARTS

A. Myrmecia (HPV 1)

Myrmecia is the term given to painful palmoplantar warts which are characterized by having a rough horny surface projecting slightly above the skin, surrounded by a horny collar.[4,5] If the cap is pared away, the wart tissue appears soft and crumbly and shows a white opaque color. Characteristic findings include small bleeding points and punctate dots. The wart is well circumscribed, with a deep flask-shaped body that presses into the dermis causing pain on walking if it occurs on a weight bearing area (Figure 2). Although usually single, multiple lesions may occur. Myrmecia are not only localized on the palms and soles, but also on the lateral aspects of the fingers and toes, under the nails, on the pulp of the digits and, rarely, on the face, scalp, and body. At the dorsal sites of the foot and hand they may be less deep, somewhat elevated, and more hyperkeratotic.

Myrmecia are frequent in children between 5 and 15 years of age, with peak incidence between 12 and 15 years.[6]

B.   Common Warts (HPV 2, 4, 7, 26, 27, 28, 29, 57)

1.   Typical Common Warts (HPV 2 or 4)

Typical common warts start as a small flesh-colored papule, often more easily felt than seen. Common warts have a dome shape, and their surface is rough, irregular, and hyperkeratotic, with minute papillary projections (Figure 3). Around the orifices of the face and in the submental and beard regions, they may appear as so-called filiform or digitate warts (Figure 4). Their size varies from a few millimeters to more than 10 mm. Not infrequently they are confluent and hypertrophic, especially in periungual location[6] (Figure 5). They are grayish, brownish, or flesh-colored. Common warts may be single, but are usually multiple. They are mostly seen on the hands and fingers, but can occur on any part of the skin, including the thin epithelia of the anal and genital regions and the vermillion of the lips.

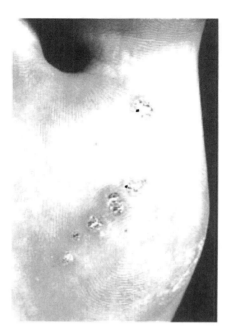

FIGURE 2 Several plantar warts (myrmecia) (HPV1), bleeding points present.

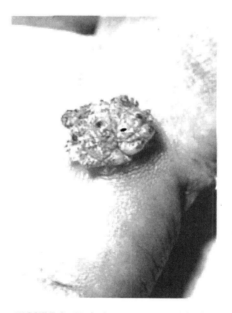

FIGURE 3 Typical common wart (HPV 2).

It was thought that most typical common warts were caused by HPV 2, but recent studies have shown that they can also be due to HPV 4 infection and other HPVs.[6-9]

2.   Mosaic Warts (HPV 2)

On the soles, common warts usually appear as mosaic warts. They are superficial, only slightly raised above the skin level, hyperkeratotic, multiple, confluent with polygonal outlines, and painless. There may be only one large plaque, but it is common to find several small warts of the same

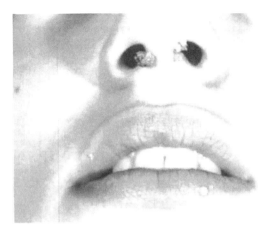

FIGURE 4 Filiform or digitate warts on the nose and a common wart on the lower lip.

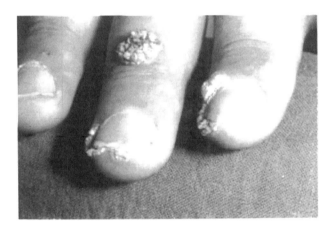

FIGURE 5 Periungual and subungual warts.

structure in its neighborhood[10] (Figure 6). Mosaic plantar warts are notorious for their longevity and resistance to treatment.

3. Endophytic Common Warts (HPV 4)

Endophytic common warts appear characteristically in palmar and plantar localizations of the foot and of the hand. As their name suggests, they are small, punctate lesions with a horny wall surrounding a central depression. They usually occur in groups and are relatively painless.

Their recognition, especially if single in the plantar location, is usually difficult, and they are often misdiagnosed for myrmecia warts,[5] although histologically they are different.[5-8] Additional helpful diagnostic criterion may be the hard keratin in common warts, in contrast to the soft keratinous masses disclosed in myrmecia.

4. "Butcher's Warts" (HPV 7)

It is well established that the incidence of warts is significantly higher in butchers, meat cutters, poulterers, and fish handlers than in the general population.[11-16] "Butcher's warts" are large, cauliflower-like, proliferative, friable warts occurring on the hands. They usually coexist with other types of common warts (Figure 7), and occur exclusively on the hands.

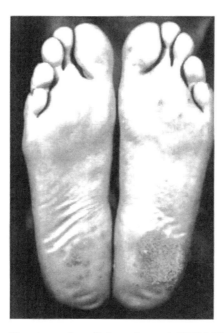

FIGURE 6   Plantar warts (so-called mosaic warts) (HPV 2 DNA present).

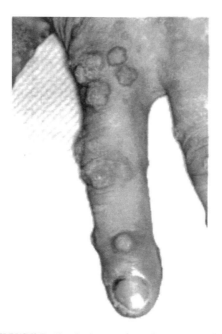

FIGURE 7   Butcher's warts (HPV 7 DNA present).

Interestingly HPV 7 could also be identified in oral warty lesions of patients suffering from a human immunodeficiency virus (HIV) infection.[17,18] De Villiers demonstrated the presence of HPV 7 DNA in lesions from both the oral mucosa and the facial skin of HIV positive patients.[18] These data warrant further studies to clarify the role of HPV 7 in immunocompetent and immunodeficient patients.

C.   Flat Warts (HPV 3, 10, 27-29, 41)

Flat (plane) warts are slightly raised above the skin level, smaller than common warts, with flatter, smoother surfaces and irregular outlines. They are multiple with the number of warts ranging from two to three to several hundreds, irregularly disseminated or grouped and confluent, not infrequently distributed in lines (Koebner phenomenon) (Figure 8). They are mainly localized on the face, dorsa of the hands, and sometimes elsewhere. On the face they are flatter, almost at the skin level, and often pigmented. On the dorsa of the hands, flat warts are somewhat more elevated, sometimes hyperkeratotic, and coalescent (Figure 9). Flat warts are more common in children and young women than in men, and very often they are found in immunocompromized individuals.[2] They often last for several years but eventually resolve spontaneously in immunocompetent patients heralded by inflammation of the warts leading to itch, erythema, and swelling. Often resolution is preceded by a sudden increase of the warts in size and numbers.[19] Flat warts respond poorly to treatment and may pose cosmetic problems.

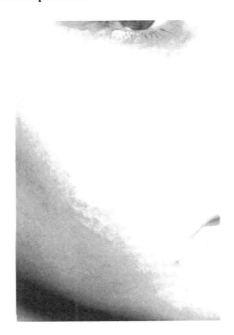

FIGURE 8   Flat warts (Verrucae planae juveniles), partially in linear arrangement (Koebner's phenomenon).

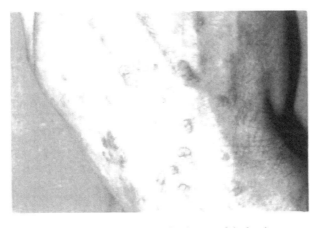

FIGURE 9   Flat warts on the dorsum of the hands.

D.   Intermediate Warts (HPV 10, 28)

Jablonska et al.[6] applied the term intermediate warts to lesions that cannot be classified as common or plane warts, as they combine clinical features of both. Even if hyperkeratotic, raised, and coalescent, they differ from common warts by flatter surface and, not infrequently, typical flat warts are found between the raised ones. The intermediate warts also appear, sometimes, in linear arrangement.[6] The clinical recognition of intermediate warts and their differentiation from early common warts may be difficult. Histology is of diagnostic significance.

E.   Epidermodysplasia Verruciformis (EV)

This rare familial disease presents with flat wartlike lesions which may be brownish or reddish or even hypochromatic resembling pityriasis versicolor. The most favored locations are face, neck, dorsa of the hands, fingers, and trunk. EV is associated with the specific EV HPVs, except for HPV3 and 10 which are present also in normal population. Development of squamous cell carcinoma of the skin is associated mostly with HPV 5 and 8, rarely with HPV 17 and 20 (see Chapter 8 by Majewski et al. in this volume).

III.   SUMMARY

Warts may occur at any location on the skin, but certain sites are favored. The morphology of skin warts is variable. Common warts have a generally dome-shaped appearance with multiple conical projections. They are often multiple and mostly found on the hands. Plantar warts are characterized by a highly thickened corneal layer, and can be classified as myrmecia or mosaic warts. Flat warts exhibit minimal or no papillomatosis. They are almost always multiple and are found most frequently on the face, on hands, and around the knees sometimes in a linear arrangement. Intermediate warts occur most often on the back of hands.

Differentiation from other skin disorders (Table 2) and between the clinical types of warts (Table 1) is important because of their differing behavior and response to treatment which in turn influences their prognosis and management. The morphology of a lesion usually, but not always, makes the diagnosis clear, but histological examination may also help to distinguish between the types.

TABLE 2   Differential Diagnosis to Viral Warts

Face, Extremities	Mollusca contagiosa, seborrhoeic keratoses, cornu cutaneum, keratoacanthoma, squamous cell carcinoma, Bowen's disease, lichen ruber verrucosus, tuberculosis cutis verrucosa, acanthosis nigricans, Darier's disease, lichen ruber (flat warts)
Palmar, Plantar Sites	Palmar and plantar keratosis, carcinoma cuniculatum
Peri-, Subungual Sites	Glomus tumors, subungual exostosis, malignant melanoma

REFERENCES

1. Orth, G, Favre, M., Croissant, O., Characterization of a new type of human papillomavirus that causes skin warts, *J. Virol.*, 1977; 76:569–80.
2. Pfister, H., Gross, G., Hagedorn, M., Characterization of human papillomavirus 3 in warts of a renal allograft patient, *J. Invest. Dermatol.*, 1979; 73:349–53.
3. Orth, G., Jablonska, S., Favre, M., Croissant, O., Jansbek-Chorselska, M., Rzesa, G., Characterization of two types of human papillomaviruses in lesions of epidermodysplasia verruciformis, *Proc. Natl. Acad. Sci. U.S.A.*, 1978; 75:1537–41.
4. Lyell, A., Miles, J. A. R., The myrmecia, *Br. Med. J.*, 1951; 28:912–16.
5. Laurent, R., Kienzler, J. L., Croissant, O., Two anatomoclinical types of warts with plantar localisation: specific cytopathogenic effects of human papillomavirus type 1 (HPV-1) and type 2 (HPV-2), *Arch. Dermatol. Res.*, 1982; 274:101–11.

6. Jablonska, S., Orth, G., Obalek, S., Croissant, O., Cutaneous warts clinical, histologic, and virologic correlation, *Clin. Dermatol.*, 1985; 3:71–82.

7. Gross, G., Pfister, H., Hagedorn, M., Gissman, L., Correlation between human papillomavirus (HPV) type and histology of warts, *J. Invest. Dermatol.*, 1981; 78:160–164.

8. Grussendorf, E., Lichtmikroskopische Untersuchungen an typisierten Virus-Warzen (HPV 1 und HPV 4), *Arch. Dermatol. Res.*, 1980; 268:141.

9. Bunney, M. H., Benton, C., Cubie, H. A., Viral Warts, *Biology and Treatment*, Oxford, Oxford University Press, 1992, 2.

10. Rasmussen, K. A., Verrucae plantares: symptomatology and epidemiology, *Acta Derm. Venerol. (Stockh)*, 1958;38 (Suppl. 39): 1–146.

11. Bosse, K., Christophers, E., Beitrag zur Epidemiologie der Warzen, *Hautarzt*, 1964; 15:80–6.

12. De Peuter, M., De Clerq, G., Minette, A., Lachapelle, J. M., An epidemiological survey of virus warts of the hands among butchers, *Br. J. Dermatol.*, 1977; 96:427–31.

13. Litt, J. Z., Warts in meat-cutters, *Arch. Dermatol.*, 1969, 100:773.

14. Rüdlinger, R., Bunney, M. H., Grob, R., Hunter, J. A. A., Warts in fish handlers, *Br. J. Dermatol.*, 1989: 120:375–81.

15. Orth, G., Jablonska, S., Favre, M., Identification of papillomaviruses in butchers warts, *J. Invest. Dermatol.*, 1981; 76:97–102.

16. Melchers, W., De Mare, S., Kuitert, E., Galama, J., Walboomers, J., Van den Brule, A., Human papillomavirus and cuteanous warts in meat handlers, *Clin. Microbiol.*, 1993; 31:2547–49.

17. Greenspan, D., de Villiers, E. M., Greenspan, J. S., de Souza, Y. G., zur Hausen, H., Unusual HPV types in oral warts in association with HIV infection, *J. Oral Path.*, 1988; 17:482–87.

18. De Villiers, E. M., Prevalence of HPV 7 papillomas in the oral mucosa and facial skin of patients with human immunodeficiency virus, *Arch. Dermatol.*, 1989; 125:1590.

19. Berman, A., Berman, J. E., Efflorescence of new warts: a sign of onset of involution in flat warts, *Br. J. Dermatol.*, 1978; 99:179–82.

Histology

I.   INTRODUCTION

Warts induced by various HPVs differ in clinical morphology and histological pattern.[1-10] Distinct HPVs are preferentially associated with specific types of warts.[2,6-14] although the clinical morphology is not always sufficient to predict HPV type. HPV 1 usually induces plantar myrmecia warts, and sometimes also hand warts, most often endophytic palmar and periungueal warts. HPV 2—responsible for common warts—may also be associated with endophytic mosaic plantar warts, and common hand warts may also be induced by HPV 4, HPV 7, and by newly characterized HPV 57. Flat warts are associated with HPV 3, HPV 10, HPV 28, HPV 27, HPV 29, and HPV 41. Thus clinical characteristics of warts do not always provide a clue to recognizing HPV type. However, there is an evident correlation between the histologic features of warts induced by main cutaneous HPVs and the type of infecting virus, and the most important marker is the specific cytopathic effect (CPE).

The cytopathic effect results from the derangement of terminal differentiation of keratinocytes infected by HPV and is associated with viral DNA replication.[15,16] In absence of CPE, the histology is inconclusive since the mere structure of the lesion is not a sufficient criterion. To get reliable information, the wart to be studied histologically must be very carefully chosen, and the biopsy must be taken from the center, and not the periphery of the lesion.

We are presenting the histological patterns of the main cutaneous HPVs which have been carefully studied and found to be characteristic and of some diagnostic importance.

II.   HPV 1-INDUCED MYRMECIA (INCLUSION) WART

The growth is endophytic, with prominent hyper- and parakeratosis and completely disorganized granular layer. The most characteristic features are eosinophilic cytoplasmic and basophilic nuclear inclusions, larger and more numerous in the upper layers of the epidermis[1,10] (Figure 1). The cytoplasm becomes progressively clarified with more prominent inclusions. In the enlarged cells, the nuclear chromatin is dense and irregular, and the nucleoli are hypertrophic. The basophilic inclusions are loaded with virions, while cytoplasmic inclusions contain low molecular peptides characteristic of this CPE.[16] It should be stressed that some keratinocytes are nonpermissive and undergo normal differentiation.

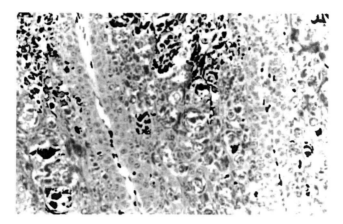

FIGURE 1   HPV 1-induced inclusion wart. Numerous large eosinophilic inclusions of bizarre shapes in the cleared cytoplasm. Nuclear basophilic inclusions in the upper layers. Between the wholly disorganized epidermal cells, strands of normally appearing nonpermissive keratinocytes. H+E, ×250.

III.   COMMON WARTS

A.   HPV 2-Induced Warts

A characteristic feature is hyperkeratosis with parakeratosis, often in columnar arrangement, papillomatosis and clarification of the cells in the upper layers with condensed keratohyalin granules of various shapes, sizes, and stainability. These upper granular cells contain virions; however, they are much less abundant than in myrmecia warts[2,10,11] (Figure 2). The study by electron microscopy *in situ* hybridization disclosed gold particles located on the viral particles in the nuclei mainly of the granular layer, starting at the third layer above the basal cells.[7]

HPV 2-induced warts may differ in structure: some are highly proliferative with branched rete ridges, while mosaic plantar warts are endophytic, but the characteristic CPE is similar, although variously pronounced. Gross et al.[9] stress some difficulties in distinguishing between cytopathic effects of HPV 2- and HPV 3-induced warts.

B.   HPV 4-Induced Warts

HPV 4 is preferentially associated with palmar hand warts, either verruca vulgaris or small endophytic lesions, usually in palmar localization. The histologic features are highly characteristic.[6,7,11] The proliferating rete ridges extend deep into the dermis (endophytic growth) and the large clarified cells with crescentic, small, peripherally located nuclei start to appear suprabasally, arranged in clusters in the squamous and granular layers. No keratohyalin granules overlay the clear cells, while the surrounding granular cells contain heavily stained very small granules of keratohyalin (Figure 3).

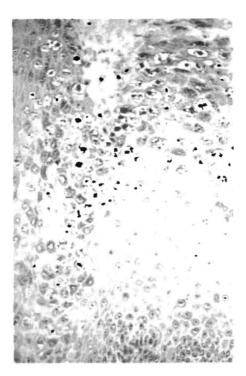

FIGURE 2 Specific cytopathic effect of HPV 2-induced wart. Vacuolized cells in the granular layer and overlying strongly stained keratohyalin granules of different sizes and shapes. H+E ×600.

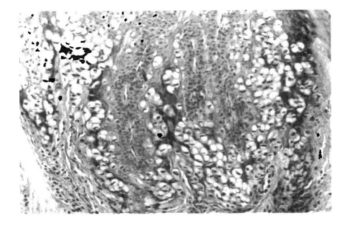

FIGURE 3 HPV 4-induced wart. Characteristic endophytic growth. Clusters of large clear cells with peripherally located crescentic nuclei. In the central parts of proliferating downward rete ridges, the squamous keratinocytes appear to be nonpermissive. The clusters of clear cells are surrounded in the granular layer by heavily stained cells containing very small keratohyalin granules. H+E ×160.

C. HPV 7-Induced Warts

This is an extremely interesting type of wart occurring almost exclusively in butchers or meat dealers,[7,11,18-24] found only in single cases of longlasting recalcitrant warts, mainly in immuno-suppressed persons.[20,25] HPV 7, referrred to as "butchers" wart virus was found associated in about 30% of warts in meat dealers.[7,19,21-24]

The warts are often hyperproliferative, with prominent hyperkeratosis and papillomatosis.[7,27] The clear cells are smaller then in HPV 4-induced lesions, with centrally located nuclei and no keratohyalin granules. They appear isolated or in small clusters, and are surrounded by heavily stained granular cells containing small keratohyalin granules. A fairly common characteristic is the presence of cytopathic effect exclusively within the rete ridges[7,11] (Figure 4). Some studies of butcher warts were performed by PCR from scrapings and therefore the pathology could not be established.[22-24]

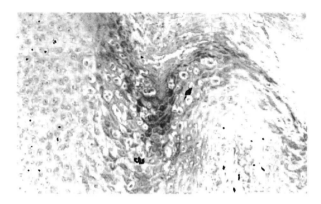

FIGURE 4 HPV 7-Induced wart. Hyperkeratosis with focal parakeratosis and prominent papillomatosis. Characteristic cytopathic effect: clear cells isolated or in small clusters, with centrally located nuclei, and no overlying keratinohyalin granules, surrounded in the granular layer by strongly stained cells. H+E, ×200.

Mucosal and cutaneous HPV 7-induced warts in HIV patients have been of an unusual clinical morphology, spiky or cauliflower-shaped, and of no characteristic histology.[25,26] HPV 7 was found only in 2 out of 654 biopsy specimens from unusually persistent multiple warts (probably in immunosuppressed persons), but in 7 of 17 total oral lesions in HIV patients.[26]

The clinico-pathological correlations of HPV 7 warts in nonbutchers have not been established.

IV. FLAT AND INTERMEDIATE WARTS

A. HPV 3-Induced Flat Warts

Stratum corneum is loose, and papillomatosis is usually slight or moderate, with broad and short rete ridges. Highly characteristic is perinuclear clarification around small basophilic, sometimes pyknotic, usually centrally located nuclei by well-defined borders of the cells (so called bird's eyes[7,9,12] (Figure 5).

B. HPV 10, HPV 27, and HPV 28-Induced Plane and Intermediate Warts

HPV 10, HPV 27, and HPV 28 may be associated with typical plane warts, but more frequently they are found in the so called intermediate warts.[11,27] These warts have clinical features of verruca vulgaris.[13,14] They are more elevated and more hyperkeratotic than plane warts, however they sometimes appear in linear arrangement (Koebner phenomenon), and regress simultaneously amid inflammatory reaction like plane warts. Most importantly, the histologic pattern has features characteristic of common warts, i.e., hyperkeratosis, focal parakeratosis, and prominent papillo-matosis, combined with the more or less pronounced cytopathic effect of HPV 3 (Figure 6).

The recognition of intermediate warts is of clinical importance because they are frequently found in an immunosuppressed population, and very often are classified as common warts.[11,13,14,28] The regression is simultaneous, similar to that of plane warts, although in heavily immunosuppressed people we have seen regression without any inflammatory reaction.

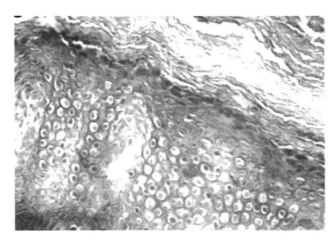

FIGURE 5   HPV 3-induced wart. Loose hyperkeratosis, superficial heavily stained granular cells. Pronounced perinuclear vacuolization in the spinous and granular layers. H+E, ×200.

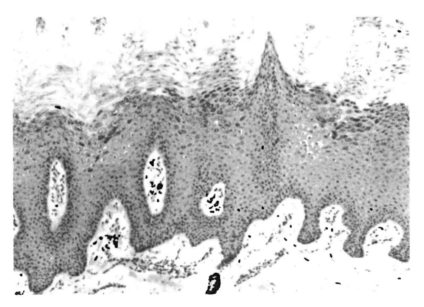

FIGURE 6   HPV 28-induced intermediate wart. Prominent hyperkeratosis with focal, partly columnar, parakeratosis. Hypergranulosis and pronounced papillomatosis. Slight perinuclear vacuolization in the upper squamous and granular layers. H+E, ×100.

V.   INCLUSION WARTS ASSOCIATED WITH NEW TYPES OF HPVS

New types of inclusion warts displaying characteristic clinical and histological features were found to be associated with recently characterized HPVs and to have distinctive cytopathic effects (CPE).

Described repeatedly in the Japanese literature since 1986, cystic warts of the sole led to discovery of new HPVs found to induce some unusual warts. A novel HPV 60 was characterized from a plantar cyst displaying specific CPE.[29] This HPV produced either cysts[30] or noncystic lesions of the sole which had a smooth surface, retaining appearance of the rete ridges. These unusual lesions were referred to as "ridged warts" distinct from other types of warts,[31,32] with the most characteristic CPE: amorphous eosinophilic intracytoplasmic inclusion bodies.

The novel HPVs, HPV 60, HPV 63, and HPV 65, were found in the warts of the sole. HPV 63, usually associated with punctate whitish endophytic warts, had CPE of a filamentous type: a heavily stained keratohyalin-like substance with filamentous brush-like structure within the vacuolated cells. This CPE differed considerably from the granular cytoplasmic inclusion bodies characteristic of HPV 1-induced warts. A homogeneous pattern of CPE was found in both HPV 60 associated warts and in the pigmented warts associated with HPV 65.[33] Egawa[34] proposed a classification of inclusion warts according to their clinical features, type of CPE, and type of associated HPVs: filamentous CPE characteristic of HPV 63-associated punctate warts and homogeneous intracytoplasmic inclusions characteristic of both HPV 60 and HPV 65 (virus related to HPV 4). The reported double infection with HPV 63 and HPV 1 within a single cell of a punctate plantar wart appears to be of special interest since the CPE was exclusively of HPV 1 type.[35] This poses the problem of a possible interference or a role of HPV 1 in transactivation of the other HPV, as reported for HPV3/10 and EV HPVs in immunosuppressed population.[28]

The cystic warts associated with novel HPVs might be due to mechanical pressure since they are mainly located beneath the weight bearing surface of the sole. Very similar epidermoid inclusion cysts harboring HPV 11 within the walls were found after subcapsular inoculation into the athymic mice of HPV 11[36] or HPV 1.[37] Cysts with characteristic EV cytopathic effect and presence of viral DNA were also obtained by subcapsular inoculation of athymic mice with EV specific HPVs.[38] Thus, such cysts might be due to unusual conditions when infected epithelial cells are surviving beneath the skin either in experimental conditions, or pushed into the dermis by pressure, as in epidermoid plantar cysts.

In a most recent study, HPV 60 DNA sequences were detected in eccrine ductile structures within the walls of epidermoid palmoplantar cysts.[39] These cysts could develop from eccrine ducts due to implantation of infected epidermis as a result of trauma.

The presence of HPV in eccrine ducts is comparable to the presence of HPV in hair follicles elsewhere on the skin, which is not an infrequent finding in EV.[15]

VI.   CONCLUSIONS

Since there is a preferential association of different cutaneous warts with distinct HPVs, and the clinical morphology is usually not sufficient to recognize the type of inducing HPV, the histological patterns, fairly characteristic of main cutaneous HPV types, might be of significance.

Testing scrapings by PCR does not provide information on the wart pathology. The importance of histological study and characterization of CPE is best evidenced in a group of novel inclusion warts. A careful examination of unusual CPEs led to the conclusion that the warts could not be induced by known HPVs, and indeed three new HPVs have been cloned, all three differing in CPEs from those of previously characterized warts.

Another problem is that several types of warts may coexist in one patient and therefore the histological and virological study should be performed in all warts differing in clinical morphology. The pathological examination is conclusive only if the specimen is well chosen, properly fixed, and if the appropriate sections are studied. However, there may be samples with no CPE, and then histological evaluation becomes impossible. In addition, by coexistence of two HPVs in a single cell, CPE of only one HPV might be present, even if the copy numbers of the HPVs are comparable. Thus, histology in all cases must be supplemented by virological study.

It should be stressed that a large number of new cutaneous HPVs has been characterized, e.g., 41, 57, etc., for which the histological correlations are not yet known.

REFERENCES

1. Lyell, A., Miles, J. A. R., The myrmecia. A study of inclusion bodies in warts, *Br. Med. J.*, 1951; 28:912.
2. Orth, G., Favre, M., Croissant, O., Characterization of a new type of human papillomavirus that causes skin warts, *J. Virol.*, 1977; 24:108.

3. Gissmann, L., Pfister, H., zur Hausen, H., Human papillomaviruses (HPV): characterization of four different isolates, *Virology*, 1977; 76:569.
4. Pfister, H., Gross, G., Hagedorn, M., Characterization of human papillomavirus 3 in warts of a renal allograft patient, *J. Invest. Dermatol.*, 1979; 73:349.
5. Grussendorf, E. I., zur Hausen, H., Localization of viral DNA - replication in sections of human warts by nucleic acid hybridization with complementary RNA of human papillomavirus type 1, *Arch. Dermatol. Res.*, 1979; 264:55.
6. Grussendorf, E. I., Lichtmikroskopische Untersuchungen an typisierten Virus-Warren (HPV 1 und HPV 4), *Arch. Dermatol. Res.*, 1980; 268:141.
7. Orth, G., Jablonska, S., Favre, M., Croissant, O., Obalek, S., Jarzabek-Chorzelska, M., Jibard, N., Identification of papillomaviruses in butchers' warts, *J. Invest. Dermatol.*, 1981; 76:97.
8. Jablonska, S., Orth, G., Glinski, W., Morphology and immunology of human warts and familial wartrs. In: Bachmann, P. A., Ed., *Leukemias, Lymphomas and Papillomas: Comparative Aspects*, London: Taylor and Francis 1981; 107.
9. Gross, G., Pfister, H., Hagedorn, M., Gissmann, L., Correlation between human papillomavirus (HPV) type and histology of warts, *J. Invest. Dermatol.*, 1982; 78:160.
10. Laurent, R., Kienzler, J. L., Croissant, O., Orth, G., Two anatomoclinical types of warts with plantar localization: specific cytopathogenic effects of human papillomavirus type 1 (HPV 1) and type 2 (HPV 2), *Arch. Dermatol. Res.*, 1982; 274:101.
11. Jablonska, S., Orth, G., Obalek, S., Croissant, O., Cutaneous warts: clinical histologic and virologic correlations, *Clin. Dermatol.*, 1985; 3:71.
12. Jablonska, S., Orth, G., Jarzabek-Chorzelska, M., Obalek, S., Glinski, W., Favre, M., Croissant, O., Epidermodysplasia verruciformis versus disseminated verrucae planae: is epidermodysplasia verruciformis a generalized infection with wart type virus? *J. Invest. Dermatol.*, 1979; 72:114.
13. Ostrow, R. S., Zachow, K. R., Watts, S., Bender, M., Pass, F., Faras, A., Characterization of two HPV-3 related papillomaviruses from common warts that are distinct clinically from flat warts or epidermodysplasia verruciformis, *J. Invest. Dermatol.*, 1983; 80:436.
14. Ostrow, R. S., Zachow, K. R., Thompson, O., Faras, A. J., Molecular cloning and characterization of a unique type of human papillomavirus from an immune deficient patient, *J. Invest. Dermatol.*, 1984; 82:363.
15. Orth, G., Favre, M., Breitburd, F., Croissant, O., Jablonska, S., Obalek, S., Jarzabek-Chorzelska, M., Rzesa, G., Epidermodysplasia verruciformis: a model for the role of papilloma viruses in human cancer, *Cold Spr. Harb. Cell Prolif. Conf.*, 1980; 7:259.
16. Croissant, O., Breitburd, F., Orth, G., Specificity of the cytopathic effect of cutaneous human papillomaviruses, *Clin. Dermatol.*, 1985; 3:43.
17. Hagari, Y., Shibata, M., Mihara, M., Shimo, S., Kurimura, T., Detection of human papillomavirus type 2a DNA in verrucae vulgares by electron microscopic *in situ* hybridization, *Arch. Dermatol. Res.*, 1993; 285:255–260.
18. Oltersdorf, T., Campo, M. S., Favre, M., Dartmann, K., Gissmann, L., Molecular cloning and characterization of human papillomavirus type 7 DNA, *Virology*, 1986; 149:247.
19. Jablonska, S., Obalek, S., Golebiowska, A., Favre, M., Orth, G., Epidemiology of butchers' warts. *Arch. Dermatol Res.*, 1988; 280 (supp):524.
20. de Villiers, E. M., Neumann, C., Oltersdsorf, T., Fierlbeck, G., zur Hausen, H., Butcher's wart virus (HPV 7) infections in nonbutchers, *J. Invest. Dermatol.*, 1986; 87:236–238.
21. Melchers, W., de Mare, S., Kuitert, E., Galama, J., Walboomers, J., Van den Brule, A. J. C., Human papillomavirus and cutaneous warts in meat handlers, *J. Clin. Microbiol.*, 1993; 31:2547–2549.
22. Keefe, M., Al-Ghamdi, A., Coggon, D., Maitland, N. J., Egger, P., Keefe, C. J., Carey, A., Sanders, C. M., Cutaneous warts in butchers, *Br. J. Dermatol.*, 1994; 130:9–14.
23. Keefe, M., Al-Ghamdi, A., Coggon, D., Maitland, N. J., Egger, P., Keefe, C. J., Carey, A., Sanders, C. M., Butcher's warts: no evidence for person to person transmission of HPV 7, *Br. J. Dermatol.*, 1994; 130:15–17.
24. Maitland, N. J., Keefe, M., Al-Ghamdi, A.,Coggon, D., Human papillomavirus type 7 and the butcher's wart, *Papillomavirus Report*, 1995; 6:33–37.
25. Greenspan, D., de Villiers, E. M., Greenspan, J. S., de Souza, Y. G., zur Hausen, H., Unusual HPV types in oral warts in association with HIV infection, *J. Oral. Pathol.*, 1988; 17:482–8.

26. de Villiers, E. M., Prevalence of HPV 7 papillomas in the oral mucosa and facial skin of patients with human immunodeficiency virus, *Arch. Dermatol.*, 1989; 125:1590.
27. Jablonska, S., Obalek, S., Favre, M., Golebiowska, A., Croissant, O., Orth, G., The m orphology of butchers' warts as related to papillomavisrus types, *Arch. Dermatol. Res.*, 1987; 279:566.
28. Obalek, S., Favre, M., Szymanczyk, J., Misiewicz, J., Jablonska, S., Orth, G., Human papillomavirus (HPV) types specific of epidermodysplasia verruciformis detected in warts induced by HPV 3 or HPV 3 - related types in immunosuppressed patients, *J. Invest. Dermatol.*, 1992; 98:936.
29. Matsukura, T., Iwasaki, T., Kawashima, M., Molecular cloning of a novel human papillomavirus (type 60) from a plantar cyst with characteristic pathological changes, *Virology*, 1992; 190:561–564.
30. Kawase, M., Honda, M., Niimura, M., Detection of human papillomavirus type 60 in plantar cysts and verruca plantaris by the in situ hybridization method using digoxigenin labeled probes, *J. Dermatol.*, 1994; 21:709–715.
31. Honda, A., Iwasaki, T., Sata, T., Kawashima, M., Morishima, T., Matsukura, T., Human papillomavirus type 60-associated plantar wart: ridged wart: *Arch. Dermatol.*, 1994; 130:1413–1417.
32. Kashima, M., Adachi, M., Honda, M., Niimura, M., Nakabayashi, Y., A case of peculiar plantar warts: human papillomavirus type 60 infection, *Arch. Dermatol.*, 1994; 130:1418–1420.
33. Egawa, K., Delius, H., Matsukura, T., Kawashima, M., de Villiers, E.-M., Two novel types of human papillomavirus, HPV 63 and HPV 65: comparison of their clinical and histological features and DNA sequencing to other HPV types, *Virology*, 1993; 194:789–799.
34. Egawa, K., New types of human papillomaviruses and intracytoplasmic inclusion bodies: a classification of inclusion warts according to clinical features, histology and associated HPV types, *Br. J. Dermatol.*, 1994; 130:158–166.
35. Egawa, K., Shibasaki, Y., de Villiers, E.-M., Double infection with human papillomavirus 1 and human papillomavirus 63 in a single cell of a lesion displaying only an human papillomavirus 63-induced cytopathogenic effect, *Lab. Invest.*, 1993; 69:583–588.
36. Kreider, J. W., Howatt, M. K., Wolfe, S. A., Bartlett, G. L., Zaino, R. J., Sedlacek, T. V., Mortel, R., Morphological transformation *in vivo* of human uterine cervix with papillomavirus from condylomata acuminata, *Nature*, 1985; 317:639–641.
37. Kreider, J. W., Patrick, S. D., Cladel, N. M., Welsh, P. A., Experimental infection with human papillomavirus type 1 of hand and foot skin, *Virology*, 1990; 177:415–417.
38. Majewski, S., Breitburd, F., Skopinska, M., Croissant, O., Jablonska, S., Orth, G., A mouse model for studying epidermodysplasia verruciformis - associated carcinogenesis, *Int. J. Cancer*, 1994; 56:1–4.
39. Egawa, K., Honda, Y., Inaba, Y., Ono, T., de Villiers, E.-M., Detection of human papillomaviruses and eccrine ducts in palmoplantar epidermoid cysts, *Br. J. Dermatol.*, 1995; 132:533–543.

14

Warts and HPV-Related Squamous Cell Tumors of the Genitoanal Area in Adults

Geo von Krogh, Gerd Gross, and Renzo Barrasso

CONTENTS

I.   ABSTRACT

Genitoanal papillomavirus infection (GPVI) induces multicentric, multifocal, and multiform lesions occurring predominantly on areas submitted to microtraumatizion during sexual activity, inclusively those of the epithelial transformational zones on the cervix uteri and in the anal canal, but also on inflamed and/or traumatized genital epithelium. The potential coexistence of other STDs must always be sought.

Comprehension that subclinical infection is extremely common has created ambiguity on an optimal ambition level for patient management. A pragmatic approach is advocated, with an emphasis on diagnosing and treating overt warts, symptomatic flat acetowhite lesions, and HPV-associated premalignant conditions such as bowenoid papulosis, Bowen's disease, Buschke-Löwenstein tumors and, above all, moderate and severe cervical intraepithelial neoplasia (CIN II-III). Psychosexual implications entail a range of emotional disturbances, in particular in long-term sufferers. In children, the potential of sexual abuse must be evaluated and the child preferably be referred to pediatric and sociomedical expertise.

Rather than screening for subclinical disease on the outer genitals, focus should be put on managing overt warts and GPVI-associated symptoms, and females above 25 years of age must be advised to attend available Pap-smear programs for CIN detection. Conventional histopathological examination of biopsy material is usually sufficient for differential diagnostic purposes. HPV virological assays have yet no place in clinical routine with the exception of *in situ* hybridization assays as tools for histopathological quality control. However, due to current sensitivity problems of convential Pap-smear methodology, adjuvant use of specific PCR DNA detection of oncogenic HPV types is disussed as a potential mean of optimizing targeted etiology-oriented smear programs.

II.   EPIDEMIOLOGICAL AND PATHOGENETIC ASPECTS

A.   The "Iceberg Dilemma"

For details on the epidemiological aspects of HPV infection, see Shoultz, Koutsky, and Galloway in Chapter 5. HPV 6 and HPV 11 are usually associated with the traditional concept of medically benign "venereal" warts (condylomata acuminata). In Western countries the incidence of patients self-checking for genitoanal warts is about 0.5–1% of sexually active 15–25 year-old people.[1-7] In sexually active males in their upper teens, rates of penoscopically detectable warts as high as 6–7% have been reported.[8] The true prevalence, however, of virologically detectable GPVI among adolescents is in the approximate upper range of 30–50%.[9-20]

Some confusion has existed regarding the differentiation between **latent** and **subclinical** infection.[21] In the present context, latent infection refers to the occurrence of a viral reservoir in the epidermal basal layer without concurrent histopathological changes, while subclinical infection entails that histopathologically demonstrable activity exists in the absence of visible warts or other symptoms.

The fact that most lesions induced by oncogenic HPV types remain undetectable by naked eye examination appears as a sociomedical paradox and an intriguing clinical dilemma. Subclinical GPVI lesions are probably as sexually contagious as condylomas, not only during adolescence but, at least in some populations, in the third and fourth decade of life as well. Several collaterally independent, yet frequently overlapping, epidemics seem to exist,[6] with acquisition of various HPV types usually coinciding with change of sexual partners.[12,16-19,22,23] Sexual partners examined at a given time, however, do not consistly have detectable HPV types in common.[24] This may be due to several factors. Many patients eliminate the infection spontaneously, while others may remain consistently or intermittently positive with episodes of either low- or high-level viral expression.[14,23]

Risk of acquiring GPVI covariates with early sexual activity, frequent partner changes, concurrent and previous other STDs, heavy smoking habits and, in the male, lack of circumcision.[25] The relative risk of acquiring multiple genital HPV infections may be as high as three for each new sexual partner and lifetime-risk as high as 80%.[26-29] An inverse relationship exists with consistent use of condoms.[8]

As a rule, multifocal epithelial alterations are induced, and the infection is generally regional rather than local.[22,30,31] Overt warts frequently coexist with subclinical lesions.[32,33] As accounted for by Syrjänen in Chapter 9, benign lesions and intraepithelial neoplasia often also coexist and are parts of a morphological spectrum of continuity. Depending on severity, the epithelial dysplasia is classified as grade I (mild), II (moderate), or III (severe). The denominations CIN, VAIN, VIN, PIN, PEIN, and AIN are used when intraepithelial neoplasia engages, respectively, the cervix, vagina, vulva, penis, perineum, or the anus.

Incidence of CIN appears to be a time-dependent phenomenon. Based on PCR-related studies of women with normal cytology attending STD-clinics, a puzzling high risk for development of transient dysplasia has been demonstrated recently. Progression to CIN II-III may occur in as many as 30–40% at two years' follow-up; however, a marked trend exists towards spontaneous regression within a 5-year period.[26-29,34,35] Short-term persistence by the same HPV type seems to be frequent but long-term persistence is rare in teen-agers and young adolescents. High-risk HPV types tend to cause persistent infections twice as frequently as low oncogenic risk types.[34] A number of the women remain consistently or intermittently HPV positive for several years,[23] suggesting that the virus retains the capability of undergoing episodes of reactivation in a subset of patients.

The cervix uteri represents a locus minoris for subsequent cancer development,[36-39] while the relative risk of irreversible malignancy is very low in remaining genitoanal areas. However, even on the cervix cancer seems to arise only in a minor fraction of cases, when HPV-related dysplasia persists and progresses over periods of at least 5–10 years and are concurrently associated with cofactors such as chronic infections,[40] chemical cocarcinogens, and/or an immunological dysfunction.[20] In this respect, the relative risk increases significantly in women over 30 years of age infected with, above all, the oncogenic HPV types 16, 18, 31, 33, and 45.[41] For further details on the pathogenesis of irreversible dysplasia and malignant transformation the reader is referred to Fuchs and Pfister in Chapter 2, K. Syrjänen in Chapter 9, and Malejczyk et al. in Chapter 11.

B. Regulatory Mechanisms for Biological Expression

For GPVI, ultimately afflicting much of the world's population, it is believed that a state of subclinical/latent infection most commonly is sustained due to down-regulatory control mechanisms exerted by tumor suppressor gene products of the keratinocytes and/or immunological surveillance mechanisms (see Chapters 9 and 11). Fluctuations often occur from a state of subclinical or latent infection to overt wart disease, or vice versa.[14,23,28,42]

As outlined in Chapter 11, several observations suggest that the cell-mediated immune response is important in the outcome of HPV infection: a high wart incidence in patients receiving immunosuppressive treatment, a weak delayed hypersensitivity to tuberculin, and a decreased number of peripheral blood T lymphocytes or reduced *in vitro* blastogenic responses of lymphocytes to mitogens.[43-46] A detrimental effect by some product(s) from HPV has been postulated as a contributing cause of faint immune reactions leading to persistent infection in immunologically otherwise healthy individuals. Partial depletion and morphological alterations of Langerhans' cells,[43-45] as well as impaired HLA-DR and ICAM-1 associated antigen presenting capacity of infected keratinocytes[43,46] have been demonstrated locally in persistent lesions. It has been postulated that specific viral proteins may mediate immunological suppression by inhibiting the IL-1 receptor and down-regulate the expression of MHC class molecules, being essential for efficacy of cytotoxic cells in tumor surveillance. The loss of HLA I class expression, however, seems to be a relatively late event in the natural history of HPV-associated malignancy.[46]

Increase of biological expression, with a high degree of recalcitrance, recurrence, and malignant transformation, occurs during immunosuppression associated with malignancies (chronic lymphatic leukemia, Hodgkin's disease),[47] with HIV infection[48-50] and in allograft recipients.[51,52] As accounted for by Majewski et al. in Chapter 8, epidermodysplasia verruciformis is associated with inherited deranged immunological homeostatic mechanisms.[6,53]

Other modes of disrupting a down-regulatory homeostasis may include lifestyle related factors, such as up-regulatory influences from tobacco smoking, alcohol consumption, and drug abuse.[54] Such factors covariate with gonorrhoea, chlamydia trachomatis, vaginal candidiasis/bacterial vaginosis, and possibly other infectious agents as well.[6,40,55,56] Dietary factors seem of little significance, perhaps with the exception of cruciferous vegetables, containing the chemical indole-3-carbinol, which has been shown to exert a papilloma virus inhibitory effect in animal experiments.[57,58]

Influence of hormonal factors, exerted by stimulation of a common receptor for progesterone and glucocorticoid on keratinocytes,[59] is also demonstrated during pregnancy when warts tend to become florid and coalescent.[60] A similar growth potential is also associated with diabetes mellitus (von Krogh, personal observations).

C.   Range of Biological Expression

1.   Genital Lesions

a.   Condylomata Acuminata.   Since the sexually transmitted nature of "classical" HPV 6/11 induced genital warts ("condylomas"; condylomata acuminata) first was demonstrated in the 1950s,[61] the magnitude of the clinical problem has increased significantly. In the U.S. the number of self-examination cases increased 4.5-fold during the period 1966–1984.[3-5] In England, the yearly incidence has increased 5-fold since 1970 and more than doubled during the decade 1983–1993.[62] At present, condylomas represent a significant burden in, above all, dermatology, STD, and gynecology clinics. The management, however, involves primary care physicians and specialists in urology, proctology, and pediatric surgery as well.[3,6,63]

The incubation period may be as short as 3–6 weeks, or as long as several years; on average two thirds of patients' sex partners are afflicted after an incubation period of a mean of 2.8 months. Age of onset parallells that of other STDs, with peak incidence being reached in the age groups 19–22 years for females and 22–26 years for males.[1,61]

b.   Subclinical Lesions.   In parallel with methodological improvements during the past decade, the cognizance of subclinical lesions has increased consequentially. It seems improbable that an increase has occurred during recent decades in the prevalence of oncogenic HPV types. Retrospective investigations on cervical smears among Australian[64] and North American[65] women, reveal that the prevalence of infection with the HPV types 16, 18, 31, 33, 35, 42, 43, 44, 45, 51, 52, and 56 remained unchanged over study periods within the range of the years 1964–1989.

Sexual contagion appears to be as high as for condylomas. Peak incidence, however, may possibly occur in even younger age groups than those of condylomas. Using Southern-blot, Rosenfeld et al.[66] detected HPV DNA, mostly of the oncogenic types, in as much as 38% of cervicovaginal lavage samples collected from sexually active females aged 13–21 years. Soares et al.[67] found the highest prevalence of HPV carriage in the age-group 16–20 years, after which a gradual decline occurred in the age-group 35–45 years of age. These data agree with that of Köchel et al.,[68] showing an age dependent pattern of HPV positivity, including that of oncogenic HPV types, with a peak prevalence during early adolescence.

As appears from the contribution by Meisels in Chapter 18, the cytological pick-up rate of cervical infection is also age-related; most biologically active lesions disappear by time. In Meisels'[69] studies, the prevalence rate was close to 6% in women up to the age of 25 years, while a gradual decline to a level of around 2–3% occurred in females above the age of 35 years. However, although the frequency of cervical lesions tends to decrease by increasing age, a clear propensity exists for women over the age of 30–35 years to be afflicted persistently with CIN III and concurrently exhibiting expression of oncogenic HPV types.[20,27,28,42]

2. Airway Lesions

A survey on airway lesions is presented by S. Syrjänen in Chapter 10. Transmission of HPV from mother to baby seems to be common. An association exists between a maternal history of genital warts and the development of laryngeal papillomas in children.[70,71] The transmission rate of HPV DNA to the airway epithelium may occur at a frequency of 30–50% during fetal passage through an infected maternal genital tract.[72,73] Mucosothrophic HPV types may also afflict the upper aerodigestive tract of GPVI-afflicted individuals when the oral cavity possibly represents a viral reservoir for orogenital transmission.[74]

The morbidity rate of the oral, laryngeal, and airway epithelium appears to be very low both in children and in adults. Laryngeal papillomas are several hundred to 1,000-fold less common than maternal infection at the time of delivery, and laryngeal papillomas in adults are also quite rare.[75] Yet, in afflicted individuals the consequences of laryngeal disease are often quite serious and require long-lasting therapeutic interventions associated with much suffering. This aspect is futher elucidated by Kashima et al. in Chapter 17.

3. Other Lesional Sites

Occassionally, mucosotrophic HPV types such as HPV 6, 11, 16, and 18 have been detected in warty lesions afflicting thin skin areas such as the nipples, intertriginous areas (the breasts, the groin, the umbilicus), the legs, and in the periungual area.[76-80] (See also Chapter 6 by de Villiers and Chapter 7 by Grussendorf-Conen). Although the relative risk of subsequent malignant transformation is low,[81,82] it is, nevertheless, in no way negligible in long-lasting lesions.[83-86] The risk is further augmented in immunosuppressed patients such as transplant recipients[87] and in HIV infected persons with CD4 counts below 200.[49,88]

III. CLINICAL FEATURES

A. Lesional Types

Lesions are multifocal, multicentric, and multiform, with individual cases never being identical. Lesions visible to the naked eye can roughly be distinguished into three types: (1) acuminate, (2) papular, and (3) flat warts. With the exception of typical condylomata acuminata, lesions do not show type-specific clinical or colposcopic features. More than one type of lesions are frequently seen in individual patients. Many times the warts coalesce into plaques, most commonly in immunosuppressed individuals and in patients with diabetes, but occasionally in healthy individuals as well, when dispersion of multiple papillae sometimes cover large surfaces ("papillomatosis").[89,90]

There is a strong inclination for HPV types 6 and 11 to induce acuminate warts, and for HPV types 16 and 18 to be present in flat and papular lesions.[91] However, this propensity is not sufficient for a differentiation on a clinical basis between individuals infected with the various HPV types. Thus, "high-risk" HPV types may be harbored in all clinical wart types,[6,63,92-94] and concurrent infection with several HPVs is common.

1. Acuminate Lesions

Acuminate lesions (Tables 1 and 2) predominate on moist and thin epithelium, such as the preputial cavity in uncircumcised men (Figure 1), the urinary meatus (Figure 2), the posterior and the medial parts of the vulva (Figure 3), the introitus and the hymenal ring (Figure 4), the vagina (Figure 5), the portio-cervix (Figure 6), the anus, and the anorectal junction (Figure 7). They may also afflict drier epithelium such as the penile shaft, where papular warts also are frequently present (Figure 8). Often they afflict intertriginous moist skin such as in the groin, the perineum, and the perianal area. Perioral condylomas may occur in immunocompetent individuals, but more frequently in HIV infected patients (Figure 9).

TABLE 1   Distribution of Genitoanal Warts in Men

	Percentage of patients affected	
Site	Oriel 1971 (*n* = 191) Mostly uncircumcised men	Chuang et al. 1984 (*n* = 246) Mostly circumcised men
Glans, fraenulum, corona	52	10
Prepuce	33	8
Urethra	23	10
Shaft of penis	18	51
Scrotum	2	1
Perineum	0	3
Anus, perianal	8	34

TABLE 2   Distribution of Genitoanal Warts in Women

	Percentage of patients affected	
Site	Oriel 1971 (*n* = 141)	Chuang et al. 1984 (*n* = 500)
Urethra	8	4
Labia majora	31	66
Labia minora, clitoris	32	
Introitus	73	37
Vagina	15	
Cervix	6[a]	8[a]
Perineum	23	29
Anus	18	23

[a] Figures up to 30-50% have been revealed in subsequent publications.[28,38,42]

These warts are papilliferous with finger-like peduncles exhibiting highly vascularized dermal cores appearing as a typical punctuated and/or fork/loop-like patterns by magnifying equipment, unless being heavily keratinized. The color is pinkish-red through reddish-white on thin epithelium, or grayish-white on more keratinized skin.

2. Papular Lesions

These are most common on fully keratinized dry parts of the genitoanal area such as the penile shaft (Figures 8 and 10), the lateral parts of the vulva, the perineum, and the perianal area. Regardless of anatomical location, acuminate warts sometimes change into more papular variants during the course of time.

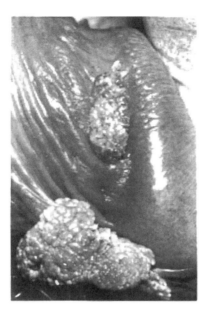

FIGURE 1 Typical acuminate condylomas afflicting predilection sites in the male (sulcus coronarius, fraenulum) of the penis.

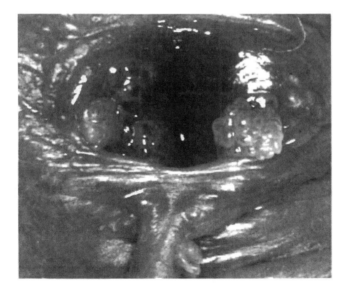

FIGURE 2 Typical acuminate warts of fraenulum as well as of the urethra lips of a male (high-power colposcopy magnification). The proximal border is clearly visible as the urethral orifice is kept overted. The proximal border may be better appreciated by using a small sized nose-speculum or an otoscopic tube. In about 5% of cases, referral to an urologist will be required to be done subsequent to treatment of other penile lesions. Testing for Chlamydia trachomatis using an ENT swab must be performed very carefully in order to avoid iatrogenic infection of the urethra, or, preferably, be delayed until meatal warts have been cured. Alternative PCR or LCR testing in urine samples for Chlamydia trachomatis is recommended.

Although the surface is relatively smooth, it may appear micropapillary when viewed through magnifying equipment, when typical punctuated dermal vessels often are appreciable (Figure 11). Exact delineation of lesions is often difficult without assistance from magnification equipment and/or acetic acid testing. The color is usually similar to that of acuminate warts, varying within the range of pinkish-red to grayish-white. On pigmented sites such as the penile shaft,

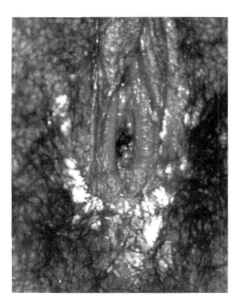

FIGURE 3 Keratinized whitish acuminate warts afflicting a predilection site in the female, the posterior part of the vulva.

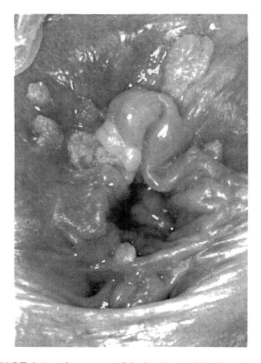

FIGURE 4 Acuminate warts of the introitus and the hymenal ring.

the labium majora, and the perineum/perianal region, the color tone is regularly more brownish. When conspicuously pigmented, bowenoid papulosis should be ruled out (Figure 12).

3.   Flat Lesions

These typically exhibit a punctuated capillary pattern at magnification unless being heavily keratinized, and sometimes reveal their presence due to subtle color deviations such as grayish-white, pinkish-red, or brownish epithelial shades similar to that originally ascribed to bowenoid papulosis.

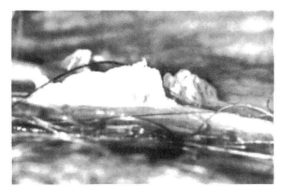

FIGURE 5 Intravaginal acuminate warts exhibiting feather-like capillaries (high-power colposcopy magnification).

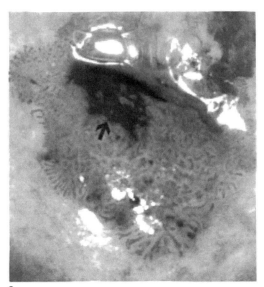
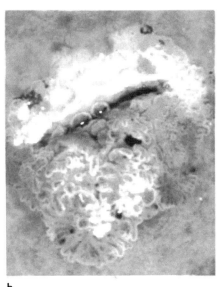

a b
FIGURE 6 a) Acuminate wart afflicting the transitional zone of the portio-cervix. Prior to acetic acid testing; the endocervical opening is surrounded by a highly characteristic lesion exhibiting typical punctuated and fork-loop-like capillary patterns. The patient attended due to postcoital bleeding; an haemorrhagia is detected close to the cervical os (arrow). b) A similar lesion as in Figure 6a subsequent to acetic acid testing (Courtesy of Eva Rylander, M.D., Department of Gyneacology, Hospital of Danderyd, Stockholm, Sweden).

Still others exhibit an undulating wavy exterior, sometimes with focal "microspikes." Yet others give rise to periodic fissuring (Figures 13 and 14).

4.   Bowenoid Papulosis

When bowenoid papulosis (BP) was first described[95] the condition was interpreted as "multicentric Bowen's disease" due to striking histological similarities with that of Bowen's disease, a condition denominated Queyrat's erythroplasia when located to the glans and foreskin. In subsequent studies, BP has been allocated as an entity clearly distinguishable from Bowen's disease (Table 3) through clinical features as well as age distribution of patients.[96,97] The presence of HPV type 16 DNA was demonstrated in about 80%,[98,99] and oncogenic HPVs of higher type numbers (18, 33, and 39) have also been demonstrated.[100,101]

BP represents a clinically appreciable form of oncogenic HPV-associated lesions that exhibit severe intraepithelial dysplasia. When clinically typical, BP is characterized by the occurrence on the outer genitoanal area in young adolescents (average age 28 years; upper range <40 years) of 2–10 mm large maculopapular lesions that are usually either erythematous, reddish-violaceous, or brownish with a

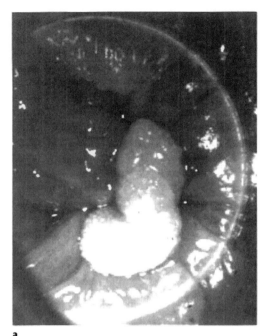 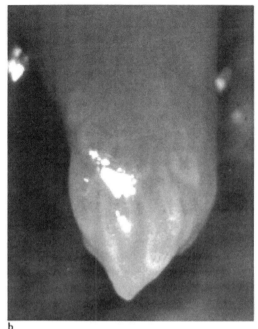

a   b

FIGURE 7 a) Intraanal acuminate condyloma as viewed through a proctoscope. Note the warty surface; viewed through colposcopic magnification typical capillary patterns are most often discernable. b) Intraanal physiologic papilla; the surface is smooth and capillaries run parallell with the surface texture. These papillae do not turn acetowhite.

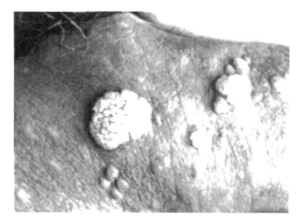

FIGURE 8 The coexistence of acuminate and papular warts on the outer aspects of the foreskin/the penile shaft.

smooth, velvety, or highly keratinized surface.[91,97,99] Clinically evident lesions are typically located on the vulva in the female and on the glans penis in the male (Figure 12a). Atypical forms also occur, for example when multiple lesions coalesce, as in the case illustrated in Figure 12b. Sometimes BP concur with benign warts and may signal their presence as recurrences after therapy.

Most frequently, the histological growth pattern is flat, but endophytic as well as exophytic variants occur.[91,99] BP may also exist as skin-colored subclinical lesions, located on thinner, moist genital epithelium which may be more common than the clinically evident forms. In settings where GPVI patients frequently are biopsied, the likelihood of encountering histologically bowenoid changes is quite high and in the magnitude of perhaps 10%.[32] The natural course has not been studied in any detail but is considered as predominantly benign. Some cases have regressed spontaneously within 1–2 years of observation; in others, the lesions have persisted for more than 10 years.

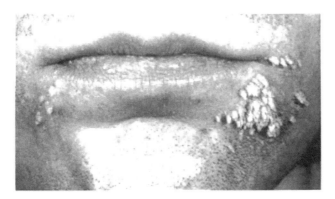

FIGURE 9 HPV 6 associated acuminate condylomas in the beard area of a 25-year-old otherwise healthy heterosexual male. Perioral warts are otherwise uncommon; when detected, underlying HIV-infection or other types of immunosuppression should be ruled out.

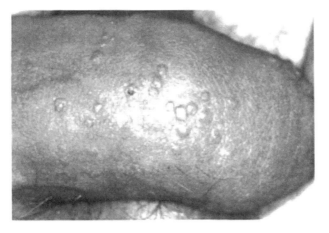

FIGURE 10 Papular warts on the penile shaft.

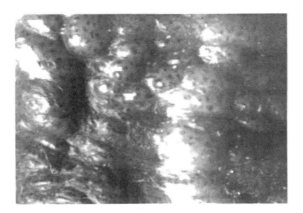

FIGURE 11 Papular warts exhibiting a typical punctuated capillary pattern as evaluated through colposcopic magnification.

5.   Bowen's Disease/Queyrat's Erythroplasia

Histologically, BP may mimic carcinoma *in situ* and cannot easily be differentiated from Bowen's disease (BD) and Queyrat's erythroplasia (QE). As a rule, however, BP vs. BD/QE can

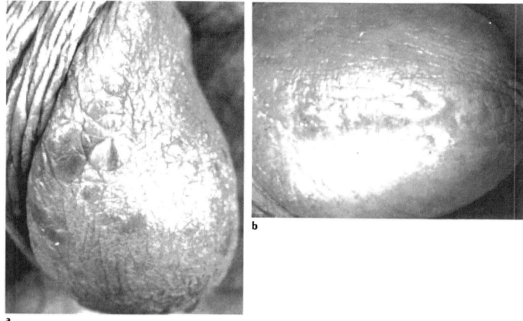

a
FIGURE 12 a) Bowenoid papulosis of the glans penis of a 28-year old male. Major clinical features for differentiation vs. Bowen's disease (Queyrat's erythroplasia) are outlined in Table 3. Other important differential diagnostic considerations include psoriasis and lichen ruber planus. These lesions are in general not precancerous and may, accordingly, be excised or destroyed surgically with a narrow margin but followed-up for 6-12 months as the recurrence rate often is high. b) Bowenoid papulosis of the glans penis of a 26-year old male, who developed an atypical form of lesions probably as a consequence of an orogenital "love-bite" by his girlfriend. In this case a linear lesion occurs as a "Koebner-phenomenon". The lesion measures 3 × 25 mm. Due to the patients' young age the lesion was not considered as premalignant (see Table 3) and was destroyed by electrodissication with a narrow surgical margine.

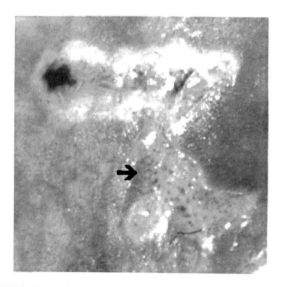

FIGURE 13 Fissured flat GPVI lesion on the inner aspect of the foreskin in a male experiencing recurrent balanoposthitis and superficial dyspareunia. Following application of acetic acid and the use of magnifying equipment ("penoscopy") a typical well demarcated GPVI lesion is detected exhibiting a fissure with a central, partially haemorrhagic groove (upper part); and typical punctuated capillaries (arrow).

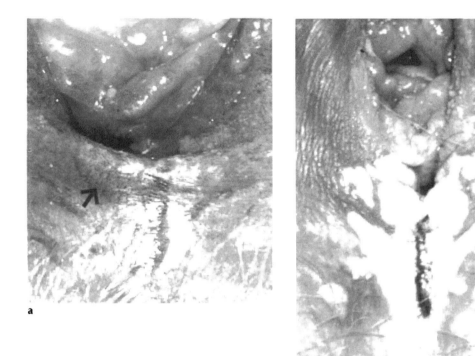

FIGURE 14 Fissured flat GPVI lesion of the posterior labial fourchette in a female experiencing recurrent vulvitis, episodes of bleeding and superficial dyspareunia. a) Magnifying equipment reveals the presence of a fissure surrounded by areas exhibiting a punctuated capillary pattern (arrow). b) The acetic acid test reveals the true extension of the GPVI lesion.

TABLE 3 Bowenoid Papulosis vs. Bowen's Disease and Queyrat's Erythroplasia Clinical Features

Clinical features	Bowenoid papulosis	Bowen's disease/Queyrat's erythroplasia
Patient's age	< 40 years	> 40 years
Lesions		
– number	multiple	solitary
– color	reddish-brown	reddish brown
	reddish blue	bright red
	pigmented	occasionally erosive
	grayish-white	
	skin coloured	
– surface	dry, sometimes peeling occasionally fissured	moist or peeling
– size	5–10 mm	> 10 mm

be distinguished on clinical grounds (Table 3), and in both lesions oncogenic HPVs such as type 16 have been detected.[102] The truly precancerous lesions of BD/QE are preferentially seen in patients over 40–50 years of age and usually show up as a solitary, nummular, slowly enlarging erythematous patch that often exhibits scaling and/or oozing (Figure 15).

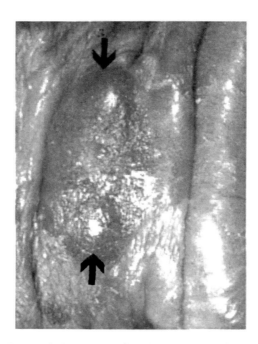

FIGURE 15 Queyrat's erythroplasia on the inner aspect of the foreskin (arrows) in a 65-year old male. The differential diagnostic aspects vs. those of bowenoid papulosis are outlined in Table 3.

Occasionally, long-lasting persistent BP may convert into BD/QE, or into frank squamous cell carcinoma.[103] It has been proposed that BP, regarded as a benign and self-limiting disease in the younger age group, in older persons incidently may transform into squamous cell carcinoma. In immunocompromised patients, the rate of malignant conversion may possibly be higher.

6.   Buschke-Löwenstein Tumor ("Giant Condyloma") and Verrucous Carcinoma

As accounted for previously, condylomata may grow exuberantly during pregnancy (Figure 16), in diabetic patients (Figure 17), or in cases of immunosuppression. Histopathologically such "giant warts" exhibit unequivocal features of benign exophytic condylomata.

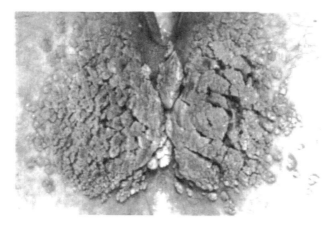

FIGURE 16 Confluent acuminate warts in a pregnant female, growing largely as a plaque covering the anal/perineal area.

In contrast, the Buschke-Löwenstein tumor (Figures 18 and 19) represents a histopathologically prominent acanthotic downgrowth into underlying dermal structures that leads to a local expansion with a semi-malignant invasion that ultimately may inflict on adjacent structures such as subcutaneous

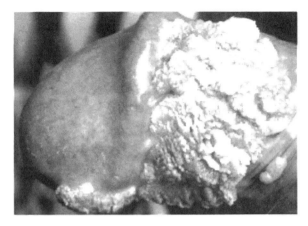

FIGURE 17 Acuminate warts in a diabetic male, coalescing as a confluent plaque afflicting the foreskin, the coronal sulcus and the fraenulum.

fat, the urethra, or the rectum. Fistula formation may occur and may be complicated by secondary bacterial infection. Sometimes, a complex histological pattern exists that may impose differential diagnostic difficulties. Thus, large areas of benign condylomas—frequently with koilocytosis—may occur but being intermixed with focal areas exhibiting atypical epithelial cells or even well differentiated squamous-cell carcinoma *in situ* features (Figure 20). Frank malignant conversion, however, is usually absent. Although regional lymph node metastasis is extremely rare, reactive inguinal lymphadenopathy, on the other hand, is not uncommon. This, together with an absence of distant metastasis in almost all cases, clearly distinguishes the condition from invasive squamous-cell carcinoma.[104-107]

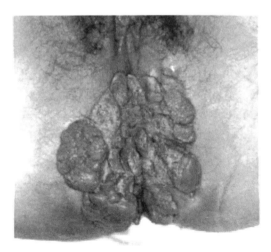

FIGURE 18 Buschke-Löwenstein tumor occupying the dorsal part of the vulva, the entire perineum and large parts of the anal region of a 35-year old woman.

This peculiar semi-malignant squamous-cell tumor was described on the penis already in 1898 by Buschke,[108] and detailed histological features were described in 1925 and in 1939 by Buschke and Löwenstein, respectively.[109] Similar tumors have subsequently also been described on the vulva,[105] and less frequently in the perineal-perianal area, in the groins, in the urethra, and in the anal canal.[104,110,111] On the penis, the tumor usually arises after years of poor hygiene and most frequently in the phimotic preputial cavity of uncircumcised men between 18 and 86 years of age.[103,110,111] These tumors tend to grow quite slowly but often enlarge to over 5 cm in diameter.

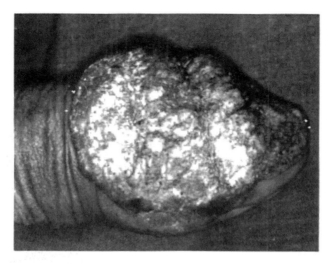

FIGURE 19 Buschke-Löwenstein tumor afflicting large parts of the glans penis and the foreskin of a 54-year-old man.

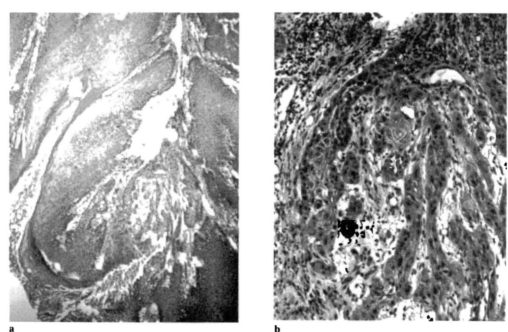

a   b

FIGURE 20 a) Histology of a penile Buschke-Löwenstein tumor, demonstrating atypical cells in a lesion expanding by downgrowth into the dermis (HE × 60). b) Magnification from (a) (HE × 120).

Most case reports refer to the semimalignant variant only. Nevertheless, a small series exists in which Buschke-Löwenstein tumors subsequently have converted into invasive and metastasing carcinomas.[112-115] The demonstration of HPV 6, and to a lesser degree of HPV 11, DNA sequences in a number of such tumors[110,116,117] underlines a pathogenetic association with HPV. Some features exhibit similarity to verrucous carcinoma, which was first described in the oropharynx by Ackermann in 1948[118] and subsequently by others.[119,120]

Verrucous carcinoma is by most authors considered as representing a well differentiated (low-grade) squamous-cell carcinoma. As for the Buschke-Löwenstein tumor, verrucous carcinomas appears as wart-like excrescences that tend to displace and destroy local tissues but that have little tendency to metastasize. The question has arisen as to whether verrucous carcinoma and the

Buschke-Löwenstein tumor should be considered as tumors of identical nature or whether they represent separate entities;[121] some investigators consider the Buschke-Löwenstein tumor to be on a continuum between a benign viral wart and a verrucous carcinoma.[110]

Verrucous carcinoma is presently used as a collective term including three clinical entities: oral florid papillomatosis, epithelioma cuniculatum, and the Buschke-Löwenstein tumor. Usually, florid papillomatosis afflicts the oropharynx and epithelioma cuniculatum afflicts the feet.[122] HPV 16 and HPV 2 DNA has occasionally been detected in oral and laryngeal verrucous carcinoma.[123,124] Although HPV DNA could not be disclosed in any sample from 13 patients with carcinoma cuniculatum when using PCR,[125] HPV 60 DNA was recently detected in so-called "ridged" plantar warts.[126,127]

The various synonyms for the Buschke-Löwenstein tumor that have been reported in the literature, including "giant condyloma," "giant malignant condyloma," and "carcinoma-like condyloma," has led to misunderstanding and confusion. The diagnosis may be difficult and requires a careful clinical examination combined with thorough histopathological investigation based on multiple biopsies sampled from several tumor areas, entailing adequate depth as well as margins. Multiple sections are necessary to differentiate between well differentiated squamous-cell carcinoma and condyloma acuminatum. In cases where the extent and exact location of the tumor are otherwise difficult to define, computerized tomography is recommended.[128]

Although the course in general is quite benign, the biologic behavior is sometimes uncertain and cannot be predicted by determination of the associated HPV type. Thus, close clinical surveillance of conspicious cases is important. Recurrences normally occur locally and demonstrate identical histological and biological behavior as that of the primary tumor. Both adjuvant local interferon gel therapy after ablation, and subcutaneous systemic low-dose interferon alpha therapy may prevent recurrences.[138] Rare observations exist on metastasis to regional lymph nodes, and exceptional cases exist with more distant metastases.[105,118,129-135] In a series accounting for 120 cases of verrucous carcinoma at various sites, lymph node metastasis was seen in 11 (9%) of patients;[132] in one review, 7 of 20 cases of verrucous carcinoma of the vulva died of the disease.[133] Anaplastic changes occur predominantly in patients previously treated with radiation.[105,118,129-131] Evidently, radiotherapy should be avoided even if local recurrences occur. Furthermore, Buschke-Löwenstein tumors and verrucous carcinomas both tend to be quite resistant to radiation.

Some observations suggest that the development, proliferation, and potential malignant conversion of the Buschke-Löwenstein tumor is related to the patient's immune status and to some yet unidentified cofactors as determinants as to whether HPV 6 or HPV 11 induced genital lesion will lead to simple condylomas, or occassionally, to a Buschke-Löwenstein tumor.[105,117,136-139]

B.   Anatomical Distribution of Lesions

The distribution **on the penis** (Table 1) differs between circumcised[3,140] and uncircumcised men.[1] In **uncircumcised** men, the preputial cavity is most often affected (i.e., the glans penis, the coronal sulcus, the frenulum and the inner aspect of the foreskin), while in the **circumcised** man the shaft of the penis is most commonly engaged.[63] Warts in the groin, the perineum, and on the scrotum are quite rare.[1-3,63]

In the **female** (Table 2), lesions often afflict the posterior fourchette, the medial and/or lateral parts of the vulva, the areas adjacent to the clitoris and/or the meatus urethrae, the perineum, the anal region, the vestibulum/introitus, the hymenal ring and the vagina.[1-3] The cervix uteri, and in particular the exocervix, are concurrently afflicted in 30–50% of cases, although infrequently with acuminate warts but rather with macular lesions.[28,38,42]

Acuminate lesions afflicting either the meatal lips of the **urinary meatus** or the **distal area of the urethra** (Figure 3) are far more common in males (10–28%) than in females (<5%). About half of the patients with meatal lip warts also have distal urethral warts that generally can be observed adequately by meatoscopy.[141-143] Warts situated proximally of the fossa navicularis in the male are rare; yet, about 5% of cases require referral to an urologist for urethroscopy.[1,3,141] **The posterior urethra** is seldom involved without simultaneous growth of anterior warts.[144,145] Because involvement beyond the distal 3 cm of the urethra is so rare, it is beyond medical liability to screen patients unless urethral dysfunctions such as haematuria, recalcitrant urethritis, or voiding problems eventuate. However, in immunosuppressed patients, urethral dissemination sometimes occurs and may occasionally become extensive,[145] when palpable masses along the penile urethra should be sought.

Extension to the **bladder** is very rare.[146-148] Malignant transformation into squamous cell carcinoma is extremely uncommon except in severely immunosuppressed patients[149] and has been associated with HPV 6/11 as well as 16/18 and 31/33.[147-150]

Anal warts (Figures 7 and 16) occur in about 1/3 of females in the perineum, the perianal area, and/or in the anus. Anal warts in males have by tradition been ascribed to homosexuality and the practice of anal sex; actually, concurrent intra-anal warts exist in as much as 70% of homosexual men with external anal warts,[6,151] when lesions frequently are found up to the dentate line. Although a spread beyond this point is rare, the lower rectum appears to be coinfected in up to 10% in selected materials on homosexual males seen in proctology units.[152] It needs to be emphasized, however, that anal warts, including those afflicting the anal canal, are not uncommon in strictly heterosexual men as well.[153-155] Digital autoinoculation from penile lesions may represent the major pathogenetic factor in these cases: this hypothesis is in agreement with the fact that in heterosexual males anal warts are often associated with concurrent or antecedant penile warts.[1,151,155]

In **children**, warts occasionally develop in the genitoanal region, most commonly perianally and less frequently in boys than in girls. Although the potential of sexual abuse always must be kept in mind, in particular in children above the age of 2–4 years, condylomas cannot be used as the sole medicolegal indicator of abuse,[156-157] because the perinatal infection rate of mucosotrophic HPVs possibly may be as high as 30–70%, as measured by PCR technique, when the birth canal of the mother is afflicted with either condylomas, or with subclinical cervicovaginal lesions.[158] Viral reactivation from vertical acquisition, after months or years of subclinical/latent infection—rather than new HPV exposure—seems to be the case in 50–70% of children with genitoanal warts[6,63,156] (See also Chapter 15).

An exact outlining of the anatomical distribution of **subclinical lesions** on the outer genitals cannot be given at this point. Although studied extensively during the past few years, using the acetic acid test and colposcopy/penoscopy combined with histopathological and/or HPV DNA hybridization analysis, some confusion still exists because recent results demonstrate that the acetic acid test sometimes gives false positive results, for example in the presence of inflammatory conditions.[32] Yet, data presented so far indicate that the distribution of subclinical GPVI lesions is an analogy to that of overt warts. Symptomatic acetowhite lesions, however, are predominantly detected on thin mucous membranes such as in the preputial cavity (Figure 13) and the posterior fourchette of the vulva (Figure 14). In some cases, flat acetowhite lesions may coexist with, or perhaps even predispose for recurrent and long-lasting balanoposthitis and vulvovaginitis.[33]

C.   Differential Diagnosis

Exophytic warts are clinically pathognomonic and easily distinguishable from "pearly penile papules" (Figure 21) as well as from sebaceous glands of the prepuce and of the vulva (Figures 22 and 23). Differentiation from physiological squamous papillae of the vestibulum/introitus of the vagina ("vaginal micropapillomatosis") is somewhat more difficult; yet, they are most often distinguishable from condylomas for their symmetrical and linear assay distribution. Moreover, they do not have the clustered and pleomorphic characteristics of classical condylomas.[159] "Condylomata lata" in secondary syphilis may be ruled out by syphilis serology and/or histopathology investigation. The gross features of BP may cause differential problems vs. fibroma, psoriasis, eczema, lichen ruber planus, lichen sclerosus and atrophicus, seborrheic keratosis, lentigo, and naevi, but are easily distinguished by routine histology. Molluscum contagiosum, occuring as multiple 2–5 mm papules, are pinkish-gray to fleshy in color with an umbilicated center. Anal warts must be differentiated from physiological intraanal papillae (Figure 7), skin tags and hemorrhoids.

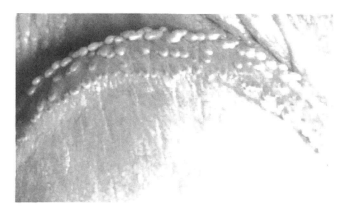

FIGURE 21 High-power magnification of the corona glandis, revealing the existence of typical "pearly penile papules," in this case occuring in three parallell rows. Their presence is highly individual; in some men they are completely absent. Such physiologcal papules do not exhibit capillary patterns typical for GPVI and remain acetonegative. Similar papules are often also present symmetrically in the distal part of the parafrenulum region.

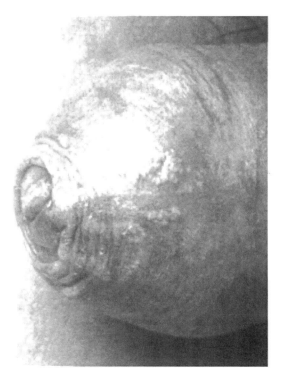

FIGURE 22 Sebaceous glands on the outer aspect of the foreskin; analogous glands also occur on the inner aspect of the foreskin. Their presence and distribution are highly individual.

As balanoposthitis or vulvovaginitis may occur concurrently with flat and macular GPVI lesions,[33] it may be wise to initiate topical anti-inflammatory therapy and subsequently reevaluate the patient when differential uncertainty exists. Vulvar candidiasis often induces fissures in the posterior vulva fourchette, giving rise to symptoms and a clinical presentation that may be hard to differentiate from GPVI. Acetowhite lesions often require biopsy for a correct diagnosis; inflammation, psoriasis, lichen ruber planus, and lichen sclerosus and atrophicus may give rise to acetowhitening as well.[33] Melanocytic naevi, seborrhoic keratosis, Bowen's disease, basal-cell carcinoma, melanoma, and cutaneous

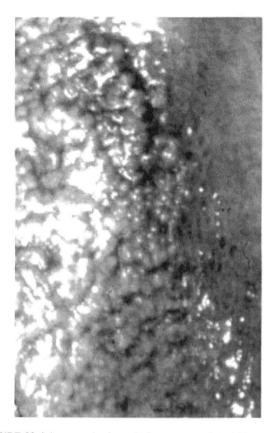

FIGURE 23 Sebaceous glands on the inner aspect of the labium minora.

Hodgkin's disease rarely impose problems in the differential diagnosis vs. verrucous carcinoma and/or Buschke-Löwenstein tumor. Sometimes, benign condylomas recently treated with podophyllotoxin and/or podophyllin reveal histologically degenerative changes such as bizarrely configurated keratinocytes with chromatin changes that mimic the pathological mitosis seen in squamous-cell carcinoma if biopsies are taken shortly after therapy.[160] Podophyllin-induced features, however, disappear within a week or two after application.

D.   Symptoms

1.   Physical Symptoms

Physical symptoms frequently occur with a fluctuating "come-and-go" course. Both benign and dysplastic GPVI lesions may induce symptoms and clinical signs within a highly variable range and severity. Symptoms may be associated either with visible warts noted by the patient, by tiny exophytic lesions being visible only by colposcopic magnification, or with flat and macular lesions that require acetic acid testing for identification.[32,33,90,161] Occasionally, edema or inguinal adenopathy may occur in males.[33] Warts may **bleed, itch,** and/or **burn** spontaneously or when submitted to traumas such as coitus (Figures 6, 13, 14). Itching and burning are also associated with episodes of **vulvovaginitis** and **balanoposthitis. Dyspareunia** may be due to **fissuring** (Figures 13 and 14).

Some symptomatic patients have previously been afflicted with visible warts that were believed to have responded successfully to therapy. Others have never noted overt warts.[33] Occasionally, symptoms appear to be related to a repetitive epidermal fissuring of flat lesions (Figures 13, 14). In females, this commonly occurs in the posterior vulvar fourchette.[161] In the male, symptoms often afflict the frenulum, the coronal sulcus and/or the foreskin of the penis.[33]

In the condition denominated **vestibular papillomatosis,** associated with multiple and often confluent papillae covering various areas of the vestibulum, as many as half of the females may be symptomatic.[90]

Recurrent and sometimes long-lasting symptoms of the outer genitals, being associated with GPVI and concurrent epithelial inflammation, have been referred to as **"papillomavirus-associated balanoposthititis"** in the male[33] and **"papillomavirus-associated vulvovaginitis"** (Figure 24 and 25) in the female.[162-164] In females, the symptomatology, including either a feeling of dryness, or recurrent episodes of discharge as well as deep dyspareunia,[163,164] partially overlaps with that of the syndrome originally denominated **"the burning vulva syndrome"**—later replaced by the terms **"vulvodynia"**[89] and **"vulvar vestibulitis"**.[163]

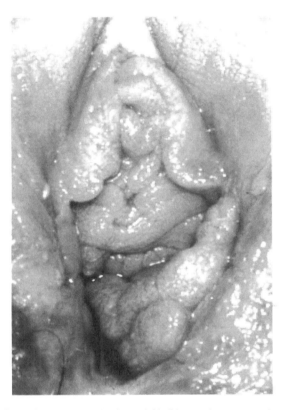

FIGURE 24 A case of "papillomavirus - associated vulvovaginitis;" hymenal remnants and parts of the vagina are covered by an HPV 16-associated hypertrophic, granulated mucosa in an otherwise healthy female who suffered from long-lasting deep dyspareunia (Courtesy of Eva Rylander, Associate Professor, M.D., Department of Gynea-cology, Danderyd Hospital, Sweden).

These conditions were previously often attributed to a presumed neurotic personality. However, there is no evidence that these women have a higher rate of psychiatric constitution than control patients.[165] As a working hypothesis, vulvodynia is believed, most commonly, to be induced by covarying exogeneous and/or endogeneous somatic causes, of which HPV represents one and various Candida species onother one.[89,166,167] Sometimes, intensive rubbing of the affected mucosa, for instance during horseback riding, biking, or sexual intercourse, may induce exacerbations of symptoms in females.[168]

Symptomatic lesions may sometimes be difficult to cure, but patients often feel helped by various methods aiming at symptomatic relief. Repetitive topical anti-inflammatory therapy, oral antibiotics, oral retinoids,[169] and/or surgical excision of fissured lesions[33] have been tried; ultimately a permanent cure is usually accomplished.

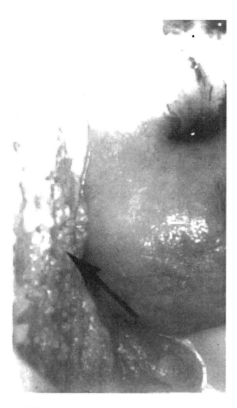

FIGURE 25 Disseminated, granulated HPV lesions covering the lateral vaginal wall in an otherwise healthy woman experiencing long-lasting periods of deep dyspareunia and a feeling of dryness (Courtesy of Eva Rylander, Associate Professor, M.D., Department of Gynaecology, Danderyd Hospital, Stockholm, Sweden).

Vulvar vestibulitis is characterized by a severe tenderness of the vestibular area, where the vagina opens onto the vulva. In some cases sexual intercourse is impossible and even insertion of a tampon is hindered. No uniform explanations has yet been forthcoming.[170] A diversity of pathological findings including that of HPV influence, indicate that the condition may be the end point of a number of pathological processes.

2.   Psychosexual and Psychosocial Implications

Genitoanal warts are of great **cosmetic and psychosexual significance.** Patients often experience them as both distasteful and disfiguring and consider them as a major hindrance to sexual performance. Available data on **psychosexual and psychosocial influences** of GPVI indicate the existence of negative effects on sexual and social life that are quite analogous to—and at least as common and pronounced—as those described for genital herpes simplex.[171-174] Psychosexual impact, possibly more frequent in females than in males, includes profound influences on sexuality, mood, social life, emotional relationship with the partner, and fear of cancer.[94,173,175-177]

In a U.S. inquiry[175] among 454 mostly female long-term sufferers, a negative impact on sexual feelings and behavior during the year of diagnosis was reported in the predominant majority of responders, including problems approaching a new partner (86%), a reduced frequency of sexual contact (72%) and decreased enjoyment of sexual life (68%). More than two thirds also reported emotional disturbances such as feeling undesirable and fearing rejection, feeling anger, shame, guilt, or depression. As much as 73% felt that the situation influenced their ability to be spontaneous and 70% reacted with some degree of isolation.

Although most of the long-term sufferers had told someone about having GPVI, including their current partner, a friend, and a family member (48–69%), one third did not rely on anyone for emotional comfort. A minority (9%) reported a need for psychotherapeutic interventions and/or help from a support group (4%). Thus, the need for support and counseling appears to be significant. In many cases health care professionals tend to underestimate sexuality related emotional problems. Reasons for changing their provider was mostly related to lack of advice on emotional issues (84%) and failure to ask questions about sexual practices (76%).

These aspects are concordant with those underscored by Filiberti et al.,[173] who found that among 52 consecutive patients, as many as 28% feared that the disease might develop into cancer and another 16% reported severe disturbances within their relationship. As much as 57% described their sexual life as worsened, often due to fear of possible reinfection from, or sexual transmission of the disease to the partner. Suggestions of using condoms were not infrequently associated with inhibited sexual desire.

The psychosocial impact in women may be even more pronounced following the finding of an abnormal cervical smear; the diagnosis of CIN and treatment of pre-invasive cervical neoplasia may induce anxiety and fear from the spectre of cancer; being monitored for the natural course rather than being immediately treated sometimes causes great distress.[178] The diagnosis also has implications for body image, questions related to future fertility, child bearing capacity, and sexual function. A deleterious effect of diagnosis and treatment of CIN upon sexual behavior and response has been accounted for by Campion et al.,[179] who found significant increase on negative feelings towards sexual intercourse or towards a regular sexual partner, decreased frequency of intercourse, as well as decreased vaginal lubrication, sexual arousal, and frequency of orgasm.

IV.   CLINICAL EVALUATION

A.   When to Investigate

The insight that biologally active GPVI afflicts an approximate 10% of the sexually active population evokes important questions and dilemmas because present resources, as well as therapeutic modalities, are limited (Figure 26). Management of patients with overt disease already puts a notable strain on the resources of dermatovenereology and gynecology. A much larger challenge is evidently ahead if subclinical cases are also to be diagnosed and treated.

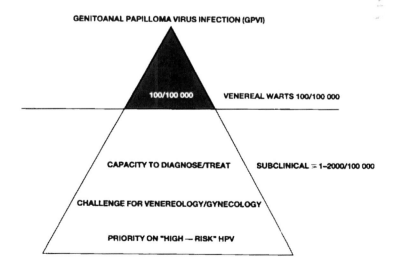

GENITOANAL PAPILLOMA VIRUS INFECTION (GPVI)

100/100 000   VENEREAL WARTS 100/100 000

CAPACITY TO DIAGNOSE/TREAT   SUBCLINICAL ≈ 1–2000/100 000

CHALLENGE FOR VENEREOLOGY/GYNECOLOGY

PRIORITY ON "HIGH → RISK" HPV

FIGURE 26 GPVI: "the ice-berg dilemma".

One important question is whether it is pertinent or practically possible to perform a screening for GPVI in all sexually active individuals attending, for example STD and gynecology clinics for routine investigation. Second, even if sufficient resourses are created for this purpose, are we really able to remove all these multifocal lesions, or should we rather observe the natural course in the majority of cases until a sponaneous, and probably immunomodulated dissappearance occurs? Third, what strategy should be used to prevent a further spread of GPVI, and in particular of the "high-risk" HPV types that are associated with subsequent development of genital cancer?

As it is not the HPV itself which is harmful to the patient, the primary task at the time being must inevitably be to focus on **lesions** being either of psychosexual importance, giving rise to symptoms, or representing significant risk of cancer sequelae. In light of available epidemiological data, routine screening for the potential presence of subclinical lesions on the outer genitals of asymptomatic individuals seems pointless and rather instead causes unnecessary fear and anguish in presumably healthy people.[6,180] Yet, it is important that every physician who handles these patients is familiar with the various methods for diagnostic optimization that exist at present, and that a thorough investigation is recommended in the following situations: (1) Genitoanal warts have been diagnosed by gross appearance—what is the full extension of multifocal disease?; (2) Symptoms are present that cannot otherwise be explained (bleeding, coital dysfunction including dyspareunia, pruritus, burning, fissures, recurrent balanoposthitis/vulvovaginitis); (3) Investigation and counseling of steady partner of a patient with GPVI; and (4) Atypical cells have been detected in a cervical smear.

A decentralized primary management by primary health care providers is a possibility in some clinical settings.[181] A number of patients, estimatedly in the range of 20–40%, may require subsequent transfer to specialist care. Occurrence of urinary meatus and anal warts often requires a specialist team including urologists and proctologists.[32] Although therapy most often will be the responsibility of dermatovenereologists, pediatric or gynecological expertise may also be required for surgical assistance Whenever sexual abuse is suspected, children with condylomas should be referred for pediatric and sociomedical expertise evaluation.[182-185]

The potential risk of cancer transformation from lesions on the outer genitals is low in patients under the age of 30–35 years and does not justify screening. On the other hand, routine vaginocervical cytology examination during Pap smear of females above the age of 25–30 years must be performed liberally, aiming at the detection of persistent CIN II - III.

B. Screening for Other STDs

Prevalence of other concurrent STDs is variable and dependent on the study population. Yet, although patients attending STD clinics should be considered a high-risk group, comparable STD rates have been reported in other settings as well.[186-188] In a large series of patients with genital warts being treated at an STD department, additional genital infection(s) have been detected in one third of men and two thirds of females.[189]

Whether chronic infections may represent a contributing pathogenic factor for cervical cancer is a matter of controversy.[40,56,190-192] STDs may possibly be surrogate markers of population-associated risk factors for HPV exposure and of no separate etiologic significance. Some STDs, however, seem to have the potential of viral activation, possibly leading to stimulation not only of wart growth and/or contributing to HPV-associated symptoms[55] but to the promotion of CIN development/progression as well.[40,56] Regardless of a pathogenetic association, however, it must be stressed that GPVI evaluation represents a significant counselling situation that should be regarded as a "golden opportunity" for implementing primary and secondary preventive strategies for other covarying STDs.[56,193-195] In symptomatic women, the prevalence of *Neisseria gonorrhoeae* is higher than that of *Chlamydia trachomatis*,[196] while in asymptomatic women the relationship tends to be reversed.[56] According to Kharsany et al.,[56] it also seems that bacterial vaginosis occurs more often in women with CIN than in those without (50% vs. 20%).

We advocate, above all, routine tests for *N. gonorrhoea, C. trachomatis, Trichomonas vaginalis*, and bacterial vaginosis, but also feel that a liberal offering of tests for syphilis, HIV, and Hepatitis B and C is required.

C.   Procedures of GPVI Investigation

The outer genitoanal area is systematically inspected for the existence of overt warts. A good light source is a prerequisite; a magnification device, preferably a colposcope, is of major advantage and represents a necessity for specialist evaluation.

Concerns have been raised on the mediocolegal dilemma of missing or underdiagnosing genital HPV disease. This aspect is significant for the diagnosis of CIN and cervical cancer but less valid for the outer genitals. It has been suggested that women with CIN may benefit from examination and treatment of clinical and/or subclinical lesions of their male partners, aiming at optimizing the cure rates of CIN.[197] This might seem rational; as is the case for clinically apparent BP,[197] these men appear to have a high frequency of severe penile intraepithelial neoplasia (PIN III) when their acetowhite lesions are biopsied.[32] However, treatment failure rates of women with CIN whose steady partners are carefully examined and treated for subclinical penile lesions do not, so far, differ from those of women whose partners remain untreated, and there appears to be no protective effect from condom use in the male against progression rates of CIN in the female counterpart.[198]

1.   Urethra Inspection

The meatus can be everted manually or using cotton wool swabs. Whenever the proximal border of urethral warts is hard to outline, "meatoscopy" is recommended, i.e., inspection with a small nose speculum or with an otoscopic (auroscopic) endpiece tube.[142,199] It is rather unusual (<5% of cases) that the border cannot be delineated by these means; if so, a urologist must be consulted for urethroscopic inspection. Warts located proximally of the fossa navicularis are usually associated with micturation problems, such as dysuria, bleeding, and/or voiding problems.[141,144] The anterior part of the urethra should be routinely palpated. If any mass is present, or if the patient has voiding problems such as reduced urinary stream or haematuria, endoscopy and/or cystourethrography should be performed for identification of intraurethral bladder papillomata. Urethrography following intravenously injected contrast medium, is recommended because this technique avoids urethral instrumentation and possible associated risk for a retrograde spread of infection.[200] Sampling for C. trachomatis with an ENT swab should preferrably be performed after therapy of meatus warts in order to avoid inducing an iatrogenic spread of warts to more proximal parts of the urethra; the alternative use of PCR or LCR methodology in first-void-urine samples is recommended in such cases.

2.   Anoscopy/Proctoscopy

Anoscopy is recommended not only when a history of anal sex is obtained but as a rule when anal warts are encountered. In order to obtain optimal therapeutic results without recurrence of disease, it is crucial to remove all visible warts at extenal and internal sites. In view of the possibility of transferring a tissue-bearing infectious virus, some authorities recommend a two-step procedure. First, the external visible lesions should be removed and the area allowed to heal before performing anoscopy. Typical acuminate warts are easily recognized even without magnification (Figure 7a). Nevertheless, they may occasionally resemble hypertrophic physiological papillae (Figure 7b), which may occur just beneath the dentate line and may be quite prominent. Such papillae do not turn white from 5% acetic acid and do not have the vascular pattern characteristic for condylomata. Inspection through the anoscope proves to be a very valuable technique for a proper evaluation of intra-anal growths.

3.   The Acetic Acid Test

The application of 5% acetic acid, combined with colposcopic magnification, has become the standard method for investigating, above all, flat and subclinical GPVI lesions. The effect—"ace-towhitening"—is due to a swelling of infected suprabasal cells, associated, above all, with over-expression of cytokeratin 10,[201] the opaqueness of acetowhite areas emanating from light reflected from turgid epitheloid cells. The reliability of the test has recently been challenged, as false positivity is common in the presence of epithelial inflammation and/or some specific dermatological conditions such as lichen sclerosus and atrophicus.[32,202,203]

The true presence of GPVI lesions is signaled by an acetowhitening that typically exhibits well demarcated, slightly elevated areas, in which a punctuated capillary pattern can be distinguished. Some GPVI lesions exhibit a central "groove," (Figures 13 and 14) in which the epidermis is quite thin and sometimes is associated with haemorrhagic epithelial breaks. In contrast, acetowhitening due to inflammatory conditions mostly exhibits ragged, irregular borders and varying degrees of underlying erythema (Figure 28).

Sometimes, GPVI and epithelial inflammation coexist ("papillomavirus-associated vulvovaginitis;" "papillomavirus-associated balanoposthitis"). When any doubt comes forth regarding the nature of acetowhitening, it might be wise to apply a topical anti-inflammatory remedy, followed by subsequent re-testing of the patient. Although some controversy exists whether topical steroid therapy potentially might stimulate proliferation of GPVI-associated lesions through activating keratinocyte steroid receptors,[59] 1–2 weeks of mild steroid-antimicrobial cream treatment, such as Dactacort®* cream, has been advocated by some authors.[32,33,63,181] In many cases, a partial clearing of the acetowhitening follows, which facilitates further clinical and therapeutic evaluation. Magnification equipment and clinical training is required and confirmatory biopsy evaluation is highly recommended for proper evaluation. Accordingly, use of the test ought to be confined to well-trained specialists.

The test is very valuable for demarcation of papular and flat warts prior to therapy (Figure 27). It may sometimes also be helpful when a protracted course of genital condylomas occurs; applied prior to surgical therapy, subclinical lesions that could potentially contribute to therapeutic failure may be identified (Figure 29). Not the least, use of the test prior to colposcopic evaluation of the cervix aiming to assist in the detection of proper areas for subsequent targeted biopsy is extremely helpful (Figure 30). Unrequired screening, on the other hand, may create fear and other psychosexual sequelae in otherwise presumptively healthy individuals (Figure 31).

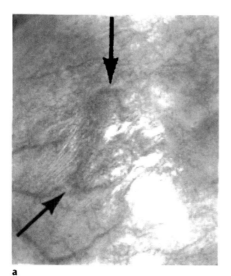 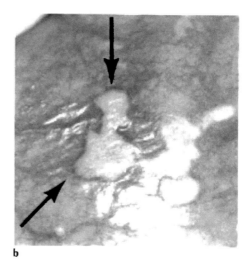

a   b

FIGURE 27 a) A slighly elevated flat lesion is seen at high power magnification prior to the acetic acid test (arrows). Punctuated capillaries are discernible. b) Same lesion as in Figure 27 a); the 5% acetic acid influence facilicates appreciation of lesional demarcation and also reveals that the infected area is much larger than was originally appreciated.

---

* Janssen Pharmaceutical B-2340, Beerse, Belgium

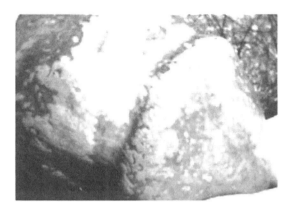

FIGURE 28 "False positive" acetowhitening, exhibiting ragged, irregular borders in a male suffering from acute balano-posthitis. Subsequent to topical anti-inflammatory therapy the acetowhitening disappeared completely.

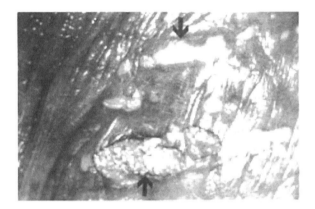

FIGURE 29 Recurrent acuminate warts have occurred on the foreskin in spite of local chemotherapy with podophyllotoxin. Prior to sugical destruction, the acetic acid test is applied. Adjacent to a visible acuminate wart several acetowhite lesions are also detected (upper area) that are surgically destructed concurrently. When using the acetic test during surgical procedures, repeated applications during the session are recommended, as the acetowhitening tend to fade or to disappear within a few minutes.

4. The Iodine Test

During estrogen influence, normal squamous epithelium of the vestibulum, the vagina, and the portio, are stained dark-brown by iodine. This reaction is due to the presence of glycogen in highly differentiated epithelium. In papillomavirus-infected, as well as in neoplastic epithelium, the glycogen content is reduced since the cells are immature. Moreover, the disturbed maturation is associated with abnormal keratinization. Therefore, when applying a 2% iodine solution ("the Schiller-test") to the region, HPV-afflicted areas will appear patchy or striped brownish-yellow in color. Intraepithelial neoplasia becomes yellowish and sharply demarcated. As for the acetic acid test, a positive outcome is not specific but nevertheless represents an indication for subsequent histological evaluation of a biopsy specimen.

5. Cytology

Cytological signs of GPVI and CIN, and the recently proposed Bethesda classification system, are accounted for by Meisels in Chapter 18. In women with vulvar GPVI lesions, almost half are concurrently afflicted by lesions of the cervix and/or of the vagina.[28,38,42] Furthermore, cervical lesions often occur without simultaneous GPVI of the outer genitals.[204]

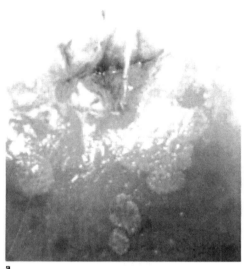
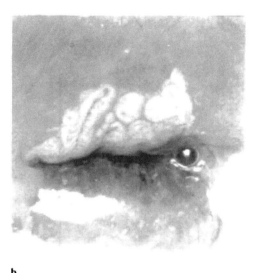

a   b

FIGURE 30 a) Physicians encountering females with GPVI must be familiar with the indentification of lesions on the portiocervix. Cytology screening (Pap-smear) represents a convenient approach; yet, high false negativity rates exist. The sensitivity for detection is considerably higher using colposcopic investigation subsequent to the application of 5% acetic acid (Figure) but specificity problems exist. (Courtesy of Eva Rylander, Associate Professor, M.D., Department of Gynaecology Danderyd Hospital Stockholm, Sweden). b) Acetowhitening on the upper lip of the cervix due to immature metaplasia.

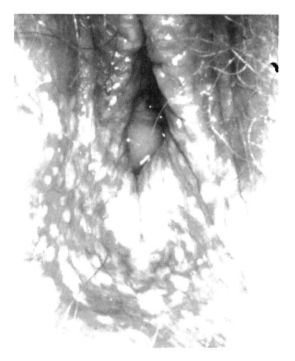

FIGURE 31 Acetowhite lesions identified on the vulva in a 20-year old presumptively healthy female attending for prescription of birth control pills. When told about the lesions "being caused by an incurable virus," she reacted with fear and emotional disturbances that influenced negatively on her ongoing sexual relationship, which was otherwise harmonious prior to the attendence.

The primary purpose of exfoliative cervicovaginal smear ("Pap smear") screening is to detect CIN lesions. Yet, the test will also identify a number of benign HPV-induced lesions through the recognition of koilocytosis, a situation that might represent either a true "false positive" Pap smear, or a false negative cytology sample presumed that the koilocytes emanate from a dysplastic cervical lesion. However, even if false negativity occurs in a proportion of CIN cases, no better alternative exists for decentralized routine screening. Current recommendations are based on cytological sampling in women older than 25–30 years of age, with rescreening every 3–5 years in negative cases.[205]

In countries where large-scale cytological screening programs have been implemented in gynecology and in general practice settings, the significant drop—up to 70%—in the rate of invasive cancer of the uterine cervix are testimonial to the efficacy of the smear programs.[206] Nevertheless, a major problem is associated with the fact that the sensitivity fluctuates within a range as broad as 55–98%, depending on the study. Several causes have been identified, including sampling and interpretational errors as well as screening policy sampling practises.[207] Accordingly, adequacy of sampling techniques and of quality control measurements for cytology reading have been discussed. Inter- and intra-observer variation for cytology readings due to monotony and fatigue factors may explain some of the deficiencies. Several automized commercial reading systems, including that of image analysis, have been proposed as quality-control measures of individual laboratories.[206]

Although great efforts are currently being made to standardize the optimal practice of cytology, many of the parameters used to achieve that goal are debatable.[207] Sampling of the appropriate area remains crucial for the sensitivity.[206] As CIN lesions arise from the cervical transformation zone (TZ), cytology is most sensitive when cellular material is obtained from this zone. TZ moves upward with age, and in most menopausal women it resides in the endocervical canal. The presence of endocervical or metaplastic cells in the smear indicates that the TZ has been sampled. However, the presence of endocervical columnar cells cannot be used as the sole criterion of an adequate Pap smear. Specimens considered satisfactory contain well-visualized squamous epithelia cells and 2 clusters of well-preserved endocervical and of at least five transformation zone cells.

The predominant screening error is caused by the nature of the screening process itself.[206] To determine the adequacy of Pap smears, some considerations regarding quality control have been suggested:[208] (1) The absence of endocervical cells or squamous metaplastic cells in women under 45 years of age suggests that the TZ has not been sampled; (2) Specimens in which cellular detail is obscured by excessive air drying, inflammation, menstruation or a lubricant are unsatisfactory, and (3) Smears obtained with the use of specialized sampling devices, such as a brush, that are composed largely or entirely of endocervical cells, are inadequate and indicate that the TZ below the endocervical canal has not been properly sampled.

Women found to have atypical Pap smears should be referred to a gynecologist for further evaluation. If only koilocytosis is detected in the smear, a gynaecologist should either be consulted, or a second smear be taken after another year. In this respect, the local policy varies.

6. The Potential Usefulness of HPV DNA Testing as an Adjuvant Screening Procedure for CIN

A significant problem with current Pap smear screening programs for CIN is the fact that we do not know which lesions will progress, regress, or remain at the same CIN stage, a dilemma apparently leading to unneccessary overtreatment at younger ages. Another major problem is a relatively low sensitivity for conventional cytology.[207,208] Furthermore, a dilemma exists on how to deal with the large number of borderline and mildly dyskaryotic smears which have a highly variable pathology; on biopsy about a third appear to arise from CIN II-III, another third from CIN I, and the remainder are normal or show very minor changes.[209] Most importantly, as recent epidemiological data indicate, the majority of CIN cases among women below 30 years of age represent transient changes, while an increased likelihood for progression exists in older women persistently infected with oncogenic high risk HPV types.[34,41,210]

The potential role of HPV DNA detection as an approach in order to optimize cytology screening procedures has been accounted for in detail by Waalboomers et al. in Chapter 19. Targeted HPV screening of females above the age of 30–35 years, in whom the risk of developing cervical cancer from persistent precursor lesions is significantly increased, might very well turn out to represent an innovative strategy to improve current cytological screening programs. As cytomorphologically abnormal cervical scrapes are heterogeneous with respect to the HPV types present, reliable HPV DNA screening procedures must focus on distinguishing multiple high- vs. low-risk HPV types. The recent development of general-primer-mediated PCR types[34,211,212] in cervical scrapes represents an important step towards the possible application of HPV DNA detection as an adjuvant to cytology readings in selected female populations, in particular if quantification techniques for amount of HPV DNA present are also implemented in order to avoid false positive results.

Also, studies on HPV-specific serology markers have demonstrated that antibody responses against several different HPV-derived epitopes are strongly associated with CIN. In several studies combinations of several HPV-specific peptides have further improved disease-specificity, and it seems likely that peptide-based serology utilizing one or several HPV-specific epitopes will become an additional tool potentially being suitable for the diagnosis of CIN and frank malignancy.[213]

7.   Colposcopy

In the 1920s and 1930s, colposcopy was the only method for the detection of precancerous lesions of the uterine cervix. With the appearance of exfoliative cytology, colposcopy was thought to be condemned to disappear. However, now the method has turned out to be of great value not only for the topographical study of neoplasia on the uterine cervix, but for the evaluation of HPV infection in all genitoanal areas as well. Its usefulness is in part to determine the site, size, and extent of the lesions, and in part to focus on representative areas for subsequent biopsies. Also, the accuracy of surgical treatment may be augmented considerably if it is performed under colposcopic control.

In the present context, only some major points will be touched on with respect to the applicability of colposcopy in the evaluation of intraepithelial neoplasia; for further information, the reader is referred to more detailed textbooks.[214-216] A comprehensive insight into the art of colposcopy requires training and experience. Nevertheless, this should not prevent any gynecologist or venereologist from mastering basic principles of this extremely valuable instrument in the clinical management of GPVI.

The acetic acid test, combined with colposcopy and when required with iodine application, is advantageous for the selection of areas for biopsy that are representative for concurrent neoplasia. On the cervix, the biopsy should be obtained from the medial part of the lesions; in general, the closer to the squamo-columnar junction of the TZ that the biopsy can be obtained, the greater is the possibility to touch on an area which represents "the worst" regarding the degree of any accompanying neoplasia.[217]

a.   Cervix Uteri.   With the exception of typical condylomata acuminata, cervical HPV-associated lesions do not show type-specific clinical or colposcopic features. Most lesions are detected by colposcopy, but often only after acetic acid application (Figure 30). However, the colposcopic features do not unequivocally allow neither a distinction between condylomas vs. CIN III nor between HPV-associated lesions and metaplasia.[218] Thus, colposcopic features of HPV-associated lesions recalls the colposcopic classification of cervical abnormalities recently approved[219] by the International Federation of Colposcopy and Cervical Pathology (IFCPC; Table 4). This terminology describes the colposcopic images that may be encountered and distinguishes between "minor" and "major" changes but without any precise diagnostic correlation. The central point of this and other types of terminology is that a focus is put on the identification of the part of the cervix which is at risk for the development of HPV-associated lesions and cancer precursors, namely the TZ.

b.   The Cervical Transformation Zone (TZ).   CIN develops inside the TZ, being characterized as that portion of the exocervix which has originally been covered by glandular epithelium and is subsequently replaced by squamous metaplasia. Thus, the caudal limit of the area is constituted by a

TABLE 4   Colposcopic Terminology

I.   Normal colposcopic findings
  Original squamous epithelium
  Columnar epithelium
  Normal transformation zone

II.a.   Abnormal colposcopic findings within the transformation zone
  Acetowhite epithelium
  Flat
  Micropapillarty or microconvoluted
  Punctation[a]
  Mosaic[a]
  Leukoplakia[a]
  Iodine-negative epithelium[a]
  Atypical vessels[a]

II.b.   Abnormal colposcopic findings outside the transformation zone,
  e.g., ectocervix, vagina
   Acetowhite epithelium[a]
   Flat
   Micropapilliary or microconvulated
   Punctation[a]
   Mosaic[a]
   Leukoplakia[a]
   Iodine-negative epithelium[a]
   Atypical vessels

III.   Colposcopically suspect invasive carcinoma

IV.   Unsatisfactory colposcopy
  Squamocolumnar junction not visible
  Severe inflammation or severe atrophy
  Cervix not visible

V.   Miscellaneous findings
  Nonacetowhite micropapillary surface
  Exophytic condyloma
  Inflammation
  Atrophy
  Ulcer
  Other

[a] Features showing minor or major change:
Minor changes
 Acetowhite epithelium
 Fine mosaic
 Fine punctuation
 Thin leukoplakia
Major changes
 Dense acetowhite epithelium
 Coarse mosaic
 Coarse punctuation
 Thick leukoplakia
 Atypical vessels
 Erosion

Source: From Stafl and Wilbanks (1991)[219]

squamo-squamous junction, where the epithelia only differ with regard to their origin (original vs. metaplastic squamous epithelia). The cephalic limit of the zone is called the squamo-columnar junction, representing the limit of the progression of the metaplastic epithelium during its attempt to reach the external os. Virtually all CIN lesions, as well as cervical cancers, originate at the squamo-columnar junction of the TZ during the metaplastic process, before the junction arrives at the os. This is why the goal of any treatment of cervical lesions will be to suppress the metaplastic and, possibly, all exocervical columnar tissue as well, in order to induce a stable junction at the os. HPV-associated lesions, including CIN, will appear inside the transformation zone and will be identified and defined by the colposcopist as an atypical TZ (ATZ). This is why the terminology of the IFCPC distinguishes cervical abnormalities inside and outside the TZ.

c.   Colposcopic Terminology.   There are three principal colposcopic criteria for defining an abnormal epithelium: (1) clinically detectable leukoplakia; (2) a white area detected only after application of acetic acid; and (3) an area not reacting to application of iodine. Two of these features may occur concurrently.

An HPV-associated lesion may appear as a leukoplakia (Figure 32) when being heavily hyper-keratotic, but this feature is not specific since some dystrophic disorders and also a well differen-tiated cervical cancer also may appear as leukoplakia. Normally, keratinized lesions only appear as white areas after the acetic acid test (Figure 30) and may contain vascular patterns defined as punctuation and mosaicism. Punctuation represents a series of fine red dots on a whitish background, while the vascular arrangement of mosaicism is seen as red "mosaic" lines and dots when the stroma is disposed as a wall or a ridge circumscribing blocks of epithelium. Additional use of a green filter on the colposcope will improve the evaluation of various capillary patterns, in particular those being conspicous for cancer, consisting of loops and bizarre networks representing sudden variations both in direction and in caliber of the vessels.

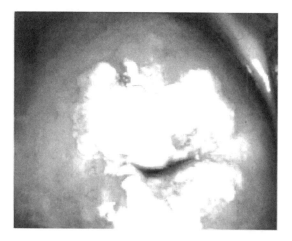

FIGURE 32 HPV-associated CIN III lesion appearing as a leukoplakia around the cervical opening and showing up as a "white spot" without prior acetic acid application. Often, such lesions exhibit a "brain-cortex"-like structure and a sharply demarcated "rolled" or "peeling" margin.

The surface of acetowhite areas may be totally flat (Figure 30), papillary (i.e., covered by finger-like projections; Figure 6) or convoluted[220] in a sulcus-like pattern (Figure 32). Acetowhite features are usually iodine-negative (Figure 33); on the other hand, sometimes iodine-negative areas occur where the acetic acid test has given a negative result. The iodine test identifies epithelia which lack glycogen, including metaplasia, dysplasia, cancer, as well as inflammatory reactive disorders. Recently, a particular feature has been described[221] as an irregular iodine uptake inside an acetowhite area. Among 6920 lesions exhibiting minor ATZ features, as much as 67% showed irregular iodine uptake but only 8% of completely iodine-negative lesions demonstrated histopathological features of condyloma or CIN. Probably, irregular iodine uptake occurring in some HPV-associated lesions is linked merely to focal HPV infection.

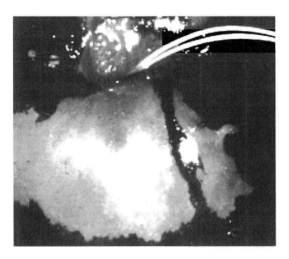

FIGURE 33 Iodine-negative areas on the lower lip of the cervix in a female carrying an IUD device (threads from copper spiral protruding from the cervical os).

It must be emphasized that acetowhite epithelium and iodine-negative areas are not colposcopically specific for abnormal tissue; a metaplastic tissue may also become white after the acetic acid test (Figure 30b), and immature metaplasia is colposcopically indistinguishable from CIN. Moreover, mature metaplastic epithelium does not contain glycogen and , like CIN, will appear as iodine-negative. If colposcopy is performed routinely, about 80% of atypical TZ detected will correspond histopathologically to a benign acanthotic nonglycogenated squamous epithelium merely,[222] representing metaplastic epithelium without any dysplastic potential.

Lack of colposcopic specificity has led to a distinction between minor and major grade abnormalities with respect to the terminology proposed by the IFCPC (Tables 4 and 5). In English speaking countries, colposcopy is generally performed only after the obtainance of an abnormal smear.[223,224] In this scenario, most acetowhite and/or iodine-negative epithelia will correspond to benign HPV-associated changes and/or CIN lesions. In Southern Europe and Germany, on the other hand, colposcopy is often performed as a supplementary tool to gynecological routine examination, performed concurrently with Pap smear sampling.[223,226] In the latter scenario, a colposcopic terminology without grading of TZ abnormalities could easily lead to a high number of unnecessary biopsies. According to the IFCPC, minor TZ changes suggest the existence of flat condyloma or CIN I, but may also correspond to benign metaplasia, while major changes mostly correspond to CIN II or III. (Tables 4 and 5) Therefore, in countries where colposcopy is performed routinely, residents and gynecologists must be taught that minor colposcopic changes do not need to be biopsied unless an associated smear is atypical.

In the group of miscellaneous lesions (Table 4) we find the only features that might be considered HPV specific. Typical condylomas can mostly be detected by the naked eye and appear as raised pink or greyish localized growths (Figure 6). Capillaries are generally detectable unless the lesions are highly keratinized. Condylomas are usually multiple and are often detected inside or outside the TZ, as well as on the vaginal walls. Colposcopically, condylomas appear as raised, irregular acetowhite lesions with finger-like projections.[225] Condylomas can be distinguished from the columnar epithelium of an ectopy or of a polyp, since these conditions do not turn acetowhite.

An acetowhite epithelium exhibiting an irregular surface and being covered by budding finger-like projections, spikes, or asperities, is defined as micropapillary or microconvoluted acetowhite epithelium. Non-acetowhite micropapillary surfaces may also be detected on the cervix, but mostly in the vagina.[225] The spikes represent elongations of the stroma towards the surface that contain a central vessel. Underlying histopathological features vary from benign condylomas to CIN III, a fact that underscores the importance of diagnostic biopsy/biopsies before treatment. Thus, cervical HPV infection may appear as several colposcopically detectable features, but the only characteristic aspect corresponding to a specific histopathology is that of condyloma acuminatum.

TABLE 5a Histological Correlations of the Colposcopic Terminology of the IFCPC: 250 Colposcopies After Abnormal Smear

Colposcopic features	Total number of cases	Histology		
		Normal	LGSIL	HGSIL
ATZ minor changes	87	21	60	6
ATZ major changes	163	3	51	109

TABLE 5b Histological Correlations of the Colposcopic Terminology of the IFCPC: 250 Routine Colposcopies

Colposcopic features	Total number of cases	Histology		
		Normal	LGSIL	HGSIL
ATZ minor changes	177	148	21	8
ATZ major changes	73	26	31	16

Note: ATZ abnormal transformation zone; LGSIL, low-grade squamous intraepithelial lesion (condyloma, CIN I); HGSIL, high-grade squamous intraepithelial lesion (CIN II-III).

Source: R. Barrasso, 1992[221]

d.   Vagina.   Colposcopic features of vaginal condylomas and of VAIN are slightly different from those of the cervix. As metaplasia does not exist in this area, the presence of acetowhite and/or iodine-negative areas are more specific signs of underlying condylomata or intraepithelial neoplasia. Moreover, features like mosaicism, linked to the existence of columnar epithelium on the cervix, are not found in the vagina. Thus, colposcopic features encountered in the vagina largely correspond to those of the cervix (leukoplakia, acetowhite areas, iodine-negative areas, typical condylomata acuminata, spiked condylomas), are relatively more specific for HPV-associated lesions. Whenever abnormal changes are detected, a biopsy is required.

8.   Evaluation of Immunosuppressed Patients

Immunosuppression, as a pathophysiological consequence of HIV-1 infection and iatrogenically as a result of transplant grafting, has been linked with a strongly increased risk of the development of HPV-associated CIN.[48-52,227] Also, among HIV-1 seropositive homosexual men, anorectal dysplasia associated with HPV infection occurs with a considerably higher incidence in HIV-seropositive than in HIV-seronegative homosexual men.[49,227,228]

a.   HIV-Positive Men.   This aspect is elucidated in detail by Palefsky in Chapter 12. Prior to the HIV epidemic, anal cancer was predominantly a disease of older women, with a female to male ratio of 2:1 to 3:1.[49,228] Since the onset of the HIV epidemic, the number of new cases of squamous cell anal cancer has increased more than seven-fold among single, never married men aged 20–49 years in the San Fransisco Bay area compared to the period spanning 1973–1978. The association with HPV is suggestive.[49,227,229] Employing techniques similar to those used for the assessment of cervical disease, anal swabs have been used to collect material for cytology and HPV DNA hybridization. HIV-associated immunosuppression appears to be an important risk factor not only for high level anal HPV infection but is associated with an increased prevalence of abnormal anal cytology and AIN as well. The relative risk increases with increasing degrees of immunosuppression. Available data indicate that while HPV infection per se is common in HIV-negative as well as in HIV-positive men practising receptive anal intercourse, development of potentially precancerous anal lesions in conjunction with anal HPV infection is largely an HIV-associated phenomenon. The risk of frank invasive anal cancer is significantly increased already 2–5 years before AIDS diagnosis.[49] Furthermore, available data suggest that precancerous changes may progress rapidly in the setting af advanced immunosuppression.

Due to the fact that many of these patients have limited survival time and that long time periods in general are required for invasive cancer to develop, the clinical significance might be disputed. However, because the incidence of anal cancer in this population clearly has increased, it has been proposed that anal cytology and anoscopy ought to be considered as a routine part of monitoring at least HIV-positive men who have absolute CD4 counts below 200–500/mm^3.[49] Individuals with normal cytology might be submitted to a re-screening on a regular basis, e. g., every 6–12 months, particularly as the immune status deteriorates. Abnormal results, including atypia, should prompt anoscopy, followed by anoscopically directed biopsy, regardless of the clinical appearance of the lesions.

Nevertheless, experience with treatment of anal disease in the setting of HIV infection is quite limited, and most clinicians tend to treat AIN and anal condylomas in HIV-positive individuals in the same manner as anal condylomas in HIV-negative individuals, i. e., with ablation of the diseased tissue.[49]

b.   HIV-Positive Women.   HPV-associated cervical disease is very common among HIV-infected women, with an odds ratio of 4.9 (95% confidence interval, 3.0–8.2) for having cervical neoplasia.[48] Several recent reports bolster a relationship between HIV-infection and an increased risk for a relatively rapid development of CIN II-III.[50,230,231] Also, when cervical cancer develops in HIV-infected females, patients are usually advanced in stage at presentation and the disease is associated with a particularly grave prognosis.[231,232]

To date, however, there has not been a significant increase in the number of reported cases of cervical cancer among these women. However, because once cervical cancer does develop in HIV-positive women its behavior seems to be more aggressive than usual, as of 1993 the Centers for Disease Control (CDC) in the U.S. has expanded the AIDS case definition to include invasive cervical cancer among HIV-positive women.[233] The current CDC guidelines for screening appears from Table 6. It might seem somewhat irrational that this type of expanded definitition has not yet also been implied for anal cancers in homosexual men.

TABLE 6   CDC Guidelines for Screening for Cervical Dysplasia in HIV-Infected Women

1. All women should receive comprehensive gynecologic examinations, including Pap smear.
2. If the initial Pap smear is normal, a second evaluation should be done in 6 months to reduce the likelihood of a false-negative inital test. If both of the initial Pap smears are negative, follow-up with annual Pap smears is adequate.
3. If severe inflammation with reactive squamous cellular changes is found, another Pap smear should be done within 3 months.
4. Dysplasia should prompt colposcopy of the lower genital tract and, if indicated, biopsies.

The sensivity of Pap smears is not diminished in HIV-seropositive individuals.[224] Based on available information, it seems reasonable to screen HIV-positive women with Pap smears on an annual to biannual basis. In addition, the clinician must be very careful to rule out disease in other anogenital areas, including the vulva, vagina, and anus, because of the possibility of multifocal HPV-associated disease.[227] Screening colposcopy may be justified in women with noncompliance to regular follow-up.[224] As with anal disease in HIV-positive men, treatment is similar to disease in HIV-negative patients; on the other hand, follow-up must be performed frequently because of the high risk of lesional recurrence and for malignant conversion.

c.   *Allograft Recipients.*   There is a 4–14-fold increase in the incidence and prevalence of HPV-associated high-grade intraepithelial neoplasia and invasive squamous tumors of the cervix in women with renal allografts.[52] A lag period of up to 5 years has been reported between the start of immunosuppressive therapy and the development of genitoanal neoplasia; the proportion of individuals affected appears to increase significantly up to 10 years, where it levels out. A strict algorithm for follow-up of these patients does yet not exist. We propose yearly screening for HPV associated dysplasia in allograft recipient.

9.   Evaluation of Children

Major aspects on clinical presentation and evaluation of genitoanal warts in children are presented by Obalek et al. in Chapter 15. This issue is touchy and not uncontroversial. When a child with genitoanal warts is encountered, it is extremely important to keep in mind that several modes of transmission must be considered, an issue that always must be addressed to the parents or the guardians. A significant number of these children have undoubtedly acquired their genito-anal HPV infection at birth by vertical transmission from the maternal genital tract.[6,63,72,156] Nonsexual horizontal spread from family members may be the cause in some of the children. Although the possibility of sexual abuse always must be borne in mind, condylomata per se cannot be considered a reliable forensic evidence of sexual abuse. Yet, in large series child abuse has been documented within a range as high as 30–50%.[156,157,234-239]

This aspect represents a clinical dilemma to which no simple solution exists. These children should—without delay—be referred to and be assessed in a multidisiplinary team and by set procedures for the consideration of sexual abuse.[182-185,240] Physical signs and psychological symptoms indicative of sexual abuse, including the concomitant presence of other STDs, must always be sought and carefully documented before any therapy is given. A biopsy should be taken as part of the routine for light microscopic confirmation of HPV etiology. The medicolegal value of additional HPV-typing has been under debate.[156] HPV types that are ordinarily associated with finger warts (HPV 1 and 2) have been detected in as much as 20–41% of genitoanal warts of children.[234-238] It seems that documented sexual abuse is rare in such cases. Nevertheless, the finding of cutaneotrophic HPVs cannot be regarded as a medicolegal proof that abuse has not taken place, as digital sexual manipulation by an abuser afflicted with finger warts theoretically might have occurred.[156] Furthermore, in cases afflicted with genitotropic HPVs such as types 6, 11, and 16, child abuse has been documented at a range as variable as 7–73%. Thus, essentially it appears that the results of typing will not alter subsequent management, whereas other evidences of sexual abuse will.

10.   Histopathology

Details on histopathological features of GPVI are accounted for by K. Syrjänen in Chapter 9 and by Meisels in Chapter 18. Major histopathological patterns include: hyperplasia with acanthotic elongation of the rete ridges, hyper- and parakeratosis, and koilocytosis, often associated with dilated vessels of corium papillae and some dermal inflammation. Koilocytes represent the only pathognomonic sign. Their presence correlates best with classical condylomas, less consistently with subclinical lesions, and on average koilocytes are absent in about half of biopsies.[33,91,92,98,99] This is particularly common in lesions associated with "high-risk" HPV types that exhibit moderate to severe dysplasia.

In situ hybridization for type specific determination of underlying HPV DNA has been suggested as a valuable tool in routine histology laboratories for increasing the accuracy of light microscopic evaluation, in particular in biopsies lacking koilocytes. Although this argument is valid, a combined appraisal of clinical features—including use of the acetic acid test and penoscopy—and conventional histological criteria will, nevertheless, for differential diagnostic purposes be satisfactory in the predominant number of routine cases. Yet, in specialized laboratories use of either *in situ* hybridization or PCR to detect HPV in lesions that are histologically ambiguous, represents a valuable adjunct quality control measurement to light microscopy.[241]

REFERENCES

1. Oriel J.D., Natural history of genital warts, *Br J Vener Dis,* 47, 1, 1971.
2. Oriel J.D., Anal warts and anal coitus, *Br J Vener Dis,* 47, 373, 1971.
3. Chuang T.-Y., Perry H.O., Kurland L.T. and Ilstrup D.M., Condyloma acuminatum in Rochester, Minn, 1950-1978. I. Epidemiology and clinical features, *Arch Dermatol,* 120, 469, 1984.
4. Chuang T.-Y., Condylomata acuminata (genital warts). An epidemiological view, *J Am Acad Dermatol,* 16, 376, 1987.
5. Koutsky L.A. and Wölner-Hanssen P., Genital papillomavirus infections: current knowledge and future prospects, *Obstet Gynecol Clin North Am,* 16, 541, 1989.
6. von Krogh G., Genitoanal papillomavirus infection: diagnostic and therapeutic objectives in the light of current epidemiological observations, *Int J STD and AIDS,* 2, 391, 1991.
7. van Ranst M., Kaplan J.B. and Burk R.D., Phylogenetic classification of human papillomaviruses: correlation with clinical manifestations, *General Virol,* 73, 2653, 1992.
8. Hippeläinen M., Syrjänen S., Hippeläinen M., Koskela H., Pulkkinen J., Saarikoski S. and Syrjänen K., Prevalence and risk factors of genital human papillomavirus (HPV) infections in healthy males: a study on Finnish conscripts, *Sex Transm Dis,* 20, 321, 1993.
9. Ley C., Bauer H.M., Reingold A., Schiffman M.H., Chambers J.C., Tashiro C.J. and Manos M.M., Determinants of genital human papillomavirus infection in young women, *J Natl Cancer Inst,* 83, 997, 1991.
10. de Villiers E.-M., Wagner D., Schneider A., Wesch H., Munz F., Miklaw H. and zur Hausen H., Human papillomavirus DNA in women without and with cytological abnormalities: results of a 5-year follow-up study, *Gynecol Oncol,* 44, 33, 1992.
11. Lauricella-Lefebre M.-A., Piette J., Lifrange E., Lambotte R., Gerard P. and Rentier B., High rate of multiple genital HPV infections detected by DNA hybridization, *J. Medical Virol,* 36, 265, 1992.
12. Rosenfeld W.D., Rose E., Vermund S.H., Schreiber K. and Burk R.D., Follow-up evaluation of cervicovaginal human papillomavirus infection in adolescents, *J. Pediatr,* 121, 307, 1992.
13. Schiffman M.H., Recent progress in defining the epidemiology of human papillomavirus infection and cervical neoplasia, *J. Natl. Cancer Inst,* 84, 394, 1992.
14. Schneider A., Kirchhoff T., Meinhardt G. and Gissman L., Repeated evaluation of human papillomavirus 16 status in cervical swabs of young women with a history of normal Papanicolaou smears, *Obstet Gynecol,* 79, 683, 1992.
15. Stellato G., Nieminen P., Aho H., Vesterinen E., Vaheri A. and Paavonen J., Human papillomavirus infection of the female genital tract: Correlation of HPV DNA with cytologic, colposcopic and natural history findings, *Eur. J. Gyneacol Oncol,,* 13, 262, 1992.
16. Bauer H.M., Hildesheim A., Schiffman M.H., Glass A.G., Rush B.B., Scott D.R., Cadell D.M., Kurman R.J. and Manos M.M., Determinants of genital human papillomavirus infection in low-risk women in Portland, Oregon, *Sex Transm Dis,* 20, 274, 1993.
17. Evans B.A., Tasker T. and MacRae K.D., Risk profiles for genital infection in women, *Genitourin Med,* 69, 257, 1993.
18. Hildesheim A., Gravitt P., Schiffman M.H., Kurman R.J., Barnes W., Jones S., Tchabo J.-G., Brinton L.A., Copeland C., Epp J. and Manos M.M., Determinants of genital human papillomavirus infection in low-income women in Washington, D. C, *Sex Transm Dis,* 20, 280, 1993.
19. Wheeler C.M., Parmenter C.A., Hunt W.C., Becker T.M., Greer C.E., Hildesheim A. and Manos M.M., Determinants of genital human papillomavirus infection among cytologically normal women attending the University of New Mexico student health care center, *Sex Transm Dis,* 20, 286, 1993.

20. Morrison E.A.B., Natural history of cervical infection with human papillomaviruses, *Clin Infect Dis*, 18, 172, 1994.

21. Morrison E.A.B., Goldberg G.L., Kadish A.S. and Burk R.D., Polymerase chain reaction, detection of human papillomavirus: quantitation may improve clinical utility, *J Microbiol*, 30, 2539, 1992.

22. Hillman R.J., Ryait B.K., Botcherby M., Walker M.M. and Taylor-Robinson D., Human papillomavirus DNA in the urogenital tracts of men with genital dermatoses: evidence for multifocal infection, *Int. J STD AIDS*, 4, 147, 1993.

23. Moscicki A.-B., Palefsky J., Smith G., Siboshski S. and Schoolnik G., Variability of human papillomavirus DNA testing in a longitudinal cohort of young women, *Obstet Gynecol*, 82, 578, 1993.

24. Ho L., Tay S.-K., Chan S.-Y. and Bernard H.-V., Sequence variants of human papillomavirus type 16 from couples suggest sexual transmission with low infectivity and polyclonality in genital neoplasia, *J. Int. Infect Dis*, 168, 803, 1193.

25. Cook L.S., Koutsky L.A. and Holmes K.K., Circumcision and sexually transmitted disease, *Am J Public Health*, 84, 197, 1994.

26. Bosch F., X., 12 th International Papillomavirus Conference 1993: a personal view of the epidermiological presentations, *Papillomavirus Report*, 4, 152, 1994.

27. Kataja V., Syrjänen K. and Mäntyjärvi R., Prospective follow-up of cervical human papillomavirus infection: life table analysis of histopathological, cytological and colposcopic data, *Eur J Epidemiol*, 5, 1, 1989.

28. Syrjänen K.J., Epidemiology of human papillomavirus (HPV) infections and their association with genital squamous cell cancer, *APMIS*, 97, 957, 1989.

29. Kataja V., Prognostic factors in cervical human papillomavirus infections, *Sex Transm Dis*, 19, 154, 1992.

30. DiBonito L., Falconieri G. and Bonifacio-Gori D., Multicentric papillomavirus infection of the female genital tract. A study of morphologic pattern, possible risk factors and viral prevalence, *Path Res Pract*, 189, 1023, 1993.

31. Rymark P., Forslund O., Hansson B.G. and Lindholm K., Genital HPV infection is not a local but a regional infection, *Genitourin Med*, 69, 18, 1993.

32. Wikström A., Hedblad M-A., Johansson B., Kalantari M., Syrjänen S., Lindberg M. and von Krogh G., The acetic test in evaluation of subclinical genital papillomavirus infection: A comparative study on penoscopy, histopathology, viology and scanning electron microscopy findings, *Genitourin Med*, 68, 90, 1992.

33. Wikström A., von Krogh G., Hedblad M-A. and Syrjänen S., Papillomavirus-associated balanoposthitis, *Genitourin Med*, 70, 175, 1994.

34. Bank L., Meeting Report; 13th International Papillomavirus Conference, Amsterdam The Netherlands, 8-13 October, 1994, *Papillomavirus Report*, 5, 183, 1994.

35. Schiffman M.H., Manos M.M., Rush B.B., Lawler P., Scott D.R., Sherman M.E., Kurman R.J., Corrigan A., Greer C.E., Zhang T., Glass A.G. and Lorincz A.T., *A Prospective Study of HPV Infection and Incident CIN*, 13th International Papillomavirus Conference, October 8-12, 1994, Amsterdam, Presentation # 31.

36. Crum C.P. and Nuovo G.J., Eds., *Genital Papillomaviruses and Related Neoplasms*, Raven Press, New York, 1991, 230 pages.

37. Schneider A., Pathogenesis of genital HPV infection, *Genitourin Med*, 69, 165, 1993.

38. Syrjänen K., Long-term consequences of genital HPV infections in women, *Ann Med*, 24, 233, 1993.

39. zur Hausen H., Disrupted dichotomous intracellular control of human papillomavirus infection in cancer of the cervix, *Lancet*, 343, 955, 1994.

40. Becker T.M., Wheeler C.M., McGough N.S., Parmenter C.A., Jordan S.W., Stidley C.A., McPherson R.S. and Dorin M.H., Sexually transmitted diseases and other risk factors for cervical dysplasia among Southwestern hispanic and non-hispanic women, *J Am Med Assoc*, 271, 1181, 1994.

41. Hildesheim A., Schiffman M.H., Gravitt P.E., Glass A.G., Greer C.E., Zhang T., Scott R.D., Rush B.B., Lawler P., Sherman M.E., Kurman R.J. and Manos M.M., Persistence of type-specific human papillomavirus infection among cytologically normal women , *J. Infect Dis*, 169, 235, 1994.

42. Syrjänen K. and Syrjänen S., Epidemiology of human papillomavirus infections and genital neoplasia, *Scand J Infect Dis*, 60, 7, 1990.

43. Viac J., Chardonnet Y., Chignol M.C. and Schmitt D., Papilloma viruses, warts, carcinoma and Langerhans' cells, *In Vivo*, 7, 207, 1993.

44. Lehtinen M., Rantala I., Toivonen A., Luoto H., Aine R., Lauslahti K., Ylä-Outinen A., Romppanen U. and Paavonen J., Depletion of Langerhans' cells in cervical HPV infection is associated with replication of the virus, *APMIS*, 101, 833, 1993.

45. Morelli A.E., Sananes C., Di Paola G., Paredes A. and Feinboim L., Relationship between types of human papillomavirus and Langerhans' cells in cervical condyloma and intraepithelial neoplasia, *Am J Clin Pathol*, 99, 200, 1993.

46. Glew S.S., Connor M.E., Snijders P.J.F., Stanbridge C.M., Buckley C.H., Walboomers J.M.M., Meijer C.J.L.M and Stern P.L., HLA expression in pre-invasive cervical neoplasia in relation to human papilloma virus infection, *Eur J Cancer*, 29, 1963, 1993.

47. Benton C., Shahidullah H. and Hunter J.A.A., Human papillomavirus in the immunosuppressed, *Papillomavirus Report*, 3, 23, 1992.

48. Mandelblatt J.S., Fahs M., Garibaldi K., Senie R.T. and Peterson H.B., Association between HIV infection and cervical neoplasia: implications for clinical care of women at risk for both conditions, *AIDS*, 6, 173, 1992.

49. Palefsky J.M., Anal papillomavirus infection and anal cancer in HIV-positive individuals: an emerging problem, *AIDS*, 8, 283, 1994.

50. Ho G.Y.F., Burk R.D., Fleming I. and Klein R.S., Risk of genital human papillomavirus infection in women with human immunodeficiency virus-induced immunosuppression, *Int J Cancer*, 56, 788, 1994.

51. Dyall-Smith D., Trowell H. and Dyall-Smith M.L., Benign human papillomavirus infection in renal transplant recipient, *Int J Dermatol*, 30,: 785, 1991.

52. Ogunbiyi O.A., Scholefield J.H., Raftery A.T., Smith J.H.F., Duffy S., Sharp F. and Rogers K., Prevalence of anal human papillomavirus infection and intraepithelial neoplasia in renal allograft recipients, *Br J Surgery*, 81, 365, 1994.

53. Majewski S. and Jablonska S., Epidermodysplasia verruciformis as a model of human papillomavirus-induced genetic cancers: the role of local immunosurveillance, *Amer J Med Sci*, 304, 174, 1992.

54. Bernard C., Mougin C. and Lab M., New approaches to the understanding of the pathogenesis of human papillomavirus induced anogenital lesions. The role of co-factors and co-infection, *J Eur Acad Dermatol Venereol*, 3, 237, 1994.

55. Cooper C. and Singha H.S.K., Condylomata acuminata in women: the effect of concomitant genital infection on response to treatment, *Acta Derm Venereol*, 65, 150, 1985.

56. Kharsany A.B.M., Hoosen A.A., Bagaratee J. and Gouws E., The association between sexually transmitted pathogens and cervical intraepithelial neoplasia in a developing community, *Genitourin Med*, 69, 357, 1993.

57. Newfield L., Goldsmith A., Bradlow H.L. and Auborn K., Estrogen metabolism and human papillomavirus - induced tumors of the larynx: chemo-prophylaxis with indole-3-carbinol, *Anticancer Res*, 13, 337, 1993.

58. Bairati I., Sherman K.J., McKnight B., Habel L.A., van den Eeden S.K., Stergachis A. and Daling J.R., Diet and genital warts: a case - control study, *Sex Transm Dis*, 21, 1993.

59. Mittal R., Tsutsumi K., Pater A. and Pater M., Human papillomavirus type 16 expression in cervical keratinocytes: role of progesterone and glucocorticoid hormones, *Obstet Gynecol*, 81, 5, 1993.

60. Kemp E.A., Hakenewerth A.M., Laurent S.L., Gravitt P.E. and Stoerker J., Human papillomavirus prevalence in pregnancy, *Obstet Gynecol*, 649, 1992.

61. Barrett T.J., Silbar J.D. and McGinley J.P., Genital warts - a venereal disease, *J Am Med Assoc*, 154, 333, 1954.

62. Department of Health, Statistical Division (2D2B), New cases seen at *NHS Genito-urinary Medicine Clinics in England*, Summary Information Form KC60, 1993.

63. von Krogh G., Clinical relevance and evaluation of genitoanal papillomavirus infection in the male, *Seminars Dermatol*, 11, 229, 1992.

64. Rakoczy P., Sterrett G. and Kulski J., Time trends in the prevalence of human papillomavirus infections in archival Papanicolaou smears: analysis by cytology, DNA hybridization, and polymerase chain reaction, *J Med Virol*, 32, 10, 1990.

65. Anderson S.M., Brooke P.K., van Eyck L., Noell H. and Frable W., J., Distribution of human papillomavirus types in genital lesions from two temporally distinct populations determined by in situ hybridization *Hum Pathol*, 24, 547, 1993.

66. Rosenfeld W.D.,Vermund S.H., Wentz S.J. and Burk R.D., High prevalence rate of human papilloma-virus infection and association with abnormal Papanicolaou smears in sexually active adolescents, *AJDC*, 143, 1443, 1989.

67. Soares V.R.X., Nieminen P., Aho M., Vesterinen E., Vaheri A. and Paavonen J., Human papillomavirus DNA in unselected pregnant and non-pregnant women, *Int J STD AIDS*, 1, 276, 1990.

68. Köchel H.G., Teichmann A., Eckardt N., Arendt P., Kuhn W. and Thomssen R., Occurrence of human papillomavirus DNA types 16 and 18 (HPV - 16/18) in cervical smears as compared to cytological findings, *Int J Gynecol Obstet*, 31, 145, 1990.

69. Meisels A., Cytologic diagnosis of human papillomavirus. Influence of age and pregnancy stage, *Acta Cytol*, 36, 480, 1992.

70. Quick C.A., Kryzyzek R.A. and Watts S.L., Relationship between condylomata and laryngeal papil-lomata, *Ann Otol*, 89, 467, 1980.

71. Chang F., Wang L., Syrjänen S. and Syrjänen K., Human papillomavirus infections in the respiratory tract, *Amer J Otolaryngol*, 13, 210, 1992.

72. Cason J., Kaye J.N., Jewers R.J., Kambo P.K., Bible J.M., Kell B., Shergill B., Pakarian F., Raju K.S. and Best J.M., Perinatal infection and persistence of human papillomavirus types 16 and 18 in infants, *J Med Virol*, 47, 209, 1995.

73. Fredericks B.D., Balkin A., Daniel H.W., Schonrock J., Ward B. and Frazer I.H., Transmission of human papillomavirus from mother to child, *Aust NZ J Obstet Gynaecol*, 33, 30, 1993.

74. Panici P.B., Scambia G., Perrone L., Battaglia F., Cattani P., Rabitti C., Dettori G., Capelli A., Sedlis A. and Mancuso S., Oral condyloma lesions in patients with extensive genital human papillomavirus infection, *Amer J Obstet Gynecol*, 167, 451, 1992.

75. Kashima H.K., Shah F., Lyles A., Glackin R., Muhammed N., Turner L., van Zandt S., Whitt S. and Shah K., A comparision of risk factors in juvenile-onset and adult-onset recurrent respiratory papil-lomatosis, *Laryngoscope*, 102, 9, 1992.

76. Aschinoff R., Li J.J., Jacobson M., Friedman-Kien A.E. and Geronemus R.G., Detection of human papillomavirus DNA in squamous cell carcinoma of the nail bed and finger determined by polymerase chain reaction, *Arch Dermatol*, 127, 1813, 1991.

77. Garven T.C., Thelmo W.L., Victor J. and Pertchuk L., Verrucous carcinoma of the leg positive for human papillomavirus DNA 11 and 18: a case report, *Hum Pathol*, 22, 1170, 1991.

78. Blauvelt A., Duarte A.M., Pruksachatkunakorn C., Leonardi C.L. and Schachner L.A:, Human papil-lomavirus type 6 infection involving cutaneous nongenital sites, *J Am Acad Dermatol*, 27, 876, 1992.

79. Yell J.A., Sinclair R., Mann S., Fleming K. and Ryan T.J., Human papillomavirus type 6 - induced condylomata: an unusual complication of intertrigo, *Br J Dermatol*, 128, 575, 1993.

80. Nathan M., Umbilical warts: a new entity? *Genitourin Med*, 70, 49, 1994.

81. Eliezri Y.D., Silverstein S.J. and Nouvo G.J., Occurrence of human papillomavirus type 16 DNA in cutaneous squamous and basal cell neoplasms, *J Am Acad Dermatol*, 23, 836, 1990.

82. Guitart J., Bergfeld W.F., Tuthill R.J., Tubbs R.R., Zienowicz R. and Fleegler E.J., Squamous cell carcinoma of the nailbed: a clinico-pathological study of 12 cases, *Br J Dermatol*, 123, 215, 1990.

83. Moy R.L., Eliezri Y.D., Nouvo G.J., Zitelli J.A., Bennett R.G. and Silverstein S., Human papillomavirus type 16 DNA in periungual squamous cell carcinomas, *J Am Med Assoc*, 12, 2669, 1989.

84. Ostrow R.S., Shaver M.K., Turnquist S., Viksnins A., Bender M., Vance C., Kaye V. and Faras A.J., Human papillomavirus 16 DNA in a cutaneous invasive cancer, *Arch Dermatol*, 125, 666, 1989.

85. Moy R.L. and Quan M.B., The presence of human papillomavirus type 16 in squamous cell carcinoma of the proximal finger and reconstruction with a bilobed transposition flap, *J Dermatol Surg Oncol*, 17, 171, 1991.

86. Pierceall W.E., Goldberg L.H. and Ananthaswamy N., Presence of human papillomavirus type 16 DNA sequences in human nonmelanoma skin cancers, *J Invest Dermatol*, 97, 880, 1991.

87. Soler C., Chardonnet Y., Allibert P., Euvard S., Schmitt D. and Mandrand B., Detection of mucosal human papillomavirus types 6/11 in cutaneous lesions from transplant recipients, *J Invest Dermatol*, 101, 286, 1993.

88. Johnson J.C., Burnett A.F., Willet G.D., Young M.A. and Doniger J., High frequency of latent and clinical human papillomavirus cervical infections in immunocomprised human immunodeficiency virus-infected women, *Obstet Gynecol*, 79, 311, 1992.

89. McKay M., Frankman O., Horowitz B.J., Lecart C., Michiletti L., Ridley C.M., Turner M.L. and Woodruff J.D., Vulvar vestibulitis and vestibular papillomatosis. Report of the ISSVD Committee on vulvodynia, *J Reprod Med*, 36, 413, 1991.

90. Welch J.M., Nayagam M., Parry G., Das R., Campbell M., Whatley J. and Bradbeer C., What is vestibular papillomatosis? A study of its prevalence, aetiology and natural history, *Br J Obstet Gynecol*, 100, 939, 1993.

91. Gross G., Ikenberg H., Gissman L. and Hagedorn M., Papillomavirus infection of the genital region: correlation between histology, clinical picture and virus type. Proposal of a new nomenclature, *J Invest Dermatol*, 85, 147, 1985.

92. von Krogh G., Syrjänen S.M. and Syrjänen K.J., Advantage of human papillomavirus typing in the clinical evaluation of genitoanal warts. Experience with the in situ deoxyribonucleic acid hybridization technique applied on paraffin sections, *J Am Acad Dermatol*, 18, 495, 1988.

93. Lassus J., Niemi K.M., Syrjänen S., Krohn K. and Ranki A., A comparison of histopathologic diagnosis and the demonstration of human papillomavirus-specific DNA and proteins in penile warts, *Sex Transm Dis*, 19, 127, 1992.

94. Voog E., and Löwhagen G-B., Follow-up of men with genital papilloma virus infection, *Acta Derm Venereol*, 72, 185, 1992.

95. Lloyd K., Multicentice pigmented Bowen's disease of the groin, *Arch Dermatol*, 101, 48, 1970.

96. Gerber G., Carcinoma in situ of the penis, *J Urol*, 151, 829, 1994.

97. Aynaud O., Ionesco M. and Barrasso R., Penile intraepithelial neoplasia, specific clinical features correlate with histologic and virologic findings, *Cancer*, 74, 1762, 1994.

98. Ikenberg H., Gissmann L. and Gross G., Human papillomavirus type-16-related DNA in genital Bowen's disease and in bowenoid papulosis, *Int J Cancer*, 32, 563, 1983.

99. Gross G., Hagedorn M., Ikenberg H., Rufli T., Dahlet C., Grosshans E. and Gissmann L., Bowenoid papulosis: presence of human papillomavirus (HPV) structural antigens and of HPV 16-related DNA sequences, *Arch Dermatol*, 121, 858, 1985.

100. Obalek S., Jablonska S., Beaudenon M.B., Walczak L. and Orth G., Bowenoid papulosis of the male and female genitalia: risk of cervical neoplaisa, *J Am Acad Dermatol*, 14, 433, 1986.

101. Rolighed J., Sörensen I.M., Jacobsen N.O. and Lindeberg H., The presence of HPV types 6/11, 13, 16 and 33 in bowenoid papulosis in an HIV-positive male, demontrated by DNA in situ hybridization, *APMIS*, 99, 583, 1991.

102. Gross G. and Mausch H. E., Bowenoid papulosis, Bowen's disease and erythroplasia of Queyrat - papillomavirus associated? *Am J Dermatopathol*, 14, 1, 67, 1992.

103. de Villez R.L. and Stevens C.S., Bowenoid papules of the genitalia: a case progressing to Bowen's disease, *J Am Acad Dermatol*, 3, 149, 1980.

104. Knoblich R. and Failing J.F. Jr., Giant condyloma acuminatum (Buschke-Löwenstein tumor) of the rectum, *Am J Clin Pathol*, 48, 389, 1967.

105. Crowther M.E., Lowe D.G. and Shepherd J.H., Verrucous carcinoma of the female genital tract: a rewiew, *Obstet Gynecol Surv*, 43, 263, 1988.

106. Schwartz R.A., Buschke-Löwenstein tumor. Verrucous carcinoma of the penis, *J Am Acad Dermatol*, 23, 723, 1990.

107. Grassegger A. Höpfl R., Hussl H., Wicke K. and Fritsch P., Buschke-Löwenstein tumor infiltrating pelvic organs, *Br J Dermatol*, 130, 221, 1994.

108. Buschke A., Condylomata acuminata, in: *Stereoskopischer Medizinischer Atlas*, Neisser A., Ed., Fischer-Verlag, Leipzig, 1896.

109. Buschke A. and Löwenstein L.W., Über Carcinomähnliche Condylomata acuminata des Penis, *Klin Wschr*, 4, 1726, 1925.

110. Bogomoletz W.V., Potet F. and Molas G., Condylomata acuminata, giant condyloma acuminata (Buschke-Löwenstein tumor) and verrucous squamous carcinoma of the perianal and anorectal region: a continuous spectrum? *Histopathology*, 9, 1155, 1985.

111. Mortensen P.H.G., The Buschke-Löwenstein tumor or verrucous carcinoma of the penis, *Aust NZ J Surg*, 57, 37, 1987.

112. Boxer J.R., and Skinner D.G., Condylomata acuminata and squamous cell carcinoma, *Urology*, 9, 72, 1977.

113. Wells M., Robertson S. and Lewis F., Squamous carcinoma arising in a giant perianal condyloma associated with human papillomavirus types 6 and 11, *Histopathology*, 12, 319, 1988.

114. Creasman C., Haas P.A., Fox T.A. and Balazs M., Malignant transformation of anorectal giant condylomata acuminatum (Buschke-Löwenstein tumor), *J Dis Col Rect*, 32, 481, 1989.

115. Feindt P., Schüder G., Kreissler-Haag D. and Feifel G., Monströser Buschke-Löwenstein-Tumor (Condylomata acuminata gigantea) mit übergang in ein invasiv wachsendes Plattenepithelkarzinom, *Chirurg*, 64, 499, 1993.

116. Lehn H., Ernst T.M. and Sauer G., Transcription of episomal papillomavirus DNA in human condyloma acuminatum Buschke-Löwenstein tumors, *J Gen Virol*, 65, 2003, 1984.

117. Boshart M. and zur Hausen H,. Human papillomavirus in Buschke-Löwenstein tumors: Physical state of the DNA and identification of a tandem duplication in the noncoding region of a human papillomavirus 6 subtype, *J Virol*, 58, 963, 1986.

118. Ackerman L.V., Verrucous carcinoma of the oral cavity, *Surgery*, 26, 670, 1948.

119. Dawson D.F., Duckworth J.K. and Bernhardt H., Giant condyloma and verrucous carcinoma of the genital tract, *Arch Pathol (Chicago)*, 79, 225, 1965.

120. Kraus F.T. and Perez-Mesa C., Verrucous carcinoma. Clinical and pathologic study of 105 cases involving oral cavity, larynx and genitalia, *Cancer*, 19, 26, 1966.

121. Robertson D.I., Maung R. and Duggan M.A., Verrucous carcinoma of the genital tract: is it a distinct entity?, *CJS*, 36, 147, 1993.

122. Aird J., Johnson H.D., Lennox B. and Stausfeld A.G., Epithelioma cuniculatum - a variety of squamous cell carcinoma, peculiar to the foot, *Br J Surg*, 42, 245, 1954.

123. Adler-Storthz K., Newland J.R., Tessin B.A., Yendall W.A. and Shillitoe E.J., *HPV2 DNA in Oral Verrucous Carcinoma*, Internatl. Workshop on Papillomaviruses, Cold Spring Harbor (Abstr.), 1986.

124. Brandsma J.L., Steinberg B.M., Abramson A.L. and Winkler B., Presence of human papillomavirus type 16 related sequences in verrucous carcinoma in the larynx, *Cancer Res*, 46, 2185, 1986.

125. Petersen C.S., Sjölin K.E., Rosman N. and Lindeberg H., Lack of human papillomavirus DNA in carcinoma cuniculatum, *Acta Derm Venereol*, 74, 231, 1994.

126. Honda A., Iwasaki T., Sata T., Kawashima M., Morishima T. and Matsukura T., Human papillomavirus type 60 - associated plantar warts, *Arch Dermatol*, 130, 1413, 1994.

127. Kashima M., Adachi M., Honda M., Niimura M. and Nakabayashi Y., A case of peculiar plantar warts. Human papillomavirus type 60 infection, *Arch Dermatol*, 130, 1418, 1994.

128. Balthazar E.J., Streiter M. and Megibow A. J., Anorectal giant condylom acuminatum (Buschke-Löwenstein tumor): CT and radiographic manifestations, *Radiology*, 150, 651, 1989.

129. Isaacs J.H., Verrucous carcinoma of the female genital tract, *Gynecol Oncol*, 4, 259, 1976.

130. Powell J.L., Franklin E.W. and Nickerson J.F., Verrucous carcinoma of the female genital tract, *Gynecol Oncol*, 6, 565, 1978.

131. Gupta J., Pilotti S. and Shan K.V., Human papillomavirus - associated early vulvar neoplasia investigated by in situ hybridization, *Am J Surg Pathol*, 11, 430, 1987.

132. Gallousis S., Verrucous carcinoma, *Obstet Gynecol*, 40, 502, 1972.

133. Sonck C.E., Condylomata acuminata mit Übergang in Karzinom, *Z Haut Geschl Krankheit*, 46, 273, 1970.

134. Andreasson B., Bock J.E. and Strom K.V., Verrucous carcinoma of the vulvar region, *Acta Obstet Gynecol Scand*, 62, 183, 1983.

135. Degfu S., O'Quinn A.G. and Lacey G.C., Verrucous carcinoma of the cervix, *Gynecol Oncol*, 25, 37, 1986.

136. Jablonska S. and Schwartz R.A., Giant condyloma acuminatum of Buschke and Löwenstein. In: *Clinical Dermatology*. 18th Ed. Demis D.J., Philadelphia: Harper and Row.

137. Malejczyk J., Majewski S. and Jablonska S., Abrogated NK-cell lysis of human papillomavirus (HPV) - 16-bearing keratinocytes on patients with precancerous and cancerous HPV-induced anogenital lesions, *Int J Cancer*, 43, 209, 1989.

138. Gross G., Roussaki A. and Pfister H., Recurrent vulvar Buschke-Löwenstein tumor-like condylomata acuminata and Hodgkin's disease effectively treated with recombinant interferon alpha-2c gel as adjuvant to electrosurgery. In: Fritsch P., Schuler G. and Hintner H. Eds., *Immunodeficiency and Skin Curr Probl Dermatol*, Basel, Karger, 1989.

139. Piepkorn M., Kumasaka B., Krieger J.N. and Burmer G.C., Development of human papillomavirus-associated Buschke-Löwenstein penile carcinoma during cyclosporine therapy for generalized pustular psoriasis, *J Amer Acad Dermatol*, 29, 321, 1993.

140. Cook L.S., Koutsky L.A. and Holmes K.K., Clinical presentation of genital warts among circumcised and uncircumcised heterosexual men attending an urban STD clinic, *Genitourin Med*, 69, 262, 1993.

141. McKenna J.G. and McMillan A., Management of intrameatal warts in men, *Int J STD AIDS*, 1, 259, 1990.

142. Thin R.N., Meatoscopy: an important technique for assessing meatal warts in men, *Int J STD AIDS*, 5, 18, 1994.

143. Nathan P.M., Thompson V.C., Sharmacharja G., Hawkswell J. and Fogarty B., A study of the prevalence of male intrameatal warts using meatoscopy in a genitourinary medicine department, *Int J STD AIDS*, 6, 184, 1995.

144. de Benedictis T.J., Marmar J.L. and Praiss D.E., Intraurethral condylomas acuminata: Management and review of the literature, *J Urol*, 118, 767, 1977.

145. Kessner K.M., Extensive condylomata acuminata of male urethra: management by ventral urethrotomy, *Br J Urol*, 71, 204, 1993.

146. Del Mistro A., Koss L.G., Braunstein J., Bennet B., Saccomano G. and Simons K.M., Condylomata acuminata of the urinary bladder, *Amer J Surg Pathol*, 12, 205, 1988.

147. Shibutani Y.F., Schoenberg M.P., Carpiniello V.L. and Malloy T.R., Human papillomavirus associated with bladder cancer, *Urology*, 40, 15, 1992.

148. Wilczynski S.P., Cook N., Liao S.Y. and Iftner T., Human papillomavirus type 6 in squamous cell carcinoma of the bladder and cervix, *Hum Pathol*, 24, 96, 1993.

149. Maloney K.E., Wiener J.S. and Walther P.J., Oncogenic human papillomaviruses are rarely associated with squamous cell carcinoma of the bladder: evaluation by differential polymerase chain reaction, *J Urol*, 154, 360, 1994.

150. Kerley S.W., Persons D.L. and Fishback J.L., Human papillomavirus and carcinoma of the urinary bladder, *Modern Pathol*, 4, 316, 1991.

151. von Krogh G. and Wikström A., Efficacy of chemical and/or surgical therapy against condylomata acuminata: A retrospective evaluation, *Int J STD AIDS*, 2, 333, 1991.

152. Samenius B., Perianal and ano-rectal condyloma acuminata, *Schweiz Rundschau Med*, 72, 1009, 1983.

153. Goorney B.P., Waugh M.A. and Clarke J., Anal warts in heterosexual men, *Genitourin Med*, 63, 216, 1987.

154. Sonnex C., Scholefield J.H., Kocjan G., Kelly G., Whatrup C., Mindel A. and Northover J.M.A., Anal human papillomavirus infection in heterosexuals with genital warts: prevalence and relation with sexual behaviour, *Br Med J*, 303, 1243, 1991.

155. von Krogh G., Wikström A., Syrjänen K. and Syrjänen S., Anal and penile condylomas in HIV-negative and HIV-positive men; clinical, histological and virological characteristics correlated to therapeutic outcome, *Acta Dermatovener*, 75, 470, 1995.

156. Lacey C.J.N., Genital warts in children, *Papillomavirus Report*, 2, 31, 1991.

157. Handley J., Dinsmore E., Maw R., Corbett R., Borrows D., Bharucha H., Swann A and Bingham A., Anogenital warts in prepubertal children; sexual abuse or not?, *Int J STD AIDS*, 4, 271, 1993.

158. Cason J., Kaye J. N. and Best J.M., Non-sexual axquisition of human genital papillomaviruses, *Papillomavirus Report*, 6, 1, 1995.

159. Garzetti G.G., Ciavattini A., Goteri G., Menzo S., De Nictolis M., Clementi M., Brugia M. and Romanini C., Vaginal micropapillary lesions are not related to human papillomavirus infection: in situ hybridization and polymerase chain reaction detection techniques, *Gynecol Obstet Invest*, 38, 134, 1994.

160. Wade T.R. and Ackerman A.B., The effects of podophyllum resin on condylomata acuminata, *Am J Dermatopathol*, 6, 109, 1984.

161. Byrne M.A., Walker M.M., Leonard J., Pryce D. and Taylor-Robinson D., Recognising covert disease in women with chronic vulval symptoms attending an STD clinic: value of detailed examination including colposcopy, *Genitourin Med*, 65, 46, 1989.

162. Bodén E., Eriksson A., Rylander E. and von Schoultz B., Clinical characteristics of papillomavirus - vulvovaginitis, *Acta Obstet Gynecol Scand*, 67, 147, 1988.

163. Turner M.L. and Marinoff S.C., Association of human papillomavirus with vulvodynia and the vulvar vestibulitis syndrome, *J Reprod Med*, 33, 533, 1988.

164. Rylander E., Eriksson A., Ingelman-Sundberg H. and von Schoultz B., Classification of colposcopic findings associated with human papilloma virus infections of cervix uteri and vagina, *Cervix LFGT*, 3, 123, 1985.

165. Jadresic D., Barton S., Neill S., Staughton R. and Marwood R., Psychiatric morbidity in women attending a clinic for vulval problems - is there a higher rate in vulvodynia?, *Int J STD AIDS*, 4, 237, 1993.

166. McKay M., Vulvodynia, *Arch Dematol*, 125, 256, 1989.

167. Marinoff S.C. and Turner M.L.C., Vulvar vestibulitis syndrome: an overview, *Am J Obstet Gynecol*, 165, 1228, 1991.

168. Rylander E., Personal communication, 1994.

169. Birley H.D.L., Luzzi G.A. Walker M.M., Ryait B., Taylor-Robinson D. and Renton A.M., The association of human papillomavirus infection with baloposthitis: a description of five cases with proposals for treatment, *Int J STD AIDS*, 5, 139, 1994.

170. Editorial, Vulvar vestibulitis, *Lancet*, 338, 729, 1991.

171. Brookes J.L., Haywood S. and Green J., Adjustment to the psychological and social sequelae of recurrent genital herpes simplex infection, *Genitourin Med*, 69, 384, 1993.

172. Catotti D.N., Clarke P. and Catoe K.E., Herpes revisited. Still a cause of concern, *Sex Transm Dis*, 20, 77 1993.

173. Filiberti A., Tamburini A., Stefanon B., Merola M., Bandieramonte G., Vantafridda V. and De Palo G., Psychological aspects of genital human papillomavirus infection: a preliminary report, *J Psychosom Gynaecol*, 14: 145, 1993.

174. Clarke P., The psychosocial effects on genital herpes, *Herpes* 1, 13, 1994.

175. American Social Health Association, Survey shows how we live with HPV, *HPV News*, 3, 1, 1993.

176. Goodkin K., Antoni M.H., Helder L. and Sevin B., Psychoneuroimmunological aspects of disease progression among women with human papillomavirus-associated cervical dysplasia and human immunodeficiency virus type 1 co-infection, *Int J Psych Med*, 23, 119, 1993.

177. Persson G., Dahlöf L.G. and Krantz I., Physical and psychological effects of anogenital warts on female patients, *Sex Transm Dis*, 20, 10, 1993.

178. Palmer A.G., Tucker S., Warren R. and Adams M., Understanding women's response to treatment for cervical intra-epithelial neoplasia, *Br J Clin Psychol*, 32, 101, 1993.

179. Campion M.J., Brown J.R., McCance D.J., Atia W., Edwards R., Cuzick J. and Singer A., Psychosexual trauma of an abnormal cervical smear, *Br J Obstet Gynaecol*, 95, 175, 1988.

180. von Krogh G., Clinical manifestations and counselling in HPV genital infection; the venereologist's role, In. *First Int. Conf. on Counselling in Sex. Transm. Viral Infect.*, Florence, Italy September 23-24, 1994.

181. von Krogh G., Genitoanal papillomavirus infection; a pragmatic approach with focus on the role of primary health care providers, *J Pediatric Obstet Gynaecol*, 20, 5, 1994.

182. American Academy of Dermatology Task Force on Pediatric Dermatology: Genital warts and sexual abuse in children, *J Am Acad Dermatol*, 11, 529, 1984.

183. Schachner L. and Hankin D.E., Assessing child abuse in childhood condylomata acuminatum, *J Am Acad Dermatol*, 12, 157, 1985.

184. Schwartz S.K. and Whittington W.L., Sexual assault and sexually transmitted diseases: detection and management in adults and children, *Rev Infect Dis*, 12 (Suppl), 682, 1990.

185. Committee on Child Abuse and Neglect, American Academy of Pediatrics: Guidelines for the evaluation of sexual abuse in children, *Pediatrics*, 87, 254, 1991.

186. Fairris G.M., Statham B.N. and Waugh M.A., The investigation of patients with genital warts, *Br J Dermatol*, 111, 736, 1984.

187. Mitchell D.M., Kellett J.K. and Haye K., Investigation of patients with genital warts presenting to dermatological and to genitourinary departments, *Br J Dermatol*, 113 (Suppl), 22, 1985.

188. Elsner P., Hartmann A.A. and Wecker I., Condylomata - acuminata - assoziierte STD-Infektionen der Urethra des Mannes, *Hautarzt*, 38, 26, 1987.

189. Kinghorn G.R., Genital warts; incidence of associated genital infections, *Br J Dermatol*, 99, 405, 1978.

190. Claas E.C.J., Melchers W.J.G., Niesters H.G.M., van Muyden R., Stolz E. and Qiunt W.G.V, Infections of the cervix uteri with human papillomavirus and Chlamydia trachomatis, *J Med Virol*, 37, 54, 1992.

191. Jha P.K.S., Beral V., Peto J, Hack S., Hermon C., Deacon J., Mant D., Chilvers C., Vessey M.P., Pike M.C., Müller M. and Gissmann L., Antibodies to human papillomavirus and to other genital infectious agents and invasive cervical cancer risk, *Lancet*, 341, 1116, 1993.

192. Sanjosé De S., Munoz N., Bosch F.X., Reimann K., Pedersen K.R., Orfila J., Auscunce N., González L.C., Tafur L., Gili M., Lette I., Viladiu P., Tormo M.J., Morero P., Shah K. and Wahren B., Sexually transmitted agents and cervical neoplasia in Columbia and Spain, *Int J Cancer*, 56, 358, 1994.

193. Byrne M.A., Turner M.J., Griffiths M., Taylor-Robinson D. and Soutter W.P:, Evidence that patients presenting with dyskaryotic cervical smears should be screened for genital-tract infections other than human papillomavirus infection, *Eur J Obstet Gynecol Reprod Biol*, 41,129 1991.

194. Andersson-Ellström A. and Forssman L., Genital papillomavirus infection in women treated for chlamydial infection, *Int J STD AIDS*, 3, 42 1992.

195. Handley J.M., Lawther H., Horner T., Bharucha H. and Dinsmore W.W., Human papillomavirus DNA detection in primary anogenital warts and cervical low-grade intraepithelial neoplasias in adults by in situ hybridization, *Sex Transm Dis*, 19, 225, 1992.

196. Hoosen A.A., Quinlan D.J., Moodley J., Kharsany A.B.W. and van den Ende J., Sexually transmitted pathogens in acute pelvic inflammatory disease, *Aft Med J*, 76, 251, 1989.

197. Gross G., Ikenberg H., de Villiers E.M., Schneider A., Wagner D. and Gissmann L., Bowenoid papulosis: a venereally transmissible disease as a reservoir for HPV 16. In: zur Hausen H., Peto R. (Eds) Origin of female genital cancer: virological and epidemiological aspects. *Banbury Report*. Cold Spring Harbor, New York (1986), pp 149–165.

198. Ward B.G. and Thomas I.L., Randomized prospective intervention study of human cervical wart virus infection, *Aust NZ J Obstet Gynaecol*, 34, 182, 1994.

199. Nathan P.M., Thompson V.C., Sharmacharja G., Hawkswell J. and Fogarty B., A study of the prevalence of male intrameatal warts using meatoscopy in a genitourinary medicine department, *Int J STD AIDS*, 6, 184, 1995.

200. Pollack H.M., de Benedictis T.J., Marmar J.L. and Praiss D.E., Urethrographic manifestations of venereal warts (condylomata acuminata), *Radiology*, 126, 643, 1978.

201. Maddox P., Szarewski A., Dyson J. and Cuzick J., Cytokeratin expression and acetowhite change in cervical epithelium, *J Clin Pathol*, 47, 15, 1994.

202. van Le L., Broekhiuzen F.F., Janzer-Steele R., Behar M. and Samter T., Acetic acid visualization of the cervix to detect cervical dysplasia, *Obstet Gynecol*, 81, 293, 1993.

203. Teresita M.A., Vulvoscopy in the diagnosis of genital mycosis, *Cervix LFGT*, 12, 35, 1994.

204. Krowchuk D.P. and Anglin T.M., Genital human papillomavirus infections in adolescents: implications for evaluation and management, *Seminars Dermatol*, 11, 24, 1992.

205. IARC Working Group on Evaluation of Cervical Screening Programmes, Screening for squamous cervical cancer: duration of low risk after negative results of cervical cytology and its implications for screening policies, *BMJ*, 293, 659, 1986.

206. Koss L.G., Cervical (Pap) smear, *Cancer*, (Suppl) 71, 1406, 1993.

207. Davila R.M., Cervicovaginal smear, true or false?, *Am J Clin Pathol*, 101, 1, 1994.

208. Canadian Society of Cytology, The adequacy of the Papanicolaou smear, *Can Med Assoc J*, 150, 25, 1994.

210. van Oortmarssen G.J. and Habbema J.D.F., Epidemiological evidence for age-dependent regression of pre-invasive cervical cancer, *Br J Cancer*, 64, 559, 1991.

211. van den Brule A.J.C., Snijeders P.J.F., Meijer C.J.C.M. and Waalboomers J.M.M., PCR-based detection of genital HPV genotypes: an up-date and future perspectives, *Papillomavirus Report*, 4, 95, 1993.

212. Cuzick J., Terry G., Ho L., Hollingworth T. and Anderson M., Type-specific human papillomavirus DNA in abnormal smears as a predictor of high-grade cervical intraepithelial neoplasia, *Br J Cancer*, 69, 167, 1994.

213. Dillner J., Antibody responses to defined HPV epitopes in cervical neoplasia, *Papillomavirus Report*, 5, 35, 1994.

214. Burghardt E., *Colposcopy Cervical Pathology—Textbook and Atlas*, George Thieme Verlag, 1984.

215. Cartier R., Practical Colposcopy, Karger Basel. Laboratoire Cartier, Second Edition, Paris, 1984.

216. Singer A., Monaghan J.M., Eds, *Lower Genital Tract Precancer*, Blackwell Scientific Publications, Cambridge, MA, U.S.; Oxford, England. 1994.

217. Reid R. and Scalzi P., Genital warts and cervical cancer VII. An improved colposcopic index for differentiating benign papillomaviral infections from high-grade cervical intraepithelial neoplasia, *Am J Obstet Gynecol*, 153, 611, 1985.

218. Barrasso R., Coupez F., Ionesco M. and De Brux J., Human papillomavirus and cervical intraepithelial neoplasia: the role of colposcopy, *Gynecol Oncol*, 27, 197, 1987.

219. Stafl A. and Wilbanks G.D., An international terminology of colposcopy: report of the nomenclature committee of the International Federation of Cervical Pathology and Colposcopy, *Obstet Gynecol*, 77, 313, 1991.

220. Coppleson M., Colposcopic features of papillomavirus infection and premalignancy in the female lower genital tract, *Obstet Gynecol Cl North Am*, 14, 471, 1987.

221. Barrasso R., Colposcopic diagnosis of HPV cervical lesions, in *The epidemiology of Cervical Cancer and Human Papillomavirus*, Munoz, N., Bosch, F.X., Shah, K.V., and Meheus, A., Eds., IARC, 67, 1992.

222. Wespi H.J., Colposcopic-histologic correlations in the benign acanthotic non-glycogenated squamous epithelium, *Colposc Gyn Laser Surg*, 2, 147, 1986.

223. Coppleson M., Pixley E., and Reid B., *Colposcopy*, C.C. Thomas, Springfield, IL, 1971.

224. Jordan J.A. and Singer A., *The Cervix*, W.B. Saunders London, 1976.

225. Roy M., Clinical spectrum of genital HPV infection in the female I. Cervix and vagina, *Clin Pract Gynecol*, 2, 42, 1989.

226. Coupez F., Colposcopie des viroses du col, *Gynécologie*, 34, 177, 1983.

227. Williams A.B., Darragh T.M., Vranizan K., Ochia C., Moss A.R. and Palefsky J.M., Anal and cervical human papillomavirus infection and risk of human immunodeficiency virus-infected women, *Obstet Gynecol*, 83, 205, 1994.

228. Palefsky J.M., Holly E.A., Gonzales J., Lamborn K. and Hollander H., Natural history of anal cytologic abnormalities and papillomavirus infection among homosexual men with Group IV HIV desease, *J AIDS*, 5, 1258, 1992.

229. Shroyer K.R., Kim J.G., Manos M.M., Greer C.E., Pearlman N.W. and Franklin W.A., Papillomavirus found in anorectal squamous carcinoma, not in colon adenocarcinoma, *Arch Surg*, 127, 741, 1992.

230. Marte C., Kelly P., Cohen M., Fruchter R.G., Sedlis A., Gallo L., Ray V. and Webber C.A., Papanicolaou smear abnormalities in ambulatory care sites for women infected with human immunodeficiency virus, *Am J Obstet Gynecol*, 166, 1232, 1992.

231. Lipsey L.R. and Northfeldt D.W., Anogenital neoplasia in patients with HIV infection, *Curr Opinions Oncol*, 5, 861, 1993.

232. Maiman M., Fruchter R.G., Guy L., Cuthill S., Levine P. and Serur E., Human immunodeficiency virus infection and invasive cervical carcinoma, *Cancer*, 71, 402, 1993.

233. Centers for Disease Control, HIV/AIDS Surveillance Report, October 1993.

234. Hanson R.M., Glasson M., McCrossin I., Rogers M., Rose B. and Thompson C., Anogenital warts in childhood, *Child Abuse Negl*, 13, 225, 1989.

235. Boyd A.S., Condylomata acuminata in the pediatric population, *Am J Dis Child*, 144, 817, 1990.

236. Gibson P.E., Gardner S.D. and Best S., Human papillomavirus types in anogenital warts of children, *J Med Virol*, 30, 142, 1990.

237. Obalek S., Jablonska S. and Favre M., Condylomata acuminata in children: Frequent association with human papillomaviruses responsible for cutaneous warts, *J Am Acad Dermatol*, 23, 205, 1990.

238. Oranje H.P., de Waard-van der Spek F.B., Vuzevski V.D. and Bilo R.A.C., Condylomata acuminata in children, *Int J STD AIDS*, 1, 250, 1990.

239. Padel A.F., Venning V.A. and Evans M.F., Human papillomaviruses in anogenital warts in children: typing by in situ hybridization, *Br Med J*, 300, 1491, 1990.

240. Herman-Giddens M.E., Gutman L.T. and Berson N.L., Association to coexisting vaginal infections and multiple abusers in female children with genital warts, *Sex Transm Dis*, 15, 63, 1988.

241. Felix J.C. and Wright T.C., Analysis of lower genital tract lesions clinically suspicious for condylomata using in situ hybridization and the polymerase chain reaction for the detection of human papillomavirus, *Arch Pathol Lab Med*, 118, 39, 1994.

15

Warts of the Genitoanal Area in Children

Slavomir Obalek, Stefania Jablonska, and Gerard Orth

CONTENTS

I. INTRODUCTION

The incidence of genital warts is steadily increasing in adults,[1] and the same trend has been recently observed in children,[2-9] in whom condylomata were previously only rarely recognized.[10,11]

II. MODE OF TRANSMISSION AND EPIDEMIOLOGY

A. Sexual Abuse as a Mode of Transmission

Sexual abuse is a possible cause of childhood condylomata associated with genital HPVs since these viruses are usually sexually transmitted. However, reported frequency of sexual abuse varies considerably depending on the series studied. In children referred for examination because of suspected molestation, almost all genital warts were due to sexual abuse. Herman-Giddens et al.[2] found historical and/or physical evidence of sexual abuse in 10 of 11 children with condylomata, and concluded that all genital warts in girls are sexually transmitted.

Gutman[12] noticed abnormal findings on physical examination in 8 of 9 girls with genital warts, and in 5 of them coexisted other vaginal infections. This author believes that in almost all children with genital warts, even younger than 3 years of age, sexual abuse could be documented. Childhood condylomata are regarded as an indicator of sexual abuse by several authors.[5,6,13-20] However, most authors who stressed that anogenital warts are sufficient grounds to pursue the possibility of sexual abuse, could establish abuse only in some: in half of the cases studied,[21,22] in 30% of children[23] or only in single cases: 7 of 73,[4] 2 of 14,[24] or 1 of 32.[3] In our last series of 25 cases, sexual abuse was suspected in 4 girls and 2 boys,[8] but was not fully documented in any. Also, Gross stresses that nonveneral transmission is much more likely than by sexual abuse.[7]

The divergent opinions are probably mainly due to the difficulties in evaluating sexual abuse. This evaluation is based on identification of perpetrator, presence of another sexually transmitted disease, physical indications (vaginal opening, sphincter tone, signs of previous trauma), and behavioral indicators. The diagnosis is made on history rather than examination, as only infrequently physical signs of abuse can be found. Thus, in a proportion of cases, sexual abuse, even if strongly suspected, cannot be proved.

Since this problem is of special importance, the evaluation of a possible sexual molestation, including also nonviolent abuse, is necessary in all cases of childhood condylomata irrespective of the inducing HPVs.

In our series of 73 children with condylomata acuminata, sexual abuse was suspected in four girls and two boys, but except for two children was not confirmed either by interview, presence of signs of abuse, and/or other sexually transmitted diseases. In these 9- and 12-year-old boys, both children and parents provided evidence of sexual abuse (anal coitus). Because of the difficulty in assessing child abuse,[14] it is quite possible that some cases may have been missed.

B.   Other Modes of Transmission of Genital HPVs

Another possible way of transmission of HPV infection to children is from mothers with cervical or vulvar condylomata during passage through the birth canal.[10,25-27] In our series, in the children born of mothers having condylomata during pregnancy, anogenital condylomata appeared at the mean age of 25 years vs. 4 years 10 months in children born of women free of condylomata during pregnancy and delivery. A possible transmission of genital HPV infection is evidenced by laryngeal papillomas appearing in early childhood in babies born from mothers with condylomata.[28] In an 18-month-old boy suffering from laryngeal papillomas, these were noticed at the age of 3 months.[25] We have observed two newborns in whom the lesions were present at the first week of life, and their mothers had cervical condylomata during pregnancy. There are anecdotal reports of congenital condylomata,[4,29] which suggested transplacental transmission.

Besides that, HPV infection may be transmitted to children by sharing beds, using the same towels and baths, by fomites,[30] or direct contact with contaminated objects and/or fingers during care of the anogenital area of the babies.[3,31] In our patients, the most likely modes of transmission of genital HPVs were nursing or contact with contaminated objects, and/or infection during the passage of the birth canal.

C.   Transmission of Cutaneous HPVs

Almost 30% of condylomata in our series found to be positive for HPV in Southern blot studies were induced by HPV2 and less frequently by other cutaneous HPVs. Children with HPV2 associated condylomata were in an older age group than those with HPV6/11 associated warts (mean 9 years 6 months vs. 4 years 10 months). Similar results were also reported by Padel.[22] Importantly, the parents of these children were free of anogenital lesions and cutaneous warts were present in family members or in children themselves. This favors transmission from hand warts either by auto- or heteroinoculation.

Although in almost all cases the same HPV types were disclosed in the parents and children, in single patients there was some discordance, or the source of infection could not be disclosed. Four mothers had hand warts induced by HPV2, HPV4, and/or HPVX, and the children contracted condylomata associated with HPV6. Neither mothers nor fathers of those children had external condylomata at the time of the study. However one mother was found to have cervical condylomata of which she was not aware, and it is conceivable that other mothers had had cervical lesions which have not been recognized. This could be explained by a high prevalence of latent anogenital and cervical infections,[23,32-34] which might be transmitted to children during pregnancy and delivery. The infection may remain subclinical[32] and/or become overt under some adverse conditions.

Contrary to that, in all children with condylomata induced by HPV2 the source of the infection were cutaneous warts. The transmission was always from warts of the parents (heteroinoculation) or of the children themselves (autoinoculation), and anogenital and cutaneous warts were associated with the same HPV types. However, some exceptional cases in our series indicate that the mere presence of cutaneous warts in family members or persons taking care of children does not provide evidence on the origin of infection in the child, as stressed also by Padel et al.[22] Similarly, the detection of genital HPVs does not preclude sexual transmission of the infection.[7,8]

III. VIROLOGICAL FINDINGS VS. CLINICAL MANIFESTATIONS

A. Virological Studies

The results of virologic studies differ in various reports depending on the series of patients. Children referred to special centers because of suspected sexual abuse had a high prevalence of genital HPVs.[2,6,35] Gibson et al.[5] reported 22 cases associated with HPV6 and HPV11 while HPV2 was detected in only one child. Cohen et al.[4] found HPV6/11 in 27 of 34 cases studied and HPV2 in 6 cases, i.e., the percentage of infection with cutaneous HPVs was comparable with our earlier findings.[3]

In our present series of 73 children, virologic studies disclosed genital HPVs in 70% of condylomata found to be positive for HPV DNA: HPV6 in 37 children and HPV11 in 5. In no case was the infection induced by potentially oncogenic HPVs16 and 18. However, there are reports on single cases of children condylomata associated with HPV16 or 16/18 coexisting with HPV6/11.[4-6,19,36]

In addition, there were 3 cases of bowenoid papulosis in small children described; two of them were confirmed by presence of HPV16. In one child, the lesions appeared in the first year of life, and the mother had had genital warts during pregnancy;[37] another 3 year-old girl was sexually abused;[38] and in the third 34-month-old girl the parents were not studied for HPV-associated lesions.[39]

In 30% of our cases was detected HPV2 (in 14 girls and 2 boys). A similar percentage of HPV2-associated genital warts in children (25–27%) was also reported by some other authors.[4,6,22] In the study of de Villiers,[40] over 50% of children's condylomata were associated with HPV57, a virus closely related with HPV2, and with HPV27. Interestingly, in two girls, we found HPV2 even in vulvar lesions.

B. Clinical Manifestations

We did not find evident clinical difference between anogenital warts associated with HPV6/11 and cutaneous HPVs. However, HPV6/11-induced warts located on or near mucosa showed features of proliferative condylomata (Figure 1), while warts localized on the skin in perianal region were somewhat more hyperkeratotic (Figures 2a and 2b).

C. Histological Patterns

The histology of children's condylomata is that of papillomas with various degrees of koilocytosis, usually less pronounced than in anogenital warts of adults (Figure 3), and in a proportion of cases absent at all. In condylomata induced by HPV2, a cytopathic effect (CPE) characteristic of HPV2 infection could be detected in serial sections, (Figure 4). The same CPE was also present in

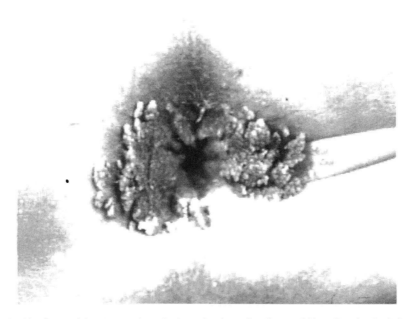

FIGURE 1   Proliferative condylomata acuminata in the perianal area in a 2-year-old boy, found to be induced by HPV6.

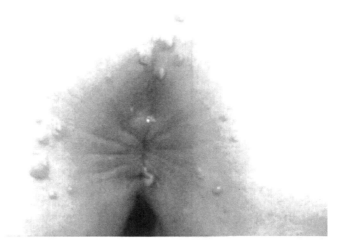

a
FIGURE 2   a) Perianal hyperkeratotic warts in a 7-year-old girl, found to be induced by HPV2. b) Palmar wart in the mother of the girl, found also to be induced by HPV2 (see Figure 2b).

cutaneous warts of the children or their parents. Thus the histologic study could provide some additional information on the HPV type.

IV.   THE ROLE OF IMMUNOLOGY

In general, children with condylomata do not show symptoms of decreased immunity. However, in immunosuppressed patients, anogenital warts may become highly proliferative resembling giant condylomata.[41] Such profuse condylomata were observed in a Japanese child treated topically with betamethasone and this was due to locally induced immunosuppression.[42]

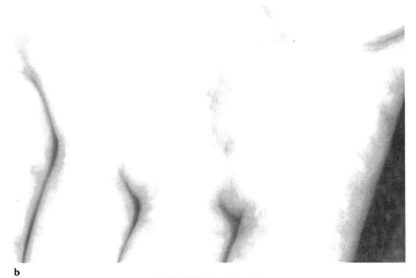

b

FIGURE 2 (continued)

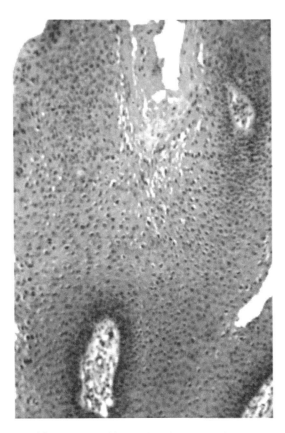

FIGURE 3 Histology of the genital wart induced by HPV11, localized at the vulva of a 3-year-old girl. Epidermal proliferation typical of papilloma with slight koilocytosis (H + E, ×120).

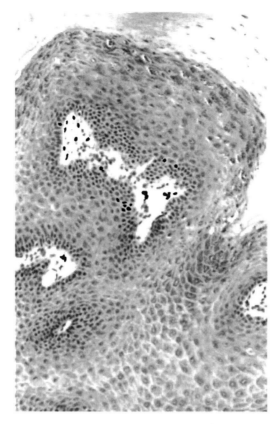

FIGURE 4 Histology of anal wart induced by HPV2 in a 3.3 year-old-girl whose mother had common hand warts. Papilloma with cytopathic effect of HPV2 type in the upper layers of the epidermis (keratohyalin granules of different sizes and shapes). H + E, ×200.

V.   COURSE OF THE DISEASE

The natural course and the duration of childhood condylomata are variable and depend on such factors as protracted sexual abuse, concomitant sexually transmitted infections, itching diseases, including intestinal parasitic infections and atopic dermatitis, lack of hygiene, etc. By recalcitrant anal warts, the source of reinfection might be condylomata localized in the anal canal. In such cases, rectoscopic examination is indicated.

VI.   MANAGEMENT AND PREVENTION

The management of childhood condylomata comprises mainly cryotherapy, scissor excision, electrocautery, and laser.[43-45] We do not use podophylline in children since it may induce dysplastic changes. Of greatest importance appears to be prevention, i.e., careful examination of persons taking care of children for anogenital and cutaneous warts, and detailed interviews of children and parents for possible sexual abuse.

REFERENCES

1. Koutsky, L. A., Galloway, D. A., and Holmes, K. K., Epidemiology of genital human papillomaviruses infection. *Epidemiol. Rev.*, 1988; 10:122.
2. Herman-Giddens, M. E., Gutman, L. T., and Berson, N. L., Association of coexisting vaginal infections and multiple abuses in female children with genital warts. *Sex. Transm. Dis.*, 1988; 15:63.

3. Obalek, S., Jablonska, S., Favre, M., Walczak, L., and Orth, G., Condylomata acuminata in children: Frequent association with human papillomaviruses responsible for cutaneous warts. *J. Am. Acad. Dermatol.*, 1990; 23:205.

4. Cohen, B. A., Honig, P., and Androphy, E., Anogenital warts in children: clinical and virologic evaluation for sexual abuse. *Arch. Dermatol.*, 1990; 126:1575.

5. Gibson, P. E., Gardner, S. D., and Best, S. J., Human papillomavirus types in anogenital warts of children. *J. Med. Virol.*, 1990; 30:142.

6. Hanson, R. M., Glasson, M., McCrossin, I., and Rogers, M., Anogenital warts in childhood. *Child Abuse Negl.*, 1990; 13:225.

7. Gross, G., Condylomata acuminata in der Kindheit-Hinweis fur sexuellen Misbrauch. *Hautarzt*, 1992; 43:120.

8. Obalek, S., Misiewicz, J., Jablonska, S., Favre, M., and Orth, G., Childhood condylomata acuminata: association with genital and cutaneous human papillomaviruses. *Pediatr. Dermatol.*, 1993; 10:101.

9. Handley, J. M., Maw, R. O., Binghan, E. A. et al., Anogenital warts in children. *Clin. Exp. Dermatol.*, 1993; 18:241.

10. Eftaiha, M. S., Amshel, A. L., and Shonberg, I. L., Condylomata acuminata in an infant and mother: report of a case. *Dis. Colon Rectum*, 1978; 21:369.

11. Ingber, A., Grunwald, M. H., and Feuerman, E. J., Perianale Condylomata acuminata bei einem 13-Monate alten Madchen. *Z. Hautkr.*, 1982; 58:1200.

12. Gutman, L. T., Sexual abuse and human papillomavirus infection. *J. Pediatr.*, 1990; 116:495.

13. Seidel, J., Zonana, J., and Totten, E., Condylomata acuminata as a sign of sexual abuse in children. *J. Pediatr.*, 1979; 95:553.

14. Schachner, L. and Hankin, D. E., Assessing child abuse in childhood condylomata acuminata. *J. Am. Acad. Dermatol.*, 1985; 12:157.

15. Sait, M. A. and Garg, B. R., Candylomata acuminata in children: report of 4 cases. *Genitour. Med.*, 1985; 61:338.

16. Rock, B., Naghashfar, Z., Barnett, N., Buscema, I., Wooddruff, D., and Shah, K., Genital tract papillomavirus infection in children. *Arch. Dermatol.*, 1986; 122:1129.

17. Shelton, T. B., Jerkins, G. R., and Noe, H. N., Condylomata acuminata in the pediatric patient. *J. Urol.*, 1986; 135:548.

18. Goldenring, J. H., Warts and diagnosis of sexual abuse. *Lancet*, 1987; 2:1018.

19. Vallejos, H., Del Mistro, Kleinhaus, S., Braunsteins, J. D., Halluer, M., and Koss, L. G., Characterization of human papilloma virus types in condylomata acuminata in children by in situ hybridization. *Lab Invest.*, 1987; 56:611.

20. Derksen, D. J., Children with condylomata acuminata. *J. Fam. Pract.*, 1992; 34:419.

21. Roussey, M., Dabadie, A., Chevrant-Breton, O., Chevrant-Breton, J., and Lemarec, C. B., Condylomata acumines chez l'enfant. *Arch. Fr. Ped.*, 1988; 45:429.

22. Padel, A. F., Venning, V. A., Evans, M. F., Quantrill, A. M., and Fleming, K. A., Human papillomaviruses in anogenital warts in children: typing by *in situ* hybridization. *Br. Med. J.*, 1990; 300:1491.

23. Hirschfeld, L. S. and Steinberg, B. M., Clinical spectrum of HPV infection in the neonate and child. *Clin. Pract. Gynecol.*, 1989; 2:102.

24. Herrera Saval, A., Rodriguez Pichardo, A., Garcia Bravo, B., and Camacho, F., Verrues ano-genitales chez les enfants. *Ann. Dermatol Venereol.*, 1990; 117:523.

25. Hajek, E., Contribution to the etiology of laryngeal papilloma in children. *J. Laryngol. Otol.*, 1956; 70:166.

26. Fredericus, B. D., Balkin, A., and Daniel, A. W., Transmission of human papillomaviruses from mother to child. *J. Obstet. Gynecol.*, 1993; 33:30.

27. Armbruster-Moraes, E., Joshinoto, L. M., Leao, E., Ioshimoto, L. M., Leao, E., and Zugaib, M., Presence of human papillomavirus DNA in amniotic fluids of pregnant women with cervical lesions, *Gynecol. Oncol.*, 1994; 54:152.

28. Mounts, P. and Shah, K. V., Respiratory papillomatosis: etiological relation to genital tract papillomaviruses. *Prog. Med. Virol.*, 1984; 29:90.

29. Tang, C. K., Shermeta, D. W., and Wood, C., Congenital condylomata acuminata. *Am. J. Obstet. Gynecol.*, 1978; 131:912.

30. Ferenczy, A., Bergeron, C. H., and Richart, R. M., Human papillomavirus DNA in fomites on objects used for the management of patients with genital human papillomavirus infections. *Obstet. Gynecol.*, 1989; 74:950.

31. Singh, K. G., Bajaj, A. K., and Sharma, R., Perianal condylomata acuminata in an infant. *Int. J. Dermatol.*, 1988; 27:181.

32. Roman, A. and Fife, K., Human papillomavirus DNA associated with foreskins of normal newborns. *J. Infect. Dis.*, 1986; 153:855.

33. Jenison, S. A., Yu, X., Valentine, J. M., et al., Evidence of prevalent genital type human papillomavirus infections in adults and children. *J. Infect. Dis.*, 1990; 162:60.

34. Schiffman, M. W., Recent progress in defining the epidemiology of human papillomavirus infection and cervical neoplasia. *J. Natl. Canc. Inst.*, 1992; 84:394.

35. Davis, A. J. and Emans, S. J., Human papilloma virus infection in the pediatric and adolescent patient. *J. Pediatr.*, 1989; 115:1.

36. Benton, E. C., MacKinlay, G. A., Barr, B. B. B., and Smith, I. W., Characterization of human papillomavirus DNA from genital warts in children. *Br. J. Dermatol.*, 1989; 121 (Suppl.):34.

37. Brenemann, D. L., Lucky, A. W., Ostrow, R. S., Faras, A. J., Volger, C., and Jenshi, L. J., Bowenoid papulosis of the genitalia associated with human papillomavirus DNA type 16 in an infant with atopic dermatitis. *Pediatr. Dermatol.*, 1985; 2:297.

38. Halasz, C., Silvers, D., and Crum, C. P., Bowenoid papulosis in a three-year-old girl. *J. Am. Acad. Dermatol.*, 1966; 14:326.

39. Weitzner, J. M., Fields, K. W., and Robinson, M. J., Pediatric Bowenoid papulosis: risk and management. *Pediatr. Dermatol.*, 1989; 6:303.

40. de Villiers, E. M., Importance of human papillomavirus DNA typing in the diagnosis of congenital warts in children. *Arch. Dermatol.*, 1995; 131:366.

41. Laraque, D., Severe anogenital warts in child with HIV infection. *N. Engl. J. Med.*, 1989; 320:1221.

42. Matsumura, N., Kumasaka, K., Maki, H., Yoshie, O., and Tagami, H., Giant condylomata acuminata in a baby boy. *J. Dermatol.*, 1992; 19:432.

43. Kraus, S. J. and Stone, K. M., Management of genital infection caused by human papillomaviruses. *Rev. Infect. Dis.*, 1990; 12(Suppl. 6):620.

44. Riva, J. M., Sedlecek, T. V., Cunnane, M. F., and Mangan, C. E., Extended carbon dioxide laser vaporisation in the treatment of subclinical papillomavirus infection of the lower genital tract. *Obstet. Gynecol.*, 1989; 73:25.

45. Cohen, B. A., Scissor excision plus electrocautery of anogenital warts in prepubertal children. *Pediatr. Dermatol.*, 1991; 8:248.

16

HPV-Related Squamous Cell Tumors of the Airways and Esophagus: Clinical Presentation

Stina Syrjänen

CONTENTS

I.   INTRODUCTION

Papillomaviruses are epitheliotrophic viruses causing hyperplastic, papillomatous, and verrucous lesions of the skin and different mucosal sites. It is currently well established that papillomas of the oral cavity and larynx are caused by HPV. However, the association of HPV with esophageal papillomas or squamous carcinomas of the airways is less convincing and further studies are needed. Classical papillomas do not usually present any major diagnostic problems. Nevertheless, small lesions exhibiting the same color as the adjacent normal tissue may easily be ignored, especially because they are symptomless. In the oral cavity, a thorough palpation of the mucosa may be helpful. In other regions of the airways, however, no data are available on the prevalence of these tiny, epithelial lesions caused by HPV. Epithelial changes in the paranasal sinuses, pharynx, larynx, and bronchus are usually not detected until they cause clinical symptoms like stuffiness, epistaxis, hoarseness, phonetic changes, or coughing.

0-8493-7356-5/97/$0.00+$.50
© 1997 by CRC Press, Inc.

This chapter describes the clinical features of the squamous cell lesions with suggested HPV-etiology in the airways and esophagus. In addition, the diagnostic evaluation and treatment of oral HPV lesions will be briefly discussed.

II.   PAPILLOMAS OF THE SINO-NASAL TRACT

Apart from the inflammatory polyps which represent the most frequent benign tumors in this region, different types of papillomas can be distinguished in the nasal cavity and paranasal sinuses.

A.   Inverted Papillomas

Inverted papillomas are uncommon benign tumors of the nasal cavity and paranasal sinuses,[1,2] comprising about one half of the sino-nasal papillomas. These lesions arise from the lateral wall of the nasal cavity and may extend into the maxillary or ethmoid sinuses (Figure 1). Inverted papillomas are usually large and bulky, exhibiting a deep red to gray color and a marked vascularity. Typical clinical symptoms entail nasal stuffiness and/or obstruction.[1,2] In contrast to in patients with inflammatory polyps, an allergic history is usually absent. The frequency of inverted papilloma has been calculated as 1/25–50 of that reported for the common inflammatory polyps.[3] In general hospitals, the incidence varies from 0.4% to 4.7% of all tumors of the nasal cavities.[4,5] Nasal inverted papilloma has been observed in all age groups, males being affected more commonly than women, the sex ratio ranging from 3:1 to 10:1.[1-5] These papillomas frequently recur (i.e., 28 to 67% of cases) in spite of a seemingly radical therapy.[6,7] They are associated with a significant risk for transformation into a squamous cell carcinoma, the risk ranging from 3 to 32% in different series.[8,9]

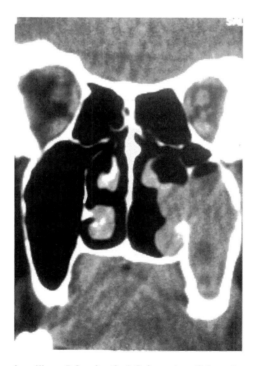

FIGURE 1   A CT-scan of a nasal papilloma deforming the inferior and medial concha nasalis. The tumor has perforated the median wall of the maxillary sinus occupying it totally. This entirely benign lesion (on light microscopy) is behaving like a malignant tumor. (With courtesy of Prof. Erkki Virolainen).

B. Fungiform Papillomas

Fungiform papillomas, regarded as a separate entity from the inverted papillomas, arise from the anterior nasal septum and rarely from the lateral nasal wall or paranasal sinuses. These lesions reveal a cauliflower-like, exophytic growth pattern and are attached to the mucosa by a broad base. Symptoms are similar to those associated with inverted papillomas, although epistaxis may be more common. The lesions recur in spite of therapy in approximately one third of the cases. Malignant transformation is rare.[10]

III. PAPILLOMAS OF THE LARYNX

The primary site of laryngeal papillomas is the true cords of the larynx.[11-14] Laryngeal papillomas show a biphasic age distribution, occuring in both young children and in adults, and therefore being distinguished as juvenile and adult-onset types.[12-14] According to their clinical presentation, they can be further classified into multiple and solitary papillomas (Figure 2).[13] Children under the age of 5 years are at the highest risk of acquiring laryngeal papillomas. In a series of 76 children, 21 (28%) presented between birth and 6 months of age and 43 (57%) appeared before 2 years of age.[14] Many patients with the juvenile-onset form continue to have the disease throughout their life, although spontaneous regression of papillomas has been described at puberty.[15] In small children, a phonetic change represents the usual first symptom. However, severe obstructive symptoms may ensue and become dramatic and sometimes life threatening. Juvenile papillomas appear as whitish to pinkish red nodules. In contrast to papillomas in the adult where solitary papillomas dominate, the existence of multiple lesions is the rule in the juvenile form.

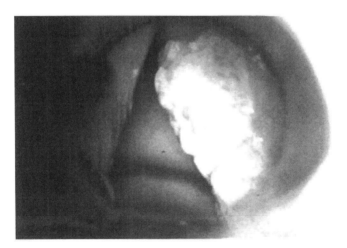

FIGURE 2   A solitary adult-type laryngeal papilloma. (With courtesy of Prof. Erkki Virolainen).

Age distribution of the adult-onset papillomas usually shows a peak between the ages of 20 and 40 years. Males are affected slightly more frequently than females.[15] Malignant conversion of laryngeal papillomas is rare.[16-28] A review of the available case reports shows that malignant neoplasms are more likely to occur in cases of severe papillomatosis with long duration and where the lesions spread throughout the respiratory tract.[16-18] Malignant transformation seems to be more common in cases with juvenile papillomas and it has been associated with irradiation.[19,20]

IV. TRACHEOBRONCHIAL PAPILLOMAS

Tracheobronchial papillomas are rare benign tumors that may occur with or without concomitant or preceeding laryngeal papillomatosis. On bronchoscopy, a solitary exophytic growth is encountered with a color ranging from pink to whitish, depending on the extent of the superficial parakeratosis. The frequency of tracheal papillomatosis was reported as being similar for both the juvenile onset (26%) and adult-onset disease (25%) by Weiss and Kashima.[21] Clinically, there is a tendency for papillomas to spread into previously uninvolved areas of the respiratory tract, including the lungs. Tracheal extension of the disease from the larynx has been reported to occur in 2 to 36% of the cases.[16,21-23] Extension into the bronchi and lungs is far less common (<1% of cases), but when this occurs, the prognosis is generally poor.[15,21,22] Manifestations of pulmonary papillomatosis were well documented by Kramer et al.[22] and these include the development of cystic or solid lung masses, usually consisting of benign squamous cell proliferation with central cavitation. Approximately 50% of the solitary adult tumors are estimated to undergo malignant transformation.

V.   HPV LESIONS OF THE ORAL CAVITY

Recent data suggest that squamous cell papilloma, condyloma acuminatum, verruca vulgaris, and focal epithelial hyperplasia of the oral cavity are associated with or caused by HPV. Furthermore, HPV DNA has been found in oral premalignant lesions including leukoplakia and lichen planus as well as in squamous cell carcinoma. However, the association seems to be weaker than that of the cervix (for review see references 22,24). So far, no reliable data exist on the prevalence and incidence of oral HPV infections except that published by Kellokoski et al.[25-27] They found HPV DNA in 2.6% of cytological scrapings taken from 334 woman with past or present genital HPV infections using a dot blot hybridization.[25] On clinical inspection, only three tiny exophytic growths similar to condyloma were diagnosed in these patients.[26] Using Southern blot hybridization, 15% of the biopsies taken from clinically normal buccal mucosa contained HPV DNA. The PCR technique increased the positivity rate of HPV DNA in these biopsies to 21.8%.

Only in one subject has the same HPV type been detected both in the genital tract and oral mucosa.[27] This finding questions oral sex as a possible transmission route of oral HPV infection. The acetic acid application on oral mucosa is of no use in diagnosis of HPV infection. In the oral cavity, acetowhite lesions reflect changes caused by nonspecific irritation rather than HPV infections. In diagnosing oral HPV infections, demonstration of HPV DNA is mandatory because gross morphology and (not infrequently) even histological appearance of HPV lesions in the oral cavity is not distinct enough.[25-27]

A.   Papillomas

Oral squamous cell papilloma is a benign tumor, which can occur at any age (Figure 3).[28,29] It usually affects the soft palate, but can sometimes be present in the dorsum, lateral borders, and frenulum of the tongue and lower lip as well (Figure 3).[28,29] Most papillomas are single and small in size (<1 cm). A slight male predominance exists and whites comprise the majority (87.5%) of patients.[29] Papillomas represent exophytic growths, appearing as a broad-based ovoid swelling, or as a pedunculated lesion. The surface may show small fingerlike projections, giving rise to a rough verrucous contour. The color varies from white to pink depending on the degree of keratinization and vascularization (Figure 4). Multiple papillomas are rare. Recurrence subsequent to radical excision is exceptional.

B.   Condylomas

Originally, oral condyloma acuminatum is regarded as a sexually transmitted disease (STD), contracted by oro-sexual contact.[30,31] As early as in 1901, Heidingsfield described a case of "Puella publica" believed to have acquired condylomata in her tongue as a result of "coitus illegitum".[32] At onset, oral condylomas usually present multiple small, white, or pink nodules, which proliferate and coalesce to form soft sessile growths.[30,31] The lesions are usually asymptomatic. Regression after a duration varying from two weeks to several months has been observed. The surface contour in most cases is more cauliflower-like than that of papillomas. Differentiation from the squamous

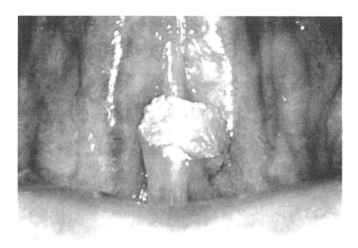

FIGURE 3 Papilloma of the mouth located in the frenulum. (With courtesy of Prof. Erkki Virolainen).

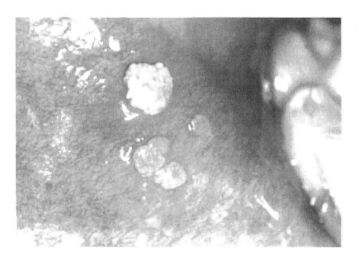

FIGURE 4 Several small papillomas on buccal mucosa. Note the different gross morphology of the three lesions which depends on the age of the lesion and level of keratinization.

cell papilloma is difficult and largely academic. According to some authors, it might be attempted on the basis of papillomatosis which shows a tendency for a sessile architecture in condylomatous lesions rather than a pedunculated form in the papilloma. The recent discovery of HPV DNA even in normal oral mucosa of both children and adults has questioned the sexual route as the only mode of HPV transmission.[25,27]

C. Common Warts

The common wart, or verruca vulgaris, is one of the most common skin lesions, especially in children. Oral warts are clinically indistinguishable from the squamous cell papillomas, appearing as whitish, sessile, papillomatous, rough-surfaced lesions.[33] Warts usually grow rapidly. They may be located at any site, although the lips and the tongue are afflicted most often. The diagnosis of a common wart in the oral cavity should be restricted to lesions showing clinical and histological characteristics of verruca vulgaris of the skin. Oral verrucas are mostly located on the lips or in the keratinized oral mucosa. Recently, oral warts containing HPV 7 DNA have been found in HIV-infected subjects (Figure 5).[34]

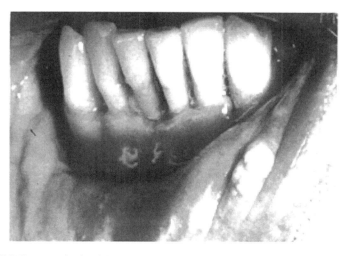

FIGURE 5 Verruca vulgaris of the lip caused by HPV type 7. The patient was HIV-seropositive.

D.   Focal Epithelial Hyperplasia (Heck's Disease)

The term focal epithelial hyperplasia (FEH) was first introduced by Archard et al. in 1965 to signify multiple nodular elevations of the oral mucosa observed among Eskimos and Indians from North and South America.[35] Since then, numerous additional cases have been reported. The highest prevelence (33.8%) has been found in Indian children in Venezuela.[36] Similar studies among the Eskimo populations have shown FEH to be remarkably frequent, the prevalence varying from 7 to 36%.[37] In contrast, very low prevalence figures have been reported in caucasian populations. A strong familial history has been suggested by several authors.[34,38] Clinically, FEH is characterized by multiple (or solitary) painless, soft papules of the oral mucosa, notably on the lower lip but sometimes extending to the vermilion border,[35-38] buccal mucosa, and the tongue (Figure 6). The lesions appear to occur predominantly in children less than 18 years of age, although an increasing number of FEH lesions has been described in adults as well.[35-38] These lesions, which often persist for several years, are totally benign and do not require therapy except for aesthetic reasons. Spontaneous regression might occur. The histologic picture is characteristic, enabling a proper diagnosis by biopsy which can be confirmed by detection of HPV 13 and 32 DNA in the sample.

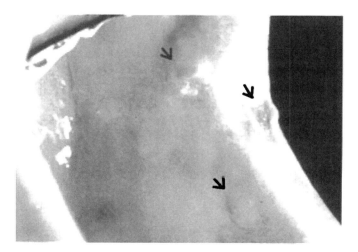

FIGURE 6   Focal epithelial hyperplasia on buccal mucosa caused by HPV type 32. Similar lesions were also found in her tongue.

E. Leukoplakia, Oral Precancer, and Cancer

While previously considered most common in the males, leukoplakias have been reported with an increasing frequency in women as well.[39,40] This shift has been attributed to the changes in the smoking habits among young women. The prevalence of leukoplakia in the world literature varies considerably from 0.4 to 11.7%.[39-41]

Although the clinical appearance of oral leukoplakia is variable, a clear distinction between homogenous and patchy white lesions is usually easy. The most common location appears to be the mandibular mucosa, while the tongue is least frequently affected. The most useful clinical classification is: leukoplakia simplex, verrucous leukoplakia, and leukoplakia erosiva.[40] Leukoplakia simplex is the most common and also the most benign form (Figure 7). The verrucous type should be considered as highly suspicious for malignant transformation.[41] The erosive form ranks as a high-risk lesion, being associated with a 30% risk for malignant transformation. However, it is to be emphasized that the clinical appearance should not be considered as a reliable predictor of malignant transformation. Therefore, a biopsy is mandatory. Histopathologic presentation entails a variety of epithelial changes ranging from benign hyperplasia to various degree of dysplastic changes including the *in situ* and early invasive carcinoma.

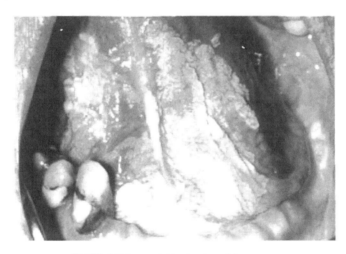

FIGURE 7 Leukoplakia simplex of the tongue.

VI. ESOPHAGEAL PAPILLOMAS

Squamous cell papillomas of the esophagus are rare tumors, usually smaller than 20 mm in diameter with distinct histological characteristics. Usually they are sessile lesions in the distal one third of the esophagus. In autopsy studies, the incidence of squamous cell papillomas vary from 0.006 to 0.04%.[42] On endoscopy, the papillomas appear as smooth, round, pink, sharply demarcated, sessile tumors. Esophageal papillomas are generally considered as benign tumors and appear as a single lesion or as multiple nonconfluent lesions. Confluent and multiple papillomas with a verrucous pattern are called esophageal papillomatosis. Esophageal papillomatosis is a rare condition which may be symptomatic (dysphagia or hemorrhage).[42]

VII. ESOPHAGEAL CANCER

One of the most intriguing features of esophageal squamous cell cancer (ESCC) is its considerable geographic variation. Data worldwide present a mosaic of varying incidence rates and sex ratios.[43-46] In most countries, incidence rates of ESCC per 100,000 are around 2.5 to 5.0 for the males and 1.5 to 2.5 for the females. In certain areas, however, the incidence rates are remarkably higher, varying up to 500-fold from one area to another, from one country to another, and between different ethnic groups even within the same country.[43-46] Epidemiological studies have identified the high risk countries for ESCC: the People's Republic of China, Singapore, Iran, Russian, Puerto Rico, Chile, Brazil, Switzerland, France, and South Africa.[43-46] In the People's Republic of China, the annual deaths due to esophageal cancer account for 27% of all cancer deaths among the males and 20% in the females, ranking among the two leading causes of cancer deaths, second only to that of stomach cancer.[45]

In general, the incidence of ESCC is higher in males than in females. This sex difference disappears in the high-incidence areas, but curiously enough, the incidence in females is generally much lower in the adjacent low-risk areas. On clinical presentation, the majority of ESCC cases are encountered in advanced age group, showing a peak between 50 and 70 years. However, in the high-incidence areas, the disease may occur 5–15 years earlier than in the general population.[46] Although the incidence and mortality rates slightly fluctuate from year to year, they do not appear to decline to any significant extent.[43-46]

REFERENCES

1. Lawson W, Le Benger J, Som P. Inverted papilloma: An analysis of 87 cases. *Laryngoscope* 99:1117, 1989.
2. Phillips PP, Gustafson RO, Facer GW. The clinical behavior of inverting papilloma of the nose and paranasal sinuses. Report of 112 cases and review of the literature. *Laryngoscope* 100:463, 1990.
3. Segal K, Atar E, Har-El G. Inverting papilloma of the nose and paranasal sinuses. *Laryngoscope* 96:394, 1986.
4. Kelly JH, Joseph M, Coroll E. Inverted papillomas of the nasal septum. *Arch. Otolaryngol.* 106:767, 1980.
5. Kristensen S, Vorre P, Elbrond O. Nasal Schneiderian papillomas: A study of 83 cases. *Clin. Otolaryngol.* 10:125, 1985.
6. Norris HJ, Papillary lesions of nasal cavity and paranasal sinuses. A study of 29 cases. *Laryngoscope* 73:1, 1963.
7. Ridolfi RL, Lieberman PH, Erlandson RA. Schneiderian papillomas: A clinico-pathologic study of 30 cases. *Am. J. Surg. Pathol.* 1:43, 1977.
8. Siivonen L, Virolainen E. Transitional papilloma of the nasal cavity and paranasal sinuses. Clinical course, viral etiology, and malignant transformation. *ORL J. Otorinolaryngol. Rel. Special.* 51:262, 1989.
9. Myers EN, Schramm VL, Barnes EL. Management of inverted papilloma of the nose and paranasal sinuses. *Laryngoscope* 91:2071, 1981.
10. Batsakis JC. The pathology of head and neck tumors. Nasal cavity and paranasal sinuses. V. *Head Neck Surg.* 2:410, 1980.
11. Quick CA, Faras A, Krzysek R. The etiology of laryngeal papillomatosis. *Laryngoscope* 88:1789.
12. Cook TA, Cohn AM, Brunschwig JP. Laryngeal papillomas: Etiology and therapeutic considerations. *Ann. Otol.* 82:649, 1973.
13. Lindeberg H, Oster S, Oxlund I. Laryngeal papillomas: Classification and course. *Clin. Otolaryngol.* 11:423, 1986.
14. Cohen SR, Geller KA, Seltzer. Papilloma of the laryngx and tracheobroncial tree in children. A retrospective study. *Ann. Otolaryngol.* 89:497, 1989.
15. Mounts P. Shaha KV. Respiratory papillomatosis: Etiological relation to genital papillomaviruses. *Prog. Med. Virol.* 29:90, 1984.
16. Dekelboum AM. Papillomas of the laryngx. *Arch. Otolaryngol.* 81:390, 1986.
17. DiMarco AF, Montenegor H, Payne CB. Papillomas of the tracheobroncial with malignant degeneration. *Chest* 74:464, 1974.
18. Friedberg SA, Stagman R, Hass GM. Papillary lesions of the laryngs in adults. A pathologic study. *Ann. Otol. Rhinol. Laryngol.* 80:683, 1971.
19. Galloway TC, Soper GR, Elsen J. Carcinoma of the laryngx after irradiation for papilloma. *Arch. Otolaryngol.* 72:289, 1960.

20. Matsuba HM, Thawley SE, Maurey M. Laryngeal epidermoid carcinoma associated with juvenile laryngeal papillomatosis. *Laryngoscope* 95:1264, 1985.

21. Weiss M, Kashima H. Traceal involvement of laryngeal papillomatosis. *Laryngoscope* 93:45, 1983.

22. Kramer SS, Wehunt WD, Stocker JT. Pulmonary manifestations of juvenile laryngotraceal papillomatosis. *Am. J. Roentgenol.* 144:687, 1985.

23. Syrjänen SM. Human papillomavirus infection in the oral cavity. In: Syrjänen KJ, Gissman L, Koss LG. Eds. *Papillomavirus and Human Disease,* Heidelberg: Springer-Verlag, 104, 1987.

24. Chang F, Syrjänen S, Kellokoski J, Syrjänen K. Human papillomavirus (HPV) infections and their associations with oral disease. *J. Oral Pathol. Med.* 20:305, 1991.

25. Kellokoski J, Syrjänen S, Yliskoski M, Syrjänen K. Dot blot hybridization in detection of human papillomavirus (HPV) infections in oral cavity in women with genital infections. *J. Oral Microbiol. Immunol.* 7:19, 1992.

26. Kellokoski J, Syrjänen S, Syrjänen K. Oral mucosal changes in women with genital HPV infection. *J. Oral Pathol. Med.* 19:142, 1990.

27. Kellokoski J, Syrjänen S, Chang F, Yliskoski M, Syrjänen KJ. Southern blot hybridization and PCR in detection of oral human papillomavirus (HPV) infections in women with genital HPV infections. *J. Oral Pathol. Med.* 21:459, 1992.

28. Greer RO, Goldman HM. Oral papillomas. Clinico-pathologic evaluation and retrospective examination for dyskeratosis in 110 lesions. *Oral Surg.* 38:435, 1974.

29. Abbey LM, Page DG, Sawyer DR. The clinical and histopatologic features of a series of 464 oral squamous cell papillomas. *Oral Surg.* 49:419, 1980.

30. Knapp MJ, Uohara GI. Oral condyloma acuminatum. *Oral Surg. Oral Med. Oral Pathol.* 23:538, 1967.

31. Doyle JL, Grodjesk JE, Manhold JH. Condyloma acuminatum occuring in the oral cavity. *Oral Surg.* 6:434, 1968.

32. Heidingfield ML. Condyloma accuminata linguata. *J. Cutan. Genitour. Dis.* 19:226, 1901.

33. Hertz RS. The occurrence of a verruca vulgaris on an intraoral skin graft. *Oral Surg.* 34:934, 1972.

34. Syrjänen S, Von Krogh G, Kellokoski J, Syrjänen K. Two different human papillomavirus (HPV) types associated with oral mucosal lesions in an HIV-seropositive man. *J. Oral Pathol. Med.* 18:366, 1989.

35. Archard HO, Heck JW, Stanley HR, Gallup NM. Focal epithelial hyperplasia: an unusual oral mucosal lesion found in Indian children. *Oral Surg.* 20:201, 1976.

36. Soneira A, Fonseca N. Sobre una lesion de la mucosa oral en los ninos Indios de la Mision Los Angeles de Tokuko. *Venezuela Odontol.* 29:109, 1964.

37. Praetorius-Clausen F. Geograpical aspects of oral focal epithelial hyperplasia. *Scand. J. Dental Res.* 39:204, 1973.

38. Buchner A, Mass E. Focal epithelial hyperplasia in an Israeli family. *Oral Surg.* 36:507, 1973.

39. Banoczy J. *Oral Leukoplasia* Nijhoff, Hague, 1982.

40. Burkhardt A, Maerker R. *A Color Atlas of Oral Cancers.* Wolf, London, 1981.

41. Pindborg JJ. *Oral Cancer and Precancer.* Henry Ling, Dorset Press, Dorchester. 1980.

42. Quitadoma M, Benson J. Squamous papilloma of the esophagus: a case report and review of the literature. *Am. J. Gastroenterol.* 83:194, 1988.

43. Waterhouse J, Muir CS, Shanmugaratman K, Powell J. *Cancer Incidence in Five Continents.* IARC Scientific Publications 42, Lyon vol III, 1976.

44. Parkin DM, Läärä E, Muir CS. Estimates of the worldwide frequency of sixteen major cancers in 1980. *Int. J. Cancer* 41:184, 1988.

45. Amstrong B. The epidemiology of cancer in the People's Republic of China. *Int. J. Epidemiol.* 9:305, 1980.

46. Silber W. Carcinoma of the esophagus: aspects of epidemiology and etiology. *Proc. Nutr. Soc.* 44:101, 1985.

17

Recurrent Respiratory Papillomatosis

Haskins K. Kashima, Brigid G. Leventhal, Keerti V. Shah, and
Phoebe Mounts

CONTENTS

Papilloma is the most common benign laryngeal neoplasm. This lesion occurs with particular predilection in the larynx, but the entire upper respiratory tract epithelium, from the nasal vestibule to the peripheral lung is at risk. Although the lesions are histologically benign, rapid regrowth threatens airway patency, and repeated surgical excisions are needed, particularly in infants and young children.

Formerly, the term *Juvenile laryngeal papillomatosis* designated this disorder, but the current preferred term is *Recurrent Respiratory Papillomatosis*, which more accurately describes the widespread extent of disease and its tendency for repeated regrowth, and encompasses the juvenile and adult disorder. Approximately one half the cases are designated *Juvenile Onset* (JO), wherein initial lesions appear from early infancy up through age 12 years. *Adult Onset* (AO) Recurrent Respiratory Papillomatosis includes those in whom initial diagnosis occurs as late as the seventh or eighth decade, although the peak incidence is during the third and fourth decades. Initial presentation of papilloma between ages 12 through 20 years is rare.

Juvenile Onset Recurrent Respiratory Papillomatosis (JO-RRP) presents with hoarseness, attributable to vocal fold lesions, which interferes with accurate apposition during phonation. The small size of the infant and pediatric larynx predisposes to upper airway obstruction in the face of rapid growth and regrowth of the papillomatous lesions, and repeated surgical excisions are often necessary.

Males and females are afflicted in equal numbers; JO-RRP has long been regarded as entering spontaneous remission at puberty, although there are insufficient data to support this view.

Adult Onset Recurrent Respiratory Papillomatosis (AO-RRP) is histologically indistinguishable from JO-RRP. Clinically, the lesions are more often solitary; upper airway obstruction occurs less frequently than in JO-RRP due, in part, to the larger adult laryngotracheal dimensions. In contrast to JO-RRP, there is distinct male predominance among AO-RRP patients.

I.   ETIOLOGY

The light microscopic appearance of respiratory papilloma is similar to that observed in genital and cutaneous warts. A viral agent had long been suspected to be the causative agent for this lesion, but it was not until the early 1980s when molecular biological techniques led to the identification of human papillomavirus (HPV) types 6 and 11 in respiratory papillomata and genital warts.[1-2] This coincidence reinforced the relevance of maternal condyloma to respiratory papilloma, as had been speculated by Hajek as early as 1956.[3] Infection by HPV-11 (also referred to as HPV-6c) has been correlated with the most severe respiratory tract disease.[4,5]

II.   EPIDEMIOLOGY

A history of maternal condyloma is elicited in 30–50% of patients with JO-RRP.[6] Transmission of HPV infection is presumed to occur during passage of the newborn through an HPV-infected birth canal. This view was supported in a review of records of 109 JO-RRP patients, where only a single instance of cesarean section was recorded.[7] A detailed questionnaire survey of subjects with Respiratory Papillomatosis indicated that the clinical triad of a first born delivered vaginally to a young mother with condyloma was present in complete or partial form in 72% of JO-RRP patients, and in 36% of AO-RRP subjects. In juvenile controls and adult controls, the triad was observed in 29 and 38%, respectively. The clinical observation that adopted children constitute a disproportionately large number of JO-RRP is in accord with the prediction of the foregoing triad. These conclusions have been supported by more recent survey results.[8]

The prevalence of genital condyloma in women of child-bearing age far exceeds the reported number of new cases of respiratory papillomatosis. The risk of transmission from a mother with HPV infection to her newborn has been estimated to be in the range of 1:80 to 1:1500.[7] A more precise definition of risk factors associating maternal condyloma with respiratory papillomatosis is needed before caesarean section can be advocated to eliminate or reduce the risk of respiratory papillomatosis in the newborn.

AO-RRP has been presumed to occur on basis of sexual contact, mainly oral-genital exposure. AO-RRP subjects reported more lifetime sex partners (P<0.01) and higher frequency of oral sex (P<0.05) than among adult controls.[9] Some cases of AO-RRP have a lifelong history of hoarseness, which suggests the alternative possibility that initial viral transmission and infection had occurred at childbirth, but that the infection remained dormant until diagnosis in adulthood.

Transmission of HPV infection through oral-pharyngeal secretions is rare. There is no documented case of RRP occurring among siblings, marital partners, or family members who are constantly exposed to secretions from papillomatosis patients.

III.   CLINICAL MANIFESTATIONS

A.   Childhood

Inasmuch as the vocal fold is usually the first and predominant site of a papilloma lesion, hoarseness is the cardinal symptom in JO-RRP as well as AO-RRP. In JO-RRP, it is not unusual for family members to remark that the voice was hoarse or "weak" from the time of initial vocal utterance. Upper airway obstructive symptoms of varying severity often worsen during intercurrent upper respiratory tract infection. In preschool children, whose airway dimensions are small, the initial presentation may occur as a sudden airway crisis, accompanying an otherwise routine respiratory tract infection.

Endoscopic excision of the papillomatous lesions restores a safe and adequate airway, but rapid regrowth of papilloma often necessitates repeated excisions. A small subset of patients requiring 100 or more endoscopic operations are not unusual.

B.   Adolescence

The numbers of multifocal lesions, the numbers of anatomic sites involved, and the severity of symptoms due to hoarseness or airway encroachment, diminish at puberty, when the adult-sized larynx is achieved. Coincident with this lessening in clinical severity, the intervals between operation lengthens. The symptoms diminish to the point that the patient ceases to consult the otolaryngologist although active papillomatous lesions may remain. An undetermined proportion of patients may achieve spontaneous remission from papilloma regrowth, but the belief that JO-RRP undergoes spontaneous remission at puberty is unwarranted; there are numerous adults with persistent papillomatosis, whose childhood onset is well-documented.

C.   Adulthood

Papillomatosis in adulthood is not usually severe. The growth rate is slower than that occurring in JO-RRP. In women, accelerated regrowth of papilloma occurs during pregnancy—particularly during the third trimester.

Respiratory papilloma have widespread anatomical distribution. The nasal vestibule, nasopharyngeal surface of the soft palate, the mid-zone on the laryngeal surface of the epiglottis, the immediate undersurface of the vestibular fold, the upper- and under-surface of the vocal folds, the carina, and bronchial spurs are sites at which the papilloma lesions commonly occur. It has been observed that these are sites at which the ciliated respiratory epithelium junctions with squamous epithelium. The squamo-ciliary junction has been suggested as a particular site of predilection for papilloma lesions.[10] Iatrogenic squamo-ciliary junctions are produced where the metaplastic squamous epithelium in the tracheostomal tract junctions with the ciliated epithelium of the trachea. Additional iatrogenic squamo-ciliary junctions are created when surgical instrumentation or manipulation causes injury to the ciliated epithelium; the resulting metaplastic squamous epithelium is surrounded by a squamo-ciliary junction, which appears to be susceptible to a new lesion site.

Intraoral papilloma have been identified on the soft palate, uvula, tonsils, and tonsillar fossae, as well as on the alveolar mucosa and tongue. Oral lesions have an association with a wider range of HPV types.[11,12] The larynx is the most commonly diseased site in the RRP.(Figure 1 A,B,D) The subglottic larynx and tracheo-bronchial tree are rarely, if ever, the site of disease in the absence of laryngeal lesions. The occurrence of tracheal, (Figure 1 C) bronchial, and ultimately pulmonary papillomatosis invariably occurs in a step-wise fashion. Papilloma are rarely observed at these sites at initial presentation. The history of tracheotomy is present in a high proportion of patients with tracheo-bronchial spread of papilloma and underscores the importance of atraumatic instrumentation and avoidance of tracheotomy.[13]

Pulmonary papilloma is manifested initially as an asymptomatic noncalcified nodule in the pulmonary parenchyma; slow enlargement and central cavitation occurs late. Pulmonary lesions may have widespread distribution, and the radiographic picture is alarming (Figure 2). The clinical course is slowly progressive; pulmonary dysfunction may be surprisingly mild, but respiratory failure and death ultimately occurs. Detailed histological examination of pulmonary lesions may disclose sites of squamous metaplasia, and unsuspected squamous cell carcinoma.[14,15]

The malignant transformation of respiratory papillomatous squamous carcinoma is unusual and occurs in less than 5% of cases. The malignancies most often occur in the larynx or lung. Neither the adult or childhood cases appear to be disproportionately at risk. Irradiation therapy and tobacco use may be factors that increase the risk for this malignant transformation.[16]

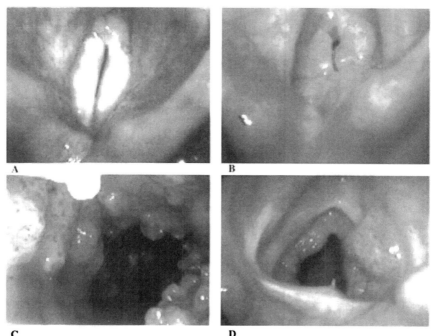

FIGURE 1 A. Adult onset (AO) - RRP. Lesions on vocal folds, bilaterally at the anterior commissure. B. Juvenile onset (JO) - RRP. Exophytic lesions on vocal folds, bilaterally. C. AO-RRP. Trachea distal to a tracheostomy. Multi-focal papilloma. Note typical vascular pattern on each lesion. D. JO-RRP. Papilloma lesions on the right vestibular (false) fold and a circumferential cuff of subglottic lesions in the subglottis. Vocal fold is lesion-free but has a synechial web.

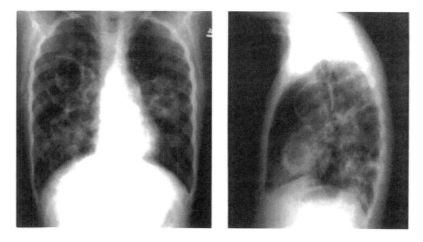

FIGURE 2 JO-RRP in a 10-year-old male. Typical pulmonary papillomatous lesions which progress from small peripheral lesions which enlarge, cavitate, undergo central liquefaction necrosis, and characteristically show air-fluid levels. The patient was *asymptomatic* at the time of this radiograph but ultimately succumbed to respiratory failure.

IV. PATHOLOGY

The typical clinical appearance of a papilloma is that of a multi-nodular growth. In one form, the solitary exophytic lesion may arise from a narrow or a broad-based stalk (Figure 3). Alternatively, the lesion may occur as a velvety, sheet-like abnormality mimicking an inflammatory reaction rather than a benign neoplasm. This type of lesion is most frequently encountered on the vocal fold, where the confluent growth spreads to involve the entire epithelium. In its most severe form, particularly in childhood, the tumor may resemble a cauliflower firmly impacting the laryngeal aperture with

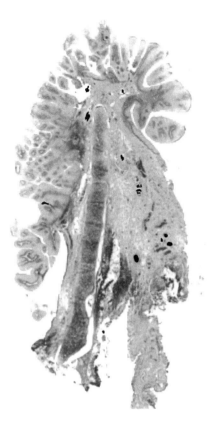

FIGURE 3   Epiglottis (midsagittal section) in AO-RRP. The papilloma arose at the squamo-ciliary junction on the laryngeal surface of the epiglottis. The pre-epiglottic space is on the right.

near-total obliteration of the airway. Many of these lesions may arise from a narrow stalk, and excision with maximal preservation of normal epithelium is possible.

The exophytic and sessile lesion types also occur in the tracheo-bronchial tree. The earliest lesions may appear as small, pale button-like lesions. A central vascular tuft is the tell-tale feature identifying these as early papilloma.

Histologically, the papilloma consists of stratified, squamous epithelium with a vascularized connective tissue stroma. There is increased proliferation of epithelial cells, with abnormal differentiation, including nuclear retention in the superficial layers. The occurrence of cells with hyperchromatic nuclei surrounded with large, clear transparent space identifies a koilocyte, a term assigned by Leo Koss and regarded as a histological feature implicating viral etiology.[17]

Steinberg et al. have observed the presence of HPV DNA in normal-appearing epithelium in RRP patients during complete clinical remission.[18] Although the disease-causing potential for this viral presence is not known, documentation of widespread distribution of HPV DNA may partially explain the basis for the relapse occurring after complete remission of variable duration and for susceptibility of traumatized epithelium to form new papilloma lesions.

V.   TREATMENT

The clinical course of RRP is predictably unpredictable. There is general consensus that AO-RRP is less severe than JO-RRP, whether based on disease extent, clinical symptomatology, or the frequency and total numbers of operations required for disease control. The cornerstone of papilloma management is endoscopic excision under magnified visualization. CO_2 laser excision of airway obstructive lesions have the twin objectives of disease elimination and maximal preservation of normal epithelium. Representative tissue specimens should be obtained at each operation to document epithelial maturation patterns. Total disease elimination is *not* the objective at every surgical intervention, particularly if there is risk of damage to normal laryngo-tracheal anatomy and function.

On the basis of our current understanding, two treatment interventions should be undertaken only after thorough consideration of the consequences and of alternative management options. Tracheotomy is a time honored technique of airway restoration, but retrospective reviews demonstrate that risk of distal spread of the papilloma into the lower respiratory tract, and at the site of tracheotomy, is increased. When the ideal treatment options (microsurgical instrumentation, laser) are not available, endotracheal intubation and transfer to a properly equipped facility is the preferred option. Irradiation therapy for treatment of histologically benign papillomatosis is generally not recommended, except in exceptional circumstances. There is no documentation as to short term efficacy, but a significant proportion of malignant transformations of histologically benign papillomatosis into invasive squamous cell carcinoma have occurred in irradiated patients.

The natural history of this disorder is that of invariable lesion recurrence and progressive compromise of the upper airway, which requires surgical intervention. Over the years, a variety of surgical techniques have been proposed and later abandoned. Endoscopic excision, preferably with magnification of the operating microscope and performed with utilization of precision microsurgical forceps and/or surgical laser, is the contemporary standard.

VI. NONSURGICAL TREATMENT ADJUVANTS

A wide variety of physical agents, caustic chemicals, antibiotics, antineoplastic agents, and, most recently, biological derivatives, have been used as adjuvants in papilloma management. Of these, the most durable has been podophyllum, which is applied topically at the time of conventional endoscopic excision.[19] Abramson and colleagues have utilized photodynamic therapy (PDT), in which a hematoporphyrin derivative (HPD) is activated by an argon pump laser.[20] The hematoporphyrin product is administered several days prior to the scheduled operation and accumulates in the papilloma where exposure to an argon laser activates HPD to release singlet oxygen and selectively destroys the papilloma. It is reported that latent HPV DNA, present in the clinically and morphologically normal laryngeal epithelium, is eliminated. This form of treatment is time consuming and, as presently administered, prohibits the patient from exposure to sunlight because of toxicity risk. PDT is a modality of promise and awaits a more suitable photo-active product and precise definition of subjects most benefited.

Of the anti-neoplastic agents, 5-fluorouracil (5-FU) has been on trial as an aerosolized application, although there were significant side effects.[21] Methotrexate, *cis*-platinum, and 5-FU, agents with proved efficacy in squamous cell carcinoma of the upper aerodigestive tract, have had limited testing in RRP and additional controlled trials are probably justified.

Vitamin A derivatives, isotretinoin and 13-*cis*-retinoic acid, have both produced a clinical response, the latter in a randomized clinical trial. The use of these agents was accompanied by significant mucocutaneous toxicity, consisting of dryness and cracking of the skin and mucosa, resulting in bleeding, and so it could not be continued on a chronic basis.[22]

Interferon in RRP has been a focus of interest beginning in the late 1970s. Initial positive response was reported from the Karolinska Institute, where seven patients all showed improvement while receiving blood bank leukocyte interferon.[23] A trial with a synthetic interferon-inducer (poly IC:LC) produced a clinical response, but with accompanying systemic toxicity.[24] Two major randomized clinical trials were conducted in the U.S. in the early 1980s. The first was a 12-month randomized crossover study utilizing lymphoblastoid interferon α-n1 interferon (Wellferon®, Glaxo Wellcome, Inc.).[25] Of the 66 patients who were entered into study, 57 patients had evaluable records. Of this number, 8 entered complete remission, based on a minimum of 4 months of papilloma-free state, verified by operative microendoscopic examination. Also, 19 additional patients achieved a partial remission, defined as a 50% reduction in an objective composite lesion score. Acute toxicity of interferon was similar to that seen during a viral infection and included fever, chills, nausea, vomiting, headache, and fatigue. The early toxic side effects are usually transient so that by week 4 of treatment, symptoms were rare.

Of the 66 patients originally entered into this study, 60 elected to continue, or restart interferon α-n1 on one of two dose schedules. Of 60 patients entered into this phase of study, 22 achieved complete remission with average duration of more than 550 days, and 25 achieved partial remission of median duration of over 400 days. 14 of 28 patients who had a tracheotomy at time of entry into study were safely decannulated.[26]

A study by Healy et al. using human leukocyte (blood bank) interferon involved 123 subjects randomized to receive interferon for one year or not to receive interferon.[27] The growth rate was significantly lower in the interferon group during the first six months, but there was return of growth despite continuation of the agent. It is relevant to cite that the maintenance dose of interferon was 2 mU/m^2 three times weekly (6 mU/m^2 per week), compared to 5 mU/m^2 3 times weekly (15 mU/m^2 per week) in the crossover study.[26] The crossover study as well as the two year study cited above both utilized an objective lesion scoring system,[28] rather than the notation of total numbers of operation during a fixed interval or the frequency of operations—an important basis for evaluating future therapeutic trials and for marking natural history.

In 1985, Zenner et al. reported 11 of 20 complete remissions and 7 of 20 partial remissions of subjects receiving α-2c interferon at a dose rate of 13.5 mU/m^2.[29] Of the nonsurgical adjuvants used to date, the interferon experience appears to be the most promising. Neither the precise interferon preparation nor the optimal dose rate and duration of administration are established.

Inasmuch as the natural history of RRP is uncertain, the following management plan has been adopted for patients with RRP.

1. Microendoscopic excision at fixed intervals tailored to the individual need (2, 4, or 6 monthly intervals) with documentation of anatomic extent, nature, and rate of papilloma regrowth to be evaluated at each operative endoscopy.
2. Consider an interferon adjuvant in patients with moderately severe disease or those with uncontrolled or progressive disease in spite of conventional microendoscopic excisions.
3. Interferon dose of administration of 5.0 mU/m^2 three times per week for a minimum of 12 months. Discontinue interferon if there is no response; continue for additional 6 to 12 months if there is partial response. Discontinue interferon after 6 to 12 months of sustained complete remission.

VII. CONCLUSION

RRP is an uncommon but important disorder with significant morbidity and mortality. Up to 5% of cases may undergo malignant transformation, and up to 5% of patients die as a consequence of this disease.

The natural history of this disease is not defined with precision. Among those entering spontaneous remission, the ultimate long term outcome is unknown. The significance of the HPV types, presently identified as the etiologic agent, needs further definition to ascertain the prognostic relevance, if any, of the specific types and sub-types. As with many disorders with recurrent growth, a staging system should be used in prospectively designed randomized clinical trials so that appropriate treatment for a given stage of disease can be competently evaluated and management guidelines can be established.

REFERENCES

1. Mounts, P., Shah, K. V., Kashima, H. K., Viral etiology of juvenile and adult onset squamous papilloma of the larynx, *Proc Nat Acad Sci U.S.A.* 79:5425, 1982.
2. Gissmann, L., Wolnik, L., Ikenberg, H., Koldovsky, U., Schnurck H. G., zur Hausen H., Human papillomavirus types 6 and 11 DNA sequences in genital and laryngeal papillomas and in some cervical cancers. *Proc Nat Acad Sci U.S.A.* 80:560, 1983.
3. Hajek, E. F., Contribution to the etiology of laryngeal papilloma in children, *J Laryngol Otol* 70:166, 1956.

4. Mounts, P., Kashima, H. K., Association of human papillomavirus subtype and clinical course in respiratory papillomatosis, *Laryngoscope* 94:28, 1984.

5. Hartley, C., Hamilton, J., Birzgalis, A. R., Farrington, W. T., Recurrent Respiratory Papillomatosis - the Manchester experience, *J Laryngol Otol* 108:226, 1994.

6. Quick, C. A., Kryzyzek, R. A., Watts, S. L., Foras, A. J., Relationship between condylomata and laryngeal papilloma, *Ann Otol Rhinol Laryngol* 89:467, 1980.

7. Shah, K., Kashima, H. K., Polk, B. F., Shah, F., Abbey, H., Abramson, A., Rarity of caesarean delivery in cases of juvenile onset respiratory papillomatosis, *Obstet Gynecol* 68:795, 1986.

8. Derkay, C. S., Task Force, Recurrent Respiratory Papillomas: Preliminary Report, December 1995.

9. Kashima, H. K., Shah, F., Lyles, A., Glackin, R., Muhammad, N., Turner, L., Van Zandt, S., Whitt, S., Shah, K., A comparison of risk factors in juvenile-onset and adult-onset recurrent respiratory papillomatosis, *Laryngoscope* 102:9, 1992.

10. Kashima, H., Mounts, P., Leventhal, B. G., Hruban, R., Sites of predilection in recurrent respiratory papillomatosis, *Ann Otol Rhinol Laryngol* 102:580, 1993.

11. Gassenmaier, A., Hornstein, O. P., Presence of human papillomaviruses in benign and precancerous oral leukoplakia and squamous cell carcinomas, *Dermatologica* 176:224, 1988.

12. Syrjänen, S. M., Syrjänen, K. J., Happonen R. P., Human papillomavirus DNA sequences in oral precancerous lesions and squamous cell carcinoma demonstrated by in situ hybridization, *J Oral Pathol* 17:273, 1988.

13. Weiss, M. D., Kashima, H. K., Tracheal involvement in laryngeal papillomatosis, *Laryngoscope* 93:45, 1983.

14. Solomon, D., Smith, R., Kashima, H. K., Malignant transformation in non-irradiated recurrent respiratory papillomatosis: report of a case and review of the literature, *Laryngoscope* 95:900, 1985.

15. Kashima, H. K., Wu, T.- C., Mounts, P., Heffner, D., Cachay A., Hyams, V., Carcinoma ex-papilloma: histologic and virologic studies in whole-organ sections of the larynx, *Laryngoscope* 98:619, 1988.

16. Walsh, T. E., Beamer, P. R., Epidermoid carcinoma of the larynx occurring in two children with papilloma of the larynx, *Laryngoscope* 60:1110, 1950.

17. Koss, L. G., Durfee, G. R., Unusual patterns of squamous epithelium of the uterine cervix: cytologic and pathologic study of koilocytic atypia, *Ann NY Acad Sci* 63:1245, 1956.

18. Steinberg, B., Topp, W. C., Schneider, P. S., Abramson, A. L., Laryngeal papillomavirus infection during clinical remission, *New Engl J Med* 388:1261, 1983.

19. Dedo, H., Jackler, R. K., Laryngeal papilloma: results of treatment with the CO_2 laser and podophyllum, *Ann Otol Rhinol Laryngol* 91:425, 1982.

20. Abramson, A. L., Shikowitz, M. J., Mullooly, V. M., Steinberg, B. M., Amella, C. A., Rothstein, H. R., Clinical effects of photodynamic therapy on recurrent laryngeal papillomas, *Arch Otol Head Neck Surg* 118:25, 1992.

21. Smith, H. G., Healy, G. B., Vaughn, C. W., Strong, M. S., Topical chemotherapy of recurrent respiratory papillomatosis, *Laryngoscope* 95:900, 1985.

22. Bell, R., Hong, W. K., Itri, L. M., McDonald, G., Strong, M. S., The use of cis-retinoic acid in recurrent respiratory papillomatosis of the larynx: a randomized pilot study, *Am J Otolaryngol* 9:161, 1988.

23. Haglund, S., Lundquist, P.-G., Cantell, K., Strander, H., Interferon therapy in juvenile laryngeal papillomatosis, *Arch Otolaryngol* 107:327, 1981.

24. Leventhal, B. G., Whisnant, J., Kashima, H. K., Levy, H., Biggers, W. P., Recurrent respiratory papillomatosis, *J Biol Response Mod* 4:525, 1985.

25. Leventhal, B. G., Kashima, H. K., Weck, P. W., et al. Randomized surgical adjuvant trial of interferon alpha-n1 in recurrent papillomatosis. *Arch Otol Head Neck Surg*, 114:1163, 1988.

26. Leventhal, B. G., Kashima, H. K., Mounts, P., Thurmond, L., Chapman, S., Buckley S., A long-term study of lymphoblastoid interferon in recurrent respiratory papillomatosis, *N Engl J Med* 325:613, 1991.

27. Healy, G. B., Gelber, R. D., Trowbridge, A. L., 1988 Treatment of recurrent respiratory papillomatosis with human leukocyte interferon: results of a multi-center randomized clinical trial, *N Engl J Med* 319:401, 1988.

28. Kashima, H. K., Leventhal, B., Mounts, P., and the Papilloma Study Group, Scoring system to assess severity in recurrent respiratory papillomatosis. Papillomaviruses: molecular and clinical aspects, in: *UCLA Symposia on Molecular and Cellular Biology, New Series*, vol 32, Howley, P. M., Broker, T. R., Eds., Alan R. Liss, New York, 1985, p. 125.

29. Zenner, H. P., Kley, W., Claros, P., et al, Recombinant interferon alpha-2c in laryngeal papillomatosis: preliminary results of a prospective multi-center trial, *Oncology* 42 (suppl 1): 15, 1985.

18

Cytology and Histology of HPV Infection of the Lower Genital Tract

Alexander Meisels

CONTENTS

This chapter describes the morphologic changes detectable by cell and tissue studies of the cervix, vagina, vulva, perineal, and perianal areas, as well as of the penis, in patients infected with the human papillomavirus (HPV). In order to put the morphological findings in HPV infections into proper perspective, it is necessary first to define the terminology to be used in this chapter.

I. TERMINOLOGY

The Papanicolaou classification has a significant historical value, but it is no longer a reliable system to communicate clinically significant information. It does not reflect current understanding of cervical neoplasia, does not provide for the diagnosis of noncancerous entities, and because of multiple idiosyncratic modifications over the years, no longer reflects diagnostic interpretations uniformly.

The subdivisions of intraepithelial lesions (mild, moderate, severe dysplasias, and carcinoma *in situ*) did not take into consideration the unity of the disease, which represents really a continuum from the morphologically mildest to the most severe changes. This reality was better served by the concept of Cervical Intraepithelial Neoplasia (CIN),[1-3] although the term "neoplasia" did not really seem to apply to a lesion which did not form a tumor.

Currently *The Bethesda System* seems to be the best possible solution. This was developed by a specially constituted Terminology Workshop convened at the National Cancer Institute, in

Bethesda, Maryland, U.S. (1988)[4] and subsequently reviewed and slightly modified at a reconvened workshop in April 1991.[5] The recommendations, which have been approved by many of the leading medical associations implicated in cytology,[6] can be summarized as follows as far as lesions related to HPV are concerned:

The 1991 Bethesda System

Adequacy of the specimen
    Satisfactory for evaluation
    Satisfactory for evaluation but limited by... (specify reason)
    Unsatisfactory for evaluation... (specify reason)
General categorization (optional)
    Within normal limits
    Benign cellular changes: See descriptive diagnosis
    Epithelial cell abnormality: See descriptive diagnosis
Descriptive diagnosis of Epithelial Cell Abnormalities

Squamous Cell

Atypical squamous cells of determined significance: Qualify[b]
Low grade squamous intraepithelial lesion encompassing: HPV[a] mild dysplasia/CIN 1
High grade squamous intraepithelial lesion encompassing: Moderate and severe dysplasia,
    CIS/CIN 2 and CIN 3
Squamous cell carcinoma

Glandular Cell

Atypical glandular cells of undetermined significance: Qualify[b]
Endocervical adenocarcinoma

---

[a] Cellular changes of human papillomavirus (HPV), previously termed koilocystosis, koilocytotic atypia, or condylomatous atypia, are included in the category of low grade intraepithelial lesion.

[b] Atypical squamous or glandular cells of undetermined significance should be further qualified as to whether a reactive or premalignant/malignant process is favored.

All these lesions have been shown to be HPV-related.[7] At this writing, HPV is considered a necessary factor in the development of cancer and its precursor lesions of the lower female genital tract and the penis.

This terminology is simple, easily reproducible from one laboratory to another, provides for uniformity of criteria, and can also be used for tissue diagnosis.

The importance of a common terminology can not be stressed enough. Without it, results from various centers cannot be compared. For the clinician, this simplification has long been obvious: management of patients with *all* intraepithelial lesions has become standardized: after colposcopy and confirmatory biopsy, when the lesion has been entirely visualized and there is no suspicion of early stromal invasion, all grades of intraepithelial lesions and HPV infections are locally destroyed.[8-10]

II.   CYTOMORPHOLOGY OF HPV INFECTION

HPV infection (low grade SIL) can confidently be diagnosed on the cell spread in the presence of the two pathognomonic signs of *koilocytosis* and/or *dyskeratosis* which we described for the first time in 1976.[11]

Koilocytes[12] (Figure 1) are intermediate or mature squamous cells characterized by a large perinuclear cavity. In the periphery, the cytoplasm is dense and often amphophilic. The limits of the cavity are sharply defined. Nuclei may be single, but are often double and sometimes multiple.

The chromatin may be well preserved in the early stages of infection but later it becomes smudged. The nuclear membrane is generally not apparent and there are no nucleoli nor inclusion bodies.

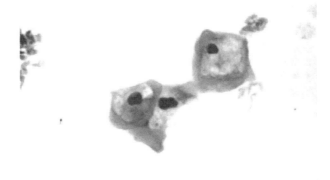

FIGURE 1   Three typical koilocytes on a cellular sample from a low grade squamous intraepithelial lesion (SIL). Note the perinuclear sharply delimited large cavity and the dense cytoplasm in the periphery.

Dyskeratocytes[13,14] (Figure 2) are mature squamous cells with a dense, refringent, orangeophilic cytoplasm, indicating the presence of keratin or its precursors. The nuclei are similar in appearance to those of the koilocytes. There is no perinuclear cavity. Dyskeratocytes are frequently shed in three-dimensional clusters, more rarely as discrete entities. Occasionally small dyskeratocytes or "miniature squamous cells" are seen. At times they are degenerated and included within vacuoles of other squamous cells. It is important to distinguish the dyskeratosis of HPV infection from the nonspecific and nonsignificant dyskeratotic change sometimes observed on "normal" cell samples. This consists of small "pearls" or a few layers of elongated cells in parallel arrangement. This nonspecific dyskeratosis is a simple surface phenomenon, unrelated to HPV infection.

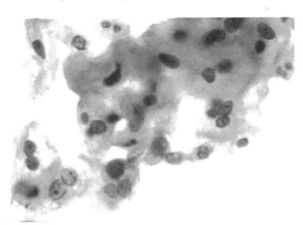

FIGURE 2   A group of characteristic dyskeratocytes from a cellular sample of low grade SIL. Note the overlapping of the mature orangeophilic squamous cells with degenerating chromatin and frequent binucleation.

Both the koilocyte and the characteristic dyskeratosis are diagnostic for HPV infection. If dyskeratosis is ignored, then many cases of HPV infection will escape cytologic detection.

Our laboratory currently screens about 150,000 gynecological samples per year. The yield of HPV infections is about 1.5%. In Germany, the prevalence of HPV infection in an asymptomatic population of about 20,000 women was found to be about 10% using DNA hybridization techniques.[15] Other studies have given similar results.[16,17] However about 80% of patients presenting visible lesions of the cervix were shown to harbor HPV.[18] When cell samples previously diagnosed as "normal" from women who tested positive for HPV were later reviewed, minute cell changes were found: mostly these consisted of binucleation, amphophilia, and "incomplete koilocytosis." Sometimes small intermediate or parabasal cells with amphophilic cytoplasm and degenerating chromatin may be observed.[19] These features by themselves are not however sufficient to justify the diagnosis of HPV infection. Overdiagnosis has as many drawbacks as underdiagnosis, particularly when dealing with a sexually transmitted disease.

III.   HISTOMORPHOLOGY OF HPV INFECTION

Four distinct but related forms of "pure" HPV infection have been identified:[13]

1. The flat condyloma (condyloma planum) (Figure 3) which we described in 1977,[13] displays koilocytes in the middle and upper layers of the epithelium. Often there are blood vessels surrounded by scanty stroma reaching upwards towards the surface. There may be dyskeratosis, keratinization, or even epidermization.
2. The "spiked" condyloma (Figure 4) is a variant of the flat lesion, characterized by small projections on the surface of the epithelium. These "spikes" contain a blood vessel surrounded by scarce stroma.
3. The papillary or exophytic form (Figure 5) is rare on the cervix, but may be found on the vulva and the penis. There is marked papillomatosis, acanthosis, and often keratinization of the superficial layers. The intermediate layers may contain koilocytes.
4. The "inverted" condyloma (Figure 6) is rare. It may have a flat, spiked, or papillary surface and grows inward, replacing the columnar epithelium of the endocervical crypts.

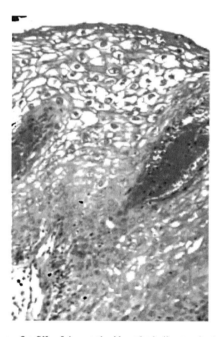

FIGURE 3   Histologic section from a flat SIL of the cervix. Note the koilocytes in the middle and superficial layers, and the blood vessels surging towards the surface of the epithelium.

By far, the flat and "spiked" lesions are the more frequently seen. Mitotic figures vary in frequency. Even in "pure" HPV infection, some mitoses may be atypical. The lesions can be polyploid or aneuploid.[20]

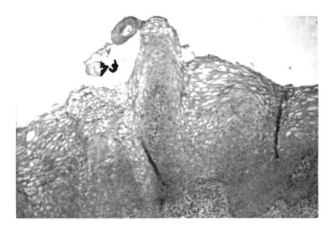

FIGURE 4 This is an example of a "spiked" low grade SIL. The spike contains a blood vessel surrounded by scant stroma.

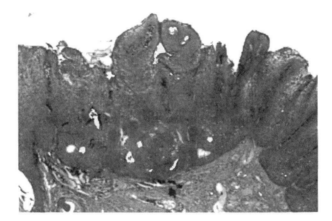

FIGURE 5 The exophytic form of low grade SIL shows papillary fronds jutting out from the surface of the cervix.

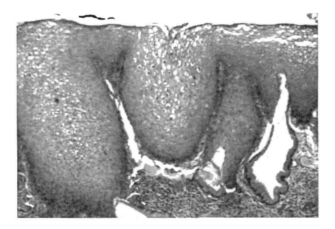

FIGURE 6 In the endophytic type of low grade SIL the abnormal squamous epithelium grows downward and replaces the columnar epithelium of the endocervical clefts and spaces.

A.   HPV and Intraepithelial Lesions

As can be expected, morphological signs of HPV infection are frequently associated with the more advanced intraepithelial lesions. There are three distinct types of association:[21]

1. The mixed association: In this lesion, changes characteristic of both HPV infection and of a more advanced lesion coexist within the same area, intimately intermixed (Figures 7 and 8). The cellular sample will contain mostly dyskeratotic cells with enlarged, darkly stained nuclei. The cellular pattern may be confused with that of an invasive keratinizing squamous carcinoma, and thus may cause "false positive" reports. We previously had called this association the "atypical condyloma."[22]
2. The horizontal association: Areas of intraepithelial lesions alternate with areas of HPV infection, either adjacent to each other (Figure 9) or at a distance. Cytological preparations will not only contain cells typical for HPV infection, but also cells with more advanced changes corresponding to the intraepithelial lesion. This is a common finding, particularly well demonstrated on cone biopsies.
3. The vertical association: There is an intraepithelial lesion in which the upper layers display changes typical of HPV infection while the deeper layers demonstrate changes characteristic for a high grade SIL (Figure 10). The cell spread in such a case may only display the cells characteristic of an HPV infection, scraped from the surface, while the more advanced deeper lesion escapes detection. It is important to realize that this particular type of association may cause "false negative" reports.

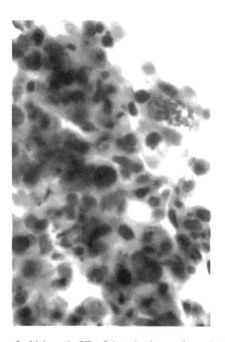

FIGURE 7   Cytologic presentation of a high grade SIL of the mixed type (formerly called "atypical condyloma"). This is a dense cluster of orangeophilic cells containing large, irregular, darkly stained nuclei. This cell pattern may be difficult to differentiate from an invasive keratinizing squamous carcinoma.

B.   The Intraepithelial Lesions

This term replaces cervical intraepithelial neoplasia, dysplasia, and carcinoma *in situ*. Cellular samples contain small intermediate or, more frequently, parabasal cells containing enlarged, irregular, hyperchromatic nuclei. The N/C ratio is increased. The cytoplasm is cyanophilic and dense. The chromatin is reticular or granular, with prominent chromatin bands and chromocenters. Small nucleoli are sometimes observed. The nuclear membrane is seen as a band of varying thickness, due to chromatin deposits on its inner aspect.

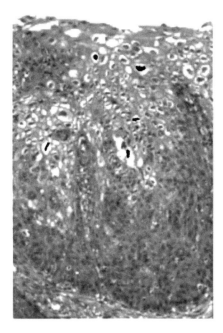

FIGURE 8 Histologic presentation of a high grade SIL of the mixed type. The middle and superficial layers contain many koilocytes with large, irregular hyperchromatic nuclei. The deeper layers also contain mostly abnormal cells.

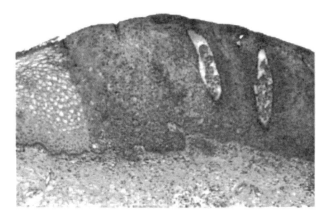

FIGURE 9 Histologic presentation of a high grade SIL of the horizontal type. On the left side, the squamous epithelium contains many koilocytes. The rest of the epithelium shows the pattern of a high grade SIL.

The cells typically occur isolated or in small groups, sometimes in chain-like arrangements. They are immature metaplastic cells with considerable nuclear atypia.

Biopsies of these lesions reveal an immature squamous epithelium in which there is little differentiation from the deep layers towards the surface. The uppermost layers may be flattened and dyskeratotic. N/C ratios are high and the nuclei are hyperchromatic with prominent chromatin detail. The overall pattern is rather homogenous. Mitoses are commonly seen and may be atypical.

1. Microinvasive Carcinoma

This is most definitely a histologic diagnosis. Although the cytologic pattern may be suggestive of early invasion, i.e., there are small nucleoli and the cells tend to aggregate in sheets, it is not diagnostic. When microinvasion is suspected, a cone biopsy becomes necessary to confirm (or infirm) the diagnosis.

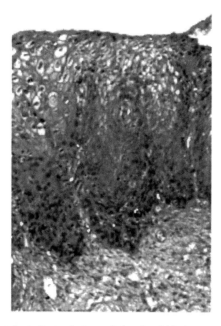

FIGURE 10 This histologic section shows the vertical association, in which the more superficial layers of the epithelium show the pattern of a low grade SIL, but the deeper layers indicate the presence of a high grade SIL.

2.   Invasive Squamous Cell Carcinoma

There are three main types:

1. Keratinizing squamous carcinoma is the one most readily diagnosed by cytology. The cellular sample contains discrete, large, irregularly shaped squamous cells which often display an abundant orangeophilic or eosinophilic cytoplasm, and an irregularly enlarged, darkly stained or pyknotic nucleus. Sometimes keratinized "pearl" formation can be seen in which concentrically arranged cells show the cytoplasmic and nuclear characteristics described above.
2. The large cell squamous carcinoma is recognized by the presence of sheets of cells slightly larger than normal parabasal cells, but with a considerably increased N/C ratio: the nucleus occupies 2/3 or more of the cell surface, as compared to 1/3 or less in normal parabasal cells. The cytoplasm is cyanophilic and the nucleus is irregularly shaped, with grossly granular or reticular chromatin, prominent chromocenters, margination of chromatin, and small to medium sized nucleoli. There is often considerable overlapping of the cells in the sheets. If these criteria are taken into consideration, differential diagnoses with cells from repair/regeneration can easily be done in most cases. In repair, there is no overlapping of the cells in the sheets, the nuclei are regular, with a fine chromatin pattern and there usually are macronucleoli; the N/C ratio is within normal limits.
3. Small Cell Squamous Carcinoma is relatively rare. It sheds cells in the size-range of neutrophils. The cytoplasm is scarce and cyanophilic, the nucleus is hyperchromatic and somewhat irregular and may contain a small nucleolus. When present in groups, there may be some molding of the nuclei, which helps differentiating these malignant cells from lymphocytes, not commonly found on routine gynecological samples.

In general cells from an invasive squamous carcinoma show more polymorphism than cells from intraepithelial lesions, with the exception of the third type of association (high grade SIL with HPV) which can easily be confused with keratinizing squamous cell carcinoma. When the tumor has grown to a large size, areas of necrosis appear, and the cell spreads show a "dirty" background, called *tumor diathesis*.

IV.   ELECTRON MICROSCOPY OF CELLS INFECTED BY HPV

Electron microscopy can be used on tissue obtained by colposcopically directed biopsies, or on cells reprocessed from Papanicolaou stained cell spreads.[23] The virions are localized within the nuclei of koilocytes and dyskeratocytes. They are round bodies measuring about 55 nm in diameter (much smaller than Herpesvirus). HPV particles may fill all interstices between the chromatin network, or occur isolated and in small numbers. About half of the samples of HPV infections contain virions visible by EM (Figure 11). With this technique, as with the immuno-peroxidase technique, only complete virions (including the protein coat) can be visualized. Only mature squamous cells are permissive, but only about one half of even the clinically obvious "genital warts" or condylomata acuminata, contain permissive cells. In nonpermissive cells, the viral DNA is present in the nucleus as either a free circular strand, called episome (HPV-6 and HPV-11), or integrated into the host DNA (HPV-16 and HPV-18), and cannot be demonstrated by electron microscopy. The fact that replication occurs only in mature squamous cells may also explain why growing HPV *in vitro* has proven to be so difficult. Present day research is based mostly on DNA obtained by cloning HPV DNA or fragments thereof in plasmids. This has been used to determine the sequence of bases in the viral DNA and to study the DNA structure in great detail. With the polymerase chain reaction amplification technique, large amounts of viral DNA have become available for further research.

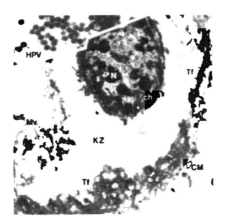

FIGURE 11 Electron microscopy of a koilocyte. The nucleus (N) is surrounded by an empty appearing cavity (KZ) and contains a large number of viral corpuscles (HPV in the inset in the upper right corner). Dense tonofilaments (Tf) surround the koilocytotic cavity.

V.   CONCLUSION

Morphologic cell and tissue studies enable us to diagnose lesions produced by HPV with a high degree of specificity. However, only a small percentage of patients who harbor the virus do develop lesions. The others escape detection by morphologic studies and can only be found utilizing molecular hybridization or amplification techniques. At the present time, treatment is available only for the eradication of lesions. There is no treatment as yet which will effectively destroy the virus in its latent form. It is therefore more important to detect minute lesions, which may only be visible under amplification (colposcopy) and can be successfully treated, than to diagnose HPV infection per se.

REFERENCES

1. Richart, R. M., Natural history of cervical intraepithelial neoplasia, *Clin. Obstet. Gynecol.*, 10, 748, 1967.

2. Richart, R. M. and Barron, B. A., A follow-up study of patients with cervical dysplasia, *Am. J. Obstet. Gynecol.*, 105, 386, 1969.

3. Richart, R. M., A modified terminology for cervical intraepithelial neoplasia, *Obstet. Gynecol.*, 75, 131, 1990.

4. National Cancer Institute Workshop, the 1988 Bethesda System for Reporting Cervical/Vaginal Cytologic Diagnoses, *J. Am. Med. Assoc.*, 262, 31, 1989.

5. The 1991 Bethesda Workshop Report, The Revised Bethesda System for Reporting Cervical/Vaginal Cytologic Diagnoses, *Acta Cytol.*, 36, 273, 1992.

6. Association of Directors of Anatomic and Surgical Pathology, Standardization of the Surgical Pathology Report, *Am. J. Surg. Pathol.*, 16, 84, 1992.

7. Schiffman, M. H., Recent progress in defining the epidemiology of human papillomavirus infection and cervical neoplasia, *J. Natl. Cancer Inst.*, 84, 394, 1992.

8. Ferenczy, A., Hilgarth, M., Jenny, J., Koss, L. G., Masubuchi, K., Noda, K., Richart, R. M., Wentz, W. B., and Wied, G. L., Editorial: The place of colposcopy and related systsems in gynecologic practice and research, *J. Reprod. Med.*, 33, 737, 1988.

9. Goppinger, A., Ikenberg, H., Birmelin, G., Hilgarth, M., Pfleiderer, A., and Hillemanns, H. G., [CO_2 laser therapy and typing of human papilloma virus in follow-up studies of cervix intraepithelial neoplasms], *Geburtshilfe. Frauenheilkd.*, 48, 343, 1988.

10. Schwartz, D. B., Greenberg, M. D., Daoud, Y., and Reid, R., Genital condylomas in pregnancy: Use of trichloroacetic acid and laser therapy, *Am. J. Obstet. Gynecol.*, 158, 1407, 1988.

11. Meisels, A. and Fortin, R., Condylomatous lesions of the cervix and vagina. I. Cytologic patterns, *Acta Cytol.*, 20, 505, 1976.

12. Koss, L. G. and Durfee, G. R., Unusual patterns of squamous epithelium of the uterine cervix: cytologic and pathologic study of koilocytotic atypia, *Ann. N.Y. Acad. Sci.*, 63, 1245, 1956.

13. Meisels, A., Fortin, R., and Roy, M., Condylomatous lesions of the cervix. II. Cytologic, colposcopic and histopathologic study, *Acta Cytol.*, 21, 379, 1977.

14. Purola, E. and Savia, E., Cytology of gynecologic condyloma acuminatum, *Acta Cytol.*, 21, 26, 1977.

15. de Villiers, E. M., Wagner, D., Schneider, A., Wesch, H., Miklaw, H., Wahrendorf, J., Papendick, U., and zur Hausen, H., Human papillomavirus infections in women with and without abnormal cervical cytology, *Lancet II*, 703, 1987.

16. Lorincz, A. T., Temple, G. F., Patterson, J. A., Jenson, A. B., Kurman, R. J., and Lancaster, W. D., Correlation of cellular atypia and human papillomavirus deoxyribonucleic acid sequences in exfoliated cells of the uterine cervix, *Obstet. Gynecol.*, 68, 508, 1986.

17. Toon, P. G., Arrand, J. R., Wilson, L. P., and Sharp, D. S., Human papillomavirus infection of the uterine cervix of women without cytological signs of neoplasia, *Br. Med. J.*, 293, 1261, 1986.

18. Lorincz, A. T., Reid, R., Jenson, A. B., Greenberg, M. D., Lancaster, W., and Kurman, R. J., Human papillomavirus infection of the cervix: relative risk associations of 15 common anogenital types, *Obstet. Gynecol.*, 79, 328, 1992.

19. Schneider, A., Meinhardt, G., de Villiers, E. M., and Gissman, L., Sensitivity of the cytologic diagnosis of cervical condyloma in comparison with HPV-DNA hybridization studies, *Diagn. Cytopath.*, 3, 250, 1987.

20. Reid, R., Fu, Y. S., Herschman, B. R., Crum, C. P., Braun, L., Shah, K. V., Agronow, S. J., and Stanhope, C. R., Genital warts and cervical cancer. VI. The relationship between aneuploid and polyploid cervical lesions, *Am. J. Obstet. Gynecol.*, 150, 189, 1984.

21. Meisels, A. and Morin, C., *Cytopathology of the Uterine Cervix*, Chicago, IL, ASCP Press, 1991.

22. Meisels, A., Roy, M., Fortier, M., Morin, C., Casas-Cordero, M., Shah, K. V., and Turgeon, H., Human papillomavirus infection of the cervix: The atypical condyloma, *Acta Cytol.*, 25, 7, 1981.

23. Casas-Cordero, M., Morin, C., Roy, M., Fortier, M., and Meisels, A., Origin of the koilocyte in condylomata of the human cervix. Ultrastructural study, *Acta Cytol.*, 25, 383, 1981.

19

Detection of Genital Human Papillomavirus Infections and Possible Clinical Implications

J. M. M. Walboomers, M. V. Jacobs, J. W. van Oostveen,
A. J. C. van den Brule, P. J. F. Snijders, and C. J. L. M. Meijer

CONTENTS

I.   INTRODUCTION

This chapter will summarize some important aspects of the relationship between HPV infection and cancer of the uterine cervix[1-4] with an emphasis on elucidating the potential role of HPV DNA detection as an approach to optimizing treatment of patients with premalignant cervical lesions and cytology screening procedures. The involvement of an infectious agent in this disease was already suggested by

0-8493-7356-5/97/$0.00+$.50
© 1997 by CRC Press, Inc.

epidemiological studies identifying sexual activity at a young age and promiscuity as risk factors for cervical cancer.[5,6]

The link to human papillomavirus was originally made by Zur Hausen in 1976 who pointed out that genital warts (condylomata accuminata) show an identical epidemiological pattern as cervical cancer and postulated that a papillomavirus could also be involved in the development of cervical cancer.[7] In the meantime, cytologists frequently reported the presence of HPV related cellular abnormalities, called koilocytes, in cytological smears of women with mainly mild morphological changes while condylomas could not be detected.[8] The first genital HPVs that were isolated from benign (condylomata) and malignant cervical lesions (cervical carcinoma) were HPV 6 and HPV 16 and 18 and were called low risk or nononcogenic and high risk or oncogenic HPVs, respectively. During the last years about 30 different genital HPVs with different oncogenic potential have been isolated (Table 1), 15 of which have been isolated from high grade cervical dysplasia or carcinomas.[9]

TABLE 1   Human Papillomaviruses Genotypes from Cutaneous and Mucosal Lesions

HPV genotypes	Lesions
Cutaneous	
1,2,3,4,5,7,8,9,10,12,14,15, 17,19,20,21,22,23,24,25,26, 27,28,29,36,37,38,41,46,47, 48,49,50,60,63,65	Cutaneous warts, flat warts, plantar warts, butchers' warts. Cutaneous plaques and papillomas in patients with EV. Skin carcinomas in renal allografts and EV patients.
Mucosal HPV	
6,11,13,16,18,30,31,32,33,34, 35,39,40,42,43,44,45,51,52, 53,54,55,56,57,58,59,61,62, 64,66,67,68	Cervical epithelial neoplasia (CIN) vulvar, penile and perianal intraepithelial neoplasias. Laryngeal papilloma. Cervical cancer, vulvar cancer, penile cancer, perianal and anal cancer. Condyloma acuminatum. Verrucous carcinoma of vulva and penis, Buschke-Löwenstein tumors.

Note: HPV 16,18,31,33,35,39,45,51,52,56,58,59,61,66,68 have been isolated or associated with cervical carcinoma

Modified from de Villiers, 1989.

Due to differences in oncogenic potential, detection of the different HPV types seems to be important.

In general, viral infections can be diagnosed by viral culture, serology (antibody response) and detection of viral particles, antigen, or nucleic acids. Since HPV cannot be cultured *in vitro*, HPV detection by nucleic acid hybridization is the best diagnostic tool at this moment. All available techniques for detection of HPV specific nucleic acids share the basic principle of hybridization: pairing of complementary single stranded DNA (RNA) resulting in the formation of double stranded hybrids. Consequently, HPV DNA present in a sample can be detected on the basis of its ability to hybridize with a probe or oligonucleotide primers. Purified HPV DNA or HPV type specific oligonucleotides provided with a (non) radioactive label may serve as probe. Labeled hybrids can be visualized either by autoradiography (exposure to an X-ray sensitive film) or by immunohistochemical staining procedures. The efficiency of hybridization is dependent on the extent of homology in nucleotide sequences between probe and target DNA, and reaction conditions including ionic strength of hybridization solution and temperature. By varying these conditions, it is possible to change the stringency of hybridization. High stringent hybridization allows only completely homologous DNAs to form hybrids, while under low-stringent conditions heterologous DNA also hybridizes. Since the detection of clinically relevant genital HPV associated lesions are discussed in other chapters in this book and HPV nucleic acid detection has been revolutionized during the last years, in the following sections we will focus on:

1. An evaluation and critical review of the most frequently used molecular biological methods. In particular, the polymerase chain reaction (PCR) method will be emphasized.[10,11] Also, future developments will be discussed.
2. HPV prevalence data in normal, premalignant, and malignant cervical epithelium.
3. The (potential) clinical value of HPV detection.

II.　MOLECULAR BIOLOGICAL METHODS FOR HPV DETECTION

In general, two types of HPV DNA detection methods are frequently applied, i.e., the direct detection of HPV DNA and the detection of HPV DNA following amplification by the polymerase chain reaction. The direct HPV DNA detection methods include genomic Southern blot hybridization, filter *in situ* hybridization, dot blot hybridization, and *in situ* hybridization.

A.　Direct HPV DNA Detection Methods without Amplification

1.　Southern Blot Analysis (SB)

Purified target DNA is electrophoretically separated on the basis of size of DNA fragments after digestion with specific restriction enzymes. Subsequently, the DNA is blotted onto a DNA binding filter and hybridized with HPV type specific probes. Since each HPV type has a specific restriction enzyme digestion pattern, the HPV hybridization signals can be interpreted by comparison to standard hybridization patterns of HPV prototypes. Both the probe used and the resulting hybridization pattern determine the outcome of the typing (Figure 1). By using low(er) stringent hybridization conditions, heterologous DNA fragments can also be detected, eventually allowing the identification of still undefined HPV types (HPV-X).

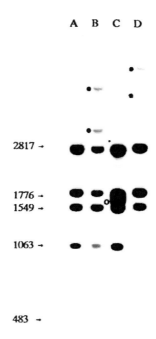

FIGURE 1　Southern blot analysis of HPV 16 postive cervical carcinoma. Normal Pstl pattern of HPV 16 DNA resulting in 2818, 1776, 1549, 1063, and 1483 base pair fragments is visible in all lanes. In lanes B and D additional bands (dotted circles) are visible indicating integration of the HPV 16 genome into chromosomal DNA. In lane C DNA fragment indicated by open circle appeared to be part of URR showing genome rearrangement.

SB is considered as the "golden standard" for HPV detection and typing. Although the technique is laborious and requires relatively large amounts of DNA (10 µg in case of low HPV copy numbers per cell), which is relevant for small tissue samples like biopsies, SB is sensitive (about 1 pg HPV DNA in 10 µg genomic DNA can be detected) and specific. The results of a comparative study in different laboratories with extensive experience using SB analysis for HPV detection and typing was recently described. Interlaboratory HPV detection agreements ranged from 66 to 97% while interlaboratory HPV typing agreement ranged from 77 to 96%. When differences regarding HPV presence and typing were combined, the results obtained by the different laboratories were in agreement for only 45% of the samples.[12] This raises the question about reliability of this technique as the golden standard and indicates that efforts in standardization are required.

The Southern blot technique can also provide information about the physical state of HPV in the sample investigated. Southern blot analysis can distinguish between episomal and integrated viral DNA as shown in Figure 1, A, C and B, and D respectively. This might be of importance for the transition of premalignant lesions to cervical cancer since episomal DNA is mainly found in benign lesions whereas integrated HPV DNA is mainly detected in cervical cancer. Also, large rearrangements in the HPV genome can be detected by Southern blot analysis (Figure 1C).

2.   Dot Blot Analysis/ViraPap/Hybrid Capture

In contrast to SB, in this method the DNA is fixed directly onto the membrane without electrophoretical separation. The method requires lower amounts of DNA (0.3–1.0 µg) and sensitivities of about 0.5–1 pg HPV DNA in 1 µg genomic DNA can be reached. There are two variants: one uses DNA probes (dot blot), the other uses RNA probes (ViraPap).

Especially the DNA/DNA dot blot procedure can only be performed reliably under high stringency conditions (and even then it is difficult to differentiate between related HPV types). The most commonly used dot blot assay is the ViraPap®/ViraType® system. The assay system makes use of RNA probes to detect HPV DNA presence (ViraPap®) and type (ViraType®) for a limited number of HPV types: 6, 11, 16, 18, 31, 33, and 35. The system can only be appropriately compared with other techniques for the seven types included in the test. Initially the system was based on radioactive probes. Recently the dot blot procedure was replaced by a liquid hybridization procedure. In this approach, HPV DNA is hybridized with HPV RNA probes in solution. The DNA/RNA complexes are captured in a tube coated with antibodies directed against DNA/RNA hybrids. These hybrids are visualized using colorimetric or chemoluminescence based detection methods. The whole procedure is called Hybrid Capture Assay (HCA; Digene, MD, U.S.) and has possibilities for quantification. In the U.S., this test is approved by the Food and Drug Administration.

3.   Filter *In Situ* Hybridization (FISH)

Cervical scrapes, without DNA extraction, are spotted directly onto a membrane followed by denaturation of the DNA.[13] HPV positive samples can be identified by hybridization with HPV specific probes. The sensitivity of the FISH was estimated to be at best half the sensitivity of the Southern blot technique. FISH is hampered by high backgroud signals and has recently recognized as inadequate for HPV epidemiological studies.

4.   *In Situ* Hybridization (ISH)

In case of the *in situ* hybridization technique, the morphology of the specimen is preserved.[14] This permits localization of HPV within the tissue and the infected cell. Pretreatment of tissue consisting of partial digestion of cellular and nuclear proteins is necessary for target DNA to become attainable for the probe. The DNA *in situ* hybridization technique has a sensitivity of 20–50 HPV genomes per cell,[15] when full-length genomic nonradioactively labeled probes are used. The requirement of biopsies makes this method unsuitable for mass screening but the possibility of determining the localization of the viral genome and analyzing its expression pattern (RNA *in situ* hybridization) is of great value in research on the pathogenesis of cervical cancer.[16] Analysis of HPV 16 DNA containing squamous and adenocarcinomas (Figure 2) showed that HPV 16 was exclusively present in neoplastic cells and not in the stroma. The definition of subclinical and latent HPV infection is still incomplete and requires clarification by highly sensitive HPV detection systems that preserve the morphology of the tissue. Previously, application of *in situ* hybridization to morphologically normal epithelium suspected to be latently infected showed no viral DNA.[17] The recently improved *in situ* PCR method,[18] which combines PCR amplification (see next section) and *in situ* hybridization might be of value to elucidate the phenomenon of subclinical or latent HPV infection.

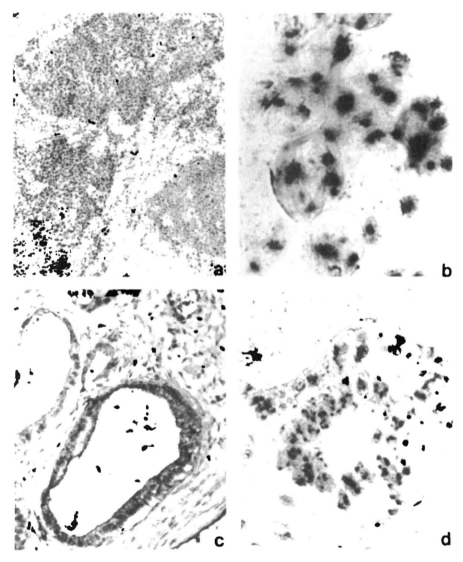

FIGURE 2   DNA *in situ* hybridization (DISH) of carcinoma of the cervix uterine: a) Low power photomicrograph of H+E stained section of squamous cell carcinoma; b) High magnification detail after DISH using standard procedures with biotinylated HPV 16 DNA probe; c) Low power photomicrograph of an H+E section of an adenocarcinoma; d) High mignification detail after DISH with HPV 16 DNA probe.

B.   HPV DNA Detection after Amplification by the Polymerase Chain Reaction

1.   Principle of PCR; Some Advantages and Disadvantages

HPV detection and typing can be strongly improved by the introduction of the polymerase chain reaction.[19,20] This method enables an *in vitro* amplification of a piece of HPV target DNA. The technique is based on specific hybridization of small pieces of complementary single stranded DNA called oligonucleotide primers, to the opposite strands of HPV DNA after heat denaturation. DNA synthesis is performed by primer extension of the free 3′ OH ends executed by a thermostabile DNA polymerase. The process includes cycles consisting of three steps of different temperature: (1) denaturation of HPV DNA (94°C); (2) primer annealing (37–70°C) and (3) primer elongation (72°C).

Usually 30–40 cycles of amplification are performed, achieving an exponential increase in the amount of HPV DNA spanned by both primers. Theoretically a millionfold increase of the amplified target DNA can be obtained after performance of 20 PCR cycles (2^{20} = 1.048576). Under optimal conditions, the PCR is able to detect one HPV DNA molecule. The amplified DNA can be detected after gel electrophoresis.

However, additional hybridization by dot, or Southern blotting using target DNA specific probes originating from the internal part of the amplified DNA, is necessary to confirm specificity. Sensitivity is at least ten times increased by this hybridization step. PCR products can also be analyzed by digestion with restriction enzymes. Some primer sets for HPV detection generate amplification products that contain unique restriction enzyme digestion patterns which can be used for HPV typing. Also the identification of novel HPV types is possible in this manner. Besides its high sensitivity and specificity, the requirement of relatively low amounts of target DNA is an important advantage of this technique. However, a prerequisite for the use of PCR in large scale HPV screening programs is the omission of the laborious DNA extraction procedure, minimizing sample-to-sample contamination. It appeared that non ionic detergent/proteinase K digestion and even freezing, thawing, and boiling of cell suspension is sufficient for succesful amplification of HPV target sequences.[21] Ironically, the major drawback of the PCR is its sensitivity, since clinical or laboratory generated contamination by environmental DNA, cloned plasmids, and PCR products may produce false positive results. Several early reports that used PCR based methods to detect HPV DNA were unreliable because of such problems and some have since been retracted.[22] "Anticontamination" or cloning site flanking primers rule out the detection of false positives from molecularly cloned HPVs (pHPV). The principle of anticontamination primers have been described by Van den Brule et al.[23]

Although these primers do not prevent contamination, they provide an extra safety barrier. Thus, application of these primers makes it possible to detect HPVs specifically in a clinical sample even in the presence of pHPVs. However, amplification products give rise to the most serious source of contamination and therefore it is advised to carry out the different PCR steps, i.e., sample preparation, electrophoresis of PCR products, and preparation of PCR solutions in three spatially separated rooms. This requires a strong laboratory discipline. An alternative manner to prevent carry over of amplification products has recently been developed, which involves the incorporation of deoxyuridine triphosphate (dUTP) and the enzyme uracil N glycosylase (UNG). Treatment of the PCR product by UNG at alkaline pH and elevated temperature destroys uracil-containing PCR products.[24] With these precautions, HPV-PCR directly performed on crude extracts are reliable to perform and can be routinely used.

2.   HPV Type Specific PCR

Since sequence data for primer selection are necessary for PCR and these data were initially only available for HPV 6, 11, 16, 18, 31, and 33, single and multiplex HPV PCRs have been developed.

In the latter case, a mixture of HPV type specific primer pairs are used in one PCR reaction, and primer pairs have been selected in such a manner that for the several HPV types different amplified fragment sizes are generated. It is easy to design HPV type specific primers by computer assisted matrix analysis (Microgenie, Gen Bank, Release # 154) for different parts of the genome. Also a ß-globine PCR can be included as an internal DNA quality control.[19] In Figure 3, the results of HPV type specific PCR and multiplex PCR for HPV 6, 11, 16, 18, 31, and 33 (lane 8) applied on cervical scrapes is shown.

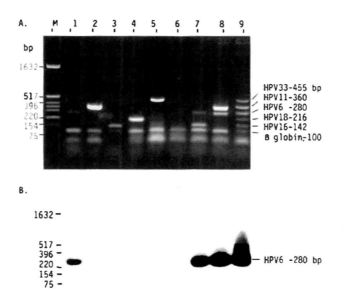

FIGURE 3 Detection of HPV genotypes. Crude cervical scrapes were analysed using the PCR with a mixture of anticontamination primer sets specific for different HPV types. Lanes 1–5, 7, and 8 contained samples from HPV-positive patients. Lane 6 contained a sample from an HPV-negative patient. In the last lane, a mixture of the DNAs of patients 1–5 is shown. The ß-globin amplification was used as an internal control. A) PCR products are shown after electrophoresis on 2% agarose gel and ethidium bromide staining; B) Southern blot analysis with an HPV 6 specific oligonucleotide probe. M:pBR322xHinfI.

In these samples, the amplified bands corresponding with the different types can be seen already after ethidium bromide staining (Figure 3A). Figure 3B shows the results after Southern blot analysis using an HPV 6 specific probe (30 oligonucleotides) originating from the internal part of the amplied product. The main advantage of multiplex PCR is that the number of PCRs can be reduced; however, multiplex PCR is hampered by a reduced sensitivity. Therefore PCR carried out with a maximum of two pairs of primers (duplex PCR) is adviced for optimal HPV detection.

3.   General or Consensus Primer Mediated HPV PCR

To carry out HPV epidemiology at a large scale, two important prerequisites are necessary to fulfill. Next to an easy sample preparation protocol, the numbers of PCRs to be carried out also has to be limited. After protocols became available to apply PCR on crude cell extracts, much attention has been paid to develop primers which amplify a broad spectrum of HPVs in one reaction. Different generalized HPV PCR methods have been described by several groups using general or consensus primers located in the L1 and E1 HPV genes, because these regions appear the most conserved as shown by sequence analysis[25] and computer assisted matrix analysis.[26]

Still, perfectly matched areas among the different HPVs were not present for primer selection. Therefore, three different approaches to adapt either the primers or the method have been introduced to overcome this problem. Adaptation includes:

1. Allowance of mismatch acceptance between primers and target DNA accomplished by reducing the stringency of primer annealing;[27,28]
2. The use of degenerate primers (a mixture of oligonucleotides showing nucleotide differences at several positions) to render them sufficiently complementary to the target HPV-DNAs,[29] and
3. The use of primers which in addition contain inosine residues at certain ambiguous base positions.[30]

Table 2 gives an overview of HPV consensus primers that have been initially selected.

TABLE 2   General or Consensus Primers for Detection of HPV DNA

ORF	Primers	Primer sequences	Length of PCR product (bp)	Localization of foreward primers for HPV 16 sequence	Reference
L1	GP5	5'-TTTGTTACTGTGGTAGATAC-3'	140–150	6624–6765	27
	GP6	5'-GAAAAATAAACTGTAAATCA-3'			
L1	MY11	5'-GCMCAGGGWCATAAYAATGG-3'	450	6582–7033	29
	MY09	5'-CGTCCMARRGGAWACTGATC-3'			
E1	IU	5'-TIIRIRIIYTAAAACGAAAGT-3'	850	1111–1962	30
	IWDO	5'-RTCRWAIGCCCAYTGIACCAT-3'			

Note: M = A + C; R = A + G: W = A + T; Y = C + T; I = Inosine.

For the ultimate identification of HPV DNA, several hybridization protocols following amplification have been proposed. In the MY 09/11 system, final HPV detection was originally carried out by dot blotting of PCR products using radioactive or biotin labeled HPV generic and HPV type specific oligomers, respectively.[29] In the IU/IWDO system described by Gregoire et al.,[30] the PCR products were radioactively labeled and hybridized against a panel of electrophoretically separated cloned HPV DNAs. In the GP 5/6 system, hybridization is carried out with an HPV cocktail probe containing the amplification products of HPV 6, 11, 16, 18, 31, and 33 under mild stringent conditions.[27,31,32]

In Figure 4, the sensitivity for HPV 6 and HPV 16 detection for the three different primer sets are shown. Using the originally described protocols, it appeared that the GP 5/6 system could detect 1 fg HPV 6 and HPV 16, and the MY 09/11 system reached a level of 100 fg and 1 pg, respectively. The IU/IWDO system reached a sensitivity of 10 fg for HPV 6 and 1 fg for HPV 16. The difference in sensitivity between the three systems is likely due to the different number of cycles performed (30 vs. 25 vs. 40) and may also reflect the different probes used. Recently, the MY09/11 system has been adapted by an increased number of cycles and the use of a cocktail probe of PCR products, internally amplified from several cloned and unknown HPVs. We favor the GP 5/6 PCR because of the shorter fragments length of generated amplification fragments (150 bp) which may be advantageous under less efficient amplification conditions such as crude cell suspensions. It is also recommended to use the GP 5/6 system for paraffin embedded tissue since in this case smaller target DNA fragments can be expected due to fixation.

Since the E6/E7 ORFs are intact and transcriptionally active in neoplastic cells, some consensus systems have also been developed, based on the amplification of regions within the E6/E7 ORFs.[33-36] Unfortunately, the E6 and E7 ORFs are heterogenous throughout the different HPVs making these systems less universal than the L1 and E1 region based universal PCR methods. Next to the three major systems described at least six other different general HPV primer systems have been described.[37-42] All these systems have their own sensitivity and specificity. Evaluation of large groups of clinical specimens will determine the value of these different assays. As previously proposed, an international HPV reference center should be organized to enable the evaluation of the specificity and sensitivity of the different developed HPV detection assays.

Comparison of different primer sets

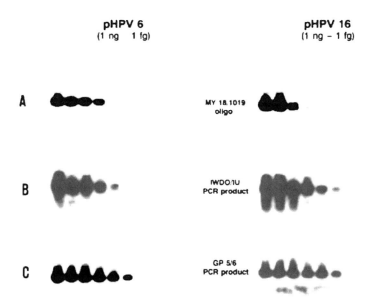

FIGURE 4   Comparison of sensitivity of three different general/consensus HPV PCRs. pHPV 6 and pHPV 16 were serial diluted (10 x) ranging from 1 ng to 1 fg. PCR was performed as follows: A) MY-PCR: mixture contained 1,5 mM MgCl2 buffer, 2,5 unit Taq polymerase, 50 pmol primer, 200 µM dNTPs. 30 cycles were performed i.e. 1 min. 95˚C, 2 min. 55˚C, 1.5 min. 72˚C. Generic probe MY 18/1019 oligo was used after 5'-end labelling; B) IWDO/IU-PCR: mixture containes 1.5 mM MgCl2 buffer, 2.5 unit Taq polymerase, 100 pmol primer, 200 µm DNTP. 25 cycles, i.e., 1 min. 94˚C, 1.5 mn in. 37˚C, 15 min. 55 C, 3 min. 72˚C. 850 bp PCR products of HPV 6 and 16 were used as probe after random-primed labeling; C) GP5/6-PCR: mixture contained 3.5 mM MgCl2, 1 unit Taq polymerase, 25 pmol primer, 200 µM dNTPs. 40 cycles, i.e., 1 min. 96˚C, 2 min. 40˚C, 1.5 min. 72˚C. Cocktail of 150 bp PCR products of HPV 6, 11, 16, 18, 31, and 33 was used as probe after random-primed labeling.

4.   **Specificity of HPV General Primer PCR Assay and Its Potential for Identifying Novel HPV Types**

An interesting observation has been made after sequencing of the GP 5/6 products of several genital HPVs. Translation of these sequences into the putative amino acid sequence according to the position of the L1 start codon and alignment of these amino acid sequences revealed the presence of a strongly conserved amino acid residue at both ends of the GP-PCR products. It appeared that all the mucosotropic HPVs contain the TRSTN amino acid sequence at the 5' part of the GP-PCR product while the conserved pentamer RHXEE was found at the 3' end.[43] These conserved sequences failed to be present in cellular sequences which were coamplified by these primers. In contrast, the internal region differing from 8 to 13 amino acid residues in length was found to be polymorphic.

Homology comparison of these unique HPV-GP-PCR sequences showed homology of more than 55% at the nucleotide level with all known sequenced mucosotropic HPV types (kindly made available to us by Dr. H. Delius and Dr. L. Gissmann, DKFZ, Germany). Much less homology was observed with cellular and other viral sequences after databank searches.

Besides confirming viral specificity, the value of HPV GP-PCR product sequencing is also substantiated by the observed homologies between GP-PCR products of different well established HPV types closely related, i.e., HPV 6 and 11 (84%), HPV 18 and 45 (80%), and HPV 33 and 58 (86%). This is in agreement with a recently established phylogenetic study which revealed similar results using larger fragments of L1 and other ORFs.[44]

Based on this knowledge, the identification of novel HPVs seems to be possible by sequence analysis of HPV-GP-PCR generated products. This means that in addition to the application of HPV detection in epidemiological studies the HPV-GP-PCR can also be an important tool for the isolation of new HPV types.

C. Evaluation of Different HPV Detection Methods

The different HPV DNA detection methods are summarized in Table 3. From these theoretical data, it appeared that PCR is superior. This is in agreement with data obtained from a case control study of cervical cancer in Spain and Columbia in which Southern blot, ViraPap, and PCR was used. In this study, HPV was detected in 40.4% of the cervical smears by PCR, while SB and ViraPap scored only 17.8 and 21.5% positivity, respectively.[45] In one study, PCR was only slightly more sensitive than SB.[46] This could be explained by the fact that in this study cervicovaginal lavages were used. These samples yield an increased DNA content, which is in favor for SB analysis. This is in agreement with the general observation that HPV type specific PCR is more sensitive, especially when the specimen size is limited.[47] Another approach to evaluate the different HPV detection methods is to analyze their significance in epidemiological studies. Several case-control studies applying FISH, Southern blot, ViraPap, or PCR have been reported. Variations between the association of HPV and cervical cancer were obtained as reflected by differences in Odds Ratios (OR) and corresponding 95% Confidence Intervals (CI). In Table 4, different case control studies on HPV are shown. From these data it appeared that the weakest association (OR 2.1 CI 1.6–2.8) was found in the Latin American study and strongest association in the Columbia (OR 77.5 CI 10.6–568.0) and Spain (OR 45.3 CI 17.9–115.0) area. It appeared that the strongest associations were found with the more sensitive HPV detection methods like Polymerase chain reaction, ViraPap, or Southern blot. The weaker associations were found with the less sensitive FISH method.[48] Since variations were still found with the most sensitive methods, additional interassay comparisons are necessary.

TABLE 3   Comparison of Different HPV DNA Detection Methods

Method	Description	Detection level	Comments
FISH[a]	Immobilization of crude cells on a filter support, followed by hybridization	>10–100 HPV copies/cell	Not applicable to solid tumor specimens. Large number of samples can be screened simultaneously. Sensitivity insufficient.
Dot Blot	Purified DNA transported to a filter support and subsequently hybridized	1–10 HPV copies/cell	High specificity, laborious.
Southern Blot	Restriction enzyme digestion step, followed by electrophoretical separation of digested DNA, follwed by transport to a filter	0.1–1 HPV copy/cell	Very high specificity, very laborious.
ISH[b]	Pretreatment to make DNA/RNA attainable for the probe	20 copies/cell	Applicable to tissue section. Preservation of morphology, laborious.
Polymerase chain reaction (PCR)	*In vitro* DNA amplification	1 HPV copy	Most sensitive DNA detection method. Specificity is dependent on primer choice.

[a] Filter *in situ* hybridization

[b] *In situ* hybridization

TABLE 4   Summary of Case-Control Studies on HPV Infection and Cervical Cancer

Study area	Cases	Controls	OR (95% CI)	HPV detection method
Latin America	759 inv cancer	1467 population and age matched	2.1 (1.6–2.8)	FISH
China	101 inv cancer	146 hospital matched for age	32.9 (7.7–141.1)	SB
Columbia	135 inv cancer	145 general population	77.5 (10.6–568.0) 10.4 (3.8–28.6) 14.6 (6.4–33.2)	ViraPap SB PCR
Spain	185 inv cancer	161 general population	26.2 (9.3–73.5) 10.1 (4.3–23.6) 45.3 (17.9–115.0)	ViraPap SB PCR

Modified from review of N. Munoz and F. X. Bosch.[48]

D.   Future Perspectives of HPV Detection by PCR

Although the three principles of primer design (degeneracy, inosine incorporation, mismatch acceptance) have been applied by different groups, further improvements will be continuously made. The ultimate goal of these improvements will be a single PCR test that detects all high risk HPV types at once at sufficient sensitivity (see also Section II C). This test requires simple and rapid detection formats for PCR generated products. Moreover, PCR primers have been adapted. In the MY11/09 system, the degeneracy of the MY11 primer has been increased (to generate MY11B) to obtain an improved PCR efficiency of poorly PCR amplified HPV types.[49] The GP5/6 PCR system has been improved by elongation of the 3' primer ends with highly conserved sequences, resulting in the primer combination GP5+/6+.[50]

In addition to the PCR reaction itself, the subsequent steps involving the detection of the PCR products are continuously amenable to modifications to obtain a simple standardized test. One aspect deals with the fact that a large number of HPV types exists, making individual typing unfeasible. Instead, it is desirable to combine HPV genotypes with a similar oncogenic potential in a single detection step. This can easily be performed by using cocktails of type specific probes to analyze PCR products. Using such an approach, the HCA has been successfully applied to detect a group of high risk HPV types at once and distinguish these types from a panel of low risk HPVs. Similarly, the group specific differentiation between high and low risk HPV types has been successfully incorporated in the GP5+/6+ PCR assay using cocktails of type specific oligonucleotide probes.[51]

Finally, the method should be suitable for application in a routine setting. Consequently, the conventional radioactive hybridization format needs to be replaced by a nonradioactive format. Also the latter option has been incorporated in the GP5+/6+ PCR system. A PCR enzyme immunoassay (PCR-EIA) utilizing one biotinylated primer, capturing the PCR products on streptavidin-coated microtiter plates, and ultimatly colorimetrically detecting DIG-labeled oligoprobes, revealed the same sensitivity and specificity as the radioactive detection assay.[52]

In addition, measurement of the quality of the sample needs further attention. Since the crude extraction methods may yield components inhibiting the PCR, it is important to judge the quality by PCR of a cellular target (e.g., ß-globin gene). Preferentially, a sample control test is included in the HPV test as an internal control, allowing assessment of both sample quality and failures of the PCR reagents. This would be the most optimal approach to prevent false negative results. In conclusion, the ongoing developments will finally result in a reproducible, quick, and routine test for HPV detection in cervical scrapes.

III.   HPV PREVALENCE RATES IN RELATION TO HISTOLOGY AND CYTOLOGY

A.   Terminology

To understand and compare the results of different studies, the relationship between different cytological and histological terms has to be explained.

Cervical lesions which may progress to invasive carcinoma were initially histologically designated as dysplasia. Dysplasia is characterized by abnormal differentiation of cervical epithelium. Gradually, lack of differentiation and increasing cellular atypia were suggested to be a hallmark for the development of cervical cancer. Dysplasia is divided into mild, moderate, and severe, depending on the proportion of the thickness of squamous epithelium with abnormal differentiation, as shown by the disturbances of tissue architecture and the presence of atypical cells. Full thickness involvement is called carcinoma *in situ*. In 1968, it was put forward by Richart[53] that the dysplastic changes represent a spectrum of the same basic change in cervical intraepithelial neoplasia (CIN-concept). It was suggested that squamous cell carcinomas of the cervix develop through a continuum of progressive consecutive CIN-lesions. Grade 1 (CIN I) represents atypical cells of the basal part of the epithelial layer up to one third of the total thickness; grade 2, one to two third; and grade 3, two third to whole thickness. Grade 3 also includes carcinoma *in situ*.

The PAP classification is used to characterize cytomorphological abnormalities in cervical smears. PAP I and II correspond with no significant morphological changes; PAP IIIa with mild to moderate dysplasia; PAP IIIb with severe dysplasia; PAP IV with carcinoma *in situ*; and PAP V with invasive carcinoma. The main drawback in histological classification and PAP smear reporting is the great inter- and intra-observer variation as scored by the pathologist. In an attempt to solve the problem of poor inter- and intra-pathologist reproducibility, the Bethesda classification system was introduced in 1988.[54] Cervical intraepithelial neoplasia (CIN) was replaced by squamous intraepithelial lesion (SIL). It was proposed to classify CIN II and III as high grade squamous intraepithelial lesions (HSIL) and CIN I by low grade squamous intraepithelial lesions (LSIL). In the proposed SIL classification, it has been suggested that low grade SILs are not necessarily precursors of cervical cancer, which either regress or persist but do not progress. In contrast, high grade SILs have been considered as one entity which may progress to cervical cancer. The relationship between PAP classification, dysplasia, CIN, and SIL is demonstrated in Figure 5.

B.   HPV Prevalence in Normal Cervical Epithelium

Both general or consensus PCRs and type specific (TS-)PCRs have been increasingly used to determine HPV prevalence rates in cytomorphological normal cervical scrapes. High variations have been found and the overall HPV prevalence ranges from 3.5 to 80%[55-57] which has led to confusion towards the role of HPV in the development of cervical cancer.[58] By now it appears that the method used and the selection of the study groups are important factors for these discrepancies. The highest reliable HPV prevalence rate (33%) was found in young women with multiple partners,[59] showing that epidemiological risk factors for cervical cancer are strongly associated with genital infections.

Melkert et al.[60] studied the HPV prevalence rate in women between 15 and 55 years old in cytomorphologically normal smears. Comparing a group of women visiting a general hospital and a group of women visiting general practitioners, it appeared in five-year-interval analysis that no age related differences existed. HPV 16 prevalence reached a maximum between 20 and 25 years but did not exceed 10%. In both populations, a gradual decrease in total HPV positivity from 25% to less than 5% was observed with increasing age. HPV 16 levels of about 1% were reached after the age of 35 years. The results of the HPV age dependency of both groups is shown in Figure 6. From these data, it seems that HPV infections can be cleared in young and asymptomatic women and are often transient.

From the HPV prevalence data in normal cytology to date, it can be concluded that the large differences are most probably due to poor definition of the cohorts studied. It seems that age and

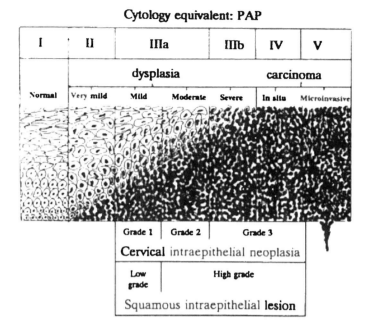

FIGURE 5 Relationship between cervical dysplasia, cervical intraepithelial neoplasia, and squamous intraepithelial lesion. The cytological equivalents according to the PAP classification are also depicted.

sexual behavior are the most important determinants of cohort definition. It is also currently assumed that in a minority of HPV 16 infected healthy women, cervical cancer can be induced after a long latency period and that also additional (co)factors are playing an important role.

C. HPV Prevalence in Premalignant and Malignant Cervical Lesions

Several combined cyto-/histological and HPV detection studies, using biopsies and cervical smears, have been carried out to investigate HPV prevalence of women with premalignant lesions. Here we have chosen to present only the data of four large representative studies in which updated HPV detection methods, i.e., Southern blot analysis and/or PCR, were used and which were performed recently.

In the Netherlands, a large study was carried out for the presence of 27 mucosotropic human papilloma virus genotypes in cytomorphologically abnormal cervical scrapes using PCR.[61] The following strategy was used. HPV general primer (GP5/6) mediated PCR was used to screen crude cell extracts for the presence of a broad spectrum of mucosotropic HPV genotypes. HPV GP-PCR positive samples were screened for HPV 6, 11, 16, 18, 31, and 33 using specific primers in the PCR. Subsequently, successive hybridization of GP-PCR products was carried out with 21 different (sub)genome HPV probes. HPV prevalence rates were determined in PAP IIIa, PAP IIIb, and PAP IV, which is equivalent to CIN I, II, and III.

Lungu et al.[62] studied a total of 276 samples including CIN I, II, and III lesions using for HPV detection PCR with L1 consensus primers and for HPV typing RFLP analysis of PCR products.

In France, Bergeron et al.[63] analyzed low (CIN I) and high CIN lesions (CIN II + III) using mainly SB technique and 13 different HPV probes. In a substantial number of specimens, PCR was also applied. Moreover, in many lesions HPV presence could also be confirmed by *in situ* hybridization.

Lorincz et al.[64] have screened for the presence of HPV DNA in cervical biopsies of CIN lesions and smears by low stringency Southern blot (590 cervical samples) subsequently. Positive samples were tested at high stringency with specific probes for HPV 6/11, 16, 18, 31, 33, 35, 42, 43, 44, 45, 51, 52, 56, and 58.

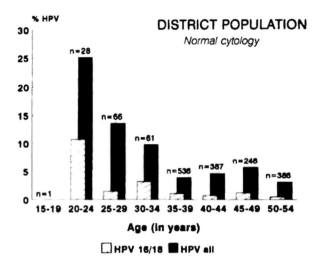

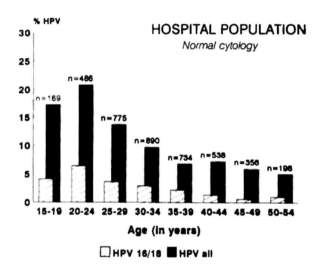

FIGURE 6   Relation HPV prevelence in cytomorphologically normal cervical smears and age as detected in a district and a general hospital population. GP 5/6 general HPV PCR in combination with HPV 16/18 TS PCR was applied. HPV all include all HPV GP-PCR positivity smears. Data are modified from Melkert et al.[60]

From all these data summarized in Table 5, it became clear that CIN represents a heterogeneous disease from a virologic point of view. The main observations are that in general the prevalence of HPV 16 increased about 2–4 times from CIN I to CIN II/III, whereas in the same lesions the prevalence of HPV 6/11, unidentified HPV types, and the presence of more than one HPV type (multiple infections) decreased.

In Table 6, HPV prevalence rates in cervical squamous cell carcinoma of seven large studies are summarized.[55,64-69] It appears that HPV prevalence rates vary between 84 and 100%. In all these studies, Southern blot and/or PCR were used. The percentage of HPV negative carcinomas is not clear because different groups applied different detection techniques. However, the association between specific HPV types and cervical cancer is very high (Table 6). The high prevalence of HPV in cervical cancer has recently been confirmed by an International Biological Study on Cervical Cancer.[69] More than 1000 specimens of invasive cervical cancer were collected from 22 countries worldwide. Using PCR, HPV DNA could be detected in 93% of the tumors. Exchange of presumed HPV negative carcinoma samples between the different groups is necessary to solve the question of

TABLE 5 A Overview of Four HPV Prevalence Studies in Women with Premalignant Cervical Diseases as Selected by Biopsies and Abnormal (>PAPIII) Cervical Smears

HPV type distribution (%) grouped to phylogenetic relationship*

First author	Classification	n	% HPV pos	LR									HR											Unknown	
				6/11	40	42	43	44	57	30	56	66	16	31	33	35	52	58	59	18	39	45	51	61	X
Bergeron[63]	Low CIN (1)	48	41 (85.4%)	-		-				4.2	6.3	-	20.8	-	4.2	2.1	2.1	4.2	-	2.1	10.4	2.1	12.5	2.1	25
SB + aPCR	High CIN (2+3)	53	49 (92.4%)	-		-				-	1.9	-	56.6	1.9	1.9	3.8	3.8	-	-	3.8	-	2	-	1.9	20.8
Lungu[62]	CIN 1	100	91 (91%)	15				1	4				16	16	-	2				3		2	-	-	19
bPCR	CIN 2	74	74 (100%)	0.4		-	-	-	-				64.8	4.1	9.5	-				5.4		1.4	1.4		4.1
	CIN 3	102	102 (100%)	-		-	-	-	-				73.1	3	6	1				2		1	1		4
Van den Brule[61,80]	PAPIIIa – CIN 1	971	694 (71.5%)	3.5	0.1	0.4	0.6			-	3.5	1.4	34.6	9.7	5.3	0.9	0.4	0.4	2.3	7.5	0.1	1.2	1.6	0.3	17.7
cPCR	PAPIIIb – CIN 2	295	253 (85.8%)	1.6		-	-	-	-	-	-	-	58.1	7.5	2.4	0.4	1.2	0.8	1.6	9.1	-	0.8	0.8	0.4	9.9
	PAPIV – CIN 3	107	107 (100%)	0.9		-	-	-	-	-	-	-	51.4	12.1	8.4	-	1.9	0.9	-	12.1	-	2.8	0.9	-	3.7
Lorincz[64]	LSIL – CIN 1	377	262 (69%)	16.7		1.1	1.1	1.3			2.1		16.2	5.0	3.4	2.7	1.9	1.3		4.0		1.1	2.4		9.3
SB	HSIL – CIN 2 and 3	261	228 (87.3%)	3.1		0.4	0	0.8			1.1		47.1	10.3	4.6	4.2	2.3	0.4		5.0		0.4	1.9		5.7

* HPV types have grouped according to phylogenetic relationship as found by van Ranst et al.[44] LR = Low Risk HPV; HR = High Risk HPV.

Note: SB = Southern blot; aConsensus PCR, Kawashima et al., *J. Invest. Dermatol.* 1990, 95, 537–542; bConsensus PCR My09/My11 + RFLP, Manos et al. 1989; cGP/TS-PCR, van den Brule et al., *J. Clin. Microbiol.* 1990, 28, 2739–2743. X = unidentified; M = multiple infection; nm = not mentioned.

TABLE 6   HPV Prevalence in Cervical Cancer

Author	n	% HPV pos	% HPV types											X	M	Area
			6/11	16	18	31	33	35	45	51	52	56	58			
Lorincz et al.[64]	153	137 (89%)	-	47.1	23.5	1.3	1.3	1.3	2.0	0.7	0.7	1.3	1.3	5.2	nm	U.S.
[a]Van den Brule et al.[80]	120	120 (100%)	-	73.3	7.5	1.7	0.8	-						5.8	17	The Netherlands
Das et al.[65]	96	94 (97.9%)	1.0	63.5	3.1	-	-	-						30.2	nm	India
Ter Meulen et al.[66]	53	47 (88.6%)	-	37.7	32.1	-	-		5.7					13.2	nm	East Africa
Resnick et al.[68]	29	29 (100%)	-	75.9	17.2	3.4	3.4		-					-	nm	U.S.
Riou et al.[67]	106	89 (83.9%)	-	54.7	12.3		6.6							10.4	nm	France
Bosch et al.[69]	932	866 (92.9%)	0.2	49.9	13.7	5.3	2.8	1.7	8.4	0.8	2.7	1.7	2.0	1.3	nm	22 countries worldwide

[a] Including additional data.

Note: X = unclassified HPV types; M = multiple infections; nm = not mentioned.

whether HPV negative cervical carcinomas exist. With respect to the HPV type distribution, HPV 16 and 18 appeared most prevalent (between 63 and 72% positivity) in all the studies. In the large international study on cervical cancer, HPV 16 was found in 50% of specimens, HPV 18 in 14%, HPV 45 in 8%, and HPV 31 in 5%. From several studies, a considerable geographic variation between HPV type distribution became evident. For example, in contrast to the majority of countries where HPV 16 prevails, HPV 18 appeared the predominant type found in Indonesia. Also, the ratio of HPV 16 and HPV 18 prevalence in a U.S. study was 2 to 1, whereas in studies in The Netherlands and India this proportion seems to be 10 to 1. Apart from these common HPVs, a significant geographic variation in HPV prevalence has also been reported for some less common HPV types. HPV 45 was apparently clustered in Western Africa, while HPV 39 and HPV 59 were almost entirely confined to Central and South America. Taken together, these results confirm a central role of genital HPVs as sexually transmitted agents in the etiology of cervical cancer worldwide.

Based on the HPV prevalence rates found in different CIN grades and cervical cancer, it was suggested by Lorincz et al.[64] to divide HPV types in four different categories, i.e., the low risk HPV 6 group (HPV 6, 11, 42, 43, and 44), the intermediate risk HPV 31 group (HPV 31, 33, 35, 52, and 58), the high risk HPV 16 group, and the high risk HPV 18 group, (HPV 18, 45, 56). Taking the data of large studies in Tables 5 and 6 together, it appears also that

1. The low risk HPV 6 group was most frequently present in low grade CIN and (almost) absent in cancer.
2. The intermediate risk HPV 31 group was frequently detected in the high grade CIN but showed a low prevalence in cervical cancer.
3. The high risk HPV 16 was almost equally associated with CIN II and III and cervical cancer.
4. The high risk HPV 18 group was found in a relatively high number of invasive cancers but was less frequently present in CIN II and III. This suggests that the HPV 18 group has to be considered as the most aggressive oncogenic type.

Using the knowledge of possible HPV involvement in the development of cervical cancer, the new classification system for premalignant lesions, i.e., squamous intraepithelial lesion (SIL) still has limitations (Bethesda classification). It was proposed to replace CIN I by low grade SIL (LSIL) with presumed little or no progression potential, while CIN II and III were considered as one entity called high SIL with a high progression potential. This hypothesis, however, is controversial. The presence of high risk HPV types in a substantial number of low SIL lesions and suggest that these lesions can also progress to invasive cervical carcinomas. This implies that LSIL lesions are heterogeneous in their clinical behavior, which is in contrast to what has been claimed by the Bethesda classification. This is also confirmed by data from follow up studies of women with HPV 16 and high risk HPV positive smears and low grade CIN lesions which show progression in a substantial number of cases to CIN III.[70-72] This is in agreement with the observation that the type of HPV infection may influence the clinical outcome of a cervical lesion, i.e., regression, persistence, or progression.[73]

A new classification system of HPVs using phylogenetic or evolutionary trees based on amino acid and nucleotide sequence alignment data of the E6 ORF has been published.[44] The genital HPV types could then be divided in three distantly related groups. It appeared that HPV 6, 11, 13, 42, 43, and 44, vs. HPV 16, 31, 33, 35, 51, 52, 56, 58, and HPV 18, 45, and 39 belong to three distinct phylogenetic trees.

Since HPV grouping based on sequence homology and biological behavior[44,64] seem to be in good agreement, this knowledge needs to be incorporated in HPV testing using PCR (see also Section II D). Although further research on the correlation between the presence of the different HPV types and disease progression is necessary in follow up studies, the classification in HPV groups with different biological behaviour instead of individual HPV typing is less confusing and will be appreciated by the clinician.

IV.   POSSIBLE CLINICAL RELEVANCE OF GENITAL HPV DETECTION

The major problem in cervical cancer is the fact that we do not know which precancerous lesions will progress, regress, or remain at the same morphological CIN grade. At the moment, it is thought that about 50% of mild dysplasias will go in regression.[74-76] Thus, using colposcopy, histology, cytology, or cervicography the clinician cannot predict the clinical outcome of the precancerous lesion of an individual woman. This results in the treatment of nearly all precancerous lesions and thus in a considerable overtreatment of women with precancerous lesions. So there is a strong need for better progression markers to predict the outcome of a precancerous lesion.

Another interesting area is screening by cytology on cervical cancer. Despite the triumph of the PAP smear, there are some important drawbacks. The complex cervical cancer detection system is prone to failures concerning the taking of the smears and interpretation by the cytologist.[77-79] False negative error rates for premalignant lesions and invasive cancer have been reported up to 50%.[77] Also interobserver variations make the results of cytological screening of cervical smears less reliable. Thus, there is a need for a more accurate screening technique for premalignant lesions and cervical cancer.

In the last decade, it has become evident that high risk or oncogenic HPV types play an important role in the development of cervical cancer.

The findings that are very important for the clinical relevance of HPV detection in cervical smears and biopsies can be summarized as follows:

1. Case-control studies from The Netherlands, Brazil, Thailand, Phillippines, Morocco, and Mali show that in at least 90% of the smears from women with cervical cancer, oncogenic HPV types can be found. When the biopsies from the HPV negative smears were tested, more than 96% of the cervical carcinomas contained oncogenic HPV types[80,81] (Muñoz et al., manuscripts in preparation). Our own experience is that the percentage of HPV negative cervical cancers is more near to 1% than 5%.
2. In all cases of carcinoma *in situ* of the cervix, oncogenic HPV types are found.[61]
3. In smears from patients with cervical dysplasia (dyskaryosis), increasing prevalence of HPV was found ranging from 70% in mild to moderate dyskaryosis to 85% in severe dyskaryosis.[61,80]
4. In women with normal smears, the prevalence of all types of HPV is age-dependent, decreasing from 20% in women with an age between 20–25 years to 4.5% in women ≥ 30 years. **Oncogenic** HPV types decrease from 7% in women between 20–25 years to ≤ 2% in women ≥ 30 years old.[60]
5. Studies from Boyes et al. (1982)[82] and Oortmarssen and Habbema (1991)[83] based on the analysis of data from the British Columbia cohort study indicate that regression of premalignant cervical lesions is age dependent with a higher proportion of regression under 34 years of age. In their computer model, Oortmarssen and Habbema estimated that at least 75% of these lesions in young women and about 30% in middle aged women will regress spontaneously. Thus, these data combined with the age dependent prevalence of HPV in cytologically normal smears and our own experience strongly suggest that a substantial number of cervical HPV infections result in an HPV associated lesion (CIN lesion). However, in young women under age of 30, more than 90% of these CIN lesions regress spontaneously whereas in middle aged women only 40% of the lesions regress.
6. Additional studies of women with normal cytology and HPV positive or negative smears show that HPV infection is the most dominant risk factor to induce cervical intraepithelial neoplasia.[84,85]
7. Retrospective and prospective studies have shown that only women with **persistent** oncogenic HPV types show progression to CIN III.[71,72] Women with abnormal cytology with low risk HPV types or HPV negative smears do not show progression during a follow up time up to 36 months.[72]
8. Studies using archival cervical smears previously taken from women who developed cervical cancer show that the same oncogenic HPV type(s) as detected in the cervical cancer biopsy can be found in these preceding smears up to at least seven years before cervical cancer diagnosis.[86]

From these findings it can be concluded that only women with persistent oncogenic HPV infection are at risk to obtain cervical cancer. Foreseeing that in the very near future a PCR based nonradioactive HPV detection method suitable for mass screening of cervical smears on oncogenic

HPV types will be available,[50-52] the following indications for HPV testing in cervical smears and biopsies can be proposed:

Abnormal Smears and Cervical Lesions

1. Determine the presence of high risk HPV types **in cytomorphologically as abnormal classified cervical smears or in cervical lesions histologically classified as ≥ CIN I**. This is important because only persistence of high risk HPV types is associated with progressive CIN lesions.[72] Thus overtreatment of CIN lesions without HPV or nononcogenic/low risk HPV types can be prevented.
2. Determine the presence of oncogenic HPV types in smears classified as **ASCUS (atypical squamous cells of undetermined significance) in the U.S. or as slight atypia or mild or moderate dyskaryosis (PAP 2/3a in The Netherlands) in Europe**. Only women with smears classified as ASCUS or PAP 2/3a which contain oncogenic HPV types should be seen by the gynecologist and when lesions are present receive treatment for their lesion, because these women have cervical lesions that will potentially show progression to cervical carcinoma.
3. Recent studies have shown that women **with HPV positive cervical lesions who have been treated by loop, laser, or excision and remain HPV positive after treatment**, even in the presence of cytomorphologically normal cervical smears, are at high risk to have recurrent disease (Reference 87 and our own observations). It appeared that demonstration of oncogenic HPV types is even more sensitive than cytology in predicting recurrent disease. Therefore, it is worthwhile to monitor these smears by HPV testing.

Screening

Furthermore, this HPV detection method can be used in combination with cytology for screening women (≥ 30 years) for cervical cancer. The combination of these two methods, which complement each other, will significantly reduce the number of false positive and false negative PAP smears leading to more accurate screening. This is based on our recent observations that:

1. Rescreening of high risk HPV positive and cytologically negative cervical smears of women ≥ 30 years yields 7–10% of smears with abnormal cytology (unpublished results).
2. In the group of women ≥ 30 years (cervical screening population in The Netherlands) with high risk HPV positive and cytomorphologically negative smears, about 10% developed severe dyskaryosis (PAP 3b) or high grade CIN in the four years follow up. However, the risk of women with HPV negative and cytomorphologically normal smears to develop CIN III in this period can be neglected.[88]

Moreover, by combining these techniques, the interval between successive screenings for women with HPV negative and cytologically normal cervical smears can be increased considerably (from 5 to 8–10 years) and will reduce costs of cervical cancer screening programs significantly.

In conclusion, results obtained so far show that the accuracy of screening for cervical (pre)malignant lesions by the combined tests is better than with morphological screening methods alone (automatically or by cytotechnicians). Studies are now in progress to further substantiate this. Finally, the advantages of combined screening on cervical cancer by cytology and HPV testing have recently extensively been discussed elsewhere.[89-91]

ACKNOWLEDGMENTS

The authors thank Miss Carla van Rijn and Miss Yvonne Duiker for excellent preparation of the manuscript and Dr. P. van der Valk for critical reading. This work was in part supported by the Dutch Cancer Society, Koningin Wilhelmina Fonds: Grants IKA-VU 91-17; IKA-VU-93-651 and the Prevention Fund, The Netherlands Grant 28-1502.

REFERENCES

1. Zur Hausen H., Human papillomaviruses and their possible role in squamous cell carcinomas, *Curr Top Microbiol Immunol* 78, 1, 1977.
2. Gissmann L. and Schneider A., The role of human papillomaviruses in genital cancer. In: *Herpes and Papillomaviruses, Their Role in the Carcinogenesis of the Lower Genital Tract*, Eds: de Palo G., Rilkes F., zur Haussen H., Raven Press, New York, vol. 31, 15, 1986.
3. Zur Hausen H., Papillomaviruses in anogenital cancer as a model to understand the role of viruses in human cancers, *Cancer Res* 49, 4677, 1989.
4. Zur Hausen H., Human papillomaviruses in the pathogenesis of anogenital cancer, *Virology* 184, 9, 1991.
5. Rotkin L. D., Adolescent coitus and cervical cancer: association of related events with increased risk, *Cancer Res* 27, 603, 1967.
6. Brinton L. A. and Fraumeni J. F., Epidemiology of uterine cervical cancer, *Chron Dis J* 39, 1051, 1986.
7. Zur Hausen H., Condylomata acuminata and human genital, *Cancer* 36, 794, 1976.
8. Meisels A. and Morin B., Human papillomavirus and cancer of the uterine cervix, *Gynecol Oncol* 12, 111, 1981.
9. De Villiers E. M., Heterogeneity of the human papillomavirus group, *J Virol* 63, 4898, 1989.
10. Mullis K. B. and Faloona F. A., Specific synthesis of DNA in vitro via a polymerase analyzed chain reaction, *Meth Enzymol* 155, 335, 1987.
11. Ehrlich H. A., Gelfland H. A. and Sninsky J. J., Recent advances in the polymerase chain reaction, *Science* 252, 1643, 1991.
12. Brandsma J., Burk R. D., Lancaster W. D., Pfister H. and Schiffman M. H., Interlaboratory variation as an explanation for varying prevalence estimates of human papillomavirus infection, *Int J Cancer* 43, 260, 1989.
13. Wagner D., Ikenberg H., Bohm N., Gissmann L., Identification of human papillomavirus in cervical swabs by deoxyribomucleic acid *in situ* hybridization, *Obstet Gynecol* 64, 767, 1984.
14. Brigati D. J., Meyerson D., Leavy J. J. et al., Detection of viral genomes in cultured cells and paraffin embedded tissue sections using biotin labelled hybridization probes. *Virology* 126, 32, 1983.
15. Walboomers J. M. M., Melchers W. J. G., Mullink H., et al., Sensitivity of in situ detection with biotinylated probes of human papillomavirus type 16 DNA in frozen tissue sections of squamous cell carcinoma of the cervix, *Am J Pathol* 31, 587, 1988.
16. Stoler M. H., Rhodes C. R., Whitbeck A., Chow L. T. and Broker T. R., Gene expression of HPV types 16 and 18 in cervical neoplasia, In: Howley P. M. and Broker T., R., Eds., *Papillomaviruses*, New York, Wiley Liss, 1, 1990.
17. Syrjänen K. and Syrjänen S., Concept of the existence of human papillomavirus (HPV) DNA in histologically normal squamous epithelium of the genital tract should be reevaluated, *Acta Obstet Gynecol Scand* 68, 613, 1989.
18. Nuovo G. J., Gallery F., MacConnel P., Becher J. and Block W., An improved technique for the in situ detection of DNA after polymerase chain reaction amplification, *Am J Pathol* 139, 1239, 1991.
19. Saiki R. K., Scharf S., Mullis K. B., Horn G. T., Ehrlich H. A. and Arnheim N., Enzymatic amplification of beta globin genomic sequences and restriction site analysis for diagnosis of sickle cell anemia, *Science* 230, 1350, 1985.
20. Saiki R. K., Gelfand D. H., Stoffel S., Scharf S. J., Higuchi R., Horn G. T., Mullis K. B. and Erhlich H. A., Primer directed enzymatic amplification of DNA with a thermostable DNA polymerase. *Science* 239, 487, 1988.
21. Van den Brule A. J. C., Meijer C. J. L. M., Bakels V., Kenemans P. and Walboomers J. M. M., Rapid human papillomavirus detection in cervical scrapes by combined general primers mediated and type specific polymerase chain reaction, *J Clin Microbiol* 28, 2739, 1990.
22. Tidy J. A. and Farell P. J., Retraction: Human papillomavirus sybtype 16b, *Lancet* II, 761, 1989.
23. Van den Brule A. J. C., Claas H. C. J., Du Maine M. et al., Use of anticontamination primers in the polymerase chain reaction for the detection of human papillomavirus genotypes in cervical scrapes and biopsies, *J Med Virol* 29, 20, 1989.
24. Longo M. C., Berninger M. S. and Hartley J. L., Use of uracil DNA glycolase to control carry-over contamination in polymerase chain reactions, *Genes* 93, 125, 1990.
25. Giri I. and Danos O., Papillomavirus genomes, From sequence data to biological properties, *Trends Genet* 2, 227, 1986.

26. Queen C. and Korn L. J., A comprehensive sequence analysis program for the IBM personal computer, *Nucleic Acids Res* 12, 581, 1984.

27. Snijders P. J. F., Van den Brule A. J. C., Schrijnemakers H. F. J., Snow G., Meijer C. J. L. M. and Walboomers J. M. M., The use of general primers in the polymerase chain reaction permits the detection of a broad spectrum of human papillomavirus genotypes, *J Gen Virol* 71, 173, 1990.

28. Van den Brule A. J. C., Snijders P. J. F., Gordijn R. L. J., Bleker O. P., Meijer C. J. L. M. and Walboomers J. M. M., General primer mediated polymerase chain reaction permits the detection of sequenced and still unsequenced human papillomavirus genotypes in cervical scrapes and carcinomas, *Int J Cancer* 45, 644, 1990.

29. Manos M. M., Wright D. K., Lewis A. J. D., Broker T. R. and Wolinsky S. M., The use of polymerase chain reaction amplification for the detection of genital human papillomavirusis, In: Furth M. and Greaves M., Eds. *Molecular Diagnostics of Human Cancer*, Cold Spring Harbor, NY, Cold Spring Harbor Press, 209, 1989.

30. Gregoire L., Arella M., Campione-Piccardo J. and Lancaster W. D., Amplification of human papillomavirus DNA sequences by using conserved primers, *J Clin Microbiol* 27, 2660, 1989.

31. Walboomers J. M. M., Brule A. J. C. van den, Snijders P. J. F., Maine M. du, Kenemans P. and Meijer C. J. L. M., Detection of genital human papillomavirus infections by the polymerase chain reaction, In: *Rapid Methods and Automation in Microbiology and Immunology*, Eds., Vaheri A., Tilton R. C. and Balows A, Springer Verlag Helsinki - Espo p. 326, 1991.

32. Walboomers J. M. M., Melkert P. W. J., Van den Brule A. J. C., Snijders P. J. F. and Meijer C. J. L. M., The polymerase chain reaction for human papillomavirus screening in diagnostic cytopathology of the cervix, In: *Diagnostic Molecular Pathology: A practical approach*, Eds: Herrington C. S., and McGee O'D., Oxford University Press, Oxford, vol. III, chapter 7, p. 152, 1992.

33. Fujinaga Y., Shimada M., Okazawa K., Fukushima M., Kato I. and Fujinaga K., Simultaneous detection and typing of genital human papillomavirus DNA using the polymerase chain reaction, *J Gen Virol* 72, 1039, 1991.

34. Evander M. and Wadell G. A., A general primer pair for amplification and detection of genital human papilloamvirus types, *J Virol Methods* 31, 239, 1991.

35. Yoshikawa H., Kawana T., Kitagawa K., Mizuno M., Yoshikura H. and Iwamoto A., Amplification and typing of multiple cervical cancer-associated human papillomavirus DNAs using a single pair of primers, *Int J Cancer* 45, 990, 1990.

36. Resnick R. M., Cornelissen M. T. E., Wright D. K., Eichinger G. H., Fox H. S., ter Schegget J. and Manos M. M., Detection and typing of human papillomavirus in archival cervical cancer specimens by DNA amplification with consensus primers, *J Natl Cancer Inst* 82, 1477, 1990.

37. Van den Brule A. J. C., Snijders P. J. F., Meijer C. J. L. M. and Walboomers J. M. M., PCR based detection of genital HPV genotypes: An update and future perspectives, *Papillomavirus Rep* 4, 95, 1993.

38. Maki H., Saito S., Ibaraki T., Ichijo M. and Yoshie O., Use of universal and type-specific primers in the polymerase chain reaction for the detection and typing of genital human papillomavirus, *JPN J Cancer Res* 82, 411, 1991.

39. Williamson A. L. and Rybicki E. P., Detection of genital human papillomaviruses utilizing a single oligonucleotide primer set, *Bio Techniques* 10, 632, 1991.

40. Snijders P. J. F., Meijer C. J. L. M. and Walboomers J. M. M., Degenerate primers based on highly conserved regions of amino acid sequence in papillomaviruses can be used in generalized polymerase chain reaction to detect productive human papillomavirus infections, *J Gen Virol* 72, 2781, 1991.

41. Rodu B., Christian C., Snyder R. C., Ray R. and Miller D. M., Simplified PCR-based detection and typing strategy for human papilloamviruses utilizing a single oligonucletide primer set, *Bio Techniques* 10, 632, 1991.

42. Tieben L. M., ter Schegget J., Minnaar R. P., Bouwes Bavinck J. N., Berkhout R. J. M., Vermeer B. J. et al., Detection of cutaneous and genital HPV types in clinical samples by PCR using consensus primers, *J Virol Methods* 42, 265, 1993.

43. Van den Brule A. J. C., Snijders P. J. F., Raaphorst P., Schrijnemakers H., Delius H., Gissmann L., Meijer C. J. L. M. and Walboomers J. M. M., General primer PCR in combination with sequence analysis to identify potentially novel HPV genotypes in cervical lesions, *J Clin Microbiol* 30, 1716, 1992.

44. Van Ranst M., Kaplan J. B. and Burk R. D., Phylogenetic classification of human papillomaviruses: correlation with clinical manifestations, *J Gen Virol* 73, 2653, 1992.

45. Guerrero E., Daniel R. W., Bosch F. X. et al., Comparison of ViraPap, southern hybridization and polymerase chain reaction methods for human papillomavirus identification in an epidemiological investigation of cervical cancer, *J Clin Microbiol* 30, 2951, 1992.

46. Schiffman H. M., Bauer M., Lorincz A. T. et al., Comparison of southern blot hybridization and polymerase chain reaction methods for the detection of human papillomavirus DNA, *J Clin Microbiol* 29, 573, 1991.

47. Melchers W., Van den Brule A. J. C., Walboomers J. M. M., et al., Increased detection rate of human papillomavirus in cervical scrapes by the polymerase chain reaction as compared to modified FISH and Southern blot analysis, *J Med Virol* 27, 329, 1989.

48. Munoz N. and Bosch F. X., HPV and cervical cancer: Review of case control and cohort studies, In: Munoz N., Bosch F. X., Shah K. V., Meheus A. (Eds), The epidemiology of human papilloma virus and cervical cancer, *IARC Publication No. 119*, Lyon, France, 251, 1992.

49. Hildesheim A., Schiffman M. H., Gravitt P. E., et al., Persistence of type specific human papillomavirus infection among cytologically normal women, *J Infect Dis* 169, 235-240, 1994.

50. Roda Husman A. M. de, Walboomers J. M. M., Van den Brule A. J. C., Meijer C. J. L. M., Snijders P. J. F., The use of general primers GP5 and GP6 elongated at their 3' ends with adjacent highly conserved sequences improves human papillomavirus detection by PCR, *J Gen Virol* 76, 1057-1062, 1995.

51. Jacobs M. V., Roda Husman A. M. de, Van den Brule A. J. C., Snijders P. J. F., Meijer C. J. L. M., Walboomers J. M. M., Group specific differentiation between high- and low-risk human papillomavirus genotypes by general primer mediated polymerase chain reaction and two cocktails of oligonucleotide-probes. *J Clin Microbiol* 33, 901-905, 1995.

52. Jacobs M. V., Van den Brule A. J. C., Snijders P. J. F., Meijer C. J. L. M., Walboomers J. M. M., A non radioactive PCR enzyme immunoassay enables a rapid identification of HPV 16 and 18 in cervical smears after GP5+/6+ PCR, *J Med Virol* 49, 223, 1996.

53. Richart R. M., Natural history of cervical intraepithelial neoplasia, *Clin Obstet Gynecol* 10, 748, 1968.

54. The 1988 Bethesda system for reporting cervical/vaginal cytologic diagnosis: Developed and approved at the National Cancer Institute Workshop in Bethesda, Maryland, December 12-13, 1988, *Hum Path* 21, 704, 1990.

55. Van den Brule A. J. C., Walboomers J. M. M., du Maine M., Kenemans P. and Meijer C. J. L. M., Difference in prevalence of human papillomavirus genotypes in cytomorphologically normal cervical smears is associated with a history of cervical intraepithelial neoplasia, *Int J Cancer* 48, 404, 1991.

56. Tidy J. A., Parry G. C. N., Ward P., et al., High rate of human papilloma virus type 16 infection in cytologically normal cervices, *Lancet* II, 434, 1989.

57. Young L. S., Bevan I. S., Johnson M. A., Blomfield P. I., Bromidge T., Maitland N. J. and Woodman E. B. J., The polymerase chain reaction: a new epidemiological tool for investigating cervical human papillomavirus infection, *B M J* 298, 14, 1989.

58. Munoz N., Bosch X. and Kaldor J. M., Does human papillomavirus cause cervical cancer? The state of the epidemiological evidence, *Br J Cancer* 57, 1, 1988.

59. Bauer H. M., Ting Y., Greer A., et al., Genital human papillomavirus infection in female university students as determined by a PCR based method. *J Am Med Assoc* 265, 472, 1991.

60. Melkert P. W. J., Hopman E., Van den Brule A. J. C., et al., Prevalence of HPV in cytomorphologically normal cervical smears as determined by the polymerase chain reaction, is age dependent, *Int J Cancer* 53, 919, 1993.

61. De Roda Husman A. M., Walboomers J. M. M., Meijer C. J. L. M., Risse E., Schipper M. E. I., Helmerhorst Th. M., Bleker O. P., Van den Brule A. J. C. and Snijders P. J. F., Analysis of cytomorphologically abnormal cervical scrapes for the presence of 27 mucosotropic human papillomavirus genotypes using polymerase chain reaction, *Int J Cancer* 56, 802–806, 1994.

62. Lungu O., Sun X. W., Felix J., Richart R. M., Silverstein S. and Wright T. C., Relationship of human papillomavirus type to grade of cervical intraepithelial neoplasia, *J Am Med Assoc* 267, 2493, 1992.

63. Bergeron C., Barrasso R., Beaudenon S., Flamant P., Croissant O. and Orth G., Human papillomaviruses associated with cervical intraepithelial neoplasia, great diversity and distinct distribution on low- and high-grade lesions, *Am J Surg Pathol* 16, 641, 1992.

64. Lorincz A. T., Reid R., Jenson A. B., Greenberg M. D., Lancaster W. and Kurman R. J., Human papillomavirus infection of the cervix: relative risk associations of 15 common anogenital types, *Obstet Gynecol* 79, 328, 1992.

65. Das B. C., Sharma J. K., Gopalkrishna V., Das D. K., Singh V., Gissmann L., et al., A high frequency of human papillomavirus DNA sequences in cervical carcinomas of Indian women as revealed by Southern blot hybridization and polymerase chain reaction, *J Med Virol* 36, 239, 1992.

66. Ter Meulen J., Eberhardt H. C., Luande J., Mgaya H. N., Chang-Claude J., Mtiro H., et al., Human papillomavirus (HPV) infection, HIV infection and cervical cancer in Tanzania, East Africa, *Int J Cancer* 51, 515, 1992.

67. Riou G., Favre M., Jeannel D., Bourhis J., Le Doussal V. and Orth G., Association between poor prognosis in early-stage invasive cervical carcinomas and non-detection of HPV DNA, *Lancet* 335, 1171, 1990.

68. Resnick R. M., Cornelissen M. T. E. Wright D. K., Eichinger G. H., Fox H. S., ter Schegget J. and Manos M. M., Detection and typing of human papillomavirus in archival cervical cancer specimens by DNA amplification with consensus primers, *J Natl Cancer Inst* 82, 1477, 1990.

69. Bosch F. X., Manos H. H., Muñoz N., et al., Prevalence of Human Papillomavirus in cervical cancer: a worldwide perspective, *J Natl Cancer Inst* 87, 796-802, 1995.

70. Campion M. J., McCance D. J., Cuzick J. and Singer A., Progressive potential of mild cervical atypia: prospective cytological and virological study, *Lancet* II, 237, 1986.

71. Gaarenstroom K. N., Melkert P., Walboomers J. M. M., Van den brule A. J. C., Van Bommel P. F. J., Meijer C. J. L. M., Human papillomavirus DNA and genotypes: Prognostic factors for progression of cervical intraepithelial neoplasia, *Int J Gynaecol Cancer* 4, 73–78, 1994.

72. Remmink A. M., Walboomers J. M. M., Helmerhorst Th. J. M, et al., The presence of persistent high risk HPV genotypes in dysplastic cervical lesions is associated with progressive disease: natural history up to 36 months, *Int J Cancer* 61, 301–311, 1995.

73. Kataja V., Syrjänen S., Mantyjävir R., Yliskoski M., Saarikoski S. and Syrjänen K., Prognostic factors in cervical human papillomavirus infections, *Sex Trans Dis* 19, 154, 1992.

74. Richart R. M. and Barron B. A., Screening strategies for cervical cancer and cervical intraepithelial neoplasia, *Cancer* 47, 1176, 1981.

75. Richart R. M. and Barron B. B., A follow-up study of patients with cervical dysplasia, *Am J Obstet Gynecol* 105, 386, 1969.

76. Nasiell K., Nasiell M. and Vaclavinkova V., Behaviour of moderate cervical dysplasia during long-term follow-up, *Obstet Gynaecol* 61, 609, 1983.

77. Koss L. G., The Papanicolaou test for cervical cancer detection: a triumph and a tragedy, *J Am Med Assoc* 261, 737, 1989.

78. National Cancer Institute Workshop, The 1988 Bethesda System for reporting cervical/vaginal cyto-logical diagnosis, *J Am Med Assoc* 262, 931, 1989.

79. Devesa S. S., Young J. L., Brinton L. A. and Fraumeni J. F., Recent trends in cervix uteri cancer, *Cancer* 64: 2184, 1989.

80. Van den Brule A. J. C., Walboomers J. M. M., Du Maine M., Kenemans P., Meijer C. J. L. M., Difference in prevalence of human papillomavirus genotypes in cytomorphologically normal cervical smears is associated with a history of cervical intraepithelial neoplasia, *Int J Cancer* 48, 404–408, 1991.

81. Eluf-Neto J., Booth M., Muñoz N., Bosch F. X., Meijer C. J. L. M., Walboomers J. M. M., Human papillomavirus and invasive cervical cancer in Brazil, *Br J Cancer* 69, 114–119, 1994.

82. Boyes D. A., Morrison B., Knox E. G., Draper G. J., Miller A. B., A cohort study of cervical cancer screening in British Columbia, *Clin Invest Med* 5, 1–29, 1982.

83. Oortmarssen G. J. van, Habbema J. D. F., Epidemiological evidence for age-dependent regression of pre-invasive cervical cancer, *Br J Cancer* 64, 559–564, 1991.

84. Koutsky L. A., Holmes K. K., Critchlow C. W. et al., A cohort study of the risk of cervical intraepithelial neoplasia grade 2 or 3 in relation to papillomavirus infection, *N Engl J Med* 327, 1272, 1992.

85. Schiffmann M. H., Bauer H. M., Hoover R. N. et al., Epidemiologic evidence showing that human papillomavirus infections causes most cervical intraepithelial neoplasia. *J Natl Cancer Inst* 85, 958, 1993.

86. Walboomers J. M. M., Roda Husman A. M. de, Snijders P. J. F., Stel H. V., Risse E. K. J., Helmerhorst Th. J. M., Voorhorst F. J., Meijer C. J. L. M., Human papillomavirus in false negative archival cervical smears: Implications for screening for cervical cancer, *J Clin Pathol* 48, 728–732, 1995.

87. Elfgren K., Bistoletti P., Dillner L., Walboomers J. M. M., Meijer C. J. L. M., Dillner J., Conization of CIN is followed by a disappearance of HPV DNA and a decline of serum and cervical mucus antibodies against HPV antigens, *Am J Ob Gyn* 174, 937, 1996.

88. Rozendaal L., Walboomers J. M. M., Van der Linden H., Voorhorst F. J., Kenemans P., Helmerhorst Th. J. M., Van Ballegooyen M., and Meijer C. J. L. M., The PCR based high risk HPV test in cervical screening gives an objective risk assessment for women with cytomorphologically normal cervical smears. Submitted.

89. Walboomers J. M. M., de Roda Husman A. M., Van den Brule A. J. C., Snijders P. J. F. and Meijer C. J. L. M., Detection of genital human papilloma virus infection, Critical review of methods and prevalence studies in relation to cervical cancer. In: Stern P., and Stanley M., (Eds), *Human Papillomaviruses and Cervical Cancer*, Oxford University Press, chapter 3, pp. 41–71, 1994.

90. Meijer C. J. L. M., Snijders P. J. F., Van den Brule A. J. C., Helmerhorst Th. J. M., Remmink A. J., Walboomers J. M. M., Can cytological detection be improved by HPV screening? In: Monsonego J. (Ed.), *Challenges of Modern Medicine;* Ares-Serono Symposia Publication, Rome: Papillomavirus in human pathology, Vol. 9, pp. 493–497, 1995.

91. Richart R. M., Screening: the next century, *Cancer* 76, 1919, 1995.

20

The Current Role of HPV Serology

Lutz Gissmann

CONTENTS

I. INTRODUCTION

Until some years ago, the information available about the humoral immune response to papillomavirus infections was very limited.[1] In the initial studies, crude extracts obtained from warts were used as antigens in serological assays. Even with virus particles purified from clinical lesions, only small collections of serum samples could be analyzed since the amount of reagents was limited and the quality of the antigen preparations was not reproducible. Nevertheless, serological data for the first time pointed to some of the important aspects of the biology of papillomaviruses, which were confirmed later when other techniques were applied. Thus, already in 1969 it was suggested by the work of Almeida and co-workers[2] that papillomaviruses infecting the skin and the mucosa are different from each other. Pfister et al.[3] demonstrated the prevalence of antibodies against HPV 8 particles in 10% of sera from asymptomatic individuals, although HPV 8-induced lesions are extremely rarely found. This report presented the first experimental evidence of a now generally accepted phenomenon, i.e., the high prevalence of clinically inapparent with certain papillomavirus infections.

II. THE USE OF GENETICALLY ENGINEERED VIRAL ANTIGENS IN SEROLOGICAL ASSAYS

After the advances of recombinant DNA technology had been applied to papillomavirus research and viral proteins were expressed by different recombinant systems, it became feasible to measure in a reproducible manner the antibodies directed to structural proteins of those HPV types which cannot be prepared from clinical lesions (e.g., the mucosotropic virus types such as HPV 16). Particularly the analysis of the humoral immune response which is directed against nonstructural (early) proteins became only feasible after the development of genetically engineered reagents.

Production of the individual papillomavirus proteins was facilitated after *in vitro* recombination of the respective genes to strong heterologous promoters followed by the introduction of such recombinant molecules into appropriate hosts such as *E.coli*, yeast, or insect cells. HPV proteins which were produced either in prokaryotic or eukaryotic vector/host systems are used as antigens in different test systems, i.e., Western blotting, ELISA, and radio-immunoprecipitation (RIPA). Recently complete virus capsids (virus-like particles: VLP) became available for serological assays that are obtained by expression of the papillomavirus structural proteins L1 and L2 in eukaryotic cells.[4] Detailed discussions of the vector/host systems as well as of the different assays which are commonly in use including their advantages and drawbacks have been published earlier.[4-7] The decision as to which technique should be given preference to the others depends on the experimental conditions and the aims of a particular study. Thus, high sensitivity and specificity of a certain assay as recently demonstrated for the HPV 16 E6- or E7-specific RIPA[8,9] may be paralleled by poor feasibility. Hence, such an assay is not suited for large scale screening or even for use in field studies under limited laboratory facilities. On the other hand, peptide-based ELISAs are very easy to perform and proved to be of high reproducibility.[8,10-12] Synthetic peptides, however, usually represent only linear epitopes of a given protein and therefore are unlikely to detect those antibodies which were formed as a response to conformational epitopes.

During the very last years, interesting results have been obtained by a number of laboratories which took advantage of the various expression systems and applied the different assays mentioned before. The published information was comprehensively reviewed elsewhere.[4,6,7,13] In this chapter, only certain more general aspects of papillomavirus serology shall be discussed.

III.   SENSITIVITY AND SPECIFICITY OF SEROLOGICAL ASSAYS

A.   Antibodies as Markers for Papillomavirus-Associated Diseases

To ascertain the significance of an HPV type-specific serological assay, the results must be correlated to the clinical record of current or past infections with this particular papillomavirus type in the test population, i.e., in patients with HPV-associated tumors and appropriate controls. In fact, antibodies against structural proteins of HPV 1, 6, 11, or 16 are more commonly detected in patients with skin warts, condylomata acuminata, laryngeal papillomas, or CIN as compared to healthy controls. It is generally accepted that these antibodies actually indicate a current and active infection by this virus.[14-19] Similarly, a positive humoral immune response to the early proteins E6, E7, and (less intensively studied) E2 of HPV 16 or HPV18 was found more frequently in cervical cancer patients than in age-matched healthy women.[8-10,20-23] The antibody prevalence is even higher in patients with HPV 16 or 18 DNA positive tumor biopsies, indicating a type-specificity of the antigen-antibody reaction measured by the individual assay.[8,9,11] The presence of E6- or E7-specific antibodies in cervical cancer patients can easily be explained by the long exposure of the immune system to virally infected cells which consistently express the E6/E7 genes and persist within such patients for many years before the tumor becomes clinically apparent.

Although less prevalent than the immune response to E6 or E7, antibodies against the HPV 16 E4 protein are also detected more frequently in cervical cancer patients as compared to healthy women.[20,24,25] The reason for this phenomenon is presently less obvious since there is evidence that the E4 protein is involved in virus particle maturation and usually virus production is absent in cervical cancer lesions. It is conceivable, however, that the presence of E4-specific antibodies indicates an ongoing HPV 16 replication in precancerous lesions which may exist besides the malignant tumor in some patients. In fact, there are reports about the detection of antibodies against papillomavirus group-specific antigens and, more recently, VLPs in sera of cervical cancer patients also suggest a current or past virus replication in those women.[26-29] Even if the biology of humoral immune responses to HPV and the significance of IgA-, IgG-, or IgM class immunoglobulins in patients' sera[10,22,23,27,28] are far from being understood, the highly significant association of a certain set of antibodies with cervical cancer may become a useful marker for this disease even as a routine laboratory diagnosis.

In contrast to the disease-related immune response as mentioned before, the significance of HPV-specific antibodies found in a small proportion of healthy individuals is not as easy to explain. Because of the plurality of human papillomaviruses which exhibit a considerable degree of amino acid homology with each other, antibodies which have developed as a response to infections by another papillomavirus type may be cross-reacting in a particular assay.[30] Only by conducting carefully designed sero-epidemiological surveys can it be evaluated whether a given assay is of low specificity or whether it actually detects past papillomavirus infections in a type-specific manner. For example, antibodies to HPV 11 late proteins in a healthy individual may indicate the history of genital warts[31,32] or laryngeal papillomas and HPV 16(18)-E6 or -E7 specific antibodies which are detected in a few healthy women may prove to be diagnostic for a persistent HPV infection. If so, it is tempting to speculate that such assays may be of value in order to identify those women who are at elevated risk for the development of cervical cancer later in life.

Despite the strong association between the detection of antibodies to the early proteins E6 or E7 of HPV 16/18 and the presence of cervical cancer as discussed before, there is a certain proportion of tumor patients who are devoid of a detectable antibody response. At present it is unclear whether the negative results are due to experimental limitations of the serological assays employed or whether some patients actually fail to develop HPV-specific antibodies. One can put forward a number of explanations, some of which have already been experimentally verified:

1. Certain epitopes of the E6 and E7 proteins are either not present in the synthetic antigens which are being used for serology (i.e., fusion proteins, synthetic peptides, *in vitro* produced proteins) or, alternatively, are not accessible to the antibodies due to the characteristics of a particular assay (Western blot, ELISA, RIPA).

   • In order to perform peptide ELISAs, linear epitopes of the HPV 16 and HPV 18 E7 proteins were mapped by a variety of methods using sera of different origin (hyperimmune sera from rabbits, mouse monoclonal antibodies, sera from human patients) and identical regions were identified.[11,33-37] Thus it seems unlikely that major linear B-cell epitopes have been missed.

   • The notion of different exposure of epitopes was supported when human sera were tested by Western blotting using the HPV E7 protein which had been fused to two different peptides of prokaryotic origin. While the reaction with the prokaryotic protein was negative, it was demonstrated that a proportion of the samples reacted differently with the fusion proteins.[20] Hence it is conceivable that, depending on the experimental system, epitopes become masked due to artificial refolding of the proteins during the experimental procedure (e.g., SDS polyacrylamide-gelelectrophoresis followed by transfer to the membrane).

   • It is assumed that by Western blot assays or ELISAs, only antibodies directed against linear epitopes are detected. In fact, when the complete HPV 16 E6 or E7 protein prepared by *in vitro* transcription/translation were used as antigen in RIPA, the number of seroreactive sera of HPV 16 positive cervical cancer patients increases to approximately 80%.[9] This data suggests that under these experimental conditions antibodies to conformational epitopes are detected, too. It is not clear, however, whether the *in vitro* product contains the genuine post-translational modifications and displays all three-dimensional epitopes which are present within the authentic protein.

2. There are variations in the B-cell epitopes of individual HPV isolates. The E7 open reading frames of 32 isolates of HPV 16 and of 26 isolates of HPV 18 were sequenced which had been obtained from cervical cancer patients or healthy individuals, respectively. Some sequence variations within the E7 ORF, depending on the geographic origin of the viral isolate, were detected but there was no mutation identified within those regions of the E7 proteins which were used as synthetic peptides. In some of the cases, the corresponding sera were available for antibody testing and there was no correlation between the E7 nucleotide sequence and the seroreactivity of the respective patient.[38,39]

3. HPV-specific antibodies develop with tumor progression. Because of the prolonged exposure to the immune system of the viral proteins which are expressed in cervical cancer cells, HPV E6- or E7-specific antibodies may develop with tumor progression and the antibody may be below the

detection limit at the time when the serum was obtained for testing. If this assumption is correct, the proportion of sero-positive cancer patients and the mean antibody titers should increase with the tumor stage. In fact, antibody levels appear to rise within stage I through stage IV cervical cancer patients.[40] When the patients were followed after radiotherapy, the antibody titers were shown to drop in the majority of cases. It remains to be evaluated whether changes in antibody levels after tumor treatment are indicative for a successful therapy and eventually may be an early marker for recurrent disease. Unlike the antibody titers, the number of cancer patients with HPV 16 or 18 DNA positive tumors that reacted with the HPV antigens proved to be independent of the tumor stage.

4. The HPV-specific antibody response is influenced by genetically determined host factors. From the data discussed so far, it can be concluded that the failure of certain cervical cancer patients to react with HPV early proteins is very likely not due to technical limitations of the assays, genetic variability of the virus, or to a short exposure of the viral proteins to the immune system. Recently, a positive and negative association between particular HLA class II haplotypes and the occurrence of cervical cancer or the presence of certain HPV types was reported.[41-46] It remains to be elucidated whether there is a correlation between HLA polymorphism and HPV seroreactivity as well.

5. Following infection with genital papillomaviruses early in life, cervical patients may be immune-tolerant. By the detection of viral antibodies directed against different HPV proteins (e.g., E4, L1) as well as of HPV DNA within oral or genital swabs, it was suggested that infection with HPV 16 may occur perinatally or during early infancy.[20,46,47] In case of HPV 6 or HPV 11, it was reported that the early infection eventually may lead to the development of laryngeal papillomatosis,[48] but the clinical consequence of infection with HPV 16 remains unclear. It is speculated, however, that in most instances papillomavirus infections early in life stay inapparent and under certain circumstances may render this particular individual tolerant. Obviously this hypothesis cannot be verified in human beings but experiments using HPV 16 transformed cells in mice showed that tolerance against the HPV 16 E7 protein can actually be induced.[49]

B. Humoral Immune Response and Latent Papillomavirus Infections

As discussed before, it is possible to test the validity of a particular assay if a positive serological reaction to a certain papillomavirus protein is correlated to a present or past infection by this HPV type. It is expected that the number of informative assays will increase in the future if appropriate sero-epidemiological studies have been conducted.

However, in cases of clinically inapparent papillomavirus infections, the specificity of a serological assay may be difficult to assess since a positive reaction cannot be verified by the presence of an HPV-associated disease within the test population. Detection of papillomavirus DNA in clinically normal tissue is possible by sensitive methods such as polymerase chain reaction (PCR) but false negative results may be obtained due to sampling problems.[50] On the other hand, the genetic similarity of the different human papillomaviruses and the multiplicity of infections which can occur within the same individual may lead to the formation of a whole variety of cross-reacting antibodies which cannot be diagnosed in a type-specific manner, especially by those assays which use whole proteins as antigens. For example, the relevance of antibodies which react with the HPV 16 E4 protein in children is difficult to assess since usually there is no clinical sign of a genital infection within those infants. HPV 16 DNA can be detected by PCR in oral or genital swabs obtained from children[20,46] but there is only a very poor correlation between seropositivity and detection of viral DNA within the same individual.[47] Hence, it is unclear whether this assay is of low specificity and antibodies against other HPV types are cross-reacting with the E4 protein or whether these antibodies are actually diagnostic for subclinical HPV 16 infection in a rather high number of young children. If so, one has to postulate that presumably this infection is normally transmitted by an asexual route either perinatally or later in life during child care.

IV. CONCLUSIONS AND PERSPECTIVES

The initial limitation in papillomavirus-serology, i.e., the restricted supply of papillomavirus antigens, has been overcome by the introduction of recombinant DNA technology. As a consequence, a large number of studies have been conducted and in many instances a significantly different response to a given viral protein between individuals with HPV related diseases and their controls have been found.[13] However, because of the low sensitivity (and sometimes also low specificity) of the currently available assays, their usefulness for routine diagnostic is as yet questionable. It remains to be elucidated whether certain combinations of viral antigens can improve the diagnostic power. Diagnosis of cervical cancer or its precursors by serology would be extremely helpful, particularly in countries with low health care standards where this disease is often the most common female cancer.

The biological significance of antibodies in healthy individuals remains unknown as long as the natural history of papillomavirus infections is poorly understood. Future research will unravel to which extent immunity against papillomavirus infections in man exists and whether it can be measured by the presence of serum antibodies. If so, HPV-serology is expected to become an important tool to monitor the efficacy of virus-specific vaccines which are currently being developed as attempts for treatment or prevention of cervical cancer.

REFERENCES

1. Spradbrow PB (1987) Immune response to papillomavirus infection. In: Syrjänen K, Gissmann L. and Koss LG, Eds, *Papillomaviruses and Human Disease* pp 334–370 Springer Verlag, Berlin.
2. Almeida JD, Oriel JD, Stannard LM (1969) Characterization of the virus found in human genital warts *Microbios*. 3, 225–232.
3. Pfister H, Nürnberger F, Gissmann L, zur Hausen H (1981) Characterization of human papillomavirus from epidermodysplasia verruciformis lesions of a patient from Upper-Volta *Int. J. Cancer* 27, 645–650.
4. Schiller JT, Roden R BS (1995) Papillomavirus-like particles *Papillomavirus Rep.* 6:121–128.
5. Gissmann L and Müller M (1994) Serological immune response to HPV In: P Stern and M Stanley (Eds), *Human Papillomaviruses and Cervical Cancer* pp 133–144 Oxford University Press.
6. Dillner J (1994) Antibodies to defined HPV epitopes in cervical neoplasia *Papillomavirus Report* 5:35–41.
7. Viscidi R, Shah KV (1992) Immune response to infections with human papillomaviruses. In: Quinn, T.C., Gallin, J.I. and Fauci, A.S. Eds, *Advances in Host Defense Mechanisms*, Vol 8, New York, Raven Press.
8. Müller M, Viscidi RP, Sun Y, Guerrero E, Hill PM, Shah F, Bosch FX, Munoz N, Gissmann L, Shah KV (1992) Antibodies to HPV 16 E6 and E7 proteins as markers for HPV16-associated invasive cervical cancer *Virology* 187, 508–514.
9. Nindl I, Benitez-Bribiesca L, Berumen J, Farmanara N, Fisher S, Gross G, Müller M, Tommasino M, Vazquez-Curiel A, Gissmann L (1994) Antibodies against linear and conformational epitopes of the human papillomavirus (HPV) type 16 E6 and E7 oncoproteins in sera of cervical cancer patients *Arch. Virol.* 137:341–353.
10. Mann VM, Loo de Lao S, Brenes M, Brinton LA, Rawls LA, Green M, Reeves WC, Rawls WE (1990) Occurrence of IgA and IgG antibodies to select peptides representing human papillomavirus type 16 among cervical cancer cases and controls *Cancer Res.* 50, 7815–7819.
11. Bleul C, Müller M, Frank R, Gausepohl H, Koldovsky U, Mgaya HN, Luande J, Pawlita M, ter Meulen J, Viscidi R, Gissmann L (1991) Human papillomavirus type 18 E6 and E7 antibodies in human sera: Increased anti-E7 prevalence in cervical cancer patients *J. Clin. Microbiol.* 29, 1579–1588.
12. Suchankova A, Krchnak V, Vagner J, Krcmar M, Ritterova L, Vonka V (1992) Epitope mapping of the human papillomavirus type 16 E4 protein by synthetic peptides *J. Gen. Virol.* 73, 429–432.
13. IARC Monographs on the *Evaluation of Carcinogenic Risks to Humans* (1995) Vol 64: Human papillomaviruses. Lyon.

14. Bonnez W, Da-Rin C, Rose RC, Reichman RC (1991) Use of human papillomavirus type 11 virions in an ELISA to detect specific antibodies in humans with condylomata acuminata *J. Gen.Virol.* 72, 1343–1347.

15. Bonnez W, Kashima HK, Leventhal B, Mounts P, Rose RC, Reichman RC, Shah KV (1992) Antibody response to human papillomavirus (HPV) type 11 in children with juvenile-onset recurrent respiratory papillomatosis (RRP) *Virology* 188, 384–387.

16. Carter JJ, Hagensee MB, Lee SK, McKnight B, Koutsky LA, Galloway DA (1994) Use of HPV 1 capsids produced by recombinant vaccinia viruses in an ELISA to detect serum antibodies in people with foot warts *Virology* 199:284–291.

17. Carter JJ, Wipf GC, Hagensee ME, McKnight B, Habel LA, Lee SK, Kuypers J, Kiviat N, Daling JR, Koutsky LA, Watts DH, Holmes KK, Galloway DA (1995) Use of human papillomavirus type 6 capsid to detect antibodies in people with genital warts *J. Infect. Dis.* 172:11–18.

18. Rose RC, Reichman RC, Bonnez W (1994) Human papillomavirus (HPV) type 11 recombinant virus-like particles induce the formation of neutralizing antibodies and detect HPV-specific antibodies in human sera *J. Gen. Virol.* 75:2075–2079.

19. Kirnbauer R, Hubbert N, Wheeler CM, Becker TM, Lowy DR, Schiller JT (1994) A virus-like particle enzyme-linked immunosorbent assay detects serum antibodies in a majority of women infected with human papillomavirus type 16 *J. Natl. Cancer Inst.* 86:494–499.

20. Jochmus-Kudielka I, Schneider A, Braun R, Kimmig R, Koldovsky U, Schneweis KE, Seedorf K, Gissmann L (1989) Antibodies against the human papillomavirus type 16 early proteinsin human sera: Correlation of anti-E7 reactivity and cervical cancer *J. Natl. Cancer Inst.* 81, 1698–1704.

21. Jha P, Beral V, Peto J, Hack S, Hermon C, Deacon J, Mant D, Chilvers C, Vessey MP, Pike MC, Müller M, Gissmann L (1993) Antibodies to human papillomavirus and to other genital infections and their relation to invasive cervical cancer risk *Lancet,* 341, 1116–1118.

22. Dillner J, Dillner L, Robb J, Willems J, Jones I, Lancaster W, Smith R, Lerner R (1989) A synthetic peptide defines a serologic IgA response to a human papillomavirus-encoded nuclear antigen expressed in virus-carrying cervical neoplasia *Proc. Natl. Acad. Sci. U.S.A.* 86, 3838–3841.

23. Lehtinen M, Leminen A, Paavonen J, Lehtovirta P, Hyoty H,Vesterinen E, Dillner J (1992) Predominance of serum antibodies to synthetic peptide stemming from HPV 18 open reading frame E2 in cervical adenocarcinoma *J. Clin. Pathol.* 45, 494–497.

24. Kanda T, Onda T, Zanma S, Yasugi T, Furuno A, Watanabe S,Kawana T, Sugase M, Ueda K, Sonoda T, Suzuki S, Yamashiro T, Yoshikawa H, Yoshiike K (1992) Independent association of antibodies against human papillomavirustype 16 E1/E4 and E7 proteins with cervical cancer *Virology* 190, 724–732.

25. Köchel HG, Monazahian M, Sievert K, Hoehne M, Thomssen C, Teichmann A, Arendt P, Thomssen R (1991) Occurrence of antibodies to L1, L2, E4 and E7 gene products of human papillomavirus types 6b, 16 and 18 among cervical cancer patients and controls *Int. J. Cancer* 48, 682–688.

26. Baird PJ (1983) Serological evidence for the association of papillomavirus and cervical neoplasia *Lancet* 2, 17–18.

27. Dillner L, Moreno-Lopez J, Dillner J (1990) Serological responses to papillomavirus group-specific antigens in women with neoplasia of the uterine cervix *J. Clin. Microbiol.* 28, 624–627.

28. Steger G, Olszewsky M, Stockfleth E, Pfister H (1990) Prevalence of antibodies to human papillomavirus type 8 in human sera *J. Virol.* 64, 4399–4406.

29. Nonnenmacher B, Hubbert NL, Kirnbauer R, Shah KV, Munoz N, Bosch FX, de Sanjose S, Viscidi R, Lowy DR, Schiller JT (1995) Serologic response to human papillomavirus type 16 virus-like particles in HPV 16 DNA positive invasive cervical cancer and cervical intraepithelial neoplasia grade III patients and controls from Colombia and Spain *J. Infect. Dis.* 172:19–24.

30. Heim K, Christensen ND, Höpfl RM, Wartusch B, Pinzger G, Zeimet AQ, Baumgartner P, Kreider JW, Dapunt O (1995) Serum IgG, IgM and IgA reactivity to human papillomavirus types 11 and 6 virus-like particles in different gynecologic patient groups *J. Inf. Dis.* 172:395–402.

31. Wikstrom A, Eklund C, von Krogh G, Lidbrink P, Dillner J (1992) Levels of immunoglobulin G antibodies against defined epitopes ofthe L1 and L2 capsid proteins are elevated in men with a history ofcondylomata acuminata *J. Clin. Microbiol.* 30, 1795–1800.

32. Bonnez W, Da Rin C, Rose RC, Tyring SK, Reichman RC (1993) Evolution of antibody response to human papillomavirus type 11 (HPV 11) in patients with condyloma acuminatum according to treatment response *J. Med. Virol.* 39;340–344.

33. Dillner J (1990) Mapping of linear epitopes of human papillomavirus type 16: the E1,E2, E3, E4, E5, E6 and E7 open reading frames *Int. J. Cancer* 46 703–711.

34. Krchnak V, Vagner J, Suchankova A, Krcmar M, Ritterova L, VonkaV (1990) Synthetic peptides derived from the E7 region of human papillomavirus type 16 used as antigens in ELISA *J. Gen. Virol.* 71, 2719–2724.

35. Tindle RW, Smith JA, Geysen HM, Selvey LA, Frazer IH (1990) Identification of B epitopes in human papillomavirus type 16 E7 open reading frame protein *J. Gen. Virol.* 71, 1347–1354.

36. Selvey LA, Tindle RW, Geysen HM, Smith JA, Frazer IH (1990) Identification of B-epitopes in the human papillomavirus 18 E7 open reading frame protein *J. Immunol.* 145, 3105–3110.

37. Müller M, Gausepohl H, de Martynoff G, Frank R, Brasseur, R, Gissmann L (1990) Identification of seroreactive regions of the human papillomavirus type 16 protein E4, E6, E7 and L1 *J. Gen. Virol.* 71, 2709–2717.

38. Eschle D, Dürst M, ter Meulen J, Luande J, Eberhardt HC, Pawlita M, Gissmann L (1992) Geographic dependence of sequence variations in the E7 gene of human papillomavirus type 16 *J. Gen. Virol.* 73, 1829–1832.

39. ter Meulen J, Schweigler AC, Eberhardt HC, Luande J, Mgaya HN, Müller M, Bleul C, Ulken V, Ikenberg H, Pawlita M, Gissmann L (1993) Sequence variation in the E7 gene of human papillomavirus type 18 in tumor and non-tumor patients and antibody response to a conserved seroreactive epitope *Int. J. Cancer* 53, 1–3.

40. Fisher SG, Benitez-Bribiesca L, Nindl I, Stockfleth E, Müller M, Wolf H, Gissmann L (1996) The association of human papillomavirus type 16 E6 and E7 antibodies with stage of cervical cancer *Gynecol. Oncol.* 61, 73–78.

41. Wank R, Thomssen C (1991) High risk of squamous cell carcinoma of the cervix for women with HLA-DQw3 *Nature* 352, 723–725.

42. Wank R, Schendel DJ, Thomssen C (1992) HLA antigens and cervical carcinoma *Nature* 356, 22–2331.

43. Helland A, Borresen AL, Kaern J, Ronningen KS, Thorsby E (1992) HLA antigens and cervical carcinoma *Nature* 356, 23.

44. Apple RJ, Erlich HA, Klitz W, Manos MM, Becker TM, Wheeler CM (1994) HLA DR-DQ associations with cervical carcinoma show papillomavirus type specificity *Nat. Genet.* 6, 157–162.

45. Gregoire L, Lawrence WD, Kukuruga D, Eisenbrey AB, Lancaster WD (1994) Association between HLA-DQB1 allels and risk for cervical cancer in African-American women *Int. J. Cancer* 57, 504–507.

46. Jenison SA, Yu X-P, Valentine JM, Koutsky LA, Christiansen AE, Beckmann AM, Galloway DA (1990) Evidence of prevalent genital-type human papillomavirus infections in adults and children *J. Inf. Dis.* 162, 60–69.

47. Klaus Mund and LG, unpublished data.

48. Shah KV, Howley PM (1990) Papillomaviruses In: Fields BN, Knipe DM, Chanock RM, Hirsch MS, Melnick JL, MonathTP, Roizman B (Eds) *Virology*, pp 1651-1678 Raven Press, New York.

49. McLean CS, Sterling JS, Mowat J, Nash AA, Stanley MA (1993) Delayed-type hypersensitivity response to human papillomavirus type 16 E7 protein in a mouse model *J. Gen. Virol.* 74:239–245.

50. Schneider A, Kirchhoff T, Meinhardt G, Gissmann L (1992) Repeated evalution of human papillomavirus 16 status in cervical swabs of young women with a history of normal Papanicolaou smears *Obstet. Gynecol.* 79, 683–688.

VII. Therapy

21

Skin Warts

Gerd Gross

CONTENTS

0-8493-7356-5/97/$0.00+$.50
© 1997 by CRC Press, Inc.

I.   INTRODUCTION

Since antiquity, the removal of warts has represented a therapeutic problem. At the beginning of the first century A.D., Celsus[1-3] recommended for the treatment of warts burning them away with the ash of wine-lees, or a mixture of alum and Sandarac resin. Other physicians tried to cure warts by the application of juices from various plants, by rubbing them with pork fat, or with a green alder stick that was then buried in muck to rot.[4-9] Perhaps some also followed the advice of Huckleberry Finn: "Say, what is dead cats good for, Huck? — Good for? Cure warts with."[10]

Nowadays patients request removal of warts for a variety of reasons. Warts on the hands or face are easily noticed by others and present a cosmetic problem to the patient. Plantar warts can be so painful that they hinder standing and walking. In addition, it is becoming common knowledge to patients that a wart is virus-induced, and thus these patients are extremely concerned that the wart will multiply and spread to other parts of the body as well as infect family members and friends.

But not every wart has to be treated. Skin warts usually regress spontaneously. It is generally stated that 35% of patients lose their warts within 2–6 months, 53% within 1 year, and 67% within 2 years.[11] On the other hand, there are a considerable number of people whose warts persist for many years in spite of aggressive therapy. Therefore, it is essential to explain all of the risks and benefits of any wart therapy before embarking on a clinical course.

This chapter is concerned basically with therapeutic modalities that are currently favored by most clinicans in ihe field. But some newer, still experimental approaches in particulary recalcitrant cases of HPV infections will also be discussed. It should be appreciated that no completely effective therapy for warts exists. The decision regarding which treatment to use depends on a number of factors, which include the size, location, and type of wart, and the immune status of the patient. In addition, the degree of pain, the risk of scarring, and the patient's commitment to the therapy all enter into the decision on which treatment modality to use.

II.   CHEMICAL TREATMENT

The majority of warts may be treated at home by the patient or his family. The need of careful instruction in the procedures to be used is a prerequisite for a successful result. Somewhat more agressive treatments need to be reserved for specialists such as the dermatologist or the surgeon.

A.   Salicylic Acid

The use of salicylic acid is an excellent first-line treatment for warts on the hands and feet. As Huber and Christophers reported,[12] salicylic acid does not affect the virus directly but, by destroying intercellular cohesiveness in the upper part of the stratum corneum, facilitates the removal of squames containing the active virus. There are numerous commercial preparations of salicylic acid in strengths varying from 10 to 40% as tinctures and plasters. Collodon-based solutions (16% salicylic acid with an equal part of lactic acid) are the most convenient preparations as they can be applied quickly and accurately and are cosmetically acceptable when used on the hands. Paints should not be applied to the facial or anogenital skin. For the treatment of extensive areas of plantar warts, salicylic acid plasters in concentrations of 20 to 40% are suitable. The success rate of these simple procedures is satisfactory. After three months of use, warts in 67% of patients with hand warts, 84% with simple plantar warts and 45% with mosaic plantar warts are completely resolved.[13] Hypersensitivity reactions are rare and resolve rapidly with the discontinuation of the treatment.

B.   Formalin

Formalin is a solution of 40% formaldehyde in water and is used in concentrations of 2 to 3%. The traditional way of treating plantar warts with formalin, particularly for warts occurring on weight-bearing areas, is to soak them in 3% formalin lotion for 10 minutes each night. These applications produce hardening and drying of the skin surface, following which the warts may be shelled out. Other remedies contain 3 to 20% in water or may be prepared in a cream base. The efficacy against plantar warts is comparable to salicylic acid.[14-16] Side-effects from formalin therapy include dryness of the skin and painful fissures as well as rare allergic contact dermatitis.

C.   Glutaraldehyde

A water-based solution of 10% glutaraldehyde has the same indication, way of action, and efficacy as formalin, but it is more powerful and more rapidly acting. It combines chemically with keratin producing brownish polymers, and like formalin it is an anhydrotic and a sensitizer. Side-effects are similar to those of formalin therapy. In addition, glutaraldehyde turns the skin brown in the treated area, and the patient must be made aware of this to avoid concern.

Salicylic acid, formalin, and glutaraldehyde can be used for home treatment.

D.   Strong Acids

Another chemical treatment for warts is the application of stronger acids, such as nitric acids or mono-, bi- and, trichloroacetic acids at concentrations of 50%. This therapy is reserved for resistant plantar mosaic warts. These acids are powerful irritants that work hydrolyzing the cellular protein, which leads to inflammation and cell death. They do not bind preferentially to the wart-infected cells and can cause destruction and produce scarring of the surrounding normal skin if not carefully applied. Therefore, these agents have to be applied by experts only. The surface hyperkeratosis is initially pared away and then a small quantity of the saturated acid is carefully applied using a pointed stick and is allowed to dry. The area is then covered with a piece of salicylic acid plaster (20 or 40%), which is left in place for several days.[17] Therapy is repeated on a weekly basis until the wart is cured. Unfortunately, the effect of this therapy is as poorly documented for the treatment of skin warts, as the topical application of Solcoderm™ (several organic acids and traces of copper in 6.6N nitric acid). In the treatment of condylomata acuminata, however, Solcoderm™ is effective.[18]

III.   CRYOTHERAPY

Cryotherapy is currently the most popular treatment for benign and malignant skin lesions, including skin warts. The two most commonly used freezing agents are carbon dioxide snow, which boils at –79°C, and liquid nitrogen (–195.8°C). Cryotherapy works mainly by destroying the host cell and stimulating an immune response to the area.[19]

A.   Carbon Dioxide Snow

Carbon dioxide snow, or dry ice, is obtained by passing carbon dioxide gas rapidly through a cylinder. It can be formed into a carbon dioxide stick with a mold, which should be smaller than the wart. Carbon dioxide snow can also be made into a slush by adding a few drops of acetone; it is applied to the wart with a cotton-tipped applicator.

B.   Liquid Nitrogen

For several reasons, the alternative use of liquid nitrogen has become more and more common for wart therapy. It does not have to be formed in any way and is simply stored in a deware holding flask. These flasks can maintain the liquid nitrogen for months. In addition, the lower temperature of liquid nitrogen, compared with carbon dioxide snow, means that the duration of treatment on the wart is shorter. Liquid nitrogen is applied to the wart with a cotton wool ball adjusted to the size of the wart. Evaporation occurs rapidly, so the ball needs to be applied immediately to the lesion. The ball should not be redipped into the liquid nitrogen after application to the skin because of the possible risk of transferring infection from one patient to another, especially if the warts have been pared down and are bleeding.[20]

During the past 3 decades, major improvements of cryotherapy technique with liquid nitrogen have taken place. Convenient, portable, hand-held spray units have been developed. Cryosprays deliver liquid nitrogen to the skin through flexible cables to and from hollow cryoprobe tips of various sizes. The liquid nitrogen is delivered more quickly, more accurately, and with greater reliability of the depth and speed of the freeze than with the cotton ball technique. This makes cryosprays suitable for eradication of warts with pronounced endo- or exophytic growth pattern. During freezing, the tip of the spray should be held 5–10 mm away from the surface of the skin and the spray directed to the center of the lesion.

In general, liquid nitrogen is applied with a cotton ball or by spraying until a frozen pale halo of 1–2 mm appears around the base of the wart, indicating that the full depth has been frozen. Duration of application obviously depends on the size of the wart. In the case of facial warts no more than about 5–10 s should be spent on the first freezing with liquid nitrogen. Flat warts in other areas may be frozen for 10–20 s. Verrucae vulgares seldom require more than 30–40 s, while large plantar warts may need 1 min. For extensive mosaic warts, a stepwise treatment of different areas is recommended, leaving untreated areas for body support between sessions. Remember, however, that longer freeze times may be associated with side-effects and do not always guarantee a cure. Rademaker et al.[21] reported a cure rate of only 58% for resistant mosaic plantar warts treated by agressive freezing under general anaesthesia.

Additionally, the use of Freon-12, dichlorodifluoromethane, for the treatment of warts has been documented by McDow and Webster.[22] Freon-12 has a boiling point of −29.79°C and can freeze the skin to −20° to −30°C, which is adequate to cause destruction of a superficial skin lesion. 90% of warts treated with this modality have been completely cured with one or two treatments.[22]

Although cryotherapy is highly successful, easily performed, and well tolerated, there are a few complications that must be considered. Scarring is rare but has been reported. Pigmentary change can occur, with hypopigmentation being a particular problem in darkly pigmented individuals. Longer freeze times have occasionally damaged peripheral nerves, with the resulting anaesthesia persisting for months.[23] Therefore, a careful discussion of possible problems with cryotherapy should be carried out prior to treatment.

IV. SURGICAL INTERVENTION

One of the oldest therapeutic approaches to the removal of warts is surgical intervention. Patients frequently request that a wart be either cut out or burned off, believing that this will be the end of the matter. However, there is still a significant recurrence rate with the surgical approach.[14] Morison[19] concluded that the removal of the bulk of the viral antigen could be responsible for an absence of an immune response following surgical removal. Other arguments against surgical intervention include the need of anaesthesia, significant post-operative pain, risk of secondary infection, and inconvenience to the patient.

Scalpel surgery is contraindicated not only because of the high recurrence rate of this technique but also because of possible cyst formation after suture, especially if the wart is located at the plantar aspect of the foot.

A. Curettage

Papillomatous common warts can be scooped off very easily with a sharp spoon curette under local anaesthesia. Haemostasis is obtained by touching the base with a silver nitrate pencil or $FeCl_3$ solution. If curettage is skillfully performed, scarring should be minimal.

B.   Electrosurgery

Certain recalcitrant warts that have been resistant to chemical treatment and cryotherapy are possible candidates for electrosurgery. Small filiform or papillomatous warts are easily removed after initial anaesthetizing of the affected area. However, electrosurgery should be avoided for treatment of plantar surfaces, where irreversible scarring may be more painful than the original warts.

The mechanism of electrosurgery is local destruction by heat.[24] As the current passes through tissue, it encounters electrical resistance, and heat is produced. Charred tissue is wiped away with a dry swab. Unfortunately, a considerable amount of heat transfer to the surrounding normal tissue is leading to local pain and scarring. Therefore, this aggressive treatment is reserved only for recalcitrant warts.

C.   Laser Surgery

Over the past 10 years, the carbon dioxide (CO_2) laser has been used more frequently for the treatment of all types of warts. The CO_2 laser in conjunction with the operating microscope provides good visualization of the field with minimal bleeding and possibly a somewhat reduced rate of recurrence. CO_2 lasers with a wavelength of 10 600 nm are useful as cutting tools, because this wavelength is strongly absorbed by cellular water, so that tissue vaporization is achieved by cellular dehydration at high temperatures.[25,26] It is possible to distinguish wart tissue from normal tissue during laser treatment, because the former gives an appearance of bubbling, whereas the normal tissue appears to melt.[27]

Published success rates of use of CO_2 laser for treatment of various warts and condylomata, including recalcitrant lesions, have been impressive in some reports, with positive outcomes around 90%;[28,29] more recent reports have shown responses around 30%.[30,31]

Other lasers in surgical intervention of recalcitrant warts are the argon and the neodymium-yttrium-aluminium-garnet (Nd:YAG) instruments. Similar success rates to CO_2 laser treatment are reported.[32-34] Whereas the results of laser vaporization are no better than those obtained by currettage and electrosurgery,[17] Nd:YAG laser hyperthermia induced regression seems to have a number of advantages, such as absence of bleeding and scarring as well as the low degree of pains together with the low costs if a Nd:YAG laser is present.

V.   PHARMACOLOGIC AGENTS

Of patients with viral warts, 60 to 80% can be cured within 3 months by conventional methods of treatment.[13] But there remains a hard core whose warts persist despite prolonged and rigorous attack. Pharmacologic agents should usually only be considered after standard therapy has failed. In each case, the possible benefits of treatment have to be weighed against the potential side-effects.

A.   Cantharidin

Cantharidin (dried extract of Spanish fly), is a powerful vesiculating agent and a proven therapy for almost all nongenital warts. It acts by blistering the skin as a result of acantholysis and death of the epidermal cells, but leaves no scarring as the basal cell layer remains intact.[35] Treatment of skin warts with a 0.7% solution of cantharidin in equal parts of acetone and flexible collodion was detailed by Epstein and Kligman.[36] Cantharidin therapy has a cure rate of approximately 80% for common, plantar, and periungual warts. The major side-effect is pain from the blister. This can be relieved by puncturing the blister with a sterile needle and then soaking the involved area. Cantharidin is used infrequently in the United Kingdom.

B.   Podophyllin and Podophyllotoxin

Podophyllin is a mixture of resins obtained from the rhizomes of *Podophyllum peltatum* and *Podophyllum emodi*. In a 25% liquid paraffin preparation, it is a powerful antimitotic agent, provoking inflammation of the skin and mucous membranes. Podophyllin has been associated with systemic toxicity, especially when used in treating genital warts. Local side-effects include erythema, swelling, tenderness, burning, and on occasion superficial erosion. Fatality has been reported with the use of the topical resin, in one incident with application to a large surface area,[37] whereas other reported cases of death have followed ingestion of the resin.[38] Nevertheless, this technique which is said to cure approximately 80 to 90% of deep plantar warts as shown by Duthie and McCallum in 1951 is not commonly used.[39]

A new alternative to podophyllin, but only for the treatment of genitoanal HPV infections, is a purified solution of podophyllotoxin. In contrast to podophyllin resin, podophyllotoxin appears to be significantly less toxic. Several studies have documented the efficacy of 0.5% podophyllotoxin applied by the patients at home for the treatment of mollusca contagiosa.[40,41] Cure rates of 53 to 94% have been reported by placebo-controlled studies with this self-administered preparation applied twice daily for 3 days. Unfortunately, the application of podophyllotoxin for the treatment of skin warts has not been documented up to now.

C.   Bleomycin

Similar cure rates have been reported using bleomycin.[42,43] Bleomycin is a cytotoxic polypeptide that is known to inhibit DNA synthesis in cells and viruses. Presumably, this interaction is due to its ability to bind to DNA, resulting in strand scission with elimination of purine and pyrimidine bases.[44] The actual mechanism by which bleomycin causes resolution of warts is still unknown.

Treatment of warts with the use of bleomycin involves intralesional injections. Bleomycin is reconstituted in normal saline solution at concentrations of up to 20 mg/ml. Intralesional injections of bleomycin are indicated in the treatment of viral warts that have failed to respond to several months of treatment with topical preparations or to cryotherapy. It is particularly useful when adequate surgical removal by curettage might pose problems, for example in periungual warts. Disadvantages to the use of bleomycin include swelling, erythema, and nail dystrophy in periungual warts.[43] Even Raynaud's phenomenon has been reported after treatment of periungual warts, although rarely being persistent.[45] In addition, one case of urticaria has been reported.[46]

D.   5-Fluorouracil (5-FU)

5-FU has a special affinity for abnormal keratinocytes and their subsequent destruction by inhibition of DNA and RNA synthesis as well as an immunostimmulatory action.[47] Topical 5-FU has been used most successfully for the treatment of verrucae planae with a cure rate of up to 80% of patients with recalcitrant disease.[47] The cure rate of other skin warts is, however, not particularly high.

E.   Retinoids

Retinoids are a class of natural or synthetic compounds structurally related to vitamin A comprising all trans retinoic acid (tretinoin), 13-cis retinoic acid (isotretinoin), and the aromatic retinoids (etretinate and acitretin). Retinoids bind to a specific cellular receptor and produce numerous effects, including alteration of epidermal proliferation and keratin differentiation as well as immunomodulatory activity. Because HPV replication appears linked to the state of keratinocyte differentiation, retinoids could potentionally block the production of new viral particles. Finally, they are capable of preventing malignant transformation, a function theoretically applicable to HPV-induced neoplasia.

Several reports have documented beneficial results with retinoids used for immunosuppressed patients with HPV disease. Both Boyle et al. and Gross et al.[48,49] found orally-given aromatic retinoids have a beneficial effect on recalcitrant common warts in immunosuppressed patients (Figure 1). Oral retinoids were also given with some success to patients with HPV 5-induced epidermodysplasia verruciformis.[50,51] Isotretinoin has been successfully used by Katz[52] in a patient with Hodgkin's disease and recalcitrant cutaneous warts. Acitretin was reported by Rogozinski et al.[53] to also be of some benefit in the treatment of three patients with common warts. But there have been no placebo-controlled controlled studies up to now.

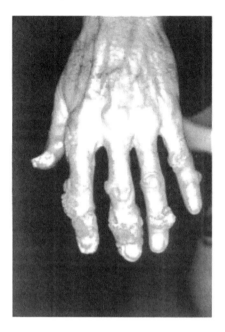

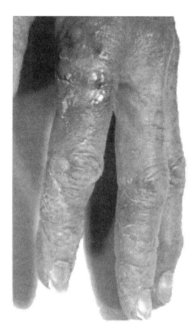

A   B

FIGURE 1   A) Common warts of the hands of a 81-year old man suffering from chronic lymphatic leukemia; B) Subtotal remission during oral therapy with etretinae.

VI.   IMMUNOTHERAPY

The susceptibility of individuals depends on the efficacy of their immune system. It has been suggested that patients with warts have some reduction of immune responsiveness and it is well established that those with immune deficiencies usually develop widespread, resistant warts.[13] In such cases it is necessary to look for treatment modalities that either stimulate a patient's own immune system or provoke a delayed hypersensitivity reaction.

A.   Dinitrochlorobenzene (DNCB)

DNCB is a potent sensitizing agent that has been used for the treatment of recalcitrant warts for nearly 20 years. The technique is to apply DNCB, 2% in acetone, to the outer aspect of the upper arm to sensitize the patient. Sensitivity usually develops within 2 weeks. The warts are then treated with a daily application of 0.1% DNCB. Succes rates of up to 90% have been reported.[54,55] The common complication is excessive irritation of the wart. The problem with DNCB sensitization is the possibilty of developing cross-reactions and contact dermatitis to other chemically related substances. Dinitrochlorobenzene does cross-react with nitrobenzene compounds, which are used in the chemical and agricultural industries. *In vitro* DNCB is mutagenic;[56] therefore, Bunney et al. recommended no longer using it in the routine treatment of warts.[17]

B.   Interferon

Interferons (IFNs) are proteins regarded as one of the natural body defenses against viral infections. These proteins also play important roles in combating tumors and regulating immunity. Interferons are not a single molecular species but consist of three families of protein molecules (α, β, and γ)[57] whose production can be induced in a number of body cells, and today they can be manufactured by recombinant biotechnology. Their mechanism of action involves antiviral, antiproliferative, antitumoral, and immunomodulatory activities, which are produced by binding to specific cell membrane receptors and altering the cellular metabolism.[58,59]

Successful results were obtained with the use of intralesional IFN-β injections in common warts, with 81% of interferon-treated lesions responding, compared with only 17% of those treated with placebo.[60] Recent studies documented even higher cure rates in treatment of common warts by systemic administration of IFN-β, and no relapse of cured warts has been observed[61,62] (Figure 2). Schoenfeldt et al.[63] reported that flat facial warts can be successfully treated with IFN-β cream.

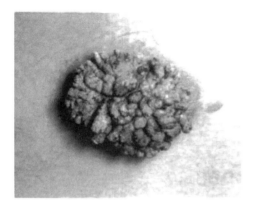 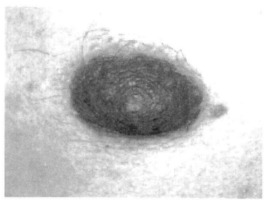

A   **B**

FIGURE 2   A) 18-year-old atopic man with common wart-like lesions of the mamilla (HPV 6 DNA positive); B) Complete healing after interferon alpha 2c therapy (dose 3 MU per subcutaneous injection, 5 times per week, 4 weeks pause; 3 cycles).

Therapy with IFN is frequently associated with mild to moderate systemic toxic side-effects characterized by a flu-like syndrome that usually starts 2 to 4 hours following the first in a series of IFN injections. In addition, patients given higher doses of IFN (>5 Mio. International Units) may experience nausea, vomiting, somnolence, anorexia, hypotension, tachycardia, and rashes.[59,61] Interferon therapy in pregnant women is currently thought to be contraindicated due to the antiproliferative and immunomodulating activity of IFNs.

Because of the toxicity and cost, IFN is unlikely to become a primary therapy of cutaneous warts. But in combination with conventional therapies, IFNs have found their place in the treatment of HPV-associated disease. Combination of IFN and retinoids could be another particularly promising therapy of HPV infections of both the mucosal and cutaneous sites.[64]

C.   Inosine Pranobex

In the recent years inosine pranobex, a molecular complex of inosine and the p-acetamidobenzoic acid salt of N-N dimethylaminoisopropanol, has been used as an immunopotentiating and antiviral agent in the treatment of viral infections. Several studies have demonstrated that orally given inosine pranobex may induce a significant regression of genital warts, particularly when given as an adjuvant to other therapeutic measurements,[17] but the use of inosine pranobex for treatment of cutaneous warts showed that the drug was no better than placebo.[65] In combination with conventional therapies such as plasters containing salicylic acid, however, good results were obtained in periungual and resistant plantar warts (personal observations, Figure 3).

VII.   PSYCHOTHERAPY

Up to the present day, the folklore concerning the removal of warts has continued to be expanded and embellished. The medical literature has likewise contributed its share of numerous anecdotal

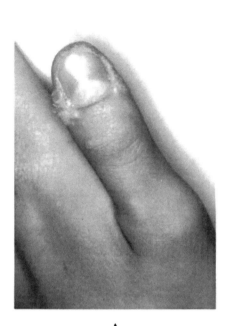
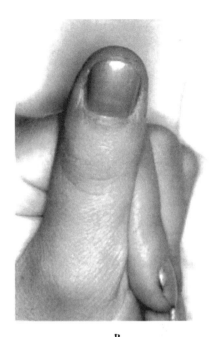

A   B

FIGURE 3   A) Periungual warts; B) Complete clearance after oral Inosine pranobex.

reports, not unlike the method of Huckleberry Finn.[10] Only in the last 2 decades several placebo-controlled studies have demonstrated improvement of warts by suggestion and hypnosis.[66-68]

A. Suggestion

Early reports on the efficacy of skin wart treatment by suggestion and charms are anecdotal. Subsequent large-scale studies have been difficult to evaluate due to lack of comparative groups receiving placebo or other treatment types. In 1965, Clarke[69] reviewed a considerable number of these reports and was dissatisfied by the methods used. He considered the cure to be attributable to suggestion in less than 1% of cases and that spontaneous regression occured in 20% of patients not receiving any therapy. This view was shared by Stankler[70] who proposed that the success of suggestion depended upon fortuitous temporal relationship between treatment and spontaneous resolution.

B. Hypnosis

The most commonly reported psychologic treatments include hypnotic suggestion and placebo intervention, including painting of warts with innocuous colored liquids and injecting placebos. Ullman and Dudek[71] claimed that patients who were good hypnotic subjects responded significantly better than those who were not easily put into a deep hypnotic state. One interesting report was by Tasini and Hackett[72] who cured, within 3 months, the widespread warts of three immunocompromised children in whom spontaneous resolution would not have been expected. A recent controlled study demonstrated that hypnotic suggestion was significantly more effective than was placebo or no treatment.[68]

VIII. RECOMMENDATIONS

As warts tend to spontaneous regression without leaving any trace, they should be treated in a gentle, nonscarring way. Any form of therapy should cause no hazard to the patient and only minimal pain, side-effects, and inconvenience. This limitation excludes certain forms of treatment such as surgical intervention leaving permanent scars, use of general anaesthesia with its small but inherent risk, and systemic application of nonspecific immunotherapies since incalculable, severe side-effects may arise.

A.   Facial Warts

Common warts on the face are best treated by freezing superficially and this is well tolerated even in children. More than one treatment is usually required, given at two or three weeks intervals. Single, large, common warts can be removed by electrosurgery under local anaesthesia. The patient must be reviewed 4 to 6 weeks afterwards because of the possibility of recurrence.

The regimen for flat (plane) facial warts especially in young children is to use no treatment. Most warts regress spontaneously and disappear without a trace. Pressure for treatment from the parents of young children should be kindly and firmly resisted. Occasionally, mild peeling agents, such as 1% salicylic acid cream or retin-A gel, applied to individual lesions, can be used to improve the cosmetic appearance.

Plane facial warts which show no spontaneous regression during about 4 months can be successfully treated with topical retinoic acid (tretinoin) or IFN-β cream. If extensive disfiguring plane warts occur in adults, the best treatment is careful freezing. But this therapy should only be given when the patient is aware of the side-effects, such as scarring, pigmentary changes, etc. Freezing is also the treatment of choice for scalp warts and for common warts on the eyelids. Common warts in the nasal vestibules can be frozen or removed by scissorsnip excision, curettage, cautery, or by electrodesiccation.

"Beard warts" represent a problem, because shaving disseminates warts rapidly and widely throughout the whole beard area. Therefore, stopping shaving will be helpful. A single, sizeable wart is best removed by electro-surgery followed by careful reexamination over the next 2 months. Multiple and smaller warts are best treated by weekly freezing.

B.   Hand Warts

The best first-line treatment for warts on the hands is the use of salicylic acid (10–40%) which is dispensed in paints, gels, pastes, or plasters. Whereas periungual warts are successfully treated with salicylic acid in combination with inosine pranobex (personal observation), resistant warts can be removed by cryosurgery or with a sharp spoon curette under local anaesthesia. The result of curettage of multiple periungual warts, however, is poor and the procedure rarely worth undertaking. As in the case of facial plane warts, plane warts of the hand will resolve in the immunocompetent host after a few years and are best left alone.

C.   Plantar Warts

In the first place, plantar warts should be treated with a salicylic acid (10–40%) or a formalin (2–3%) preparation to pare away the keratin cap of the warts. A combined treatment of freezing at intervals of 3 weeks with nightly applications of a salicylic acid paint between freezing might hasten the resolution of the warts. The application of mono-, bi- or, trichloroacetic acids at concentrations of 50% is a further useful therapy for resistant plantar mosaic warts.

Hot water treatments are a useful therapy for plantar warts. The wart is soaked in 45–48°C common salt-water for 5 to 10 minutes after 3 days applications of 60% salicylic acid-preparations.

D.   Extensive or Recalcitrant Warts

Recalcitrant warts that have been resistant to chemical treatment or cryotherapy are possible candidates for electro- or lasersurgery (CO_2, argon, Nd:YAG). Even during pregnancy, laser treatment represents the treatment of choice if there is no response to cryotherapy. Intralesional injections of bleomycin are indicated in the treatment of warts that have failed to respond to several months of treatment with topical preparations or to cryotherapy. Intralesional or systemic injections of IFN-α or IFN-β can be of value in recalcitrant common warts (Figure 2), and orally-given aromatic retinoids have a beneficial effect in immunosuppressed patients with multiple warts (Figure 1) and severe cutaneous dysplasia or

TABLE 1 Standardized Therapy of Skin Warts

	Limited Disease
Topical	salicylic acid-preparations (10–40%)
	formalin (2–3%)
	glutaraldehyde (10%)
	mono-, bi-, trichloroacetic acid (5%)
	podophyllin (15%)
	5-FU (5%)
	retinoic acid
Surgery	scissor-snip excision
	curettage
	cryotherapy
Psychotherapy	
	Extensive or Recalcitrant Warts
Surgery	cryotherapy, electrocauter, lasersurgery
	(CO_2, argon, Nd:YAG)
Topical	bleomycin
	5-FU
	IFN-β intralesional
	DNCB
	retinoic acid
Systemic	retinoids (etretinate, acitretin)
	IFN-α, IFN-β
	inosine pranobex
Psychotherapy	hypnotic suggestion, placebo intervention

squamous cell malignancy. Topical 5-FU (5%) has been used successfully for the treatment of chronic verrucae planae juveniles. All these therapies during pregnancy are contraindications.

When faced with apparently normal patients with really resistant warts, it is always useful to reassess their medical history and immunological status. Viral warts are often resistant to standard therapies in patients immunosuppressed by disease or drugs. After immunosuppression has started, patients should be monitored regularly for the development of cutaneous or genital lesions. All immunosuppressed groups should be constantly reminded about the real dangers of excessive ultraviolet light exposure as this itself adds to the immunosuppressive effect. As mentioned, in immunosuppressed patients orally-given aromatic retinoids have a beneficial effect on recalcitrant common warts. Although IFN-α has proved to be useful for the treatment of the AIDS-associated Kaposi's sarcoma, it does not appear to have a single role as a single agent for the treatment of HPV associated disease. Perhaps the greatest value of IFN will be when it is used in combination with other antiviral agents or with conventional ablative therapy.

IX. SUMMARY

The many different treatment possibilities for the eradication of skin warts provides evidence that no ideal therapy has been found. Most therapies have been aimed at removing the warts rather than controlling or stopping viral expression. Commonly used therapies include chemical destruction, cryotherapy, electrocauter, and lasersurgery, pharmacologic agents, and immunotherapy (Table 1). Although the various methods described herein are usually successful therapies, they are all associated with treatment failures and side-effects.

The decision regarding which treatment to use depends on a number of factors, which include the size, location, type of wart, and the immune status of the patient. In addition, the degree of pain, the risk of scarring, and the patient's commitment to the therapy all enter into the decision on which treatment modality to use. The physician also has to consider that warts tend to spontaneous regression. In the healthy individual, two thirds of warts resolve without therapy within 2 years. Therefore, treatments causing only minimal pain, minimal side-effects, and other inconvenience must have first priority. Finally, it should be taken into account that the treatment of skin warts should be inexpensive.

REFERENCES

1. Celsus AC. *De Medicina*. Book V 28, 14 B-E. English translation by WG Spencer. London, Heinemann, vol. 2, pp. 160–3, 1961.
2. Wilson E. On the dermo-pathology of Celsus. *Br Med J* 1963;2:446–9.
3. Rosenthal T. Aulus Cornelius Celsus. His contribution to dermatology. *Arch Dermatol* 1961;84:129–34.
4. Turner D. *Diseases of the Skin of the Hands. De Morbis Cutaneis*. pp. 278–89, 1712.
5. Zwick KG. Warts disappearing without topical medication. *Arch Dermatol* 1932;25:508.
6. Sulzberger MB, Wolf J. The treatment of warts by suggestion. *Med Rec* 1934;140:552.
7. De la Mare W. *Come Hither*. London, Constable, pp. 690–1, 1936.
8. Rolleston JD. Dermatology and folklore. *Br J Dermatol* 1940;52:43–57.
9. Bett WR. Wart I bid thee begone. *Practitioner* 1951;166:166–77.
10. Twain M. *The Adventures of Tom Sawyer*. London, Penguin Books Ltd., p. 46, 1986.
11. Massing AM, Epstein WL. Natural history of warts. A two year study. *Arch Dermatol* 1963;87:306–10.
12. Huber C, Christophers E. Keratolytic effects of salicylic acid. *Arch Dermatol* 1977;257:293–7.
13. Bunney MH, Nolan M, Williams D: An assessment of methods of treating viral warts by comparative treatment trials based on a standard design. *Br J Dermatol* 1976;94:667–79.
14. Vickers CF. Treatment of plantar warts in children. *Br Med J* 1961; 2:743–5.
15. Anderson I, Shirreffs E. Treatment of plantar warts. *Br J Dermatol* 1963;75:29–32.
16. Lyell A. The management of warts. *Br Med J* 1966;2:1576–9.
17. Bunney MH, Benton C, Cubie HA. *Viral Warts. Biology and Treatment*. Oxford, Oxford University Press, 1992.
18. Brokalakis J, Goumouzas A, Varelzidis A. Topical treatment of condylomata acuminata with Solcoderm. *Dermatalogy* 1984;168:49–51.
19. Morison WL. *In vitro* assay of immunity to wart virus. *Br J Dermatol* 1975;93:545–52.
20. Jones SK, Darville JM. Transmission of virus particles by cryotherapy and multi use caustic pencils: a problem to dermatologists. *Br J Dermatol* 1989;121:481–6.
21. Rademaker N, Meyrich-Thomas RH, Munro DD. The treatment of resistant plantar warts with aggressive cryotherapy under general anaesthesia. *Br J Dermatol* 1987;116:557–600.
22. McDow RA, Webster MM. Use of freon in treating verruca lesions. *J Fam Pract* 1987;25:73.
23. Sonnex TS, Jones RL, Weddell AG, Dawber RPR. Long term effects of cryosurgery on cutaneous sensations. *Br Med J* 1985;290:188–90.
24. Jackson R, Laughlin S. Electrosurgery. *Dermatol Clin* 1984;2:233.
25. Goldmann L. Effects of new laser systems on the skin. *Arch Dermatol* 1973;108:385.
26. Fuller TA. Fundamentals of lasers in surgery and medicine. In: Dixon JA, Ed, *Surgical Application of Lasers*, Chicago, Year Book Medical Publishers, 1983.
27. McBurney EI, Rosen DA. Carbon dioxide laser treatment of verrucae vulgares. *J Dermatol Surg Oncol* 1984;10:45.
28. Apfelberg DB, Rothermel E, Widtfeldt A, et al. Preliminary report on use of carbon dioxide laser in podiatry. *J Am Assoc* 1984;74:509.
29. Mueller TJ, Carlson BA, Lindy MP. The use of carbon dioxide surgical laser for the treatment of verrucae. *J Am Podiatr Assoc* 1980;70:136.
30. Apfelberg DB, Druker D, Maser MR et al. Benefits of CO_2 laser for verrucae resistant to other modalities of treatment. *J Dermatol Surg Oncol* 1989;15:371.
31. Street ML, Roenigk RK. Recalcitrant periungual verrucae: the role of carbon dioxide laser vaporization. *J Am Acad Dermatol* 1990;23:115–20.
32. Pfau A, Abd-el-Raheem A, Bäumler W, Hohenleutner U, Landthaler M. Nd:YAG laser hyperthermia in the treatment of recalcitrant verrucae vulgares (Regensburg's Technique). *Acta Derm Venerol* 1994;74:212–4.
33. Carlson BA, Pyrcz R. Human papilloma virus-induced lesions: their treatment and the evolution of an alternative laser application. *Cur Podiatr Med* 1989;9:9–12.

34. Dixon JA, Gilbertson JJ. Cutaneous laser therapy. *West J Med* 1985;143:758-63.
35. Coskey RJ. Treatment of plantar warts in children with a salicylic acid-podophyllin-cantharidin product. *Pediatr Dermatol* 1984;2:71.
36. Epstein WL, Kligman AM. Treatment of warts with cantharidin. *Arch Dermatol* 1958;77:508-11.
37. Ward JW, Clifford WS, Monaco AR, et al. Fatal poisoning following podophyllin treatment of condylomata acuminata. *South Med J* 1954;47:1204.
38. Cassidy DE, Drewry J, Fanning JP. Podophyllin toxicity: A report of a fatal case and a review of the literature. *J Toxicol Clin Toxicol* 1982; 19:35.
39. Duthie DA, McCallum DI. Treatment of plantar warts with elastoplast and podophyllin. *Br Med J* 1951;2:216.
40. Syed TA, Lundin S, Ahmad M. Topical 0.3% and 0.5% podophyllotoxin cream for self-treatment of *molluscum contagiosum* in males. A placebo-controlled, double-blind study. *Dermatology* 1994;189:65-68.
41. Von Krogh G, Rylander E. *GPVI-Genitoanal Papilloma Virus Infection. A Survey for the Clinician.* Karlstad, Sweden, Conpharm AB, pp. 133-46, 1989.
42. Bunney MH, Nolan MW, Buxton PK, et al. The treatment of resistant warts with intralesional bleomycin: a controlled trial. *Br J Dermatol* 1984;110:197-207.
43. Hayes ME, O'Keefe EJ. Reduced dose of bleomycin in the treatment of recalcitrant warts. *J Am Acad Dermatol* 1986;15:1002-6.
44. Kuo MT, Haidle CW. Characterization of chain breakage in DNA induced by bleomycin. *Biochem Biophys Acta* 1974;335:109.
45. Epstein E. Persisting Raynaud's phenomenon following intralesional treatment of finger warts. *J Am Acad Dermatol* 1985;13:468.
46. Willoughby DV. Personal communication in "Bleomycin and warts". Instructional Cassette. Ottawa, Bristol Myers, 1978.
47. Lee S, Kim JG, Chu SI. Treatment of verruca plana with 5% 5-fluoroacil ointment. *Dermatology* 1980;160:383.
48. Boyle J, Dick DC, Mackie RM. Treatment of extensive virus warts with etretinate (Tigason) in a patient with sarcoidosis. *Clin Exp Dermatol* 1983;8:33-6.
49. Gross G, Pfister H, Hagedorn M, Stahn W. Effect of oral aromatic retinoid (RO10-9359) on human papillomavirus-2-induced common warts. *Dermatology* 1983;166:48-53.
50. Lutzner MA, Blanchet-Bardon C. Oral retinoid treatment of human papillomavirus type 5-induced epidermodysplasia verruciformis. *N Engl J Med* 1980;302:1091-3.
51. Weiner SA, Meyskens FDI, Sarwit EA et al. Response of human papillomavirus-associated diseases to retinoids (vitamin A derivatives). In: Howley PM, Broker TR, Eds, *Papillomaviruses. Molecular and Clinical Aspects,* New York, Alan Liss, pp. 249-55, 1985.
52. Katz RA. Isotretinoin treatment of recalcitrant warts in an immunosuppressed man. *Arch Dermatol* 1986;122:19-20.
53. Rogozinski T, Geiger JM, Czarnetzki BM, Jablonska S. Acitretin in the treatment and prevention of viral, premalignant and malignant skin lesions. *J Dermatol Res* 1989;1:91-3.
54. Bruckner D, Price N,, Immunotherapy of verrucae vulgares with dinitrochlorobenzene. *Br J Dermatol* 1978;98:451-5.
55. Dunagin WG, Millikan LE. Dinitrochlorobenzene immunotherapy for verrucae resistant to standard treatment modalities. *J Am Acad Dermatol* 1982;6:40.
56. Summer KH, Goggelmann W. 1-Chloro-2,4-dinitrobenzene depletes glutathione in rat skin and is mutagenic in *Salmonella typhimurium. Mutat Res* 1980;77:91.
57. Interferon nomenclature. *Nature* 1980;286:110.
58. Stadler R, Mayer da Silva A. Bratzke B et al. Interferons in dermatology. *J Am Acad Dermatol* 1989;20:650.
59. Baron S, Tyring SK, Fleischmann RW et al. The interferons. Mechanisms of action and clinical applications. *J Am Med Assoc* 1991;266:1375-1383.
60. Nimura M. Intralesional human fibroblast interferon in common warts. *J Dermatol* 1983;10:217.
61. Gross G. Interferon bei Erkrankungen der Haut und der angrenzenden Schleimhäute. In: Niederle N, von Wussow P, Eds, *Interferone. Präklinische und klinische Befunde.* Berlin, Springer, pp. 358-94, 1990.

62. Schöfer S, Sollberg S. Systemische Behandlung vulgärer Warzen mit beta-Interferon. *Hautarzt* 1991;42:396–98.
63. Schoenfeld A, Ovadia J, Stein L, et al. Treatment of flat facial warts with interferon-beta cream. *J Dermatol Surg Oncol* 1987;13:299–301.
64. Gross G. New drugs for human papillomavirus infections. In: Burgdorf WHC, Katz SI, Eds, *Dermatology: Progress and Perspectives. The Proceedings of the 18th World Congress of Dermatology*, New York, June 12-18, 1992, pp. 236–40.
65. Benton EC, Nolan MW, Kemmett D, Cubie HA. Trial of inosine pranobex in the management of cutaneous viral warts. *J Dermatol Treat* 1991;1:295–7.
66. Surman OS, Gottlieb SK, Hackett TP et al. Hypnosis in the treatment of warts. *Arch Gyn Psychiatry* 1973;28:439.
67. Spanos NP, Stenstrom RJ Johnston JC. Hypnosis, placebo, and suggestion in the treatment of warts. *Psychosom Med* 1988;50:245.
68. Spanos NP, Williams V, Gwynn MI. The effect of hypnotic, placebo and salicylic acid. *Psychosom Med* 1990;15:109–14.
69. Clarke GHV. The charming of warts. *J Invest Dermatol* 1965;15–21.
70. Stankler L. A critical assessment of cure of warts by suggestion. *Practitioner* 1967;198:690–4.
71. Ullman M, Dudek S. On the psyche and warts II: hypnotic suggestion and warts. *Psychosom Med* 1960;22:68–76.
72. Tasini MF, Hackett TP. Hypnosis in the treatment of warts in immunodeficient children. *Am J Clin Hypno* 1977;19:152–4.

22

Genitoanal Lesions

Gerd Gross, Geo von Krogh, and Renzo Barrasso

CONTENTS

I. INTRODUCTION

Anogenital HPV induced clinical lesions are difficult to treat and recur with great frequency. The extent of the HPV infection is difficult to determine. Small lesions are often overlooked. Subclinical infections are only detectable using a colposcope or another magnifying method after the application of acetic acid. Furthermore, the presence of latent viral DNA in apparently normal surrounding tissue may contribute to the high recurrence rate of genital warts even after ablative surgery[1-13] ranging between about 38 to 81% (Table 1). The course of papillomavirus infections varies considerably. Some lesions grow rapidly, others persist without any change in growth, others still regress spontaneously over several weeks, and some regress over a long period of time. Clinical, subclinical, and latent HPV infections can exist simultaneously and can change from one to the other. It is widely assumed that the host cellular immune response is of key importance in the course and outcome of HPV infection. Possible causes for recurrent disease may be that the virus left after surgery reinfects and replicates in the proliferative surrounding epithelium. Often removal of warty tissue is incomplete or multifocal occult HPV infection occurs, which is a common finding in the anogenital region.

HPV infections of the lower genital tract, with a single site or multiple sites infected, behave as a sexually transmitted disease and should be treated as such, applying the principals recommended by the WHO for the control of venereal diseases.[14] These include encouraging the use of condoms to prevent onward transmissions, as well as medical examination when lesions are noticed and promoting examination of sexual partners. This, together with a recommendation to avoid multiple partners, is part of a general health education program being fundamental to HPV infection control.

TABLE 1   Influence of Adjuvant IFN on the Recurrence Rate of Recalcitrant Condylomata Acuminata (Controlled Studies)

Ablative therapy	Recurrence rate in %		IFN type	Application form	Study	References
	No IFN	IFN				
CO_2-laser	38	18.5	alpha 2b	perilesional	Vance and Davis 1990	(1)
CO_2-laser	45	21	alpha 2b	perilesional	Davis and Noble 1992	(2)
Electrocautery	78	40	nat beta	gel	Gross et al. 1990	(3)
CO_2-laser Cryotherapy Electrocautery	75	54	rec beta	gel	Gross et al. 1994	(4)
Surgery/ Electrocautery	64	nd			Duus et al. 1985	(5)
CO_2 laser	57	nd				
CO_2 laser	81	42	alpha 2b	sc cyclic	Hohenleutner et al. 1990	(6)
CO_2 laser	77	48	alpha 2b	sc cont.	Petersen et al. 1991	(7)
Cryotherapy	60	70.4	alpha 2a	sc cont.	Handley et al. 1991	(8)
Cryotherapy	61.2	72.3	alpha 2a	sc cont.	Handley et al. 1992	(9)
CO_2 laser	38	46	alpha 2a	sc cont.	International Condyloma Collaborative Study Group 1993	(10)
Cryotherapy	73	69	alpha 2a	sc cont.	Eron et al. 1993	(11)
CO_2 laser	32	38	alpha 2b	sc cont.	Nieminen et al. 1994	(12)
CO_2 laser	63	41	alpha 2a	sc cyclic	Gross et al. 1996	(13)

Note: nat = natural; rec = recombinant; sc = subcutaneous; cont. = continuous.

Successful treatment requires an accurate determination of the extent of both condylomatous and subclinical components of the disease. In women, colposcopy or cervical smear for cytological examination should be performed; cervical investigational methods may vary according to local traditions (see Chapter 14, pp. 288–292). Other sexually transmitted diseases should be excluded in search of reliable symptoms and factors of potential pathogenetic relevance. Furthermore, exclusion of syphilis, hepatitis, and HIV should be insured by serology testing. In all cases, the consorts should be examined and treated if necessary. There is some controversy as to when HPV infections have to be treated. Although, condylomata acuminata have a far less prominent oncogenic potential than flat lesions, especially those of the cervix uteri, some risk exists, especially in long standing giant warts of the Buschke-Löwenstein's type. Genital warts are infectious since they harbor infectious virus particles which can be easily transmitted to the sexual partners. Visible warts should therefore always be treated. This is not the case with subclinical and latent infections where the decision about management is more difficult (see also Chapter 14).

II. ESTABLISHED TREATMENTS

The various modes of treatment are listed in Table 2. The decision as to which treatment modality to use must be individualized and depends on the type, size, location, extension, symptoms, and the presence of any dysplasia[1] of the clinical lesions. Limited disease, including solitary small sized condylomas, has to be differentiated from extensive disease, widespread lesions, or recalcitrant as well as exuberantly growing genital warts.

TABLE 2   Established Treatment Modalities of Anogenital HPV Infections

Cytotoxic Agents

Podophyllin
Podophyllotoxin
Trichloroacetic Acid
5-Fluorouracil

Surgery

Scissor excision, curretage
Electrosurgery
Cryotherapy (liquid nitrogen, cryoprobe)
Laser therapy (CO_2-laser, Neodynium-YAG-laser)

Medical Treatments

Interferons

A. Topical Treatment Using Cytotoxic Agents

1. Podophyllin

Since more than 50 years ago, podophyllin has been a popular front-line treatment for genital warts because it is relatively inexpensive. Podophyllin is a crude resin extract taken from the roots of the Mayapple or Podophyllum plant (either the North American Podophyllum peltatum or the Indian Podophyllum emodi). Its efficacy, as based on a short-term follow-up study of primary cure rates of penile warts afflicting American military troops, was first described by Kaplan in 1942.[15] Several subsequent reports have focused on major short-comings of podophyllin, due to an often high degree of local irritancy, lack of satisfactory long-term efficacy, and significant risks of systemic toxicity and local mutagenic influences.[16-20] Podophyllin is an impure, nonstandardized substance, composed of various amounts of at least four cytotoxic chemicals known as lignans (Figure 1).[17] The most potent cytotoxic agent of these chemicals is podophyllotoxin (Table 3), which is present in greater concentration in resin from podophyllum emodi. Other components of podophyllin are quercetin and kaempherol, which have neither cytotoxic nor therapeutic properties, but are instead mutagenic and could, accordingly, be potentially adjuvant oncogenic cofactors in genital HPV-associated lesions.[20] Podophyllin is applied as a 20 to 25% solution in ethanol or tincture of benzoin. Podophyllin is a highly aggressive treatment that can cause severe local side effects such as burning, swelling, and ulcerations. For this reason, it must always be applied under careful medical supervision and must be washed off 4 to 6 hours after application. One of the many disadvantages of podophyllin is its unreliable stability and, because it is a natural root extract from Podophyllum plants which merely is semi-quantatively controlled with regard to content, the ingredients may vary significantly between various batches. Furthermore, degradation of the biologically active lignans into inactive isomers often occurs within some days to a few weeks.[17,21]

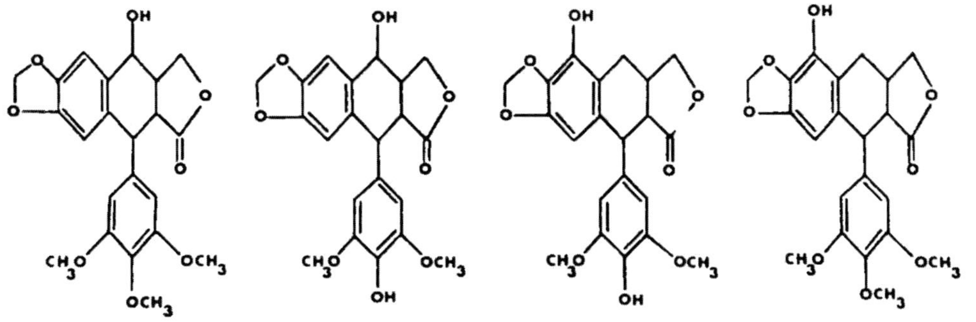

	podophyllotoxin	4'-demethyl-podophyllotoxin	α-peltatin	β-peltatin	total resin content
P. peltatum	+	–	+	+	20%
P. emodi	+	(+)	–	–	40%

FIGURE 1   Lignans: the therapeutically active ingredients of the Podophyllum plants.

TABLE 3   Composition of 25% Podophyllum Resin and 0.5% Podophyllotoxin

	25% Podophyllum Resin[a]	0.5% Podophyllotoxin
Podophyllotoxin mg/ml	25–100	5
Other lignans mg/ml[b]	2–25	0
Quercetin, Kaempherol	Yes	No
Systemic absorption	High	Minimal
Known stability	No	Yes
Patient applied	No	Yes

[a] Content varies with species and source.

[b] Alpha-peltatin, beta-peltatin, and 4-demethylpodophyllotoxin.

Normally, treatment must be repeated once—or maximally twice—a week, and due to the potential risk of irritation of the skin applications should be made by a physican or a specially trained nurse. Furthermore, potential systemic toxicity of podophyllin is another major problem and drawback of the remedy, since applied in large volumes on florid warts severe systemic toxicity symptoms have occasionally been observed. In a few instances, toxicity has caused fatal outcome due to CNS influence and cardiovascular crisis.[17,22-33]

More than 0.5 ml of 20% podophyllin should not be applied at any time (Figure 2). Use of podophyllin during pregnancy is contraindicated. Furthermore, due to its oncogenic and teratogenic potential, podophyllin should not be applied to the vagina or to the cervix. It is surprising that podophyllin treatment remains a popular method for treating condylomata acuminata despite the fact that recurrences are likely to occur. In an overview of Kraus and Stone,[34] an average primary cure rate of 50% (range 22–78%) was reported, but recurrence rates were as high as 74%. In prospective trials examining the long term efficacy at 3 months from 20% podophyllum peltatum or emodi preparations against penile warts in noncircumcised men, it has been clearly documented that the efficacy is considerably lower than was claimed originally. Only 22% of the men were cured after a single application and a second course of treatment for residual warts showed a cumulative effect of 38%.[21] In additional studies comparing podophyllin with surgical excision, although the primary clearance rates were 77% for podophyllin and 93% for surgery, significantly more patients experienced recurrences from therapy with podophyllin (65%) than from surgical exicision (29%).[35]

Thus, podophyllin treatment suffers, above all, from the disadvantages of a rather low clinical efficacy but also from heavy demands on the medical and nursing staff and inconvenience to the patient, where the cost-beneficy aspects of such therapy deserves questioning.[36-38]

Safety and Precaution. Podophyllin solutions should not be stored for more than a month. Application more frequently than once weekly is not recommended. Patients must be instructed to wash away the remedy within 4-6 hours. Prescription for self-treatment should never be done. Maximum volume for topical use should not exceed 0.9 ml preparations based on *P. peltatum* and 0.4 ml for *P. emodi*-based remedies (Figure 2). Podophyllin should not be given during pregnancy. Females must use a reliable contraceptive method, or abstain from sexual intercourse during the days of active therapy.[17,36]

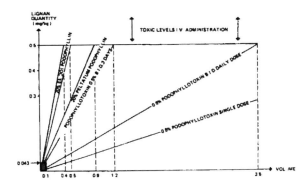

FIGURE 2 Reciprocity between various volumes (ml; abscissa) of 20% podophyllin and 0.5% podophyllotoxin preparations and corresponding lignan content (mg/kg), with reference to 70 kg of body weight. The figure demonstrates that the cumulative quantity of podophyllotoxin, (0.043 mg/kg), associated with a regimen based on repeated application of 100 μl of 0.5% preparations (5 mg/ml) twice daily for three days, falls far below the amount sufficient to elicit any clinically evident systemic toxic influence when given **intravenously** as a single dose. This volume is quite sufficient to treat even relatively large/numerous genital warts. Only in a few cases are larger volumes required, and it is very rare that more than 0.2 ml is needed. In extreme cases afflicted with very extensive warts somewhat larger doses may be required. According to our experience, more than 0.5 ml is hardly ever needed even in such patients. As appears from the figure, this volume corresponds to a podophyllotoxin dose still far below any critical level of systemic toxicity when 0.5% podophyllotoxin is used. This is not the case when 20% podophyllin, based on a *P. emodi* preparation is applied to such warts (von Krogh, 1982).

2.   Podophyllotoxin

Podophyllotoxin is a purified active ingredient of podophyllin that in several studies has appeared as the most biologically active of the lignans.[18,39,40] Although isolated as early as 1947 by Sullivan and King,[41] purified podophyllotoxin was only recently made available for use in the treatment of genital warts.The drug binds to tubulins, which are essential for mitotic cell division, preventing tubulin polymerization into microtubules,[42,43] Observed biological effects include, above all, mitotic arrest of eukaryotic cellular division in metaphase, but also nucleoside transport inhibition.[39,42,43] Therapeutic influence is possibly also associated with detrimental influence on epidermal capillaries.[39] Whether or not there is a concurrent influence on local immune functions and viral replication is yet not fully understood. On one hand, podophyllotoxin reduces lymphocyte reactivity to mitogens. On the other hand, induction of IL-2 production and of macrophage proliferation has been reported.[44,45] The therapeutic effect is associated with a necrotic involution of condylomas that is maximal 3–5 days after initial administration. Histopathologically, drug influence is demonstrable for up to 1(–2) weeks, presenting as a degenerative keratinocyte damage and/or the occurrence of abnormal bizarre mitotic figures that may occasionally be confused with epithelial dysplasia.[41] Thus, any biopsy evaluation from podophyllin/podophyllotoxin treated areas should be avoided until two drugfree weeks have passed. No long-term risk of dysplasia is associated with the regimen.[46]

In a series of studies on penile warts, a very low, and toxicologically highly safe concentration, 0.5%, of podophyllotoxin (Figure 2), was found to be very effective against penile condylomas in uncircumsized men when self-applied as an ethanolic solution twice daily for 3 days.[17,18,36] After a single three-day course, preputial cavity warts were cured in 70% of the cases. Altogether 49% of the patients got completely wart-free after one three-day course, and the cumulative cure rate was 82% when self-treatment was repeated once more. These studies showed that efficacy, as evaluated by a 3 month follow-up period, did not differ significantly whether a 1.0% or a 0.5% podophyllotoxin solution was used, or whether applications were performed twice or thrice daily (Table 4). The long-term efficacy (≥ 3 month follow-up) was significantly superior (p < 0.001) to that following use of freshly prepared 20% podophyllin.[17] Favourable results from self-treatment with various 0.5% podophylloxin preparations have subsequently been reported by others as well (Table 4).

In the urinary meatus and on the penile shaft, efficacy tends to be less impressive than under the foreskin.[17,18] Yet, in subsequent studies[47,48] it has been demonstrated that even such warts may resolve completely in about half of the cases and 80% of the original wart bulk may disappear when 3–4 repeated three-day courses are given at 4–7 days of drug-free intervals. In the trials accounted for by Beutner et al.,[47] 109 circumsized males with warts predominantly on the penile shaft (88%) were randomly allocated to 0.5% podophyllotoxin or placebo. Therapy was self-administered in treatment courses of twice daily application for 3 consecutive days followed by a 4-day drug-free period. Patients were administered a minimum of two and a maximum of four such treatment courses. None of the 53 placebo patients but 45% of the (25/56) podophyllotoxin-treated patients were completely wart-free during the study. At the end of the treatment period, 74% and 8% of treated warts in the active or placebo groups, respectively, were no longer present.

No local irritation was reported by von Krogh[17] in 49% of the patients. Another 46% experienced a slight burning and/or tenderness in association with the occurrence of superficial erosions and some erythema on days 3 to 5 after initiated treatment. Only 5% experienced some pain in association with necrosis of extensive warts. In analogy to that of surgery, such "adverse effects" should be considered as part of the therapeutic effect. Most importantly, podophyllotoxin-associated erosions heal considerably faster than those following surgical procedures.[37,49] Once or twice daily applications of 0.5% podophyllotoxin repeated for up to 4–5 days has also been evaluated. However, although favorable cure rates were accomplished (Table 4) this approach tends to induce rather unpleasant and often unacceptable local adverse reactions.[50] It was also shown that efficacy is significantly lower when applied only once daily compared to twice daily (Table 4).

TABLE 4   Summary of Clinical Trials of Patient-Applied Podophyllotoxin for the Treatment of Genital Warts

Author/Reference	Sex	Podophyllotoxin concentrations	Type of treatment cycles	Number of treatment cycles	% Cured (no of patients)
von Krogh (17)	male	1.0% sol	TID x 3 d	1	44(20/46)
		1.0% sol	BID × 3 d	1	63(17/27)
		0.5% sol	TID × 3 d	1	38(11/29)
		0.5% sol	BID × 3 d	1	49(35/71)
Edwards et al. (51)	male	0.5% sol	BID × 3 d	1–6	88(28/32)
von Krogh (50)	male	0.5% sol	OD × 4 d	1	35(18/51)
		0.5% sol	BID × 4 d	1	70(26/37)
		0.5% sol	OD × 5 d	1	42(14/33)
		0.5% sol	BID × 5d	1	63(15/26)
Beutner et al. (47)	male	0.5% sol	BID × 3 d	1–4	44(25/56)
von Krogh and Hellberg (56)	female	0.5% cream	BID × 3 d	1–3	76(34/44)
Strand et al. (57)	male	0.5% sol	BID × 3 d	⎫	69(20/29)
		0.3% cream	BID × 3 d	⎬ 1–4	68(21/31)
		0.15% cream	BID × 3 d	⎭	57(17/30)
von Krogh and Rosén (59)	male	0.5% sol	BID × 3 d	⎫	84(74/88)
		0.3% cream	BID × 3 d	⎬ 1–4	81(74/91)
		0.15% cream	BID × 3 d	⎭	71(64/90)
	female	0.5% sol	BID × 3 d	⎫	88(53/60)
		0.3% cream	BID × 3 d	⎬ 1–4	87(52/60)
		0.15% cream	BID × 3 d	⎭	81(48/59)

In a number of single-blind prospective trials (Tables 4 and 5) comparing patient-applied podophyllotoxin with clinic-applied podophyllin resin, the effect of multiple treatment courses has also been evaluated by others.[38,51,55,56] These studies generally confirm a superior efficacy from podophyllotoxin compared to that of podophyllin. Mazurkiewicz and Jablonska[52] noted a wart-free state in 68% (17/25) of podophyllotoxin men treated with 0.5% podophyllotoxin solution and in 38% (7/24) of resin-treated patients after one to two courses (Table 5). The corresponding figures given by Lassus[38] were 77% (37/48) for self-treatment with 0.5% podophyllotoxin solution and 44% (23/52) for 20% podophyllin treatment. Edwards et al.[51] noted complete resolution of warts in 88% (28/32) of self-treated patients vs. 63% (12/19) of resin-treated patients. This conclusion is not in concordance with that of Kinghorn et al., showing identical effects from podophyllin and podophyllotoxin. However, the latter study was not accounting for long-term efficacy evaluation. A highly satisfactory degree of efficacy and tolerance from multiple self-treatment courses of podophyllotoxin against genitoanal warts has been reported from a British multicenter study based on 303 uncircumcized males.[54]

In most of these reports it has been confirmed that local reactions tend to be considerably lower than those reported after podophyllin.

Self-treatment with 0.5% podophyllotoxin-ethanol has also been tested as repeated three-days courses against vulvar warts. Results are analogous to those reported for circumcized males.[58] Approximately half of the podophyllotoxin-treated women experienced mild and tolerable local erosions causing some burning and/or pain.

In order to investigate whether improvements may be accomplished, as measured as a maintenance of efficacy but further reducing the frequency and severity of local side effects, von Krogh et al. compared ethanolic solutions of 0.5% and 0.25% podophyllotoxin vs. that of placebo against penile warts.[55] While the placebo solution exerted a marginal influence, a primary cure was documented in 72% (13/18) and 81% (13/16) of altogether 34 men self-treating their warts with

TABLE 5   Podophyllotoxin 0.5% B.I D. for 3 Days vs. Podophyllin in the
Treatment of Genital Warts

	Duration (weeks, w)	% Cure rates	Study
Podophyllotoxin	4 w	77 (37/48)	Lassus (38)
Pod 20%, 1/week		44 (23/52)	
Podophyllotoxin	6 w	88 (28/32)	Edwards et al. (51)
Pod 20%, x 1/week		63 (12/19)	
Podophyllotoxin	6 w	79 (11/14)	Mazurkiewicz and Jablonska (52)
Pod 25%, x 1/week		38 (5/13)	
Podophyllotoxin	5 w	86 (83/97)	Kinghorn et al. (53)
Pod 25%, x 2/week		72 (26/36)	

0.25% or 0.50% podophyllotoxin, respectively. Follow-up investigations (range 5–23 weeks) revealed some degree of relapse in nine men (38%), when warts occurred on previously untreated sites in 33% and in another 44% on podophyllotoxin-treated sites as well as on adjacent sites. Analysis of the debulking potential of podophyllotoxin on the original warts showed that 0.25% podophyllotoxin cured 85% (184/217) and the 0.5% preparation eradicated 96% (130/135) of the original warts. Side effects, generally being mild to moderate, did not differ between the two drug concentrations, a fact signifying that use of podophyllotoxin concentrations below 0.5% should certainly be considered in further investigations.

Podophyllotoxin-ethanol applications seem convenient in the self-treatment of penile warts. Less-accessible vulvar, perineal, and anal warts, however, might potentially be reached more feasibly by cream preparations, allowing the assistance of tactile aid from the patient's own fingers for the application procedure. This has been successfully demonstrated in subsequent studies[56-58] that signal further refinements for self-therapy with podophyllotoxin in the future (Table 4).

In a double-blind, placebo-controlled study,[56] self-treatment with a 0.5% podophyllotoxin cream was evaluated by von Krogh and Hellberg among women afflicted solely with outer vulvoanal warts (Table 4). Twelve women received treatment with placebo cream and another 44 women with active substance, administered twice daily in 3-day courses once weekly for up to 3 weeks. Placebo lacked therapeutic influence. After the first course of therapy the initial wart bulk was reduced by 73%. Primary cure rates from podophyllotoxin cream were 43, 66, and 91% after 1, 2, and 3 treatment cycles, respectively. Within a 3-month follow-up period, 6 (14%) patients who were originally considered cured exhibited some degree of relapse. A permanent cure occurred in 77% of the 44 women. A slight-to-moderate tenderness, burning, and/or pain was noted by 60% of the women.

The optimal concentration of podophyllotoxin-cream formulations for genital warts is yet to be determined. However, in recent trials of 0.15%–0.3% podophyllotoxin cream preparations and solutions[57,58] a trend has been documented that is in favor of a somewhat higher efficacy when using 0.3% of the drug, while the 0.15% formulations tend to induce somewhat less local irritancy. So far, it seems that future use of 0.3% cream might be most favorable with regard to efficacy, although the 0.15% cream potentially may be of value in highly sensitive areas, such as the anal verge and other intertriginous areas, where a minimization of side effects possibly may be of major importance.

While some therapies come into use via "breakthroughs" other useful therapies evolve. Patient-applied podophyllotoxin is becoming widely available and has increasingly become recognized as a valuable first-line therapy for external genital warts.[60] Currently available podophyllotoxin preparations* have a highly satisfactory shelf-life stability, which is certainly not the case for podophyllin preparations (Table 6). The low toxic potential for podophyllotoxin has initiated a change in the

---

* Wartec®, Warticon®, Perstorp Pharma, Lund, Sweden; Condyline®, Nycomed Pharma, Oslo, Norway.

generic name to "podofilox"[47] in the U.S.* By its very nature, evaluation continues. With further evalution, improvement in commercial products can be anticipated. Commercial registration of cream as well as gel formulations are currently in process.

TABLE 6   Some Major Concerns Regarding Comparison Between Podophyllin and Podophyllotoxin

20% podophyllin - disadvantage	0.5% podophyllotoxin - advantages
Nonstandardized, unstable remedy	Standardized, stable remedy
Local toxicity high and unpredictable	Local toxicity low and predictable
Systemic toxicity risk consiberable	Systemic toxicity risk negligible
Mutagenic properties	No mutagenic properties
Low efficacy	High efficacy
Office treatment required	Home treatment feasible

Safety and Precaution.   An optimal regimen for use of podophyllotoxin preparations entails application twice daily for three days. No washing off is required between applications. When large warts occur, ethanol solutions of podophyllotoxin may induce unpleasant stinging when warts necrotize on day 2–3 of therapy. If phimosis should occur in an uncircumcised male, the patient requires medical supervision and assistance until the condition resolves, which usually happens within a few days. Any local discomfort is otherwise easily suppressed by topical anti-inflammatory remedies. Podophyllotoxin should not be given during pregnancy. Females must use a contraceptive or abstain from penetrative sexual activity.

3.   Trichloroacetic Acid

This caustic agent is applied as an ethanolic solution at weekly intervals at concentrations of 50–85%. Although the efficacy has been poorly documented, it is clear that, similar to podophyllin, numerous treatments are usually required. Since there is no report on toxicity, trichloracetic acid may be used during pregnancy. The overall efficacy has been purely documented and especially its efficacy against cervical and vaginal HPV-associated lesions is not yet fully clarified, although there are reports on an 80% cure rate in benign HPV infections of the cervix when using 85% trichloracetic acid.[61-63] In contrast to podophyllotoxin, however, trichloracetic acid is painful already at the moment of applications, and, thus, must be applied by a specialist. Furthermore, relatively deep skin erosions may develop unless applications are performed with great care.

4.   5-Fluorouracil

The pyrimidine antagonist 5-fluorouracil (5-FU), acting via inhibition of nucleic acid synthesis, is a powerful cytotoxic drug and has been tried with varying success as a 5% cream** for the treatment of resistant genital warts of the vulva and the penis, and especially of urethral warts in men. Side-effects are common and include painful epithelial erosions, sometimes accompanied also by intolerable post-treatment pain. For this reason, and because efficacy has been highly variable with a cure range of 33–100% after daily applications for up to eight weeks, primary use of 5-FU cannot be regarded justified on the outer genitoanal area.[64]

Localized areas of bowenoid papulosis have been successfully treated with 5-FU cream twice daily for 1–2 weeks (von Krogh, personal observation). Also, a 5-FU cream may be tried against lesions of the urinary meatus; these warts disappear in up to 70–90% of cases when the cream is applied after each voiding for 2–3 weeks. On this site, medication can be confined to a limited area, and ulcerations emanating from therapy cause, in general, merely a tolerable dysuria.[64]

---

* Condylox®, Oclassen Pharmaceuticals, Inc., San Rafael, CA, U.S.

** Fluoro-uracil cream®, Hoffman - La Roche AG, Basel, Switzerland.

Furthermore, intraurethral instillations of the cream may be performed using a syringe when extensive intraurethral growths are encountered.[65-67] In such cases, the patient must be monitored carefully for the potential development of urinary retention.

Also, 5-FU has been found to be valuable for treating vulvo-vaginal warts. Ferenczy applied 2.5 grams of the cream intravaginally for five subsequent evenings and found that the failure rate against condylomata was as low as 3.5% subsequent to two separate treatment courses.[68] When the drug is used in the vagina, the vulvar area should be protected by zinc oxide cream to avoid erosive vulvitis.

Various schedules have been suggested for treatment of vulvar warts. Krebs[69] reported a 41% cure rate when 5-FU cream was applied twice weekly at two subsequent nights for ten weeks, while Pride[70] found a cure rate of 68% after 1–3 treatment cycles when 5-FU was applied twice daily for one week per cycle, followed by a rest period for another 7–10 days.

5-FU cream has also been tried as prophylactic treatment after surgery on vulvo-vaginal warts. Krebs[71] inserted the cream intravaginally once every two weeks for six months subsequent to surgical treatment of vaginal warts. Of the 5-FU treated women, only 13% developed recurrences vs. 38% of women who were not 5-FU treated. Similarly, a significant reduction of the recurrence rate for vulvar warts has been reported by Reid et al.,[72] who used 5-FU applications twice weekly for up to six months subsequent to laser ablation.

Safety and Precaution.   The 5-FU should not be used during pregnancy. Local side effects are common and often pronounced and may require repetitive monitoring.

B.   Surgery

In spite of available topical chemotherapeutics effective in clinical HPV infections, surgical methods still have a major place in therapy. As for chemical therapy, surgical methods are based on the destruction of tissue and comprise scalpel surgery, the scissor-snip method, sharp currettage, electrosurgery, cryo-therapy and laser-therapy. Which of the different types of surgical aproaches is used depends on the clinical picture and the location of disease. Often, however, local traditions and the practice of individual physicians are more important.

All surgical methods more or less require analgesia which is mostly provided by local infiltration anaesthesia or when larger areas are afflicted by general anaesthesia. Recently progress has been achieved by a new local anaesthetic cream containing lidocaine and prilocaine (EMLA®),* which is valuable for reduction of pain produced by electrosurgery or CO_2 laser treatment of circumscribed vulvar or penile lesions. Its use is especially favourable in children suffering from genitoanal warts.[73]

1.   Scissor Excision, Curettage, and Electrosurgery

Scissor excision under local anaesthesia is effective in cases of circumscribed perianal and intraanal warts.[74] This method can also be used to remove well circumscribed papular lesions such as bowenoid papulosis. The technique is suitable especially for limited disease and solitary small sized lesions. It causes only minimal pain and minimal damage to adjacent tissues. Infiltration of anaesthesia into the affected skin area leads to separation and elevation of the lesions which then can be easily removed individually using scissors (Figure 3). Bleeding is easily controlled by diathermy.

The use of a sharp spoon-curette under local anaesthesia is another simple surgical approach which is useful in pedunculated or filiform warts of the perianal and inguinal areas. This method, combined with electrocautery, leads to acceptable results at anal and genital skin sites. The procedure, however, is not suitable for genital warts of the prepuce, of the glans penis, of the introitus vaginae, the vagina, the cervix, or the anus.

---

* Astra Pharmaceuticals, AB, Södertälje, Sweden.

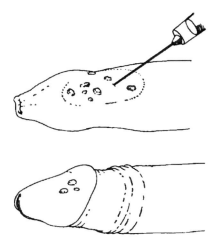

FIGURE 3A In circumscribed lesions, surgery is perfomed using infiltration anaesthesia applied subepidermally. Separation of warts is achieved and individual lesions can be removed by scissor-snip excision, curettage, electrocautery, or CO₂ laser. Infiltration anaesthesia may be performed on the penile shaft, on the foreskin and also on the penis.

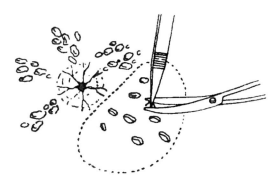

FIGURE 3B Infiltration anaesthesia of the perianal and the vulvar area is best performed with adrenalin as an adjuvant in order to promote haemostasia. Separation of individual warts will facilitate an accurate removal of the warts and sparing of uninvolved skin bridges. The application of EMLA® cream prior to infiltration anaesthesia is very advantageous in order to minimize pain from the needle-stick.

Electrosurgery is a surgical procedure in which an electrosurgical generator is used to convert household alternating current (60 Hz) into high-frequency alternating current (500 Hz to 3.3 MHz). This current is passed through a monopolar electrode to cut or coagulate tissue. The active electrode is a fine wire for cutting and an electrode of either different size for coagulation. Electrosurgery can be employed for both limited and extensive disease, widespread lesions, and recalcitrant anogenital warts as well as exuberating growing giant condylomata acuminata (electroresection) followed by curettage or CO₂ laser.

2.   Diathermy Loop in Cervical Intraepithelial Neoplasia (CIN)

The application of electrosurgical principles and techniques to the treatment of CIN eleminates most problems raised by scalpel (cold knife) and laser conization, such as postoperative bleeding for cold knife cone and high equipment costs for laser cone. For these reasons, loop excision is actually considered the treatment of choice for CIN.[75] The physical process by which electrosurgical cutting occurs is thought to be identical to that by which CO₂ lasers cut tissue. Similarly to the CO₂ laser, the diathermy loop can cut and coagulate simultaneously. The treatment is usually performed under local aneasthesia rendering the loop technique usuable for outpatient treatment. Advantages of this technique are low rate of recurrences[76] and of complications such as bleeding and stenosis.[77] Furthermore, loop excision allows a thorough histologic control of the entire transformation zone. Microscopic analysis of specimens removed by loop excision has shown that target biopsies taken before therapy usually tend to underestimate the true nature and extent of dysplastic cervical lesions by one or two degrees in about 10% of cases investigated.[78] Indications for diathermy loop excision are all histologically confirmed CIN cases with or without visible junctions. In lesions with an exocervical squamo-columnar junction, excision until a depth of 7 mm is sufficient, since this is the maximal depth of CIN within glandular tubes. CIN-lesions extending onto the cervix or even to the vagina should be treated by laser. The same is true for CIN without detectable junctions in postmenopausal women. Since a loop excision deeper than 15 mm is rather difficult, in these patients, laser or cold knife conization should preferentially be used.

Safety and Precaution. The disadvantage of both electrocoagulation and loop excision is the difficulty in knowing the extent of the warty tissue to be destroyed. Excessive coagulation may lead to necrosis of tissue resulting in unnecessary fibrosis and scarring. A hazard is that of fire or explosion if electrosurgery is conducted in the presence of alcohol, oxygen, or bowel gazes (methane). The same is also true for CO_2 laser therapy. Safety features in modern electrosurgery equipment prevent the delivery of dangerous amounts of electricity via the active electrode in cases of malfunction.

The use of disposible or sterilized electrodes is highly recommended to prevent transmission of virus via the electrode. With extensive electrocoagulation, as with CO_2 laser surgery, a smoke-plume is generated. As HPV DNA has been recovered from the smoke, an evacuator is urgently indicated for both CO_2 laser and electrosurgery procedures. All the members of the treatment team should wear surgical masks and eye protection.

In order to obtain optimal results without recurrence of disease it is crucial to remove all visible lesions at external and internal sites. In view of the possibility of transmitting tissue bearing infectious virus material, however, it is highly recommended to procede in a two step manner. The visible external lesions must have been removed thoroughly before using endoscopy, such as urethroscopy or anoscopy. If visible lesions are present in the anal canal, they are then removed in a second step. Some authorities, however, would still recommend single step procedures.

3.   Cryotherapy

Cryotherapy combines physical factors, vascular damage, and immunological reactions. It turns pure water in the cell solution into intracellular ice crystals, leading to destruction of the cells.[79] Cryotherapy has a number of advantages compared to other available surgical modalities. The technique is simple, inexpensive, nontoxic, and it is tolerated well by the patient. In general, two main freezing agents for treatment of genital HPV infections exist: liquid nitrogen, which produces cold at −196°C and which is usually applied by a special system as a spray directly to the lesion, and nitrous oxide gas leading to cold of about −88°C delivered through cryoprobe tips. In circumscribed warts, liquid nitrogen can also be applied by dipping cotton-tipped applicators into liquid nitrogen held in a small thermos. There are cryosurgery closed probe systems available which are specially prepared for therapy of portiocervical lesions. In general, most warts have to be retreated at intervals of 1–2 weeks and more than 10 applications may be necessary until the warts are finally cured.

4.   Clinical Application of Cryotherapy

Comparing the results of various clinical studies using cryosurgery, a cure rate of about 70% and a recurrence rate of genital warts after cryosurgery of 21–40% has been established.[82] In a controlled recent multicenter study, however, there was no difference between cryosurgery, laser-surgery, and electrocautery with regard to recurrence rates, reaching 75%.[4]

For women, cryotherapy has its special niche, since it is a safe method for pregnant women suffering from genital warts. A number of authors advocate, however, the principle of avoiding any treatment in the second half of pregnancy and would rather not treat until after delivery because of the risk of bleeding and of secondary infections from cryo-, CO_2-laser, and electrosurgical therapy. Nevertheless, in a series of 52 treatment sessions on females with genital warts during the last two trimesters of pregnancy, cryosurgery was found to be both safe and efficient.[80] After 2–4 sessions of cryosurgery, all patients recovered completely. This was also true in 90 women treated for cervical lesions. No side effects in terms of premature delivery or fetal injury was observed.[81] According to Ferenczy, cryotherapy is also very useful for CIN.[82] Complication rates were very low and the therapeutic success rates were calculated after refreezing persistent CIN lesions in up to 97% of cases.[82] Large cervical lesions and lesions extending into the endocervical canal, however, responded worse to this treatment. In general, cervical lesions bear the risk of vasomotor symptoms and uterine cramps, observed especially in prolonged cryotherapy sessions. As a consequence, lesions of the cervix, especially CIN lesions measuring more than 3 cm in diameter, should not be treated by cryosurgery.

Safety and Precaution.   Local anaesthesia is necessary because most patients experience pain after cryotherapy. Following intensive cryosurgery, urtication, edema, and frequent blister formation can be expected,[79] leading to a profuse watery discharge in a high proportion of patients, sometimes lasting up to three weeks. Another disadvantage is that the time required until final cure is rather long. Daily bathing is allowed and application of a mild antiseptic dressing is suggested. Antihistamines, analgesics or cold compresses are needed if large areas have been treated. Some physicians believe that topical steroid therapy should be avoided due to a potential disease activation but this aspect is controversial. The principal critic to cryosurgery, however is the lack of control of depth destruction, since removal of treated tissue is not visualized during treatment.

5.   Laser Surgery

Laser is an acronym for light amplification by stimulated emission of radiation. Any medical laser is able to focus an immense amount of monochromatic optical energy to a well-defined surface. The CO_2 laser emits light energy at a wavelength of 10.600 nm, which is in the intrared portion of the spectrum. This light beam superheats intra- and extracellular water to 100°C, resulting in evaporation of the cell and subsequent formation of steam. In many gynecology and dermatology clinics, the CO_2-laser has become the method of treatment preferred in the management of neoplastic diseases associated with HPV of the cervix, vagina, vulva, penis, urethra, and anus.[83] This is due to a number of advantages such as great precision, clean incisions, minimal tissue damage— especially to the surrounding tissue—little postoperative swelling, good haemosthasis, fine scar formation and few complications such as minimal pain, reinfections, and wound secretions.

The cost of the equipment and safety requirements are important disadvantages associated with CO_2-laser therapy. As for cryotherapy, however, the main limitation of laser ablation is the lack of histologic control. With regard to cervical lesions, this means the need for high colposcopic expertise of gynecologists. Both treatment of missed early invasive cancer as well as incomplete treatment is of special importance in CIN and other genitoanally located dysplastic lesions. The depth of tissue destruction can be carefully controlled by adjusting the powersetting (which should be of at least 20 W), and regulating the diameter of the light spot, as well as the speed of beam motion. A focused CO_2-laser beam of about 0.1mm in diameter penetrates into the tissue, enabling the laser to be used as a cutting instrument, whereas the defocused beam of up to 2 mm spot size only causes vaporization of superficial cell layers with a coagulation zone of about 0.3 mm. Within this zone, vessels up to a diameter of 0.5 mm are sealed. The endpoint of removal is ascertained under visual control. Ferenczy and coworkers have suggested to extend laser treatment 1–2 cm beyond grossly apparent CIN lesions since latent virus is often present in adjacent epithelial tissue.[84] However, the efficacy of this protocol in eradicating HPV infection has not been proven.

Due to its use for both cutting and vaporization, the CO_2-laser is an instrument with a wide spectrum of applications in HPV associated lesions of the anogenital region. The postoperative regimen will comprise baths and creams. Healing will be obtained within one to three weeks, depending on the lesional surface and location.

The recently developed CO_2 laser swift lase™ operating principle enables ablation of surface ultrathin char-free epithelial layers of about 200 microns per second if a CO_2 laser beam of 10 watts and a spot size of 0.5 mm is used: two rotating mirrors provide very fast uniform scanning of a large circular area. This technique has been already applied successfully in vulvar lesions[85] and also in dermatologic disorders (Figure 4) (Gross, in preparation).

The question as to whether anaesthesia is required or not depends mainly on the site and on the extent of the disease to be ablated. Whereas cervical and vaginal lesions are often treated without anaesthesia, external lesions of both sexes and those of the anal canal regularly require anaesthesia, either local (EMLA®), regional (infiltration), or general.

Neodymium (Nd-YAG) laser emits a beam of 1060 nm which is worse absorbed than visible light and therefore penetrates more deeply into the skin.[83] Again, the depth of coagulation can be controlled by laser power, spot size, and exposure time. As bleeding does not occur during Nd-YAG laser therapy, this laser is especially recommended for treatment of HIV-positive patients suffering from genital HPV infections. Furthermore, this instrument is of great value for urologists. The beam is transmitted by a flexible light-guidance system and can be used for therapy of urethral lesions. The main advantages of this laser application are the effectiveness of tumor destruction, closure of blood vessels and lymphatic vessels of the tumor, no anaesthesia requirement, and short operation times.

6.   Clinical Application of Lasers

Laser treatment, especially CO_2-laser, has applications in the treatment of both very flat lesions and of large and hard-to-treat lesions in any part of the genitoanal tract of both sexes.[83,86] Giant condylomata acuminata can be easily destroyed either by CO_2-laser[87,88] or by Nd-YAG-laser.[89] In order to exclude malignancy, at least one punch-biopsy has to be taken for histology and virus typing before treatment.

There is an endless list of reports on successful therapy of genitoanal warts using the CO_2-laser with cure rates between 43–90% and recurrence rates of 5–10%.[90] Critical analysis of these studies, however, has led to the assumption that in many of the cases reported, treatment had to be repeated several times, and a number of patients involved in such studies suffered from condylomata acuminata of short duration and mostly without any complications. There are few controlled studies comparing CO_2-laser surgery with other therapies. One series by Duus and co-workers[5] compared CO_2-laser surgery, conventional surgery, and electrocautery and found no significant differences in the cure rates of the lesions (43% with laser vs. 36% with surgery/electrosurgery; Table 1). Condylomata recurred within the originally treated area in all patients except one. Ferenczy compared laser treatment with topical applications of 5-FU with cure rates of 69% for the laser treated group vs. 90% for the 5-FU group.[68] Combining laser therapy with topical 5-FU led to a 90% cure rate vs. 69% for laser treatment alone.[68] In a recent comparative multicenter study there was no difference in the recurrence rate of genital warts of about 75% after either laser treatment, electrocautery, or cryotherapy.[4]

7.   Cervical Lesions (CIN) and Intraepithelial Neoplasia of the Vulva (VIN), Vagina (VAIN), and Penis (PIN)

CIN, which extends into the stroma ≤ 5 mm, is treated with the CO_2-laser either by evaporization, excisional biopsy, or a combination of both.[91] It is mandatory that prior to vaporization, colposcopy directed biopsies should be taken of the clinically most abnormal epithelium. Most patients in an ambulatory setting are treated by a colposcope- or an operating microscope-guided CO_2-laser instrument without anaesthesia. Vaporization is performed at 40–60 W of power, utilizing 2–4 mm spots in order to vaporize rapidly large tracts of tissue. Laser vaporization should be achieved down to a 5–7 mm depth in order to treat CIN in cervical glands. The cutting technique is especially

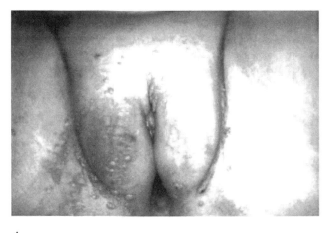

A

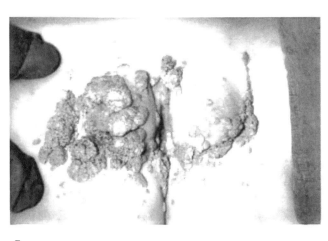

B

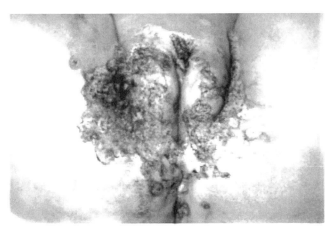

C

FIGURE 4 Vulvar condylomata acuminata in an 18-month-old girl (A) Small papular lesions located at the labia majora before electrocauterization; (B) Recurrent disseminated condylomata acuminata at the vulva; (C) CO_2 laser swift lase ablated vulvar areas prior to topical interferon beta gel therapy.

intended to remove CIN lesions expanding into the endocervical canal and also cervical invasive carcinoma. This operation is normally performed in general anaesthesia. The spot of the laser beam should be reduced for excisional purposes to 0.2 mm. The advantages of laser excision conization are rare occurrence of hemorrhage, reduced risk of postoperative stenosis, and reduced risk of necrosis in comparison with electrocauterization.[92] Neither destructive nor excisional methods are able to completely eradicate HPV induced or neoplastic changes. As the failure rate is at least 2 to 10%, consequent follow-up over at least 12 months is mandatory. Laser surgery seems superior to cryo-therapy in treating cervical lesions larger than 3 cm in diameter.[82] Although cure rates for CIN have been calculated as being as high as 90–97% after 1 to 3 settings, it is likely that recurrence rates are as high as those observed in laser surgery of genital warts.

CO$_2$-laser is a perfect tool for the treatment of intraepithelial neoplasia of the vulva (VIN), the vagina (VAIN), and the penis (PIN). This is especially true for multifocal pigmented VIN III and PIN III, which is frequently seen in young patients (pigmented bowenoid papulosis). Surgical therapies such as CO$_2$-laser enables to preserve the normal anatomy and function of the vulva and the penis. As shown by Townsend and co-workers, 31 out of 33 women suffering from VAIN III were completely cured of all disease.[93] However, 14 of these patients required 2–5 treatment sittings. Similar results were reported by Baggish and Dorsey,[94] who treated 35 women with VIN with a failure rate of 9%, 26 of the patients requiring 3 or more treatments. Stanhope and co-workers[95] and Kaufmann and Friedrich[96] report very similar results. Extensive disease, however, regularly requires multiple treatment courses, often leading to disagreeable and sometimes unacceptable discomfort for patients. Similar to therapy of CIN III, one of the main disadvantages of CO$_2$-laser treatment of VIN III is the risk of missing early invasive carcinoma despite multiple pre-therapy biopsies.[97] This problem is of particular significance in hair-bearing areas, where surgical excision of any VIN III should be performed either using scalpel or laser-excision, followed by suturing. Excision is necessary because penetration of intraepithelial disease into the hair follicles and sebaceous glands may occur, when superficial laser vaporization may be insufficient to clear all HPV foci.[86,92] Bowenoid papulosis in the male (PIN III) is also responsive to CO$_2$-laser therapy, as shown by Landthaler et al.[98] Again, the most prominent advantage of laser therapy of bowenoid lesions in the male is that mutilation of the penis can be avoided.

Safety and Precaution.　　Potential hazards associated with laser therapy in general refer primarily to injuries of the eye. While CO$_2$-laser is more apt to damage the cornea, the sclera, or surrounding skin, the Nd-YAG laser can injure the retina. Eye protection using special protective lenses is therefore mandatory for patients, physicians, and personnel. As with electrosurgery, CO$_2$-laser surgery must be flanked by a smoke evacuator because the plume of steam represents a definite health hazard for patients and the medical team. HPV DNA has been isolated from laser plume in cases in which verrucae have been treated.[99] Using PCR technique, genetic material emanating from potentially more harmful viruses such as HIV,[100] as well as of intact bacteria,[101] has also been reported.

C.　Interferon (IFN)

As GPVI exists predominantly in a subclinical or latent form, none of the currently used chemical or surgical therapeutic modalities, aiming at eradication of visible lesions, are devoid of risk of later recurrences after primary successful treatment. The issue of latency of HPV DNA in epithelial cells,[84] particularly its relevance to therapy in prevention of recurrences, is one example in which molecular biology may influence therapeutic protocols in the future. It is evident, that besides intracellular and intercellular growth control mechanisms,[102] immunological control of HPV infections plays an important role as indicated by the frequency of warts in immunocompromised individuals. Furthermore, derived from *in vitro* studies it has become likely that both local and systemic immunosurveillance are of importance in HPV infections.

Stimulation of tumor specific immunity seems to depend on a proper processing and presentation of tumor specific antigens. This process entails expression of HLA-DR antigens, when primarily T-cells, macrophages, and Langerhans' cells are being activated. Stimulation of these immune reactions is mediated in part by chemical signals that include various cytokines. Successful immune response to viral infections involves a complex cascade of events that include presentation of viral antigens to the immune system, proliferation of antigen-specific lymphocytes, and activation of a diverse array of cytokines. Viral infection of target cells normally causes the release of cytokines such as interferons (IFNs), tumor necrosis factor (TNF), interleukin I (IL-1), II (IL-2), and others.

1. Clinical Experiences with IFN in Anogenital Condylomata Acuminata

The nature of HPV induced genital lesions makes IFN administration a logical therapeutic approach. The antiviral effects of IFN should potentially limit viral replication in the new or regenerating epithelium. The antiproliferative or cell cycle inhibitory effects could possibly decrease the growth of transformed epidermal cells. These measures, in combination with the immunomodulatory effects of IFN, should promote a clearing up of visible lesions.

IFNs can be given topically as gels or creams, or by intralesional or parenteral injections given either intramuscularly, subcutaneously, or intravenously. IFN-therapy can be given as monotherapy, or as an adjuvant therapy together with other treatment modalities such as surgery.

2. Topical Administration of IFN Gel

Topical application has the potential advantage of being free of symptomatic side effects, especially systemic toxicity; only low doses are theoretically necessary. A further therapeutic advantage would be that treatment could possibly be achieved in such patients with whom systemic immunotherapy is not optimal, as, for instance, in transplant recipients. However, despite a number of optimistic open studies using IFN alpha and IFN beta gels,[103-108] no beneficial effects of IFN were demonstrated as compared to placebo.[109] Probably, available preparations do not deliver adequate quantities of IFN to the papillomavirus infected epidermal basal cell layers.

3. Intralesional IFN Treatment

In contrast to topical administration of IFN containig gels, intralesional therapy has been shown to be relatively effective both in a number of controlled and uncontrolled studies.[110-114] However, as the intralesional administration of IFNs has no beneficial effects on noninjected lesions, this therapy has no significant advantage in comparison to conventional therapies against widespread lesions. For example, papillomas located in the urethra or the anal canal, far from the injection site, do generally not respond. Also, subclinical GPVI may be missed and, in part, account for recurrence rates among treated lesions being as high as $\geq 40\%$ in some studies. Additional major disadvantages of this treatment are that it requires frequent visits and causes repetitive pain, as multiple local injections are usually required. Furthermore, the effect is far lower in immunocompromised HIV positive patients.[115] Nevertheless, intralesionally administered recombinant IFN alpha 2b has recently been licensed in the U.S. by the Food and Drug Administration for treatment of anogenital warts.

4. Parenteral IFN Treatment

Theoretically, parenteral administration of IFNs should influence all HPV infected epithelial cells. According to animal experiments, injection of IFN accomplishes an initial bolus in the circulation, followed by a rapid fall. Some of the IFN is bound by different cell receptors and various organs, and some is excreted through the kidneys. In addition to the antiviral effects, there is a direct IFN effect on the HPV positive cells and an indirect effect via the cellular immune system.[116,117]

In contrast to initial uncontrolled studies which have led to some enthusiasm regarding the clinical effect of parenteral administration of IFNs in anogenital HPV disease,[118-120] placebo-controlled studies have yielded controversial results. This has become especially apparent in a multicenter study employing subcutaneous injections of recombinant IFN alpha 2a in daily doses of 3.0 or 9.0 M.U. three times weekly for 4 weeks (continuous therapy),[121] and a multicenter placebo-controlled double-blind trial comparing 50 μg or 100 μg of recombinant IFN gamma (i.e., about 1 M.U. and 2 M.U. IFN gamma) for seven days followed by a four-week break for up to four cycles (cyclic therapy).[122,123] In contrast to the IFN alpha 2a study which failed to demonstrate superiority of any of the two IFN groups over the placebo group (response rates of 34% and 25%, respectively vs. 30%), 50% (1 MU group), and 45% (2 MU group) of patients receiving IFN gamma in the cyclic manner and 27% of the patients who received placebo were responders (p<0.01). These results indicate that low doses of recombinant IFN gamma given cyclically for up to four cycles, have a therapeutic potential in anogenital warts. Nevertheless, it remains unclear whether the type of IFN, the total dosage, or the treatment regimen was responsible for the different results obtained in these controlled IFN alpha and IFN gamma trials. This is underlined by another recently published randomized placebo-controlled trial using subcutaneous continuous injections of IFN-alpha 2a at daily doses of 1.5 M.U., which again did not show any difference in efficacy between the IFN-alpha 2a and the placebo treatment groups.[124] As in the previous IFN-alpha 2a study, duration of treatment was 4 weeks and the regimen consisted in subcutaneous injections 3 times a week.

The disadvantages of the parenteral low dose cyclic therapy are that long periods of therapy are usually required, and a notable lack of efficacy exists in immunocompromised patients such as in HIV-positive patients and in drug addicts.[125]

In addition to the clinical data using IFN gamma for genital HPV induced warts, *in vitro* experiments have shown that IFN gamma and TNF alpha[126] and other cytokines influence HPV and suppress the expression of the oncogenes HPV 16 E6 and E7 selectively in nonmalignant cells: TGF beta 1 and 2,[127,128] epidermal growth factor (EGF), leukoregulin and IFN gamma.[129,130] This could lead to future therapeutic concepts for also using IFN gamma for HPV associated intraepithelial neoplasia.

5.   Adjuvant IFN Treatment

A promising treatment comprises IFN administered either topically, intralesionally, perilesionally, or systemically when given concurrently with or after surgical procedures. A number of controlled studies have been performed comparing surgical debulking of condylomata acuminata by cryotherapy, electrocautery, or CO_2 laser with and without combination with adjuvant IFN (Table 1).

It is obvious that adjuvant IFN injections given perilesionally after CO_2 laser ablation may lead to significant reductions of the recurrence rates.[1,2] The same is true for the topical adjuvant IFN gel therapy. In some studies, it has been observed that during the first three months after surgery alone, recurrence rates ranged between 75 and 78%, whereas recurrences for IFN beta gel when used as a topical adjuvant ranged between 40 and 54%.[3,4] In contrast to the disappointing effects of topical IFN used as a single-therapy against genital warts, application of IFN beta hydrogel after destruction of the epithelial barrier by CO_2 laser, electrocautery or cryotherapy leads to lower recurrence rates of lesions.[4] Topical application of IFN is likely to prevent reinfection of basal keratinocytes during secondary healing following ablation of the epidermis, thus preventing regrowth of warty tissue. "CO_2-laser-peeling," using the CO_2 laser swift laser, may lead to further decrease the recurrence rate, especially in combination with an IFN containing gel. This method can be used in very extensive flat and papular condylomas, and may even be given to children with anogenital warts (Figure 4) (Gross, in preparation).

The analysis of the published controlled studies in patients with condylomata acuminata treated with systemic IFN therapy as an adjuvant to ablative therapies (cryotherapy, electrocautery, CO_2 laser) shows that recurrence rates for surgery alone, range between 32%[12] and 81%[6] (Table 1). Interestingly, there are only three trials in which the recurrence rates could be decreased by adjuvant IFN therapy[6,7,13] The different results of these studies are probably due to the different therapy regimens used. This is especially obvious when comparing two studies where subcutaneous injections of IFN alpha 2a, given as adjuvant to CO_2 laser therapy, have led to contradictory results.[10,13] In contrast to one study where no superiority could be shown of adjuvant IFN alpha 2a given subcutaneously in a continuous form (3 MU IFN alpha 2a thrice a week during 4 weeks; total dosage 36 MU),[10] in a more recent study[13] a significant decrease in the recurrence rate (41% in the IFN alpha 2a treated group vs. 63% in the placebo-treated group) could be shown (Table 1). The latter trial consisted of subcutaneous injections of 1 MU IFN alpha 2a given cyclically, i.e., 3 cycles consisting of 5 days therapy with a 4-week interval between the cycles. The importance of the noncontinuous cyclic therapy regimen is underlined by the study of Hohenleutner et al.[6] (Table 1), where the recurrence rate could also be significantly reduced by combination of laser with IFN alpha 2b. Again, a low-dose cyclic regimen was administered, i.e., two courses with 1 MU IFN alpha 2b subcutaneously daily for 6 days with a 2-week interval between the courses.

6.   IFN in HPV Associated Neoplasia of the Cervix Uteri, Vulva, Vagina and Penis

As with benign anogenital HPV induced lesions, controlled studies have so far not been able to confirm the optimistic results obtained in uncontrolled studies using topical IFN as well as peri- and intralesional IFN injections in patients with CIN grade I to III, VIN III, and VAIN I-II.[131-138] A double-blind placebo controlled trial of IFN alpha N1 given parenterally did not show any significant therapeutic effect on HPV infection of the cervix and vagina, neither on low nor moderate grades of CIN and VAIN.[139] The dose used in this trial was 1.5 M.U. subcutaneously, three times per week for the first week, followed by 3 M.U. three times per week for a further six weeks.[139] This result is in contrast to open studies using recombinant IFN alpha or recombinant IFN gamma.[140-143] Also, the encouraging results of earlier open studies with direct IFN injections into HPV lesions associated with intraepithelial neoplasia of the vulva and the penis could not be confirmed in a controlled study performed by Frost et al.[144]

7.   Side Effects of IFN Therapy

Side effects as well as clinical effects of IFN therapy are clearly dose-dependent. The most common adverse effects are flu-like symptoms which are seen a few hours after IFN administration. Thus, it is suggested that IFN may not be pyrogenic itself, but might act through induction of other fever-promoting mediators such as IL-1 and prostaglandins, the production of which is activated by IFN.[145] Leukopenia and thrombocytopenia are transcient, and it appears that these effects are also strictly dose-dependent since bone marrow cellularity appears to be completely preserved.[146] These side effects are well tolerated and last only for the first 2–3 days of treatment. Occasionally, mild temporary elevation of liver function tests also occur. An increase in triglyceride levels and a decrease in high density lipoprotein cholesterol levels have been seen in some patients treated with intramuscular injections of IFN alpha, but without any immediate clinical sequelae. A more dangerous side effect can be that IFN may aggravate autoimmune phenomena, probably through enhanced cytotoxicity. Consequently, patients should be tested for the absence of autoantibodies before being admitted and during, as well as at the end, of IFN therapy.

III.   NEW STRATEGIES

A particularly promising treatment seems to be the combination of IFN alpha and retinoids comprising all-trans retinoic acid (Tretinoin), 13-cis retinoic acid (Isotretinoin), and the aromatic retinoids (Etretinate and Acitretin). Although not fully satisfactory as a monotherapy in HPV infection and HPV associated cancer and precancer,[3,147] retinoids and IFN alpha applied simultaneously have shown promising results against genital warts[148] and even against squamous-cell carcinoma of the skin and cervical cancer.[149,150] Clinical studies will answer the question of whether retinoids combined with which cytokines will be optimally efficacious in HPV diseases. Retinoic acid effects proliferation and differentiation of preneoplastic and neoplastic Hela cells, derived from HPV type 18 DNA positive cervical cancer cells which express HPV 18 E6 and E7 proteins associated with oncogenic activity.[151] In cell culture experiments it has been shown that there is a synergistic antiproliferative effect when various retinoids are applied with various cytokines. Overall, IFN alpha had more inhibitory activity on proliferation than had IFN gamma, TNF alpha, transforming growth factor beta (TGF), epidermal growth factor (EGF), and IL-1.[152] Recently published data obtained from *in vitro* experiments of IFN alpha effecting inhibition of growth, transformation, and expression of HPV 16 E7 in human keratinocytes raises the question of whether some IFN alpha subtypes alone produce regression of HPV-induced lesions through a specific inhibition of the expression of the HPV 16 oncogene E7.[153] The combination of the antiproliferative effect of retinoids together with this oncogene inhibitory effect and the antiproliferative, immuno-stimulatory, and immunopotentiating activity of IFN alpha suggests that this might indeed be a promising treatment both for chronic HPV infections of mucous membranes and the skin and also for HPV-related cancer and precancer.

There are further ongoing trials with orally and locally active cytokine inducers which could be used in the future both to combat established disease susceptible to IFN and even for chemoprophylaxis. Favorable results of a study using such a cytokine inducer, the low-molecular-weight imidazoquinolinamine derivative 1-(2-methylpropyl)-1H imidazo 4,5- quinolin-4-amine (imiquimod, previously described as R-837), in the treatment of condylomata acuminata have been presented recently.[154]

IV.   PSYCHOSEXUAL COUNSELING

Recent studies emphasize the importance of properly informing patients about potential misconceptions of the HPV disease,[155,156] a process that should be initiated as a natural part of the communication during the clinical evaluation procedure. In this context, it must also be realized that even though the papanicolaou (PAP) smear is considered an innocuous medical procedure, it may entail significant mental sequelae.[157,158] If the provider allows sufficient time for communication and shows an empathetic and nonjudgmental attitude, patients may be guided through the range of possible embarassment and potential physical consequences of the infection. Providers should let patients know that the process for emotional adjustment requires time. Acknowledging and discussing the negative feelings that patients are almost certain to have, and reassuring them that the infection is ultimately managable represent crucial steps for adequate counseling.[156] The individual patient may often be comforted by repetitive information about the very high prevalence of and the generally quite benign natural history of GPVI in order to establish a balanced attitude towards their own disease, and in particular if the relatively low risk of subsequent genital cancer development is being stressed.

In view of recent observations on cofactors for the potential development of cervical cancer, however, it can never be inproper to emphasize that the risk can be minimized by adequate clinical evaluation and management. In fact, some cocarcinogenic factors appear to include controllable chronic local infections such as gonorrhoea, chlamydia, and trichomoniasis as well as bacterial and/or candidal vaginosis.[159-161]

However, it must be realized that although patients' cognitive and emotional perspectives often follow an appropriate intuitive process of recognition, people tend to consider losses in the domain of emotions as highly significant, and also worry with an intensity disproportionate to the actual danger.[162] Accordingly, a continuous reinforcing process is frequently required for the accomplishment of emotional stability. One erroneous thinking matter of major concern is that, due to the sometimes very long incubation time, the presence of GPVI in one partner of a sexual relationship does not imply that the partner has been unfaithful. This aspect needs to be actively elucidated by the caregiver. Screening with the acetic acid test, or by cytological and/or virological means in males whose partners have CIN, does not rely on a strict rationale. Neither does the introduction of condom use in a steady relationship seem to have any influence on the CIN progression rate of the female counterpart.[163] Yet, it should not be disregarded that a thorough examination of the male counterpart, combined with an individualized counseling of the couple may have significant positive psychosexual implications.

The aspect of current uncertainty regarding the secondary preventive value of condom use should be discussed with the individual patient. Within the framework of a steady ongoing relationship, it might be wiser to focus on the couple's psychosexual well-being rather than advising the male to use a condom for perhaps many months because it seems reasonable to believe that HPV transmission between the partners may have already taken place when the index patient appears for consultation. On the other hand, that the use of a condom might possibly have some protective value for the partner when the tumor bulk is large cannot be dismissed. Quite clearly, it seems sagacious to recommend the use of barrier protection with any new sexual contacts until treatment and controls for condylomas have been completed, a message that concurs with that of protecting oneself from other STDs in the future.

V. SUMMARY AND FUTURE ASPECTS

There is no optimal "once-only" therapy available for HPV induced clinical lesions of the anogenital tract. Choice of therapy should depend not only upon the site and extent of the disease but also on the function of cell mediated immunity and the compliance of the patient. The final cure of visible lesions, i.e., healing with no recurrence of treated lesions, is frequently not easily achieved by any of the single therapeutic modalities known so far. A combination of therapies, however, has proved to frequently be more effective than any single modality alone (Table 7).

TABLE 7   Therapy of Genitourinary and Anal HPV Infections

Limited Disease	
Topical	Podophyllotoxin 0.15–0.5% solution, cream, gel (penile and vulvar warts)
	5-FU cream (5%) (special indication: urethral warts)
	TCA (85%) (special indication: pregnancy)
	IFN alpha intralesional
Surgery	Scissor, curretage
	CO_2-laser
	Cryosurgery
Extensive Disease Recalcitrant Genital Warts	
Surgery	CO_2-laser, cryosurgery, electrosurgery
Topical	5-FU cream (5%) (vulvovaginal, urethral warts)
Systemic[a]	IFN alpha, beta, gamma (sc, low doses, cyclic therapy preferably as adjuvant therapy)
Combinations	Surgery + IFN[a] (sc, il, gel)
	Surgery + 5-FU (5%)
	Oral Retinoids + IFN alpha (sc, low dose)

[a] Not yet standardized.

Nevertheless, most patients may be managed quite simply merely through a few sessions of topical chemotherapy and/or surgery. Administration of 20–25% podophyllin, long considered the therapy of first choice, is associated with low efficacy and a significant toxicity risk that severely limits its routine applicability. Instead, for penile and vulvar warts the alternative use of self-treatment with ethanolic preparations of 0.5% podophyllotoxin applied b. i. d. for three days is advocated, a safe regimen that will either cure or significantly improve most patients within a few weeks when given as 1–4 courses at 5–7 days of drug-free intervals. Alternative cream and gel formulations of podophyllotoxin have also been developed, and recent results indicate that drug concentrations in the range of 0.15–3.0% might be of optimal benefit.

The use of 5-fluorouracil cream has a limited niche in the treatment of meatal, urethral, and vulvovaginal warts. Simple surgical techniques, including excision, curettage, and diathermy, may be used primarily when a few and small lesions are present and are generally recommended when topical chemotherapy has failed. Surgery is in general the therapy of choice for anal and cervical lesions, and for warts during pregnancy. During pregnancy, caustic wart destruction with trichloroacetic acid can also be used.

So far, the use of IFNs in the treatment of genital HPV infections has remained controversial. Some recent controlled studies, however, implicate the importance of the therapy regimen,[4,6,13] especially if IFN is given parenterally. Apparently low doses of about 1–3 MU are superior to higher doses. Both as monotherapy and as adjuvant therapy, IFN given cyclically lead to significantly better results than IFN given continuously. Local adjuvant IFN gel therapy is especially recommended in practice to prevent recurrence of condylomas after ablation-therapy using laser, cryotherapy, or electrocautery.

Recently, extensive attempts have been made to develop HPV-specific vaccines and to establish a vaccine program against HPV. Such a vaccine could be of therapeutic significance, since it could be used both as immunoprophylaxis and as immunotherapy of benign papillomatous growths due to HPV infections and also of HPV-related cancers and precancerous lesions (see Chapter 23). This is the challenge of the future. But there is still a long way before we can start clinical trials using HPV vaccine in patients. A combination of IFN with retinoids, as well as the use of cytokine inducers active orally or topically, are further strategies which may help to optimize therapy of HPV associated disease—either benign or even malignant.

REFERENCES

1. Vance JC, Davis D, Interferon alfa-2b injections used as an adjuvant therapy to carbon dioxide laser vaporization of recalcitrant anogenital condylomata acuminata. *J Invest Dermatol* 955, 146, 1990.

2. Davis BE, Noble MJ, Initial experience with combined interferon alpha and carbon dioxide laser for the treatment of condylomata acuminata. *J Urol,* 197, 627, 1992.

3. Gross G, Interferons in genital HPV disease: In Gross G, Jablonska S, Pfister H, Stegner HE Eds. *Genital Papillomavirus Infections.* Berlin, Heidelberg, New York: Springer-Verlag, 393, 1990.

4. Gross G, Rogozinski T, Schöfer H, et al. Recombinant interferon beta gel as an adjuvant in the treatment of recurrent genital warts: results of a placebo-controlled double-blind study in 120 patients. *J Interferon Res* 14S1, 151, 1994.

5. Duus BR, Philipsen T, Christensen JD et al. Refractory condylomata acuminata: a controlled clinical trial of carbon dioxide laser vs. conventional surgical treatment. *Genitourin Med* 61, 59, 1985.

6. Hohenleutner U, Landthaler U, Braun-Falco O, Postoperative adjuvante Therapie mit Interferon-alfa-2b nach Laserchirurgie von Condylomata acuminata. *Hautarzt.* 41, 545, 1990.

7. Petersen CS, Bjerring P, Larsen J, et al. Systemic interferon alfa-2b increases the cure rate in laser-treated patients with multiple persistent genital warts: a placebo-controlled study. *Genitorurin Med* 67, 99, 1991.

8. Handley JM, Horner T, Maw RD, Dinsmore WW, Subcutaneous interferon alpha 2a combined with cryotherapy vs cryotherapy alone in the treatment of primary anogenital warts: a randomised observer blind placebo-controlled study. *Genitourin Med* 67, 297, 1991.

9. Handley JM, Maw RD, Horner T et al. Non-specific immunity in patients with primary anogenital warts treated with interferon alpha plus cryotherapy or cryotherapy alone. *Acta Dermatol Venereol (Stockh)* 72, 39, 1992.

10. The Condylomata International Collaborative Study Group. Randomized placebo-controlled double-blind combined therapy with laser surgery and systemic interferon-alpha 2a in the treatment of anogenital condylomata acuminata. *J Infect Dis.* 167, 824, 1993.

11. Eron LJ, Alder MB, O'Rourke JM et al. Recurrence of condylomata acuminata following cryotherapy is not prevented by systemically administered interferon. *Genitourin Med* 69, 91, 1993.

12. Nieminen P, Aho M, Lehtinen M et al. Treatment of genital HPV infection with carbon dioxide laser and systemic interferon alpha 2a. *Sex Transm Dis* 21(2), 55, 1994.

13. Gross G, Roussaki A, Baur, S et al. Systemically administered interferon alpha-2a prevents recurrence of condylomata acuminata following CO_2 laser ablation: the influence of the cyclic low-dose therapy regimen. Results of a multicenter double-blind placebo-controlled clinical trial. *Genitourin Med* 72(1), 71, 1996.

14. Genital human papillomavirus infections and cancer: memorandum from a WHO meeting. *Bull WHO.* 65, 817, 1987.

15. Kaplan JW, Condylomata acuminata. *N Orleans Med* 94, 388, 1942.

16. von Krogh G, and Ruden A-K, Topical treatment of penile condylomata acuminata with colchicine at 48-72 hours intervals, *Acta Dermatovenerol* 60, 87, 1979.

17. von Krogh G, Podophyllotoxin for condylomata acuminata eradication, *Acta Derm Venerol* Suppl 98, 1, 1981.

18. von Krogh G, Penile condylomata acuminata: an experimental model for evaluation of topical treatment with 0.5%-1.0% ethanolic preparations of podophyllotoxin for three days, *Sex Transm Dis* 8, 179, 1981.

19. von Krogh, Topical treatment of outer genital warts. *Cervix Lower Fem Gen Tract.* 10, 125, 1992.

20. Sand Petersen C, Weismann K, Quercetin and Kaempherol: an argument against the use of podophyllin? *Genitourin Med* 71, 92, 1995.

21. von Krogh G, Topical treatment of penile condylomata acuminata with podophyllin, podophyllotoxin and colchicine. A comparative study. *Acta Dermatol Venereol (Stockh)* 58, 163, 1978.

22. Ward JW, Clifford WS, Monaco AR, Bickerstaff HJ, Fatal systemic poising following podophyllum treatment of condyloma acuminatum. *South Med J* 47, 1204, 1954.

23. Chamberlain MJ, Reynolds AL, Joeman WB, Toxic effect of podophyllum application in pregnancy. *Br J Med* 3, 391, 1972.

24. Schirren CG. Schwere Allgemeinvergiftung nach örtlicher Anwendung von Podophyllin Spiritus bei spitzen Kondylomen. *Hautarzt.* 17, 321, 1966.

25. Montaldi DH, Giambione JP, Courey NG, Taefi P, Podophyllin poisoning associated with the treatment of condylomata acuminata: a case report. *Am J Obstet Gynecol* 119, 1130, 1974.

26. Slater GE, Rumack BH, Peterson RG. Podophyllin poisoning. Systemic toxicity following cutaneous application. *Obstet Gynecol* 52, 94, 1978.

27. Stoehr GP, Peterson AL, Taylor WJ. Systemic complications of local podophyllin therapy. *Ann Intl Med* 89, 362, 1978.

28. Karol MD, Conner CS, Watanabe AS, Murphey KS. Podophyllum: suspected teratogenicity from topical application. *Clin Toxicol* 283, 1980.

29. Campbell A. N., Accidental poisoning with podophyllin, *Lancet* I, 206, 1980.

30. Filley CM, Graff-Radford NR, Lacy R, et al. Neurological manifestations of podophyllin toxicity. *Neurol* 32, 308, 1982.

31. Cassidy DE, Drewry J and Fanning JP, Podophyllum toxicity: A review of a fatal case and a review of the literature, *J Toxicol-Clin Toxicol* 19 (1), 35, 1982.

32. West WM, Ridgeway NA, Morris AJ and Sides PJ, Fatal podophyllin ingestion, *Southern Med J* 75(10), 1269, 1982.

33. Conard PF, Hanna N, Rosenblum M, Gross JB, Delayed recognition of podophyllin toxicity in a patient receiving epidural morphine. *Anaesth Analg* 191, 1990.

34. Kraus SJ, Stone KM, Management of genital infection caused by human papillomaviruses. *Rev Infect Dis* 12 (Suppl 6), 620, 1990.

35. Jensen SL, Comparison of podophyllin application with simple excision in clearance and recurrence of perianal condylomata acuminata. *Lancet* 2, 1146, 1985.

36. von Krogh G, Podophyllotoxin in serum: absorption subsequent to three-day repeated application of a 0.5% ethanolic preparation on condylomata acuminata, *Sex Transm Dis* 9, 26, 1982.

37. Beutner KR and von Krogh G, Current status of podophyllotoxin for the treatment of genital warts, *Seminars Dermatol* 9, 148, 1990.

38. Lassus A, Comparison of podophyllotoxin and podophyllin in treatment of genital warts, *Lancet* 2, 512, 1987.

39. von Krogh G and Maibach HI, Cutaneous cytodestructive potency of lignans. I. A comparative evaluation of influence on epidermal and dermal DNA synthesis and on dermal microcirculation in the hairless mouse, *Arch Dermatol Res* 274, 9, 1982.

40. von Krogh G and Maibach HI, Cutaneous cytodestructive potency of lignans. II. A comparative evaluation of macroscopic-toxic influence on rabbit skin subsequent to repeated 10-day applications, *Dermatologica* 167, 70, 1983.

41. Sullivan M, King L, Effects of resin of podophyllin on normal skin, condylomata acuminata and verrucae vulgares. *Arch Dermatol Syph* 56, 30, 1947.

42. Loike JD and Horowitz SB, Effects of podophyllotoxin and VP-16-213 on microtubule assembly in vitro and nucleoside transport in HeLa cells, *Biochemistry* 15, 5435, 1976.

43. Mansono-Martinez R, Podophyllotoxin poisoning of microtubules of steady-state. Effect of substoichiometric and superstoichiometric concentrations of the drug, *Mol Cell Biochem* 45, 3, 1982.

44. Brigati C, and Sander B, CHP-8.6, a highly purified podophyllotoxin, efficiently suppresses in vivo and in vitro immune responses, *J Immunopharmacol* 7, 285, 1985.

45. Zheng Q-Y, Wiranowska M and Sadlik JR, Purified podophyllotoxin (CPH-86), inhibits lymphocyte proliferation but augments macrophage proliferation, *Int J Immunopharmac* 9, 539, 1987.

46. Lassus J, Nieminen K-M, Syrjänen S, et al. A comparison of histopathologic diagnosis and the demonstration of human papillomaspecific DNA and proteins in penile warts, *Sex Transm Dis* 19, 127, 1992.

47. Beutner KR, Conant MA and Friedman-Kien A, Patient-applied podofilox for treatment of genital warts, *Lancet* 1, 831, 1989.

48. Kirby P, Dunne A, King DH and Corey L, Double-blind randomized clinical trial of self-administered podofilox solution vehicle in the treatment of genital warts, *Am J Med* 88, 465, 1990.

49. von Krogh G, Topical treatment of HPV lesions of the external genitalia, *Cervix* 10, 125, 1992.

50. von Krogh G, Topical self-treatment of penile warts with 0.5% podophyllotoxin in ethanol for four or five days, *Sex Transm Dis* 14, 135, 1987.

51. Edwards A, Atma-Ram A, Thin RN, Podophyllotoxin 0.5 vs. podophyllin 20% to treat penile warts. *Genitourin Med* 64, 263, 1988.

52. Mazurkiewicz W, Jablonska S, Clinical efficacy of condyline (0.5% podophyllotoxin) solution and cream vs. podophyllin in the treatment of external condylomata acuminata. *J Dermatol Treatment* 1, 123, 1990.

53. Kinghorn GR, McMillan A, Mulcahy F, Clarke S, Lacey C, Bingham JS, An open comparative study of the efficacy of 0.5% podophyllotoxin lotion and 25% podophyllin solution in the treatment of condylomata acuminata in males and females. *Int J STD AIDS* 4, 194, 1993.

54. Pickering RW, The treatment of condylomata acuminata - results of a questionnaire survey, *Br J Sex Med* 210, 1989.

55. von Krogh G, Szpak E, Andersson M and Bergelin I, Self-treatment using 0.25%-0.5% podophyllotoxin ethanol solutions against penile condylomata acuminata: a placebo-controlled comparative study, *Genitourin Med* 70, 105, 1994.

56. von Krogh G. and Hellberg D, Self-treatment using a 0.5% podophyllotoxin cream of external genital condylomata acuminata in women. A placebo controlled double-blind study, *Sex Transm Dis* 19, 170, 1992.

57. Strand A, Brinkeborn RM, Siboulet A, Topical treatment of genital warts in men, an open study of podophyllotoxin cream compared with solution. *Genitourin Med* 71, 387, 1995.

58. Sand Petersen C, Agner, T, Ottevanger V, Larsen J, Ravnborg L, A single-blind study of podophyllotoxin cream 0.5% and podophyllotoxin solution 0.5% in male patients with genital warts. *Genitourin Med* 71, 391, 1995.

59. von Krogh G and Rosén B, Wartec Cream Clinical Expert Report (Conpharm AB, Glunten, 751 83 Uppsala). Unpublished Manuscript.

60. Mohanty KC, The cost effectiveness of treatment of genital warts with podophyllotoxin, *Int J STD AIDS* 5, 253, 1994.

61. Swerdlow DB and Salvati EP, Condyloma acuminatum, *Dis Colon Rectum* 14, 226, 1971.

62. Willcox RR, How suitable are available pharmaceuticals for the treatment of sexually transmitted disease? II. Conditions presenting as sores or tumours, *Br J Vener Dis* 53, 340, 1977.

63. Malvija VK, Deppe G, Pluszczynski R, Boike G, Trichloroacetic acid in the treatment of human papillomavirus infection of the cervix without associated dysplasia. *Obstet Gynecol* 70, 72, 1987.

64. von Krogh G, 5-Fluoro-uracil cream in the successful treatment of therapeutically refractory condylomata acuminata of the urinary meatus, *Acta Dermatovenereol* 56, 297, 1976.

65. Dretler SP, Klein I, The eradication of intraurethral condylomata acuminata with 5-fluorouracil cream. *J Urol* 113, 195, 1975.

66. Wein AJ, Benson GS, Treatment of urethral condylomata acuminata with 5-FU cream. *J Urol* 9, 413, 1977.

67. Cetti NE, Condyloma acuminatum of the urethra: problems in eradication. *Br J Surg* 71, 57, 1984.

68. Ferenczy A, Comparison of 5-Fluoro-uracil and CO_2 laser for treatment of vaginal condylomata. *Obstet Gynecol* 64, 773, 1984.

69. Krebs HB, Treatment of extensive condylomata acuminata with topical 5-fluorouracil. *South Med J* 83, 761, 1990.

70. Pride GL, Treatment of large lower genital tract condylomata acuminata with topical 5-fluorouracil. *J Reprod Med* 35, 384, 1990.

71. Krebs HB, Prophylactic topical 5-fluorouracil following treatment of human papillomavirus-associated lesions of the vulva and vagina. *Obstet Gynecol* 68, 837, 1986.

72. Reid R, Greenberg MD, Lorincz AT et al. Superficial laser vaporization and adjunctive 5-fluorouracil therapy of human papillomavirus-associated vulvar disease. *Obstet Gynecol* 76, 439, 1990.

73. Rylander E, Sjöberg I, Lilleborg S, Local anaesthesia of the genital mucosa with a lidocaine/prilocaine cream (EMLA®) for laser treatment of condylomata acuminata. A placebo-controlled study. *Obstet Gynecol* 75, 302, 1990.

74. Thomson JP, Perianal and anal condylomata acuminata. In: Todd IP Ed. *Operative Surgery Colon, Rectum and Anus.* London: Butterworth (Publ) 376, 1977.

75. Wright TC, Ganon S, Richart R. et al. Treatment of CIN using the loop surgical excison procedure. *Obstet Gynecol* 79, 173, 1992.

76. Prendiville W, Cullimore J, Norman S, Large loop excision of the transformation zone (LLETZ). A method of management for women with cervical intraepithelial neoplasia. *Br J Obstet Gynecol* 96, 1055, 1989.

77. Luesley DM, Cullimore J, Redman CWE, Loop diathermy excision of the cervical tranformation zone in patients with abnormal cervical smears. *Br Med J* 300, 1690, 1990.

78. Wright TC, Richart RM, Ferenczy A, Comparison of specimens removed by CO_2 laser conisation and the loop electrosurgical excision procedure. *Obstet Gynecol* 79, 147, 1992.

79. Torre D. In: Zacarian SA (Ed.) *Instrumentation and Monitoring Devices in Cryosurgery.* Cryosurgery for skin cancer and cutaneous disorders. St. Louis: CV Mosby Co (Publ), 31, 1985.

80. Bergman A, Matsunaga J, Bhatia NN, Cervical cryotherapy for condylomata acuminata during pregnancy. *Obstet Gynecol* 69, 47, 1987.

81. Matsunaga J, Bergman A, Bhatia NN, Genital condylomata acuminata in pregnancy: effectiveness, safety and pregnancy outcome following cryotherapy. *Br J Obstet Gynecol* 94, 168, 1987.

82. Ferenczy A, Comparison of cryo- and carbon dioxide laser therapy for cervical intraepithelial neoplasia. *Obstet Gynecol* 66, 793, 1985.

83. Baggish MS, Improved laser techniques for the elimination of genital and extragenital warts. *Am J Obstet Gynecol* 153, 545, 1985.

84. Ferenczy A, Mitao M, Nagai N, et al. Latent papillomavirus and recurring genital warts. *N Engl J Med* 313, 784, 1985.

85. Levavi H, Ovadia J, Swift laser scanner—A new modality in laser treatment of the vulva: effect on post-operative pain. Presented at the 8th World Congress of Cervical Pathology and Colposcopy - May 1993, Chicago IL, USA.

86. Ferenczy A, Laser therapy of genital condylomata acuminata. *Obstet Gynecol* 63, 703, 1984.

87. Apfelberg DB, Maser MR, Lash H, Druker D, CO_2 laser resection for giant perianal condyloma and verrucous carcinoma. *Ann Plastic Surg* 11 (5), 417, 1983.

88. Hohenleutner U, Landthaler M, Braun-Falco O, et al. Condylomata acuminata gigantea (Buschke-Löwenstein Tumor): Behandlung mit dem CO_2 Laser und Interferon. *D Med Wschr.* 119, 985, 1986.

89. Bahmer FA, Tang DE, Payeur-Kirsch M, Treatment of large condylomata of the penis with the neodymium-YAG laser. *Acta Dermatovenereol (Stockh.)* 64, 631, 1984.

90. Landthaler M, Laser therapy of anogenital papillomavirus infections - The view of the dermatologist. In: Gross G, Jablonska S, Pfister H, Stegner HE (Eds.) *Genital Papillomavirus Infections.* Berlin, Heidelberg, New York,: Springer-Verlag (Publ). 341, 1990.

91. Anderson MC, Hartley RB, Cervical crypt involvement by intraepithelial neoplasia. *Obstet Gynecol* 55, 546, 1980.

92. Larsson G, Alm P, Grundsell H, Laser conization vs. cold knife conization. *Surg Gynecol Obstet* 154, 59, 1982.

93. Townsend DE, Levine RU, Crum DP, Richart RM, Treatment of vaginal carcinoma in situ with the carbon dioxide laser. *Am J Obstet Gynecol* 143, 546, 1982.

94. Baggish MS, Dorsey JH, Carbon dioxide laser for combination excisional-vaporization conization. *Am J Obstet Gynecol* 151, 23, 1985.

95. Stanhope CR, Phibbs Gd, Stuart GC, Reid R., Carbon dioxide laser surgery. *Obstet Gynecol* 61 (5), 624, 1983.

96. Kaufman RH, Friedrich EG, The carbon dioxide laser in the treatment of vulvar disease. *Clin Obstet Gynecol* 28 (1), 220, 1985.

97. Caglar H, Tamer S, Hreschchyshyn MM, Vulvar intraepithelial neoplasia. *Obstet Gynecol* 60, 346, 1982.

98. Landthaler M, Haina D, Brunner R, et al. Laser therapy of bowenoid papulosis and Bowen's disease. *J Derm Surg Oncol* 12, 1253, 1986.

99. Garden JM, O'Banion MK, Shelnitz LS, et al. Papillomavirus in the vapor of carbondioxide laser-treated verrucae. *J Am Med Assoc* 259, 1199, 1988.

100. Baggish MS, Polesz BJ, Joret D, Williamson P, Refai A, Presence of human immunodeficiency virus DNA in laser smoke. *Laser Surg Med* 11, 197, 1991.

101. Mullarky MB, Norris CW, Goldberg ID, The efficacy of the CO_2 laser in the sterilization of skin seeded with bacteria: survival at the skin surface and the plume emissions. *Laryngoscope* 95, 186, 1985.

102. zur Hausen H, Human papillomaviruses in the pathogenesis of anogenital cancer. *Virol* 184, 9, 1991.

103. Ikic D, Bosnic N, Smerdel S, Double-blind clinical study with human leukocyte interferon in the therapy of condylomata acuminata. *Proceedings of the Symposium on Clinical Use of Interferon, Zagreb.* 167, 1975.

104. Möller BR, Johannesen P, Osther K et al. Treatment of dysplasia of the cervical epithelium with an interferon gel. *J Obstet Gynecol* 62, 625, 1983.

105. Marcovici R, Peretz BA, Paldi E, Human fibroblast interferon therapy in patients with condylomata acuminata. *Isr J Med Science* 19, 104, 1983.

106. Vesterinen E, Meyer B, Cantell K et al. Topical treatment of flat vaginal condyloma with human leukocyte interferon. *Obstet Gynecol* 64, 535, 1984.

107. De Virgilis C, Crippa L, Leopardi O et al. The role of beta-interferon in the therapy of female genital viral diseases. *Intl J Immunol* 3, 147, 1987.

108. Schneider A, Papendick U, Gissmann L, Interferon treatment of human genital papillomavirus infections: importance of viral type. *Int J Cancer* 40, 610, 1987.

109. Keay S, Teng N, Eisenberg M et al. Topical interferon for treating condylomata acuminata in women. *J Infect Dis* 185, 934, 1988.

110. Eron LJ, Judson F, Tucker S et al. Interferon therapy for condylomata acuminata. *N Engl J Med* 315, 1059, 1986.

111. Vance JC, Bart BJ, Hausen PC et al. Intralesional recombinant alpha-2 interferon for the treatment of patients with condyloma acuminatum or verruca plantaris. *Arch Derm* 122, 272, 1996.

112. Friedman-Kien A, Eron LJ, Conant M et al. Natural interferon alfa for treatment of condylomata acuminata. *J Am Med Assoc* 259 (4), 533, 1988.

113. Reichmann RC, Oakes D, Bonnez et al. Treatment of condyloma acuminatum with three different interferons administered intralesionally. A double-blind placebo-controlled trial. *Ann Intl Med* 108, 675, 1988.

114. Welander LE, Homesley HD, Smiles KA, Peets EA, Intralesional interferon alfa-2b for the treatment of genital warts. *Am J Obstet Gynecol* 162 (2), 348, 1990.

115. Douglas JM, Rogers U, Judson FN, The effect of asymptomatic infection with HTLV-3 on the response of anogenital warts to intralesional treatment with recombinant alpha-2-interferon. *J Infect Dis* 154, 331, 1986.

116. Maluish AE, Ortaldo JR, Sherwin SA et al. Changes in immune function in patients receiving natural leukocyte interferon. *J Biol Resp Modif* 2, 418, 1983.

117. Sen GC, Biochemical pathways in interferon-action. *Pharmacol Ther* 24, 235, 1984.

118. Weck PK, Brandsma JL, Whisnant JK, Interferons in the treatment of human papillomavirus diseases. *Cancer Metast Rev* 5, 139, 1986.

119. Reichmann RC, Human papillomaviruses and interferon therapy. In: Galasso GJ, Whitley RJ, Merigan TC (Eds.) *Antiviral Agents and Viral Diseases of Man.* Raven, New York. 310, 1990.

120. Schoenfeld A, Schattner A, Crespi M, et al. Intramuscular human interferon beta injections in treatment of condylomata acuminata. *Lancet* 1, 1038, 1984.

121. The Condylomata International Collaborative Study Group. Recurrent condylomata acuminata treated with recombinant interferon alpha 2a: a multicenter double-blind placebo controlled clinical trial. *J Am Med Assoc* 265, 2684, 1991.

122. Gross G, Recombinant interferon gamma in condylomata acuminata. *J Am Med Assoc* 266, 2706, 1991.

123. Gross G, Degen KW, Fierlbeck G, et al. Recombinant interferon gamma in anogenital warts: results of a multicenter placebo-controlled clinical trial. *J Interferon Res* 11 S 1, 76, 1991.

124. The Condylomata International Collaborative Study Group. Recurrent condylomata acuminata treated with recombinant interferon aplha 2a: a multicenter double-blind placebo-controlled clinical trial. *Acta Dermatovenereol (Stockh)* 73, 223, 1993.

125. Gross G, Roussaki A, Ikenberg H, Drees N, Genital warts do not respond to systemic recombinant interferon alpha-2a treatment during cannabis consumption. *Dermatologica* 1831, 203, 1991.

126. Rösl F, Lengert M, Albrecht J, et al. Differential regulation of the JE gene encoding the monocyte chemoattractant protein (MCP-1) in cervical carcinoma cells and derived hybrids. *J Virol* 68, 2142, 1994.

127. Braun L, Dürst M, Mikumo R, Guipposo P, Differential response of nontumorigenic and tumorigenic human papillomavirus type 16-positive epithelial cells to transforming growth factor beta. *Cancer Res* 50, 7324, 1990.

128. Woodworth CD, Notario V, di Paolo JA, Transforming growth factor beta 1 and 2 transcriptionally regulate human papillomavirus (HPV) type 16 early gene expression in HPV-immortalized human genital epithelial cells. *J Virol* 64, 4767, 1990.

129. Yasumoto S, Taniguchi A, Sohma K, Epidermal growth factor (EGF) elicits down-regulation of human papillomavirus type 16 (HPV-16) E6/E7 mRNA at transcriptional level in an EGF-stimulated human keratinocyte cell line: functional role of EGF-responsive silencer in the HPV-16 long control region. *J Virol* 65, 2000, 1991.

130. Woodworth CD, Lichti U, Simpson S, et al. Leukoregulin and gamma-interferon inhibit human papillomavirus type 16 gene transcription in human papillomavirus immortalized human cervical cells. *Cancer Res* 52, 456, 1992.

131. Ikic D, Krusic J, Cupak S et al. The use of human leukocyte interferon in patients with cervical cancer and basocellular cancer in the skin. *Proceedings of a Symposium on Clinical Use of Interferon, Zagreb.* 167, 1972.

132. Byrne MA, Möller BR, Taylor-Robinson D et al. The effect of interferon on human papillomavirus associated with cervical intraepithelial neoplasia (CIN). *Br J Obstet Gynecol* 93, 1136, 1982.

133. De Palo G, Stefanon B, Rilke F et al. Human fibroblast interferon in cervical and vulvar intraepithelial neoplasia associated with papillomavirus infection. *Int J Tiss React* 6, 523, 1984.

134. De Palo G, Stefanon B, Rilke F et al. Human fibroblast interferon in cervical and vulvar intraepithelial neoplasia associated with viral cytopathic effects. *J Reprod Med* 30, 404, 1985.

135. Choo YC, Seto WH, Hsu S et al. Cervical intraepithelial neoplasia treated by perilesional injection of interferon. *Br J Obstet Gynecol* 93, 372, 1986.

136. Schneider A, Kirchmayer R, Wagner D. Efficacy trial of topically applied gamma-interferon in cervical intraepithelial neoplasia. In: Gross G, Jablonska S, Pfister H, Stegner HE (Eds.) *Advances in Modern Diagnosis and Therapy.* International Symposium on Genital Papillomavirus Infections, Hamburg. 1989 (Abstract 48).

137. Neis KJ, Tesseraux M, Claußen C et al. Lokale Therapie cervikaler intraepithelialer Neoplasien mit natürlichem beta-Interferon. *Arch Gynecol* 245, 550, 1989.

138. Iwasaka T, Hayashi Y, Yokoyama M, et al. Interferon alpha treatment for cervical intraepithelial neoplasia. *Gynecol Oncol* 37, 96, 1990.

139. Dunham AM, McCartney JC, McCance DJ, Taylor RW, Effect of perilesional injection of alpha-interferon on cervical intraepithelial neoplasia and associated human papillomavirus infection. *J Roy Soc Med* 83, 490, 1990.

140. Gross G, Roussaki A, Schöpf E, et al. Successful treatment of condylomata acuminata and bowenoid papulosis with subcutaneous injections of low-dose recombinant interferon alpha. *Arch Derm* 122, 749, 1986.

141. Yliskoski M, Syrjänen K, Syrjänen S, et al. Systemic alpha interferon (Wellferon) treatment of genital human papillomavirus (HPV) type 6,11,16 and 18 infections: Double-blind, placebo-controlled trial. *Gynecol Oncol* 43, 55, 1991.

142. Slotman BJ, Helmerhorst TJM, Wijermans PW et al. Interferon-alpha in treatment of intraepithelial neoplasia of the lower genital tract: a case report. *Eur J Obstet Gynecol Reprod Biol* 27, 327, 1988.

143. Gross G, Roussaki A, Papendick U, Efficacy of interferons on bowenoid papulosis and other precancerous lesions. *J Invest Derm* 955, 152, 1990.

144. Frost L, Skajaa K, Hvidman LE, et al. No effect of intralesional injection of interferon on moderate cervical intraepithelial neoplasia. *Br J Obstet Gynecol* 97, 626, 1990.

145. Bocci V, Possible causes of fever after interferon administration. *Biomedicine* 32, 159, 1980.

146. Dianzani F, Interferon treatments: how to use an endogeneous system as a therapeutic agent. *J Interf Res* 109, 1992.

147. Weiner SA, Meyskens FDI, Sarwit EA et al. Response of human papillomavirus-associated diseases to retinoids (vitamin A derivates). In: Howley PM, Broker TR (Eds.) *Papillomaviruses, Molecular and Clinical Aspects* New York: Alan Riss (publ.). 249, 1985.

148. Olsen EA, Kelly FF, Vollmer RT, Comparative study of systemic interferon alfa-n1 and isotretinoin in the treatment of resistant condylomata acuminata. *J Am Acad Derm* 20, 1023, 1989.

149. Lippmann SM, Parkinson DR, Itri LM, et al. 13-cis-retinoid acid and interferon alpha-2a: Effective combination therapy for advanced squamous cell carcinoma of the skin. *J Natl Cancer Inst* 84 (4), 235, 1992.

150. Lippmann SM, Kavanagh JJ, Paredes-Espinoza M, et al. 13-cis-retinoic acid plus interferon alpha-2a: Highly active systemic therapy for squamous cell carcinoma of the cervix. *J Natl Cancer Inst* 84, 241, 1992.

151. Bartsch D, Boye B, Baust C, et al. Retinoic acid-mediated repression of human papillomavirus 18 transcription and different ligand regulation of the retinoic acid receptor beta gene in non-tumorigenic and tumorigenic HeLa hybrid cells. *EMBO* 11 (6), 2283, 1992.

152. Bollag W, Peck R, Frey JR, Inhibition of proliferation by retinoids, cytokines and their combination in four human transformed epithelial cell lines. *Cancer Letters* 62, 167, 1992.

153. Khan MA, Tolleson WH, Gangemi JD, Pirisi L, Inhibition of growth, transformation and expression of human papillomavirus type 16 E7 in human keratinocytes by alpha interferons. *J Virol* 17, 3396, 1993.

154. Beutner K, Spruance S, Douglas J, et al. Double-blind, vehicle-controlled, randomized multicenter trial of 5% Imiquimod cream for the treatment of genital and perianal warts. *Second Internatl. Congress of Papillomaviruses in Human Pathology.* Paris, 6-8 August 1994 (Abstract).

155. Filiberti A, Tamburini A, Stefanon B, et al. Psychological aspects of genital human papillomavirus infection: a preliminary report, *J Psychosom Gynaecol,* 14, 145, 1993.

156. American Social Health Association. Survey shows how we live with HPV. *HPV News* 1993, 3, 1.

157. Palmer AG, Tucker S, Warren R, and Adams M, Understanding women's response to treatment for cervical intra-epithelial neoplasia, *Br J Clin Psychol* 32, 101, 1993.

158. Campion MJ, Brown JR, McCance DJ, et al. Psychosexual trauma of an abnormal cervical smear, *Br J Obstet Gynaecol* 95, 175, 1988.

159. Becker TM, Wheeler CM, McGough NS, et al. Sexually transmitted diseases and other risk factors for cervical dysplasia among Southwestern hispanic and non-hispanic women, *J Am Med Assoc* 271, 1181, 1994.

160. Cooper C and Singah HSK, Condylomata acuminata in women: the effect of concomitant genital infection on response to treatment, *Acta Dermatovenereol* 65, 150, 1985.

161. Kharsany ABM, Hoosen AA, Bagaratee J, and Gouws E, The association between sexually transmitted pathogens and cervical intra-epithelial neoplasia in a developing community, *Genitourin Med* 69, 357, 1993.

162. Redelmeier DA, Rozin P, Kahneman D, Understanding patient's decisions. Cognitive and emotional perspectives. *J Am Med Assoc* 270, 72, 1993.

163. Thomas I, Wright G, and Ward B, The effect of condom use on cervical intraepithelial neoplasia grade I (CIN I), *Aust N Z J Obstet Gynaecol* 30, 326, 1990.

23

Prospects for Vaccination

Joakim Dillner

CONTENTS

The intriguing possibility that vaccination or immunotherapy based on viral antigens could be used for prevention or therapy of HPV-associated anogenital cancers is theoretically appealing since the HPV-carrying cancers express transforming proteins which they are dependent on for continued growth and that can act as tumor rejection antigens. Effective papillomavirus vaccination has also been possible in several animal systems. This article reviews the immunobiology of HPV as well as some of the several different strategies that may be possible for immunological control.

I. THE IMMUNOBIOLOGY OF PAPILLOMAVIRUSES

A. Cell-Mediated Immune Responses

Several lines of indirect evidence indicate that cell-mediated immunity is important in the control of papillomavirus infection. Enhanced papilloma proliferation and increased frequency of HPV infections is observed in therapeutically immunosuppressed patients or in immunodeficiencies specifically involving cell-mediated immunity,[1,2] as well as among patients with HIV infection.[3] Patients with established warts frequently have a depressed cellular immune system.[2,4] The presence of HPV 16 or HPV 18 in cervical intraepithelial neoplasia correlates to a decreased number of Langerhans cells.[5] HPV infections are found up to 9 times more often among renal transplant recipients compared to the general population[6] and these patients also have an increased incidence of CIN lesions.[7] Decreased numbers of CD4+ cells are observed in CIN lesions,[8] and patients with HPV carrying CIN or cervical cancer have a decreased natural killer cell activity.[9]

0-8493-7356-5/97/$0.00+$.50
© 1997 by CRC Press, Inc.

protein expressed in bacteria which give rise to relatively poor titers of neutralizing antibodies.[21,48] Nevertheless, subunit vaccines containing L1 protein[22] or L2 protein[48,49] have been reported to confer some immunity against infection with bovine papillomavirus or cottontail rabbit papilloma-virus, respectively.

Also for HPV 11, neutralizing monoclonal antibodies react with epitopes present only on intact, but not on disrupted virions.[44] It is not clear whether the HPV neutralizing epitopes are merely sensitive to conformational changes or if they are even composite epitopes composed of antigenic sites present on more than one capsid protein monomer, brought into proximity in the assembled particle.

Recombinant proteins expressed in bacteria are often insoluble and are unlikely to adopt a native conformation following purification. Also, proteins expressed in prokaryotic expression systems do not undergo post-translational modifications. When individual HPV capsid proteins are expressed in mammalian cells, however, they will display conformation-dependent epitopes found on intact virions.[50] An important development was the work of Zhou et al.,[51] who used vaccinia virus constructs expressing both the L1 and L2 proteins of HPV 16 and observed the assembly of viral capsids lacking viral DNA (virus-like particles) following infection of epithelial cells with this construct.

Now, several systems exist for *in vitro* propagation of HPV particles. Mouse xenograft systems for HPV propagation have been successfully applied to HPV 11 and HPV 1.[44,52] Organotypic raft cultures of HPV 31-infected keratinocytes have been shown to differentiate *in vitro* and sustain the production of infectious HPV particles following culturing in the presence of tetradecanoylphorbol acetate.[53] Small amounts of HPV 16 particles can also be produced by grafting the HPV 16-carrying CIN-derived cell line W12 onto nude mice.[54] These achievements enable the production of some infectious HPV particles and may provide systems for testing of HPV antibodies for neutralizing activity.

Several well characterized animal model systems for PV immunization exist, but they are based on cutaneous-type PVs that may have very different biology and interactions with the immune system than the genital-type PVs. It is therefore most interesting that an animal model based on a malignancy-associated genital rhesus monkey PV, closely related to HPV 16, has been established.[55] Although many lessons can be learned from the interesting vaccination experiments on animal models such as CRPV and BPV, HPV vaccines would ultimately need to be tested in an HPV model system.

An additional question pertinent to genital HPV vaccines is whether a response of neutralizing IgG in serum would be sufficient for protection or if protection would require the generation of locally produced neutralizing antibodies secreted into the cervical mucus. Since such antibodies would be of the sIgA class, additional questions arise as to whether a route of immunization that favors IgA responses, such as the oral route or even topical application at the cervix, should be applied. Local IgA antibodies against PV antigens are readily detectable in cervical mucus and are preferentially found among CIN and condyloma patients.[56-58]

It should be mentioned that conventional vaccine formulations using inactivated viral particles are not feasible for human use. Since the viral DNA is oncogenic, vaccines for human use containing the oncogenic genes of the viral DNA would not fulfill basic safety requirements. Indeed, a low percentage of dogs vaccinated with a viral DNA-containing canine papillomavirus vaccine were reported to develop papillomavirus-carrying squamous cell carcinomas at the vaccine inoculation site.[47]

The prime candidate for a prophylactic vaccine is the use of the virus-like particles (VLPs). When the L1 major capsid protein is expressed at sufficiently high levels in eukaryotic cells, the capsid proteins will self-assemble into capsids that lack the viral DNA, but are morphologically indistinguishable from native virions.[59-66] A series of studies have shown that VLPs contain the conformationally sensitive neutralizing epitopes of the intact virion[60,63,65] and that immunization with VLPs induces equally high titers of neutralizing antibodies as does immunization with native virions.[61] In the classical animal model system, CRPV, immunization with CRPV VLPs leads to full protection against challenge even with high doses of virus (5×10^{10} virions).[65] Passive transfer of purified IgG from VLP-immunized rabbits to naive rabbits conferred protection against CRPV challenge, confirming that the protection is antibody-mediated.[65] Equally striking results where VLPs have induced protection have also been obtained in other animal systems.[66] Thus, VLPs are likely to fulfill both requirements for efficacy and safety. There are a number of questions that need to be considered before clinical trials of VLP-based vaccines can commence, however.

1. The Route of Immunization

Since HPV is a local genital infection, protective antibodies would have to be present locally in the genital tract. Locally produced antibodies are of the IgA class and it is therefore possible that routes of immunization that favors IgA production, such as the oral route or even intravaginal route of immunization, might result in better protective efficacy. However, in the canine oral papillomavirus (COPV) system, full protection against a mucosal papillomavirus could be achieved by intradermal immunization of the dogs.[67] Also, in the spectacularly successful history of the preventive viral vaccines, the vaccines that are being used employ routes of immunization that favor development of systemic IgG responses, even for viruses such as picorna viruses that enter the body through mucosal surfaces.

2. The Viral Types to Include in the Vaccine

In a recent world-wide survey of HPV types in over 1000 cervical cancers,[68] 93% of all cervical cancers were HPV-positive, HPV16 was found in 50%, and the 4 most common types (HPV16, 18, 31, and 45), were found in 77% of cancers. The question of whether to vaccinate against multiple HPV types is a balance between issues of cost and effectiveness. Since HPV16 is so dominant, the primary focus of vaccination efforts will probably be to obtain an optimally effective HPV16 vaccine. Although the existence of unique neutralizing epitopes that are not even shared between the closely related HPV types 6 and 11[60] suggests that the extent of cross-protection between viral types will be limited, it is actually not known to what extent cross-protection might be induced between antigenically related HPV types. For issues of whether additional HPV types apart from HPV16 should be included in a vaccine, it will be most important to obtain data on the degree of cross-protection between the oncogenic HPV types. Measurements of cross-protective activity of antisera have hitherto had to rely on surrogate measures, such as inhibition of VLP binding to cell surfaces.[69] The best surrogate marker is the inhibition of VLP hemagglutination assay[70] that has been shown to correlate quite well with neutralizing activity in the CRPV system.[70] Recently, an assay for measurement of HPV16 neutralizing antibodies was developed. The assay uses HPV16 VLPs produced in mammalian cells containing episomal BPV genomes. The HPV16 VLPs recovered from these cells will have packaged the BPV genome, and their infectivity can therefore be measured by a standard BPV focus-forming assay (R. Roden and J. T. Schiller, personal communication).

3. Whom to Vaccinate

A prophylactic HPV vaccine must be administered before the infectious event that progresses to malignancy occurs. Early serological studies and PCR-based studies indicated the existence of widespread, even nonsexually transmitted HPV infections (discussed in Reference 27). However, even before the link to genital HPV infection was demonstrated, many epidemiologic studies had provided firm evidence that cervical cancer is a sexually transmitted disease.[71] Also, several recent studies using validated, type-restricted HPV serological assays and well controlled PCR technology have failed to detect any evidence of serum antibodies to genital-type HPVs or of cervical HPV DNA among sexually inexperienced women.[27,74,75,76] When adolescent sexually inexperienced women have neither HPV DNA nor serum HPV antibodies, the still debated issue of whether perinatal infections exist (that neither induce a lasting seroconversion or a persistent cancer-causing infection) would seem to be of academic interest only and of no relevance to vaccination strategies.

Once sexual activity has commenced, the rate of HPV acquisition is rapid. In one of our longitudinal cohort studies, no teenage girls with 0 or 1 partner had antibodies against HPV 16 or 33, whereas 54% of teenage girls with more than 5 lifetime sexual partners had seroconverted against either of these viruses.[75,76] Thus, a vaccine trial targeting teenage girls seeking contraceptive advice should be able to answer questions of vaccine efficacy with a limited length of follow-up.

There are several alternative possibilities for a prophylactic HPV vaccine. *DNA vaccination* is a recent, powerful technique that enables the induction of both antibody responses and cytotoxic T-cell responses.[77] A DNA plasmid containing the coding gene for the protein of interest is injected intramuscularly. Since the immunogen is produced intracellularly, it is both correctly folded and posttranscriptionally modified and will also be correctly degraded into peptides that will be loaded onto MHC class I molecules using the normal peptide transporting pathways. In these respects, DNA vaccines resemble live attenuated vaccines. Major advantages of DNA vaccines are their low cost and stability. A major concern regarding DNA vaccines is the possibility that they might integrate into the host cell DNA and disturb the host cell function. Although several studies have failed to find evidence of plasmid integration,[77] possible long-term risks of large-scale vaccination with DNA vaccines are hard to estimate.

Live virus expression vectors have also been considered. The most widely used system, vaccinia virus, has been used to produce VLPs of several HPV types, e.g., HPV 16.[51] However, vaccinia viral disease can be severe in immunocompromised patients and long-term risk and biosafety aspects are again hard to predict.

There is increasing interest in the use of vectors based on alpha RNA viruses, since such viruses are well characterized, infect a variety of host cells, and do not replicate through a DNA intermediate.[78] A system using conditionally infectious Semliki Forest Virus (SFV), where the released viral particles are noninfectious and have to be activated into infectivity by *in vitro* protease treatment, is of special interest because of its high level of biosafety.[79] HPV16 VLPs have been produced using recombinant Semliki Forest Virus expressing the HPV16 capsid proteins.[66,80]

Subunit vaccines using bacterially expressed capsid protein have been generated for CRPV and were shown to be effective, although the neutralizing antibody titers were low.[81,82] Also, vaccination with bacterially derived L2 protein of BPV4 induced protective immunity against experimental challenge with BPV4.[83]

Synthetic peptides have not been extensively investigated as immunogens for protective immunity, since it is well known that immunization with intact virus predominantly induces neutralizing antibodies against highly conformationally dependent epitopes.[84] Also, immunization using denatured full-length major capsid protein results in a predominant antibody response against immunodominant epitopes located on the inside of the virion.[85] We have systematically evaluated the ability of overlapping HPV16 L1 and L2 peptides to induce virion-reactive antibodies.[86] A total of 13 peptides that induced antibodies reactive with intact HPV16 capsids, at titers up to 1:150,000, were identified. For the four most promising peptide immunogens, we identified the corresponding potentially surface-exposed regions of the CRPV L1 protein by alignment of the HPV16 and CRPV L1 sequences. Three CRPV L1 synthetic peptides were found to induce CRPV-neutralizing antibodies (F. Breitburd and J. Dillner, unpublished observation), although the neutralizing antibody titer was considerably lower than what was obtained using VLP immunization. Antibodies against 3/3 tested synthetic BPV-2 peptides have also been found to induce clumping of viral particles.[87] Synthetic peptides would have a number of advantages as a vaccine, such as low cost, stability, and safety. These aspects are especially important for preventive vaccines targeting a disease which is most common in poor countries.

C.   Vaccines to Aid Regression

As detailed above, most of the available evidence indicate that it is the cellular immunity that determines the rate of regression rather than the antibody response. Several lines of evidence suggest that this cellular immunity is primarily mediated by CD4+ cells: The majority of infiltrating T-cells seen in regressing CIN lesions are CD4+ cells;[13,14] a CD4+ cell-mediated delayed type hypersensitivity reaction against HPV infected cells has been demonstrated in mouse models;[88] and an HPV type-dependent increased risk to develop cervical neoplasia is associated with certain HLA classII alleles.[89] However, most efforts to develop a therapeutic HPV vaccine have not tried to mimic the immune response seen during natural infection, but have focused on experimental induction of CD8+ cytotoxic T cells (CTLs) since this approach has been very successful in many experimental systems (see below). Since HPV-carrying cancers typically appear two decades after infection, it could be asked if it is feasible to try to stimulate an immune response that was not evoked during the previous 20 years of infection. The rationale for trying to stimulate a cytotoxic T-cell (CTL) response artificially has come from consistent findings that the cytotoxic T-cells require a considerably higher amount of antigenic stimulation for activation than for recognition of target cells. In other words, a tumor that expresses minute amounts of antigen at the cell surface may not express sufficient amounts of antigen to activate an efficient CTL response, but may very well be efficiently recognized by a CTL response once it has been activated.[90]

In mouse model systems, it has been possible to efficiently induce rejection of syngeneic HPV 16-carrying tumors by vaccination using either nonmalignant cells expressing the HPV 16 E7 or E6 protein[91,92] or by using a recombinant vaccinia virus expressing the E6 and E7 proteins,[93] demonstrating that both E6 and E7 can act as tumor rejection antigens. Unfortunately, both these vaccination strategies involve introducing the DNA of the viral oncogenes into the recipient. Since the oncogenic functions of the viral oncogenes have been extensively mapped using sitedirected mutagenesis,[94] it has been possible to construct truncated or mutated nononcogenic E6 and E7 genes. Live viral vectors or DNA vaccines containing such nononcogenic E6 and E7 genes constitute attractive alternatives for therapeutic vaccines.

A new strategy for eliciting CTL-mediated immunity using nonhazardous peptide immunogens has been developed.[90] The mechanisms by which the host cell degrades endogenous cellular or viral proteins and present them to CTL cells as peptides bound in the groove of the MHC class I molecule are now elucidated.[95] Whereas the peptides that are presented in MHC class II molecules for recognition by T helper cells largely are derived from exogenous antigens that are taken up by the cell, degraded into peptides in the lysosomal pathway and then presented in the class II molecules at the cell surface, the peptides that are presented in MHC class I for recognition by CTLs seem to be exclusively derived from endogenous proteins that are degraded into peptides and loaded onto MHC class I molecules already in a pre-Golgi compartment.[95] Experiments with the murine lymphoma mutant cell line RMA-S has underscored the importance of peptide in maintenance of the structure of MHC class I molecules. This cell line has a defect in peptide transport to the place of assembly of class I molecules, resulting in a markedly reduced expression of class I molecules at the cell surface.[96] The few class I molecules present on RMA-S cultured at physiological temperature share the phenotype of class I molecules without peptide in their peptide binding groove.[96] Culturing of RMA-S cells, or some of its more recently described human counterparts, in the presence of a synthetic peptide with class I binding ability results in a marked increase of expression of class I molecules at the cell surface, which can be measured by immunofluorescence[90,97] or ELISA.[98] The mechanism of this phenomenon is most likely stabilization of "empty" class I molecules by binding of the exogenously added peptide. The assay allows a simple and efficient investigation of the ability of a given peptide to associate with MHC class I.[97] By systematically testing overlapping synthetic peptides from the protein of interest, the peptides with optimal class I-binding ability can be readily identified. Although the ability of a peptide to bind to MHC class I does not necessarily imply that it can also bind to the T cell receptor and elicit a CTL response,[99] the class I binding is clearly a requirement.

The development of technology for direct elution of class I binding peptides from the class I-peptide complexes has also tremendously increased the strength of this type of technology. By amino acid sequencing of MHC-binding peptides (from class I or from class II) the identification of major T cell epitopes can be made without prior knowledge of what protein the target peptides are derived from.[100,101] Sequencing of the total pool of class I-binding peptides has also revealed the existence of specific amino acid motifs among class I binding peptides,[102] the knowledge of which considerably facilitates the search for specific class I binding peptides derived from proteins with a known amino acid sequence, such as the viral transforming proteins.

Vaccination using free peptide with optimal MHC class I binding ability has been possible both for inducing tumor rejection of adenovirus-carrying tumors[103] and for inducing protective immunity against Sendai virus infection.[104] Since the HPV carrying cancers express the E6 and E7 viral transforming proteins, which they are dependent on for their continued growth, stimulation of a CTL response using peptides mimicking endogenously degraded E6 and E7 peptides with MHC class I binding ability that also constitute CTL epitopes seems to be a comparatively straightforward vaccination approach. When peptides with ability to induce CTL responses are identified by virtue of their HLA class I binding ability, so-called cryptotopic or subdominant epitopes may be identified.[105] During natural infection, the immune response focuses against immunodominant epitopes and a response against the subdominant epitopes are not induced. However, when subdominant epitopes are used for immunization by themselves, an effective CTL response may well be induced.[105] The identification of immunogenic subdominant epitopes is theoretically advantageous, since viruses may have evolved to escape CTL attack against immunodominant epitopes. Indeed, HPV16 substrains with a mutation in a HLA B7-binding motif are preferentially found among B7-positive individuals.[106] HPV CTL-inducing peptides have been identified in a series of pioneering studies by Martin Kast and co-workers. The epitopes with the ability to bind to the mouse class I alleles K^b and D^b in the E6 and E7 genes of HPV 16 were mapped by testing overlapping peptides tested in a RMA-S assay. Vaccination with a peptide containing the strongest class I binding peptide from E7 induced protective immunity against challenge with a syngeneic HPV 16-carrying tumor cell line.[105] Subsequently, the E6 and E7 peptides with affinity for human class I alleles were mapped. For HLA A2.1, an assay based on the RMA-S-like peptide processing defective human lymphoblastoid cell line T2 was used,[107] whereas an *in vitro* peptide displacement assay using purified class I molecules was used to measure binding affinity of the E6 and E7 peptides to five major classI A alleles (A1, A2.1, A3, A11, and A24).[108] Finally, the 3 E7-derived peptides with the highest affinity for the HLA A2.1 molecule were shown to both elicit peptide-specific CTLs in *in vivo* vaccinated A2.1-transgenic mice and to elicit peptide specific CTLs from the peripheral blood mononuclear cells of healthy A2.1-positive donors by *in vitro* peptide stimulation.[109] The peptide-specific CTL clones were able to lyse the A2.1-positive, HPV16-carrying cervical carcinoma cell line CaSki, suggesting that these peptides represent naturally processed human CTL epitopes of HPV16.[109] Also for E7 of HPV11 it has been possible to elicit CTLs with the ability to lyse E7-expressing cells, using *in vitro* stimulation with HLA A2.1-binding peptides.[110] Although the class I-binding immunogenic peptides elicit CTL responses in an HLA-restricted fashion, immunization with a cocktail of peptides corresponding to the most common alleles expected to provide a high population coverage.[108] Simultaneous immunization of A2.1-transgenic mice with several peptides did induce CTL responses against the different peptide in the immunizing cocktail, suggesting that vaccination with class I-binding peptides does not require prior HLA typing, but might be accomplished using a standard multiple peptide cocktail.[109] Similar therapeutic vaccination approaches are being pursued for other tumor antigens, notably melanoma antigens.[111,112] However, the first preliminary results that are coming out of the first clinical trials of therapeutic peptide vaccination are disappointing compared to the impressive results from mouse vaccinations. Much work remains to be done on optimization of immunization protocols for synthetic peptide CTL epitope vaccination of humans. By contrast, it is clear that *in vitro* stimulation of human PBMCs using synthetic peptide CTL epitopes regularly induces peptide-specific CTLs.[109,110,112] Somewhat surprisingly, no attempt to exploit this using the powerful technique of adoptive transfer of CTLs[113] has yet been reported.

III. CONCLUSION

Every year, about half a million women worldwide acquire HPV-associated cervical cancer. Experimental evidence strongly supports the idea that the HPV infection is a necessary risk factor in the etiology of this cancer. Also for a number of other cancers (notably anal and vulvar cancer), there is substantial evidence that HPV infection is an important risk factor. Results from animal studies have clearly shown that vaccine strategies that readily achieve protective immunity and are acceptable from a safety aspect have been found. There is therefore good reason to believe that HPV vaccination would have a tremendous public health impact. The field of preventive HPV vaccination should be moving into field trials evaluating vaccine efficacy and cost within the near future.

In the field of therapeutic vaccination, HPV is increasingly being used as a target of investigations on how to optimize exciting and innovative immunotherapeutic strategies.

REFERENCES

1. Reid, T. M. S., Fraser, N. G., and Kernohan, I. R., Generalized warts and immune deficiency, *Br. J. Dermatol.,* 95, 559, 1976.
2. Morison, W. L., Cell-mediated immune response in patients with warts, *Br. J. Dermatol.,* 93, 553, 1975.
3. Laga, M., Icenogle, J. P., Marsella, R., Manoka, A. T., Nzila, N., Ryder, R. W., Vermund, S. H., Heyward, W. L., Nelson, A., and Reeves, W. C., Genital papillomavirus infection and cervical dysplasia-Opportunistic complications of HIV infection, *Int. J. Cancer,* 50, 45, 1992.
4. Kienzler, J. L., Lemoine, M. T. H., Orth, G., Jibard, N., Blanc, D., Laurent, R., and Agache, P., Humoral and cell-mediated immunity to human papillomavirus type 1 (HPV-1) in human warts, *Br. J. Dermatol.,* 108, 665, 1983.
5. Hawthorn, R. J. S., Murdoch, J. B., MacLean, A. B., and MacKie, R. M., Langerhans cell and subtypes of human papillomavirus in cervical intraepithelial neoplasia, *Br. Med. J.,* 297, 643, 1988.
6. Halpert, R., Fruchter, R. G., Sedlis, A., Butt, K., Boyce, J. G., and Sillman, F. H., Human papillomavirus and lower genital neoplasia in renal transplant patients, *Obstet. Gynecol.,* 68, 251, 1986.
7. Alloub, M. I., Barr, B. B. B., McClaren, K. M., Smith, I. W., Bunney, M. H., and Smart, G. E., Human papillomavirus infection and cervical intraepithelial neoplasia in women with renal allografts, *Br. Med. J.,* 298, 153, 1989.
8. Tay, S. K., Jenkins, D., Maddox, P., Campion, M., and Singer, A., Subpopulations of Langerhans' cells in cervical neoplasia, *Br. J. Obst. Gynecol.,* 94, 10, 1987.
9. Malejczuk, J., Majewski, S., Jablonska, S., Rogozinski, T. T., and Orth, G., Abrogated NK-cell lysis of human papillomavirus (HPV)-16-bearing keratinocytes in patients with pre-cancerous and cancerous HPV-induced anogenital lesions, *Int. J. Cancer,* 43, 209, 1988.
10. Tagami, H., Oku, T., and Iwatsuki, K., Primary tissue culture of spontaneously regressing flat warts. *In vitro* attack by mononuclear cells against wart-derived epidermal cells, *Cancer,* 55, 2437, 1985.
11. Oguchi, M., Komura, J., Tagami, H., and Ofuji, S., Ultrastructural studies of spontaneously regressing plane warts: Langerhans cells show marked activation, *Arch. Dermatol. Res.,* 271, 55, 1981.
12. Berman, A. and Winkelmann, R. K., Involuting common warts, *J. Am. Acad. Derm.,* 3, 356, 1980.
13. Aiba, S., Rokugo, M., and Tagami, H., Immunohistologic analysis of the phenomenon of spontaneous regression of numerous flat warts, *Cancer,* 58, 1246, 1986.
14. McKenzie, J., King, A., Hare, J., Fulford, T., Wilson, B., and Stanley, M., Immunocytochemical characterization of large granular lymphocytes in normal cervix and HPV associated disease, *J. Pathol.,* 165, 75, 1991.
15 Shah, K. and Howley, P. M., Papillomaviruses, In: *Virology* 2nd edition Eds B. N. Fields, D. M. Knipe, Raven Press (New York), 1651, 1990.
16 Wank, R. and Thomssen, C., High risk of squamous cell carcinoma of the cervix for women with HLA-DQw3, *Nature,* 352, 723, 1991.
17 Han, R., Breitburd, F., Marche, P. N., and Orth, G., Linkage of regression and malignant conversion of rabbit viral papillomas to MHC class II genes, *Nature,* 356, 66, 1992.
18. Connor, M. E. and Stern, P. L., Loss of MHC class-I expression in cervical carcinomas, *Int. J. Cancer,* 46, 1029, 1990.

19. Cromme, F. V., Airey, J., Heemels, M. T., Ploegh, H. L., Keating, P. J., Stern, P. L., Meijer, C. J. L. M., and Walboomers, J. M. M., Loss of transporter protein, encoded by the TAP-1 gene, is highly correlated with loss of HLA expression in cervical carcinomas, *J. Exp. Med.*, 179, 335, 1994.

20. Kidd, J. G., The course of viurs induced rabbit papillomas as determined by virus, cells and host, *J. Exp. Med.*, 64, 63, 1938.

21. Ghim, S., Christensen, N. D., Kreider, J. W., and Jenson, A. B., Comparison of neutralization of BPV-1 infection of C127 cells and bovine fetal skin xenografts, *Int. J. Cancer*, 49, 285, 1991.

22. Campo, M. S., Vaccination against papillomavirus, *Cancer Cells*, 3, 421, 1991.

23. Evans, C. A., Weiser, R. S., and Ito, Y., Antiviral and antitumor immunologic mechanisms operative in the Shope papilloma-carcinoma system, *Cold Spring Harbor Symp. Quant. Biol.*, 27, 453, 1962.

24. Kreider, J. W., Studies on the mechanism responsible for the spontaneous regression of the Shope papilloma, *Cancer Res.*, 23, 1593, 1963.

25. Cubie, H. A., Serological studies in a student population prone to infection with human papilloma virus, *J. Hyg. Camb.*, 70, 677, 1972.

26. Pyrhönen, S. and Johansson, E., Regression of warts. An immunological study, *Lancet*, 1, 592, 1975.

27. Dillner, J., Serology of Human Papillomavirus, *Cancer J.*, 8, 264, 1995.

28. Dillner, J., Dillner, L., Utter, G., Eklund, C., Rotola, A., Costa, S., and DiLuca, D., Mapping of linear epitopes of human papillomavirus type 16: The L1 and L2 open reading frames, *Int. J. Cancer*, 45, 529, 1990.

29. Dillner, J., Mapping of linear epitopes of human papillomavirus type 16: The E1, E2, E4, E5, E6 and E7 open reading frames, *Int. J. Cancer*, 46, 703, 1990.

30. Muller, M., Gausepohl, H., de Martynoff, G., Frank, R., Brasseur, R., and Gissmann, L., Identification of seroreactive regions of the human papillomavirus type 16 proteins E4, E6, E7 and L1, *J. Gen. Virol.*, 71, 2709, 1990.

31. Yaegashi, N., Jenison, S. A., Batra, M., and Galloway, D. A., Human antibodies recognize multiple distinct type-specific and cross-reactive regions of the minor capsid proteins of human papillomavirus types 6 and 11, *J. Virol.*, 66, 2008, 1992.

32. Dillner, J., Dillner, L., Robb, J., Willems, J., Jones, I., Lancaster, W., Smith, R., and Lerner, R., A synthetic peptide defines a serologic IgA response to a human papillomavirus-encoded nuclear antigen expressed in virus-carrying cervical neoplasia, *Proc. Natl. Acad. Sci. U.S.A.*, 86, 3838, 1989.

33. Höchel, H. G., Monazahian, M., Sievert, K., Höhne, M., Thomssen, C., Teichmann, A., Arendt, P., and Thomssen, R., Occurrence of antibodies to L1, L2, E4 and E7 gene products of human papillomavirus types 6b, 16 and 18 among cervical cancer patients and controls, *Int. J. Cancer*, 48, 682, 1991.

34. Jochmus-Kudielka, I., Schneider, A., Braun, R., Kimmig, R., Koldovsky, U., Schneweis, K. E., Seedorf, K., and Gissman, L., Antibodies against the human papillomavirus type 16 early proteins in human sera: Correlation of anti-E7 reactivity with cervical cancer, *J. Natl. Cancer Inst.*, 81, 1698, 1989.

35. Muller, M., Viscidi, R. P., Sun, Y., Guerrero, E., Hill, P. M., Shah, F., Bosch, F. X., Munoz, N., Gissmann, L., and Shah, K. V., Antibodies to HPV-16 E6 and E7 proteins as markers for HPV-16 associated invasive cervical carcinoma, *Virology*, 187, 508, 1992.

36. Dillner, J., Lenner, P., Lehtinen, M., Eklund, C., Heino, P., Wiklund, F, Hallmans, G., and Stendahl, U., A population-based seroepidemiological study of cervical cancer, *Cancer Res.*, 54, 134, 1994.

37. Heino, P., Eklund, C., Fredriksson-Shahnazarian, V., Goldman, S., Schiller, J.T., and Dillner, J., Serum IgG antibodies against human papillomavirus type 16 capsids are associated with anal epidermoid carcinoma, *J. Natl. Cancer Inst.*, 87, 437, 1995.

38. Wikström, A., van Doornum, G. J. J., Kirnbauer, R., Quint, W. G. V., and Dillner, J., A prospective study on the development of antibodies against human papillomavirus type 6 among patients with condyloma acuminata or new asymptomatic infection, *J. Med. Virol.*, 46, 368, 1995.

39. Ley, C., Bauer, H. M., Reingold, A., Schiffman, M. H., Chambers, J. C., Tashiro, C. J., and Manos, M. M., Determinants of genital human papillomvirus infection in young women, *J. Natl. Cancer Inst.*, 83, 997, 1991.

40. Gustafsson, L. and Adami, H. O., Natural history of cervical neoplasia: Consistent results obtained by an identification technique, *Br. J. Cancer*, 60, 132, 1989.

41. zur Hausen, H., Viruses in human cancers, *Science*, 254, 1167, 1991.

42. Jenson, B., Rosenthal, J. D., Olsson, C., Pass, F., Lancaster, W.. D., and Shah, K., Immunologic relatedness of papillomaviruses from different species, *J. Nat. Cancer Inst.*, 64, 495, 1980.

43. Dillner, L., Heino, P., Moreno-Lopez, J., and Dillner, J., Antigenic and immunogenic epitopes shared by human papillomavirus type 16 and bovine, canine and avian papillomaviruses, *J. Virol.*, 65, 6862, 1991.

44. Christensen, N. D., and Kreider, J. W., Antibody-mediated neutralization *in vivo* of infectious papillomaviruses, *J. Virol.*, 64, 3151, 1990.

45. Lorincz, A. T., Reid, R., Jenson, A. B., Greenberg, M. D., Lancaster, W. D., and Kurman, R. J., Human papillomavirus infection of the cervix: Relative risk associations of 15 common anogenital types, *Obstet. Gynecol.*, 79, 328, 1992.

46. Olson, C., Animal papillomas Historical aspects, In: *The Papovaviridae* Eds. N. Salzman and P. Howley Plenum (New York), 2, 39, 1987.

47. Bregman, C. L., Hirth, R. S., Sundberg, J. P., and Christensen, E. F., Cutaneous neoplasms in dogs associated with canine oral papillomavirus vaccine, *Vet. Pathol.*, 24, 477, 1987.

48. Christensen, N. D., Kreider, J. W., Kan, N. C., and DiAngelo, S. L., The open reading frame L2 of cottontail rabbit papillomavirus contains antibody-inducing neutralizing epitopes, *Virology*, 181, 572, 1991.

49. Jarrett, W. F. H., Smith, K. T., O'Neil, B. W., Gaukroger, J. M., Chandrachud, L. M., Grindlay, G. J., McGarvie, G. M., and Campo, M. S., Studies on vaccination against papillomaviruses: Prophylactic and therapeutic vaccination with recombinant structural proteins, *Virology*, 184, 33, 1991.

50. Ghim, S. J., Jenson, A. B., and Schlegel, R., HPV-1 L1 protein expressed in cos cells displays conformational epitopes found on intact virions, *Virology*, 190, 548, 1992.

51. Zhou, J., Sun, X. Y., Stenzel, D. J., and Frazer, I. H., Expression of Vaccinia recombinant HPV 16 L1 and L2 ORF proteins in epithelial cells is sufficient for assembly of HPV virion-like particles, *Virology*, 185, 251, 1991.

52. Kreider, J. W., Patrick, S. D., Cladel, N. M., and Welsh, P. A., Experimental infection with human papillomavirus type 1 of human hand and foot skin, *Virology*, 177, 415, 1990.

53. Meyers, C., Frattini, M. G., Hudson, J. B., and Laimins, L. A., Biosynthesis of human papillomavirus from a continuous cell line upon epithelial differentiation, *Science*, 257, 971, 1992.

54. Sterling, J., Stanley, M., Gatward, G., and Minson, T., Production of human papillomavirus type 16 virions in a keratinocyte cell line, *J. Virol.*, 64, 6505, 1990.

55. Ostrow, R. S., McGlennen, R. C., Shaver, M. K., Kloster, B. E., Houser, D., and Faras, A. J., A rhesus monkey model for sexual transmission of a papillomavirus isolated from a squamous cell carcinoma, *Proc. Natl. Acad. Sci. U.S.A.*, 87, 8170, 1990.

56. Dillner, L., Bekassy, Z., Jonsson, N., Moreno-Lopez, J., and Blomberg, J., Detection of IgA antibodies against human papillomavirus in cervical secretions from patients with cervical intraepithelial neoplasia, *Int. J. Cancer*, 43, 36, 1989.

57. Snyder, K. A., Barber, S. R., Symbula, M., Taylor, P. T., Crum, C. P., and Roche, J. K., Binding by immunoglobulin to the HPV 16-derived proteins L1 and E4 in cervical secretions of women with HPV-related cervical disease, *Cancer Res.*, 51, 4423, 1991.

58. Dillner, L., Fredriksson, A., Persson, E., Hansson, B. G., Forslund, O. and Dillner, J., Antibodies to human papillomavirus-derived antigens in cervical secretions from condyloma patients, *J. Clin. Microbiol.*, 31, 192, 1993.

59. Zhou, J., Sun, X.-Y., Davies, H., Crawford, L., Park, D. and Frazer, I. H., Definition of linear antigenic regions of the HPV16 L1 capsid protein using synthetic virion-like particles, *Virology*, 189, 592, 1992.

60. Christensen, N. D., Kirnbauer, R., Schiller, J. T., Ghim, S. J., Schlegel, R., Jenson, A. B. and Kreider, J. W., Human papillomavirus types 6 and 11 have antigenically distinct strongly immunogenic conformationally dependent neutralizing epitopes, *Virology*, 205, 329, 1994.

61. Kirnbauer, R., Booy, F., Cheng, N., Lowy, D. R. and Schiller, J. T., Papillomavirus L1 major capsid protein self-assembles into virus-like particles that are highly immunogenic, *Proc. Natl. Acad. Sci. U.S.A.*, 89, 12180, 1992.

62. Kirnbauer, R., Taub, J., Greenstone, H., Roden, R., Durst, M., Gissman, L., Lowy, D. R. and Schiller, J. T., Efficient self-assembly of human papillomavirus type 16 L1 and L1-L2 into virus-like particles, *J. Virol.*, 67, 6929, 1993.

63. Rose, R. C., Reichman, R. C. and Bonnez, W., Human papillomavirus type 11 recombinant virus-like particles induce the formation of neutralizing antibodies and detect HPV-specific antibodies in human sera, *J. Gen. Virol.*, 75, 2075, 1994.

64. Carter, J. J., Wipf, G. C., Hagensee, M. E., McKnight, B., Habel, L. A., Lee, S. K., Kuypers, J., Kiviat, N., Daling, J. R., Koutsky, L. A., Watts, D. H., Holmes, K. K. and Galloway, D. A., Use of human papillomavirus type 6 capsids to detect antibodies in people with genital warts, *J. Inf. Dis.*, 172, 11, 1995.

65. Breitburd, F., Kirnbauer, R., Hubbert, N. L., Schiller, J. T., and Orth, G., Immunization with virus-like particles from cottontail rabbit papillomavirus (CRPV) can protect against experimental CRPV infection, *J. Virol.*, 69, 3959, 1995.

66. Schiller, J. T. and Roden, R. B. S., Papillomavirus-like particles, *Papillomavirus Report*, 6, 121, 1995.

67. Bell, A. J., Sundberg, J. P., and Ghim, S. J., A formalin-activated vaccine protects against mucosal papillomavirus infection: A canine model, *Pathobiology*, 62, 194, 1994.

68. Bosch, F. X., Manos, M. M., Munoz, N., Sherman, M., Jansen, A. M., Peto, J., Schiffman, M., Moreno, V., Kurman, R., Shah, K. V., and Group, I. B. S. O. C. C. S., Prevalence of Human Papillomavirus in cervical cancer: A worldwide perspective, *J. Natl. Cancer Inst.*, 87, 796, 1995.

69. Roden, R. B., Kirnbauer, R., Jenson, A. B., Lowy, D. R., Schiller, J.T., Interaction of papillomaviruses with the cell surface, *J. Virol.*, 68, 7260, 1994.

70. Roden, R. B. S., Hubbert, N. L., Kirnbauer, R., Breitburd, F., Lowy, D. R., Schiller, J. T., Papillomavirus capsids agglutinate mouse erythrocytes through a proteinaceous receptor, *J. Virol.*, 69, 5147, 1995.

71. Ponte´n, J., Adami, H. O., Bergström, R., Dillner, J., Friberg, L. G., Gustafsson, L., Miller, A. B., Parkin, D. M., Spare´n, P., and Trichopoulos, D., Strategies for global control of cervical cancer, *Int. J. Cancer*, 60, 1, 1995.

72. Rylander, E., Ruusuvaara, L., Wiksten-Almströmer, M., Evander, M., and Wadell, G., The absence of vaginal HPV 16 DNA in women with no experience of sexual intercourse, *Obstet. Gynecol.*, 83, 534, 1994.

73. Fairley, C. K., Chen, S., Tabrizi, S. N., Leeton, K., Quinn, M. A., and Garland, S. M., The absence of genital human papillomavirus DNA in virginal women, *Int. J. STD AIDS*, 3, 414, 1992.

74. Andersson-Ellström, A., Hagmar, B., Johansson, B., Kalantari, M., Wärleby, B., and Forssman, L., Human papillomavirus DNA in cervix only detected in girls after coitus, *Int. J. STD & AIDS*, in press.

75. Andersson-Ellström, A., Dillner, J., Hagmar, B., Schiller, J., and Forssman, L., No serological evidence for non-sexual spread of HPV 16, *Lancet*, 344, 1435, 1994.

76. Andersson-Ellström, A., Dillner, J., Hagmar, B., Schiller, J., Sapp, M., Forssman, L., and Milsom, I., Comparison of development of serum antibodies to HPV16 and HPV33 and acquisition of cervical HPV DNA among sexually experienced and virginal young girls. A longitudinal cohort study, *Sex. Transm. Dis.*, 23, 234, 1996.

77. Fynan, E. F., Webster, R. G., Fuller, D. H., Haynes, J. R., Santoro, J. C., and Robinson, H. L., DNA vaccines: Protective immunization by parenteral, mucosal, and gene-gun inoculations, *Proc. Natl. Acad. Sci. U.S.A.*, 90, 11478, 1993.

78. Liljeström, P. and Garoff, H., A new generation of animal cell expression vectors based on the Semliki forest virus replicon, *Biotechnology*, 9, 1356, 1991.

79. Berglund, P., Sjöberg, M., Garoff, H., Atkins, G. A., Sheahan, B. J., and Liljeström, P., Semliki Forest virus expression system: Production of conditionally infectious recombinant particles, *Biotechnology*, 11, 916, 1993.

80. Heino, P., Dillner, J., and Schwartz, S., Human papillomavirus type 16 capsid proteins expressed from recombinant Semliki Forest Virus self-assemble into virus-like particles, *Virology*, 214, 349, 1995.

81. Lin, Y. L., Borenstein, L. A., Selvakumar, R., and Wettstein, F. O., Effective vaccination against papilloma development by immunization with L1 or L2 structural protein of cottontail rabbit papillomavirus, *Virology*, 187, 612, 1992.

82. Christensen, N. D., Kreider, J. K., Kan, N. C., and DiAngelo, S. L., The open reading frame L2 of cottontail rabbit papillomavirus contains antibody-inducing neutralizing epitopes, *Virology*, 181, 572, 1991.

83. Campo, M. S., Grindlay, G. J., and O´Neil, B. W., Prophylactic and therapeutic vaccination against a mucosal papillomavirus, *J. Gen. Virol.*, 74, 945, 1993.

84. Christensen, N. D., Kreider, J. W., Cladel, N. M., Patrick, S. D., and Welsh, P. A., Monoclonal antibody-mediated neutralization of infectious human papillomavirus type 11, *J. Virol.*, 64, 5678, 1990.

85. Lim, P. S., Jenson, A. B., Cowsert, L., Nakai, Y., Lim, L. Y., Jin, W., and Sundberg, J. P., Distribution and specific identification of papillomavirus major capsid protein epitopes by immunohistocytochem-istry and epitope scanning of synthetic peptides, *J. Infect. Dis.*, 162, 1263, 1990.

86. Heino, P., Skyldberg, B., Lehtinen, M., Rantala, I., Hagmar, B., Kreider, J. W., Kirnbauer, R., and Dillner, J., Human papillomavirus type 16 capsids expose multiple type-restricted and type-common antigenic epitopes, *J. Gen. Virol.,* 1995.

87. Cason, J., Kambo, P. K., Jewers, R. J., Chrystie, I. L., and Best, J. M., Mapping of linear B cell epitopes on capsid proteins of bovine papillomavirus: Identification of three external type-restricted epitopes, *J. Gen. Virol.,* 74, 2669, 1993.

88. Chambers, M. A., Stacey, S. N., Arrand, J. R., and Stanley, M. A., Delayed-type hypersensitivity response to human papillomavirus type 16 E6 protein in a mouse model, *J. Gen. Virol.,* 75, 165, 1994.

89. Apple, R. J., Erlich, H. A., Klitz, W., Manos, M. M., Becker, T. M., and Wheeler, C. M., HLA DR-DQ associations with cervical carcinoma show papillomavirus type-specificity, *Nature-Genetics,* 6, 157, 1994.

90. Kast, W. M. and Melief, C. J. M., *In vivo* efficacy of virus-derived peptides and virus-specific cytotoxic T lymphocytes, *Immunol. Letters,* 30, 229, 1991.

91. Chen, L., Thomas, E. K., Hu, S. L., Hellström, I., and Hellström, K. E., Human papillomavirus type 16 nucleoprotein E7 is a tumor rejection antigen, *Proc. Natl. Acad. Sci. U.S.A.,* 88, 110, 1991.

92. Chen, L., Mizuno, M. T., Singhal, M. C., Hu, S. L., Galloway, D. A., Hellström, I., and Hellström, K. E., Induction of cytotoxic T lymphocytes specific for a syngeneic tumor expressing the E6 oncoprotein of human papillomavirus type 16, *J. Immunol.,* 148, 2617, 1992.

93. Meneguzzi, G., Cerni, C., Kieny, M. P., and Lathe, R., Immunization against human papillomavirus type 16 tumor cells with recombinant vaccinia viruses expressing E6 and E7, *Virology,* 181, 62, 1991.

94. Edmonds, C. and Vousden, K. H., A point mutational analysis of human papillomavirus type 16 E7 protein, *J. Virol.,* 63, 2650, 1989.

95. Neefjes, J. J., Schumacher, T. N., and Ploegh, H. L., Assembly and intracellular transport of major histocompatibility complex molecules, *Curr. Opin. Cell. Biol.,* 3, 601, 1991.

96. Townsend, A., Öhlen, C., Bastin, J., Ljunggren, H. G., and Kärre, K., Association of class I major histocompatibility heavy and light chains induced by viral peptides, *Nature,* 340, 443, 1989.

97. Ljunggren, H. G., öhlön, C., Höglund, P., Franksson, L., and Kärre, K., The RMA-S lyphoma mutant: Consequences of a peptide loading defect on immunological recognition and graft rejection, *Int. J. Cancer,* suppl. 6, 38, 1991.

98. Dillner, J., Enzyme immunoassay detection of upregulation of MHC class I expression by synthetic peptides from human papillomavirus type 16 E6 and E7 regions, *J. Immunol. Meth.,* 167, 195, 1994.

99. Stauss, H. J., Davies, H., Sadovnikova, E., Chain, B., Horowitz, N., and Sinclair, C., Induction of cytotoxic T lymphocytes with peptides in vitro: Identification of candidate T-cell epitopes in human papillomavirus, *Proc. Natl. Acad. Sci. U.S.A.,* 89, 7871, 1992.

100. van Bleek, G. M. and Nathenson, S. G., Isolation of an endogenously processed immunodominant viral peptide from the class I H-2Kb molecule, *Nature,* 348, 213, 1990.

101. Rudensky, A. Y., Preston-Hurlburt, P., Hong, S. C., Barlow, A., and Janeway, C. A., Sequence analysis of peptides bound to MHC class II molecules, *Nature,* 353, 622, 1991.

102. Falk, K., Rotzschke, O., Stefanovic, S., Jung, G., and Rammensee, H. G., Allele-specific motifs revealed by sequencing of self-peptides eluted from MHC molecules, *Nature,* 351, 290, 1991.

103. Kast, W. M., Offringa, R., Peters, P. J., Voodouw, A. C., Meloen, R. H., Van der Eb, A. J., and Melief, C. J. M., Eradication of adenovirus E1 induced tumors by E1A-specific cytotoxic T lymphocytes, *Cell,* 59, 603, 1989.

104. Kast, W. M., Roux, L., Curren, J., Blom, H. J. J., Voordouw, A. C., Meloen, R. H., Kolakofsky, D., and Melief, C. J. M., Protection against lethal Sendai virus infection by *in vivo* priming of virus-specific cytotoxic T lymphocytes with a free synthetic peptide, *Proc. Natl. Acad. Sci. U.S.A.,* 88, 2283, 1991.

105. Feltkamp, M. C. W., Smits, H. L., Vierboom, M. P. M., Minnaar, R. P., de Jongh, B. M., Drijfhout, J. W., ter Schegget, J., Melief, C. J. M., and Kast, W. M., Vaccination with cytotoxic T lymphocyte epitope-containing peptide protects against a tumor induced by human papillomavirus type 16-transformed cells, *Eur. J. Immunol.,* 23, 2242, 1993.

106. Ellis, J. R. M., Keating, P. J., Baird, J., Hounsell, E. F., Renouf, D. V., Rowe, M., Hopkins, D., Duggan-Keen, M. F., Bartholomew, J. S., Young, L. S., and Stern, P. L., The association of an HPV16 oncogene variant with HLA-B7 has implications for vaccine design in cervical cancer, *Nature Med.,* 1, 464, 1995.

107. Kast, W. M., Brandt, R. M. P., Drijfhout, J. W., and Melief, C. J. M., Human leukocyte antigen -A2.1 restriced candidate cytotoxic T lymphocyte epitopes of Human Papillomavirus type 16 E6 and E7 proteins identified by using the processing-defective human cell line T2, *J. Immunother.*, 14, 115, 1993.

108. Kast, W. M., Brandt, R. M. P., Sidney, J., Drijfhout, J. W., Kubo, R. T., Grey, H. M., Melief, C. J. M., and Sette, A., Role of HLA-A motifs in identification of potential CTL epitopes in human papillomavirus type 16 E6 and E7 proteins, *J. Immunol.*, 152, 3904, 1994.

109. Ressing, M. E., Sette, A., Brandt, R. M. P., Ruppert, J., Wentworth, P. A., Hartman, M., Oseroff, C., Grey, H. M., Melief, C. J. M., and Kast, W. M., Human CTL epitopes encoded by human papillomavirus type 16 E6 and E7 identified through in vivo and in vitro immunogenicity studies of HLA-A*0201-binding peptides, *J. Immunol.*, 154, 5934, 1995.

110. Tarpey, I., Stacey, S., Hickling, J., Birley, H. D. L., Renton, A., and McIndoe, A., Human cytotoxic T lymphocytes stimulated by endogenously processed human papillomavirus type 11 E7 recognize a peptide containing a HLA-A2(A*0201) motif, *Immunology*, 81, 222, 1994.

111. Wölfel, T., Schneider, J., Meyer zum Bueschenfelde, K. H., Rammensee, H. G., Rötzschke, O., and Falk, K., Isolation of naturally processed peptides recognized by cytolytic T lymphocytes on human melanoma cells in association with HLA-A2.1, *Int. J. Cancer*, 57, 413, 1994.

112. Celis, E., Tsai, V., Crimi, C., DeMars, R., Wentworth, P. A., Chesnut, R. W., Grey, H. M., Sette, A., and Serra, H. M., Induction of anti-tumor cytotoxic T lymphocytes in normal humans using primary cultures and synthetic peptide epitopes, *Proc. Natl. Acad. Sci. U.S.A.*, 91, 2105, 1994.

113. Melief, C. J. M., Tumor eradication by adoptive transfer of cytotoxic T lymphocytes, *Adv. Cancer Res.*, 58, 143, 1992.

Index

A

AaPV, 50, 58–59, 61

Acanthomas, 16, 250

Acanthosis and latent HPV infections, 154–155, 157, 160, 161

Acetic acid testing
  for cervical lesions, 267, 408
  and colposcopy, 288, 290
  for genitoanal lesions, 276, 283–286, 295, 390
  and oral HPV infections, 316

Acetowhite lesions, 157, 171, 260, 276, 285, 286

Acid treatment of warts, 377

Acitretin treatment, 380, 385, 407

Acrochordon, 7

Actinic keratosis, 123–125, 134, 138–139

Acuminate warts. *See* Condylomata acuminata

Adaptins and E5 oncoproteins, 27

Adenocarcinomas, 74, 185

Adenoviruses, 47

Adult-onset recurrent respiratory papillomatosis (AO-RRP), 89, 323–324, 327

AIN, 155, 159, 231–234, 261, 292, 401

Alces alces papillomavirus, 50, 61

Alcohol, 106, 182, 192

Alveolar carcinoma, 185

Amniotic fluid and HPV infection, 192

Amphiregulin, 214

AmPV, 51

Anaerobic bacteria and HPV lesions, 47

Anaesthesia for treatment of lesions, 398–399

Anal cancer and HPV infection, 231–234, 293, 425

Anal cytology procedure, 232

Anal-intraepithelial neoplasia (AIN), 155, 159, 231–234, 261, 292, 401

Anal lesions, 275, 276

Anaplastic carcinoma, 185

Anchorage independence assay, 140

Aneuploid cells, 31, 334

Animal papillomaviruses, 47–53

Anisokaryosis, 153

Anogenital lesions. *See* Genitoanal papillomavirus infections

Anoscopy, 232–233, 283

Antelope, pronghorn, papillomavirus (AaPV;PrPV*+), 57

Antibodies, HPV
  and animal studies, 56–59
  anticapsid, 217
  cross-reactive, 368
  to early proteins, 366
  group specific, 56–69, 121
  in healthy individuals, 367

monoclonal, 56–59, 121–122, 140, 211
  production by B lymphocytes, 205
  responses of, 192, 342, 366–368, 418
  and vaccine development, 217

Antigenic epitopes, 207–208, 367

Antigen presenting cells (APC), 142, 205–211

Antigens, papillomavirus, 154–155, 168, 184, 205–209, 365–366, 404

Antilocapra americana papillomavirus (PrPV*+), 50

Antisense transcripts in genital cancers, 30

AO-RRP, 89, 323–324, 327

AP1, 19–20, 140

Apoptosis, 138

Armadillo, hairy, papillomavirus (CvPV), 48, 57

Artiodactyla and papillomavirus-induced lesions, 50–51, 53, 61

ASCUS, 359

Asian lions and papillomaviruses, 56

ATPase and E5 proteins, 27–28

Atypical mitotic figures, 153

Atypical squamous cells of undetermined significance (ASCUS), 359

Autocrine stimulation, 209, 214–215

Autoinoculation of HPVs, 191

Autoradiography, 342

Azathioprine treatment, 125

B

Balanoposthitis, 277–279, 284–285

Basal cell carcinoma, 123–126, 134, 143, 277

Basement membrane, 157

Basophilic intranuclear inclusions, 9

B cells, 121

BD. *See* Bowen's disease

Bear, Zodiac, papillomavirus (UaPV), 49

Beaver cutaneous papilloma (CcPV), 51, 57

BePV, 51

Betel chewers, 106, 190

Bethesda System of nomenclature, 159–160, 285, 331–332, 352

Bladder, lesions of the, 276

Bladder carcinoma, 105

Bleomycin treatment, 380, 385

B7 molecules and anti-HPV immune responses, 209

Bobcat oral papilloma (FrPV), 49, 57

BoPV, 53

Bos taurus papillomavirus (BPV). *See* Bovine papillomavirus

Bovine papillomavirus (BPV)
  and antibodies, 57, 418
  and early genes, 16
  genetic stability of, 59, 70
  nomenclature of, 51, 54–55, 61

T - #1067 - 101024 - C0 - 254/178/21 [23] - CB - 9780849373565 - Gloss Lamination